=FOOT DISORDERS=

Medical and Surgical Management

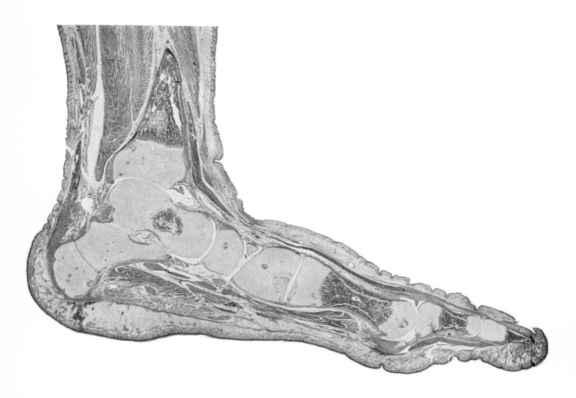

FRONTISPIECE

=FOOT DISORDERS=

Medical and Surgical Management

Nicholas J. Giannestras, M.D.

Department of Orthopaedic Surgery
University of Cincinnati, College of Medicine
Cincinnati, Ohio

Chairman, Section of Fractures and Orthopaedics
Good Samaritan Hospital
Cincinnati, Ohio

465 Illustrations and 3 in Color

LEA & FEBIGER

Philadelphia   1967

Dedication

To the patients without whose patience
I would not have gained the experience
and knowledge required to write this book.

Library of Congress Catalog Card Number 67:13888

PRINTED IN THE UNITED STATES OF AMERICA

Contributors

Frank H. Bassett, III, M.D.
Associate Professor of Orthopaedic Surgery
Duke University Medical Center
Durham, North Carolina

Mack L. Clayton, M.D.
Associate Clinical Professor of Orthopaedic
*   Surgery*
University of Colorado School of Medicine
Denver, Colorado

Paul H. Curtiss, M.D.
Professor of Orthopaedic Medicine and
*   Surgery*
Ohio State University School of Medicine
Columbus, Ohio

Kenneth C. Francis, M.D.
Associate Professor of Orthopaedics
University Hospital
New York University Medical Center
New York, New York

Alexander Garcia, M.D.
Assistant Professor of Clinical Orthopaedic
*   Surgery*
College of Physicians and Surgeons
Columbia University
New York, New York

Sawnie R. Gaston, M.D.
Assistant Professor of Clinical Orthopaedic
*   Surgery*
College of Physicians and Surgeons
Columbia University
New York, New York

Leon Goldman, M.D.
Professor of Dermatology
University of Cincinnati
College of Medicine
Cincinnati, Ohio

Michael Harty, B.M., M.Ch., M.A.
Associate Professor of Anatomy
University of Pennsylvania
School of Medicine
Philadelphia, Pennsylvania

Leonard Marmor, M.D.
Associate Professor of Orthopaedic Surgery
University of California, Los Angeles
Los Angeles, California

Alton Ochsner, Jr., M.D.
Associate Professor of Clinical Surgery
Tulane University School of Medicine
New Orleans, Louisiana

James C. Parkes, M.D.
Annie C. Kane Fellow
New York Orthopaedic Hospital
Columbia Presbyterian Medical Center
New York, New York

Jack K. Wickstrom, M.D.
Professor and Chairman of Orthopaedic
*   Surgery*
Tulane University School of Medicine
New Orleans, Louisiana

Foreword

DESPITE our modern means of locomotion, the correct management of foot disabilities is just as important today as at any time in history. Both the military and civilian population have the right to demand that expert fundamental foot care be given by well-trained orthopaedic surgeons. Too often, the management of the human foot is relegated to the untrained or the least experienced.

The footsore patient of the future will be greatly benefitted if the tenets of this book find their proper application through its students.

Doctor Giannestras has brought together an illustrious group of co-authors. They have brought to life a scholarly and distinguished text that not only reflects thoughtful clinical orthopaedic surgical practice, but beautifully encompasses foot embryology, anatomy, physiology, medicine, pathology—and even philosophy. Particularly emphasized are the details of management in the patient-physician relationship that so frequently spell success or failure in treatment.

Among the outstanding attractions of this book are the excellent line drawings and x-ray reproductions.

In the introduction, Doctor Giannestras states "This book is not intended for the orthopaedist who has been in practice for fifteen years or more. It is intended to be an easy reference for the newly established orthopaedic surgeon or the resident training in orthopaedics."

It would, in my estimation, behoove all orthopaedic surgeons, regardless of their station or training, to read this entire book. If they do, they will be better orthopaedic surgeons.

Doctor Giannestras has always been a student and teacher of the best in orthopaedic surgery. His common sense and logic, coupled with practicality and easy readability of his new text, do him and his co-authors proud.

FRANK E. STINCHFIELD

New York, New York

6

Preface

In most books, the Preface is used by the author to set forth various excuses for writing a particular book. Frankly, I have no excuse. I wrote this book because I enjoyed doing so, and it is my fervent hope, as well as the publisher's, that you, the reader, will both benefit from and enjoy its contents.

It would be remiss of me, however, not to take this opportunity to thank the contributors to the book who have made it much more authoritative and interesting than I could have done alone. As can be seen from the list of contributors on the flyleaf, I have surrounded myself with men of great clinical experience and knowledge and therefore have attempted to present to you a wide scope of combined experience. Each of these men has contributed quite appreciably in his own field of interest to the book and therefore, to each of them, I wish again to express my appreciation.

My sincere thanks also go to Mr. Eric Sovere, my photographer, who was tireless in his attempt to reproduce the clinical material by the best photographic means available; Mr. William R. Filer and Mr. Thomas Campbell, the artists whose talents so greatly enhance the text; Mrs. Lenore Brandt, who researched the entire orthopaedic literature published in the English language during the past ten years; Mrs. Margaret Parks, Mrs. Carmen Stevens, and Miss Kathy Osborne who worked so assiduously and diligently to prepare, type and retype each of the chapters and to keep the entire correspondence file so well organized; Mrs. Margaret Markham who edited this book; Miss Mary Johnstone who compiled the index, and to my patient wife who put up with the necessary disruption of a normal home when two of its rooms were progressively commandeered for the plethora of x-rays, illustrations, manuscripts and other paraphernalia necessary in the compilation of a book as well as the proof reading that she performed every night.

Last but not least, my sincere thanks to Mr. Richard P. Sullivan of Lea & Febiger who gave me "carte blanche" and simply asked that a book on the diseases and surgery of the foot be produced which would be acceptable to the profession, irrespective of the cost.

NICHOLAS J. GIANNESTRAS
Cincinnati, Ohio

Contents

Introduction

THE *remark* "Be good to your feet, they outnumber people two to one" is a very apt one. With the modern shoe styles, particularly among the females and our present method of living, our feet are not shod as they should be nor do we exercise them as they need to be with the result that the foot problems have multiplied. Fortunately, *many foot problems can be successfully treated by conservative means.*

It is not my intent that this book be an encyclopedia of all the types of therapy and surgical procedures which have been described in the medical literature. The contents recorded herein have been carefully selected after extensive investigation and painstaking evaluation by the contributors and me as the methods of treatment and the surgical procedures which have withstood the test of time and have been the most successful in the experience of the majority of the orthopaedic surgeons. This book is not intended for the orthopaedist who has been in practice for fifteen years or more because he has definite ideas as to what procedures are most effective in his experience. It is intended to be an easy reference book for the newly established orthopaedic surgeon, the resident training in orthopaedics, for the many excellent general surgeons who, either by choice or by necessity, must frequently treat orthopaedic foot problems, and for the interested physician, be he pediatrician or general practitioner, who wishes to avail himself of some knowledge of foot problems in general.

The first portion of this book deals with the treatment of the disorders of the foot in the child, whether congenital, familial or acquired. Conservative therapy, administered during the formative years, can frequently result in a normal or a nearly normal functioning asymptomatic foot. However, without a basic knowledge of the development, the physiology, the anatomy and the concept of what a normal foot is, the problems pertaining thereto will not be as easily understood. Therefore, it is strongly recommended that these first few chapters be carefully perused. I cannot urge strongly enough that when information concerning a particular problem is being sought, the entire chapter be read, since in many instances more than one method of therapy is presented. *By reading the entire chapter a better idea of the specific problem will be gained.*

In the adolescent stage different problems present themselves. Although to some, the methods of therapy may at times seem radi-

11

cal, experience has proved beyond any doubt not only in my hands, but in those of various other well-organized clinical groups, that these methods and these procedures are based on sound principles.

In the adult other clinical entities manifest themselves. These deserve more than passing interest, for though many of them may appear to be of secondary import to the average orthopaedist, they are most disabling to the patient, who may unfortunately have developed one of these so-called minor foot ailments. How often has the statement been made, "Doctor, when your feet hurt, you hurt all over." Many of the acquired static foot problems occur most frequently in the female. However, as long as Dame Fashion controls M'Lady's footwear, one cannot prevent the development of these deformities, but it behooves the orthopaedic surgeon to have an excellent repertoire of therapies to correct the problems and to make the patient comfortable. Moreover, in the adult these most frequently require surgical intervention and therefore a very careful selection of recommended operative procedures is presented. In all operations whether in the child, the adolescent, or the adult, postoperative care is fully and carefully documented, since this phase of the therapy is equally as important as the surgical procedure itself.

In the composition of this book an attempt has been made to title the chapters and to present the contents therein in such a manner as to facilitate rapid reference to a particular problem. This may at times make for repetition, particularly regarding some specific surgical procedure, *e.g.,* triple arthrodesis. On the other hand, the reader will not be required to refer to several chapters to secure the information he desires.

No attempt has been made to describe the method of preparation of the skin prior to surgery; the use of the tourniquette and the contraindications of its employment; the treatment of soft tissues with gentleness and care; the use of an instrument when sponging the wound; the use of the hands to hold the instruments rather than to insert the hand or fist into the wound, gentleness in traction, and last but *most important,* avoidance of infection. To the reader I would say, "If your infection rate, including suture infections, is over 1 per cent, you have no business practicing orthopaedic surgery and you had better sit back, take stock of yourself and find out what you are doing incorrectly." It is hoped that by the time the reader absorbs the contents of this book, he will have been exposed to sufficient orthopaedic surgery to understand what I have written in this paragraph.

Finally, dear reader, remember *"There is no minor surgery."*

=1=

Development and Physiology

One cannot well understand the function of the human foot, either from the point of view of disease or of locomotion, without first examining the evolutionary background of this important portion of the human body.

Over the centuries, the foot has undergone many changes and one can liken these changes to the progressive stages in the development of the automobile. In both instances, each improvement in the original crude model has resulted in a progressive advancement in locomotion. At the same time, because the form and function of the foot normally contribute to a major degree to body locomotion as a whole, it is essential that the foot be regarded in relation to the entire body, rather than being considered as a separate unit.

DEVELOPMENT

To begin with, embryologists have implied that there is a definite homology between the fins of the fishes and the extremities of the terrestrial vertebrates. They have cited as an example the lobefin of the barramunda, an existent Australian lungfish. The lobefin has a stout, fleshy base containing musculature as well as discrete bony segments which extend from the body into the fin structure. These osseous segments bear a direct relation to the units contained in the vertebrate limbs. Furthermore, such changes in the fins have paralleled the changes in the air-breathing apparatus in the evolution from fish to amphibian and finally, the changes which ultimately permitted the aquatic animal to emerge onto dry land and survive under new conditions.

Gregory, one of the more knowledgeable embryologists in the field of anthropoid development, suggested that the pentadactylate foot pattern of the amphibian (Fig. 1-1) is the starting point in the terrestrial development of all types of vertebrate feet irrespective of the marked dif-

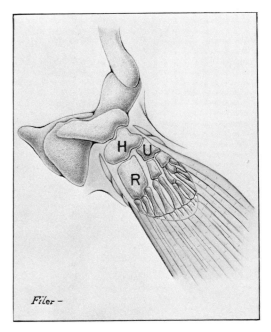

Filer —

Fig. 1-1. Hypothetical origin of foreleg from the primitive lobe-fin of the sauripterus (Redrawn from Gregory)

ferences which exist within the reptilian, avian, and mammalian species as we know them at the present time. Nor is it to be supposed that the early, land-visiting creatures were efficient in their struggle with gravity. As an example, the movements of the Australian lungfish on land are clumsy and sprawling. It uses its lobefins chiefly for pushing in order to assist the wriggling motions of the body by which it propels itself forward. Therefore, by analogy, the early land-visiting creatures gradually developed locomotor extremities of such strength and proportions as to raise the body off the ground. With this major improvement, they were able to achieve longer and longer periods of living on land and, eventually, air-breathing, land-living reptiles made their appearance.

During the Cretaceous period of the Mesozoic era the first mammal-like quadrupedal reptiles, the Theraspids, came on the scene. Fossil remains of the Theraspids reveal such distinctive characteristics as to give ample confirmation of the relationship of these reptiles to the beginning of mammalian life and to the development of the mammalian foot. If one were to study Gregory's diagrammatic pattern of the am-

phibian hind leg (Fig. 1-2), one would find that the flat, loosely joined foot had incompletely ossified tarsal units characteristic of its aquatic ancestry. Furthermore, since the legs were extended widely from the sides of the body, the feet were used chiefly as a means of pushing the body over the land surface. Actually, it was during the transition stage of the amphibian foot to the reptilian that important changes began to take place. A gradual flexion developed both at the knee and the ankle with improvement in the design of the component muscles and bones. This enabled the animal to raise its body from the ground and thus improve its method of locomotion. It also permitted the feet to become weight-bearing structures although they were still of the sprawling type.

Further improvement in the limb structure occurred in the more active vertebrates through a change in the position of the thighs. The thighs were moved forward and parallel with the axis of the body as well as beneath it. This, in turn, brought the feet into an anteroposterior alignment and further helped in the development of the human foot as we now know it. The fibulare (Fig. 1-2) became enlarged through its change in position and developed into the os calcis. The inter-medium developed into the talus; the navicular originated from the tibiale and proximal centrale through fusion. The first, second, and third tarsalia developed into the medial, middle, and lateral cuneiforms and the fourth and fifth tarsalia became the cuboid. The remaining bony units or cartilaginous tarsal units of the reptilian foot, according to most paleontologists, were resorbed. The five metatarsal bones persisted in the mammalia-like Theraspid group as did the phalanges and they are in an anatomical relationship similar to that of the osseous structures in the present human foot: five metatarsals, two phalanges for the hallux, and three phalanges for the remaining four lateral pedal digits. As an interesting sidelight, the accessory schaphoid, as we know it at the present time, is also designated as the os tibiale externum in spite of the fact that it is located on the medial aspect of the foot. It is one example of the radical

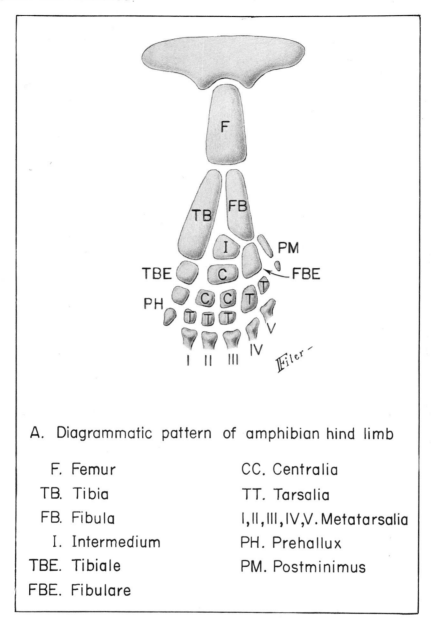

A. Diagrammatic pattern of amphibian hind limb

F. Femur	CC. Centralia
TB. Tibia	TT. Tarsalia
FB. Fibula	I,II,III,IV,V. Metatarsalia
I. Intermedium	PH. Prehallux
TBE. Tibiale	PM. Postminimus
FBE. Fibulare	

Fig. 1-2.   Osseous origin of the human foot.

OS CALCIS	—	From the Fibulare through change of position.
TALUS	—	From the Intermedium.
NAVICULAR	—	From the Tibiale and Proximal Centrale through Fusion.
MEDIAL CUNEFORM	—	From the First Tarsalium.
MIDDLE CUNEIFORM	—	From the Second Tarsalium.
LATERAL CUNEIFORM	—	From the Third Tarsalium.
CUBOID	—	From the Fourth and Fifth Tarsalia.
FIVE METATARSALS	—	From Five Metatarsalia.

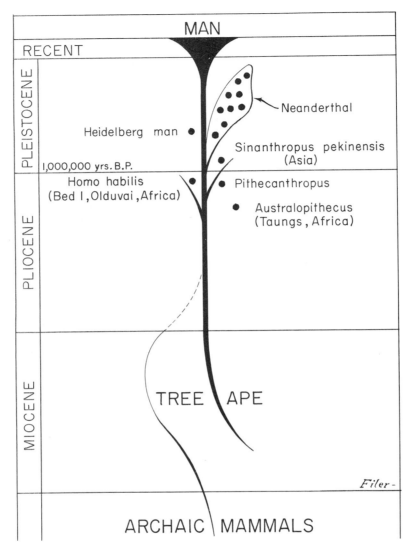

Fig. 1-3. Human evolution and fossil evidence of the development of homo sapiens through the various periods

changes which have gradually taken place in the development of the human foot.

As the primitive mammal developed, there was a general refinement of the skeletal parts of the foot with the tarsal bones coapting and interlocking in such a manner as to form a firm, efficient, functioning unit. Furthermore, as the early primates developed at the beginning of the Eocene period, the first metatarsal bone became independently mobile and prehensile as well as structurally stronger than the other metatarsals in order to accommodate the arboreal functions demanded of it. The Eocene primate is known as the Notharctus and is believed to have been a quadruped with both hands and feet adapted for grasping. He also possessed many of the characteristics of the lemur, one of the most primitive of the modern primates. His os calcis had become well developed, as had the talus. The former was advantageously located beneath the latter for effective leverage. Tarsal flexibility had been transferred to the metatarsal and to the phalangeal area with the midtarsal region becoming more rigid, thus supplying better stability to the entire foot.

The proanthropoid and the anthropoid changes of the primitive mammal began in the Oligocene epoch, approximately 39 million years ago, progressed in the Miocene epoch, about 28 million years ago. During this time the dryopithecus or "tree ape" developed and advanced during the Pliocene period, about 12 million years ago, reaching his ultimate refinement in the Pleistocene period, approximately 1 million years ago (Fig. 1-3). It was during the latter half of the Pleistocene era, approximately 50,000 to 75,000 years ago, that the Neanderthal race developed. Examination of almost complete skeletons of this race has proved conclusively, that in the course of gradual evolution, terrestrial bipedism evolved slowly as the proanthropoid quadruped gave up his arboreal mode of living.

Recent findings by Dr. L. S. B. Leakey and by Drs. M. H. Day and J. R. Napier in Bed I, Olduvai Gorge, Tanganyika, have materially altered previous opinions as to the evolvement of the biped animal. One of the most important discoveries was that of a hominoid fossil foot. The bones of this foot include the five metatarsal shafts and all of the tarsal bones. Day and Napier reported that the posterior part of the calcaneum was damaged and that the styloid process of the base of the fifth metatarsal was absent as well as all of the metatarsal heads and the phalanges. However, it is obvious when one looks at the photograph (Fig. 1-4) that it has many of the principal morphological features of the early human foot. To quote Day and Napier, "The presence of an articular facet between the bases of the first and second metatarsal demonstrates unequivocally the absence of hallucial divergence which characterizes the non-human primate feet. The articulation of the bases of the first, second, and third metatarsals with the distal tarsal row is also typical of *Homo sapiens*, the second metatarsal being wedged between, and bearing facets for the anterior extremities of the medial and lateral cuneiform bones."

Further evaluation of this foot demonstrates that it possesses the structure or structures which are associated with bipedal propulsion. A personal communication from J. R. Napier adds the following information: "The fossil foot is clearly of

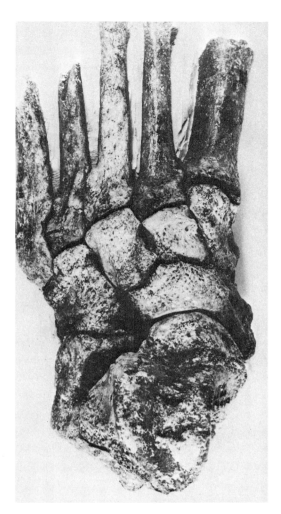

Fig. 1-4. Articulated fossil foot from Bed 1, Olduvai Gorge, Tanganyika, estimated to be approximately 1,750,000 years old and pre-dating the Neanderthal Man. Note the striking resemblance to the present human foot. There is no hallucial divergence of the first metatarsal. (Napier, courtesy of Nature)

an adult, in addition to which there is quite a severe degree of osteoarthritis present in the joints, as you may see from the photographs. Some of the other material, *e.g.*, the hand and lower jaw, found on the same site at Olduvai was of a young adult. With reference to geological age, this is not an easy thing to answer. I think most authorities would put Bed I at Olduvai in the early Pleistocene, at a post-Villefranchian date. In terms of years before the present, potassium-argon dating estimate has now been confirmed by dating using a new tech-

nique called fission-track-dating, and I
think we can take it that the earliest known
members of this *Homo habilis* group were
of the order of 1.75 million B.P. (before
the present)". Relatively speaking, the
Neanderthal man can thus be considered
to represent a rather advanced stage of
Homo sapiens.

There are wide gaps in the evolutionary
sequences of the human foot. However,
one has but to apply the principles of
Wolf's law to reinforce further the concept
of these developmental changes and the
general developmental growth of bones
since it states: "Bones in their external contour and internal architecture conform to
the intensity and direction of the stresses
to which they are habitually subjected."
Thus, the pre-human or anthropoid foot assumed its present terrestrial form or nature
by the enlargement of the os calcis and of
the surrounding soft tissues to become the
posterior end of a weight bearing lever;
the first metatarsal increased in size, power,
and mobility as compared with the other
metatarsals; the lateral four metatarsals
gradually derotated, and the toes became
shorter. These changes can readily be seen
in a gorilla's foot.

However, there are three characteristics
of the true human foot which differ from
the anthropoid and require further clari-
fication: 1) The pro-anthropoid and the
anthropoid foot had, and still have, a flattened inner border in contrast to the arched
construction of the present human foot. 2)
The primitive prototype was muscular and
flexible, whereas the current form is rigid
and ligamentous with only a minimal
amount of musculature contained within
it to directly control any of its functions.
3) The position of the hallux has changed
to facilitate adduction and this transformation has led to a loss of free mobility. In
this instance both Morton's analysis of
leverage stresses and the principles of
Wolf's law help to explain these structural
changes and differences.

Morton states, "Since the foot is distinctly
recognized as a special organ of terrestrial
leverage, we may seek to answer this question by first studying stresses as they affect
a lever, using for this purpose a block,
the dimensions of which correspond to the

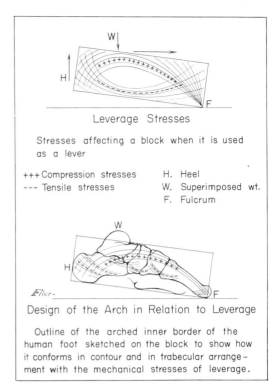

Leverage Stresses

Stresses affecting a block when it is used
as a lever

+++ Compression stresses   H. Heel
--- Tensile stresses   W. Superimposed wt.
                                F. Fulcrum

Design of the Arch in Relation to Leverage

Outline of the arched inner border of the
human foot sketched on the block to show how
it conforms in contour and in trabecular arrangement with the mechanical stresses of leverage.

Fig. 1-5. Stresses affecting a block when it is
used as a lever and outline of the arched inner
border of the human foot sketched on the block
to show how it conforms in contour and in
trabecular arrangement with the mechanical
stresses of leverage.

length and the height of the foot (Fig.
1-5). The lifting force is exerted at one
end (H is the heel); weight, W, is superimposed at a position corresponding to that
of the ankle; the lower corner of the opposite end is employed as the fulcrum, F,
representing the position of the heads of
the first and second metatarsal bones.
When H is lifted, the force, passing through
the substance of the block, is directed upward and forward in a curved direction
toward the point, W; from there it curves
forward and downward upon the fulcrum.
If the stresses involved in this movement
of force are marked on the side of the
block, they appear in two sets: a) As compression stresses. (Indicated by the sym-
bols +++). b) As tensile stresses or
breaking strains. (Indicated by the sym-
bols ---). Each step follows opposing
marks and each crosses the other toward
the extremities of the lever. If an outline

of the bones forming the inner border of the human foot be drawn on the block (Fig. 1-5), their contour will seem to follow the arc of compression stresses. In other words, the arching of the inner border of the foot conforms with this movement of force in the manner stated in Wolf's law".

Interestingly enough, if one were to section the foot longitudinally through the os calcis, talus, navicular, and first metatarsal, and were to study the arrangement of the trabeculae in these bones, one would find the trabecular distribution to be along the lines of leverage stresses. They are not placed, however, as a long continuous arc, but arranged as "small secondary systems" with the dorsal and the plantar ligamentous structures supplying the continuity of the dorsal arc and the plantar fascia forming the reverse minus arc. A typical example of bone remodeling by these forces can be easily demonstrated by a comparative study of the os calcis of the gorilla, of the Neanderthal man, and of the present-day human being. In the gorilla, the superior surface of the os calcis is tilted at an angle of 70 to 73 degrees. In the Neanderthal fossils the angle is greater. In man, the articular surface is practically horizontal. This gradual change not only involved the os calcis, as the biped position was assumed, but also led to a rearrangement of the position of all the bones of the foot. In addition, the ligamentous structures increased in strength to give the necessary support and rigidity to the foot. Despite these changes, the human foot still contains all of the muscles which are needed for grasping. They are present as the small muscles of the foot.

PHYSIOLOGY

It is only through an adequate knowledge of both the development and the physiology of the foot that one can gain a better understanding of the pathologic changes and the deformities resulting from poor structural configuration.

In the physiological position of the foot in a person standing erect, the heels are together and the foreportions of the feet are separated sufficiently to maintain adequate stability in relation to the lateral balance of the body. The angle of separation varies from approximately 5 to 15 degrees in the child, to 25 to 35 degrees in the adult. During locomotion, however, this angle is diminished. The transmission of the body weight occurs through the legs which serve as two symmetrical columns and on into the foot through the midpoint of the trochlear surface of the talus. The weight is then transmitted to the ground through the various bony components of the foot represented posteriorly by the os calcis and anteriorly by the heads of the five metatarsals.

There is an old and incorrect concept that there exists a metatarsal arch with the weight being borne by the first and fifth metatarsal heads anteriorly. Actually, *there is no metatarsal arch*. This has been substantiated not only by Morton's work, but also by roentgenograms of the human foot during standing, whether normal or pronated (but not deformed), which demonstrate the fact that there is *no* metatarsal arch and that the weight is distributed evenly on the plantar surface of all five metatarsal heads (Fig. 1-6). Furthermore, the weight borne by the heel is equal to the weight borne by all five metatarsals.

The foot is *not* a tripod as it has often been considered in the past. If the foot were a tripod, its functions of stance, balance, locomotion, and propulsion would not be carried on as so smoothly co-ordinated an activity. Much more could be written about the various aspects of the foot in walking and in running, as well as about the effect of proper muscle balance. However, at best, much of this work is inferential thus far. Some investigators have devoted a major portion of their work to the study of the kinesiology of the human foot and some of their contributions are very interesting, but even they differ in their opinions as to the functions of certain joints, ligaments and muscles when a person is standing, walking or running.

When the foot functions as passive support, as in standing, the muscles and ten-

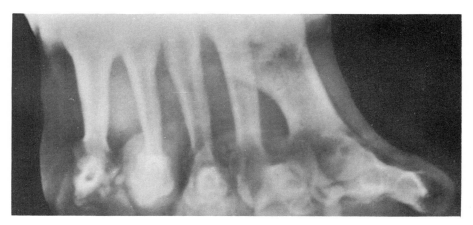

Fig. 1-6. Roentgenogram of forefoot in standing position. Note that all five metatarsal heads participate in weight-bearing. There is **no** metatarsal arch. The same conformation is also present when the weight is borne on the forefoot as in high heel shoes or in the forward thrust phase of a step.

dons contribute little if any supportive power. The ligaments and the plantar fascia are the main supporting components and since they are, at best, poorly adapted for this function, any disturbance or deformity of the osseous structures or malposition of the foot places an undue strain on these fibroelastic elements. This causes the feet to become fatigued and leads to symptomatic disturbances. It is for this reason that people who must stand for long periods of time develop foot problems.

Ligamentous structures are under the least amount of strain when the bones of the foot are so aligned that each of the tarsals and metatarsals fits into its proper supportive position; thus when the superimposed body weight falls upon the foot, it falls upon a compact mass which is relatively rigid and non-yielding but is held together by the ligamentous structures. The standing position, in which the foot points directly forward or with minimal out toeing, is the one in which this functional locking is most effective and the ligaments are under the least amount of strain. When the foot is held in a position of external rotation, producing an inversional strain on the foot, the bones are no longer in the compact mass. An undue strain is, therefore, placed on the ligamentous structures, leading to fatigue, pain and loss of the physiologic efficiency of the foot.

During the walking phase of locomotion the foot acts as a lever, and its function changes from a passive to an active or kinetic one. In a normal individual, the muscles of the leg and foot then take over the maintenance of the pedal, as well as the body, equilibrium since this is primarily a muscular function. An analysis of the various phases of this portion of function of the human foot is not within the scope of this chapter. Schwartz and his co-workers, even after some extensive and excellent oscillographic studies, have summarized the entire problem by concluding that successive steps are not duplicates of each other, and that no individual studies by them demonstrated precisely the same gait pattern in the right foot as compared to the left. When they presented their findings in 1964, they stated that each individual person presented many variables. They had found, "no quantitative, positive definition of normal gait". What is considered to be a normal gait can best be defined as one in which there is an absence of any visual demonstrable abnormality.

The more important physiologic functions of the foot can therefore be concisely summarized as follows:

1) The talus is involved only in the extension (dorsiflexion) and flexion (plantar flexion) action of the foot and is held relatively rigidly in the ankle mortise. It does not contribute to inversion or eversion movements of the foot. Inversion and eversion take place through the subtalar joints.

2) The joints through the mid-tarsal region of the foot demonstrate only a slight degree of dorsal and plantar movement and also contribute only slightly to the inversion and eversion motions of the foot.

3) The metatarsophalangeal joints function in the forward thrust phase of walking. In running they are the primary receptors of the propulsive forces.

4) The ligaments of the foot and the plantar fascia supply structural stability in all positions of weight bearing and are the prime contributors to the maintenance of the rigidly arched contour of the foot.

5) The muscles of the leg and the foot play the role of "stays" in the maintenance of foot balance. In practically all of the medical literature, muscular control or muscular balance is cited as the predominant factor in the maintenance of foot balance. This is not entirely correct. The muscles lend only postural stability. Foot balance, as such, is dependent on both ligamentous and muscular components. Any appreciable defect in either component will be manifested by unbalanced posture, despite the integrity of the other component. Weakness of the muscles, due to paralysis, inevitably leads to deformity in spite of the normal ligamentous and osseous structures. On the other hand, damage to the bones and ligaments and consequent disturbance of the structural stability of the foot, leads to an increased weight load upon the muscles of the affected foot with resultant disturbance in posture and balance.

6) In the function of walking, running or standing, there is equal distribution of weight on all five metatarsal heads, and there is no structure such as a "transverse metatarsal arch". There is transverse arching in the mid-tarsal region of the foot as well as through the tarsometatarsal joints, but it does not involve heads.

BIBLIOGRAPHY

BASMAJIAN, J. V.: Weight-Bearing by Ligaments and Muscles. Canad. J. Surg. 4:166 (Jan.) 1961. Man's Posture. Arch. Phys. Med. Rehabilit. 46:26 (Jan.) 1965.

BASMAJIAN, J. V. AND STECKO, G.: The Role of Muscles in Arch Support of the Foot. J. Bone Joint Surg. 45A:1184 (Sept.) 1963.

DAY, M. H. AND NAPIER, J. R.: Hominid Fossils from Bed I, Olduvai Gorge, Tanganyika—Fossil Foot Bones. Nature 201:967, 1964.

GREGORY, W. K.: Man's Place Among the Anthropoids. New York, Oxford University Press, Inc., 1934.

HOOTEN, E. A.: Up From The Ape. New York, The Macmillan Co., 1946.

KINGSLEY, J. S.: The Vertebrate Skeleton. Philadelphia, The Blakiston Co., 1925.

LEAKEY, L. S. B. Personal Communication. (March) 1965.

LEWIS, O. J.: The Homologies of the Mammalian Tarsal Bones. J. Anat., 98:2, 1964, London.

MANN, R. AND INMAN, V. T.: Phasic Activity of Intrinsic Muscles of the Foot. J. Bone Surg. (Amer.) 46:469 (April) 1964.

MORTON, D. J.: The Human Foot. New York, Columbia University Press. 1936.

NAPIER, J. R.: Personal Communication from the Unit of Primatology and Human Evolution. Department of Anatomy. Royal Free Hospital School of Medicine. London, W.C. 1, U.K. 21st June, 1965.

SCHWARTZ, R. PLATO, HEATH, A. L., MORGAN, D. W. AND TOWNS, R. C.: A Quantitative Analysis of Recorded Variables in the Walking Pattern of "Normal Adults". J. Bone J. Surg. 46A:324 (March) 1964.

SONNTHE, C. F.: Morphology of the Apes. London, Bale, 1924.

=2=

Anatomy

MICHAEL HARTY, M.A., M.B., M.CH., F.R.C.S.

While researchers seek smaller and smaller submicroscopic particles and ponder their functional significance, the science of clinical medicine and surgery must still center around gross anatomy. The current emphasis on the physiological and biochemical aspects of the basic sciences has thrown anatomy into a less prominent role, but *ignorance of anatomy is perhaps the greatest single handicap to a surgeon.* Readers of this book will have covered gross anatomy in considerable detail, perhaps in the dim, distant past, and the gross anatomical minutiae are readily available in a number of textbooks. *The primary object of this section is, therefore, the application of the appropriate anatomy to the clinical problems encountered.*

Unlike the hand, which is designed essentially for grasping, the foot is fundamentally a weight-bearing organ. As an instrument of support and locomotion, the human foot excels that of all other animal species. Man's normal and comfortable foot is so well adapted for independent weight bearing and locomotion that it allows full and unimpeded utilization of the hands

under cerebral control. The foot is well adapted to provide a variety of functions. It allows elasticity on weight bearing and during locomotion. It can accommodate to practically any surface irregularity under foot and it is the most readily available footstool for adding three inches to our height. The versatility and speed of foot movements can be well appreciated while running on irregular ground. The whole foot behaves as if it were articulated by a ball-and-socket joint, but by combining three separate joints that act harmoniously, we achieve an extraordinarily smooth range of movements.

Varied anatomical nomenclature has been a source of contention to clinicians, and even anatomists, since the introduction of the Basle Nomina Anatomica (B.N.A.) of 1895. Today we feel and hope that we have reached a final agreement in the Nomina Anatomica Parisiensia (P.N.A.) of 1955. Although the anatomists claim to have a standard nomenclature and use it, many years must elapse before this terminology will be familiar to many senior clinicians. For this reason some of the older

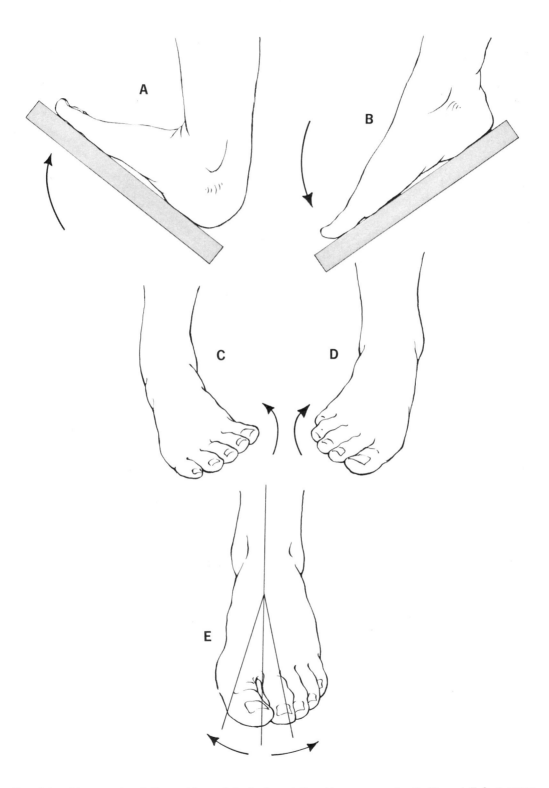

Fig. 2-1. Movements of the ankle and foot. A and B ankle movements, C. D. and E foot movements

and better known terms are also given in parenthesis.

The terms recommended for ankle and foot movements by the American Academy of Orthopaedic Surgeons (1965) and the International Congress of Anatomists, Paris, 1955 and New York, 1960, are illustrated diagramatically (Fig. 2-1).

Ankle Movements:
    A. EXTENSION (dorsi flexion)
    B. FLEXION (plantar flexion)

Foot Movements:
    C. INVERSION (supination)
    D. EVERSION (pronation)
    E. ADDUCTION OF FOREFOOT
        Left
        ABDUCTION OF FOREFOOT
        Right

Inversion includes supination, adduction and a slight amount of flexion. Eversion embraces the movements of pronation, abduction and extension.

SKELETAL SYSTEM

The skeletal system of the foot plays not only an important functional role, but is also involved in many of the problems encountered in clinical practice. It consists of seven closely articulated tarsal bones interlocking firmly with five metatarsals. These, in turn, articulate with the phalanges of the toes (Fig. 2-2). Of the seven tarsal bones only one, the talus, articulates with the tibia and fibula to form the morticed ankle joint. The tarsal bones fan outwards and forwards from the posterior tubercles of the calcaneus (os calcis) posteriorly (Fig. 2-3). The talus, the navicular, and the medial cuneiform form the medial margin of the fan; the lateral margin is formed by the calcaneus and the cuboid. Each of the first, second, and third metatarsal bones articulates at its proximal end with the medial intermediate and lateral cuneiform respectively, whereas the distal tarsal bones articulating with the fourth and fifth metatarsals have fused to form the cuboid (Fig. 2-3).

The plantar surface of the tarsal bones and proximal metatarsals forms a curved tunnel directed forward and slightly laterally. It is utilized by the neurovascular bundle and the long flexor tendons to gain safe passage to the anterior foot. The convexity of the dorsum of the foot corresponds to this tunnel. Its lateral margin is formed by the posteromedial tubercle of the calcaneus, the cuboid ridge, and the

fifth metatarsal base. The medial side is outlined by the base of the first metatarsal, the medial cuneiform, the tuberosity of the navicular, and the sustenaculum tali, projecting from the medial side to the calcaneus. This tunnel also provides a loose fascial plane for possible spread of infection from the sole to the lower leg or vice versa (Fig. 2-4).

The tarsometatarsal and intermetatarsal joints are of the gliding variety. Their motions, though limited by the strong dorsal and plantar interosseous ligaments, give considerable flexibility to the forefoot, enabling it to adapt itself to irregularities of the surface on which it rests. The mutual interlocking of these joints tends to restrict lateral and medial deviation or displacement of the forefoot. The combination of the long second metatarsal with the short intermediate cuneiform reinforces the locking mechanism of the tarsometatarsal joint (Lisfranc's) (Fig. 2-2). The transverse tarsal joint is bounded at the proximal end by the head of the talus and calcaneus, and distally by the navicular and cuboid. The medical compartment or talonavicular is basically a ball-and-socket joint, and the lateral or calcaneocuboid is a saddle joint (Fig. 2-2). A large part of the inversion and eversion of the foot occurs at this midtarsal joint. To a slighter extent there is some flexion and extension.

Calcaneus (Os Calcis)

The calcaneus is the largest tarsal bone. Not only does it form the shorter and less yielding posterior limb of the longitudinal arches of the foot, but it also carries most of the body weight transmitted by the tibia. Since the body of the calcaneus is

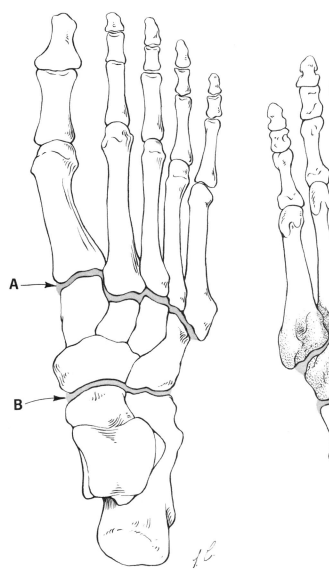

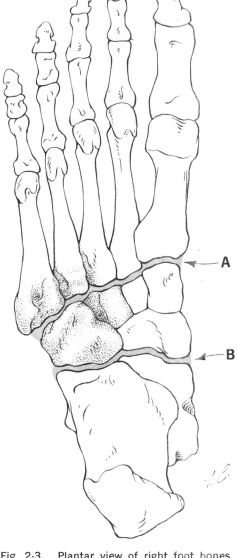

Fig. 2-2. Dorsal view of right foot bones. A. tarsometatarsal joints of Lisfranc, B. midtarsal joint of Chopart

Fig. 2-3. Plantar view of right foot bones

formed by a thin shell of cortical bone enclosing relatively sparse trabeculae, compression fractures of the calcaneus are, therefore, not uncommon. As a result of these various factors the maintenance of a good post-reduction position may at times be difficult. The posterior surface of the calcaneus has two facets separated by an irregular horizontal ridge for the attachment of the tendo calcaneus or tendo achillis (Fig. 2-5). A bursa separates the

superior facet from the tendo calcaneus which may also have another bursa on its superficial or posterior aspect. Sometimes in physically active persons, such as professional dancers and runners, these bursae join to produce a tendon sheath (justifying the term tenovaginitis of the tendo calcaneus). The inferior facet gives firm attachment to the fibrofatty subcutaneous tissue of the heel. The larger medial and smaller lateral tubercles provide anchorage

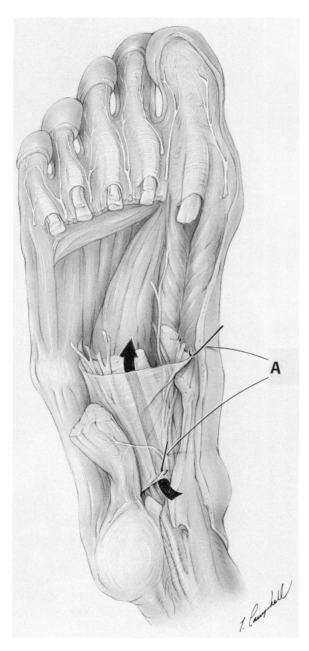

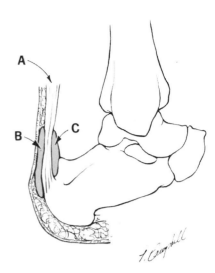

Fig. 2-5. Posterior tubercle of calcaneus to show bursae around tendo calcaneus, A. tendo calcaneus, B. subcutaneous bursa, C. subtendinous bursa

for the strong plantar fascia which may become partly calcified to form the well known calcaneal spur.

The calcaneus supports the talus by either two or three articular facets. The sustentaculum tali projects from the medial side of the calcaneus. Superiorly it provides an articular facet for the talar head; inferiorly it is grooved by the tendon of flexor hallucis longus; anteriorly it gives firm attachment to the spring ligaments and medially the tip is covered by the tendon of the flexor digitorum longus (Fig. 2-6 and 13). The anterior, articular, saddle-shaped facet of the calcaneus for the cuboid reaches the level of the talonavicular joint. Together they constitute the transverse tarsal joint.

Fig. 2-4. Fascial tunnel to the sole of the right foot, indicated by arrow. A. fascia retracted

Talus (Astragalus)

The body of the talus is covered superiorly by the trochlear articular surface which carries the body weight to the foot. This surface is wider anteriorly than posteriorly (Fig. 2-7). Medially and laterally the articular cartilage prolongs distally to articulate with the medial and lateral malleoli, respectively. The neck of the talus—

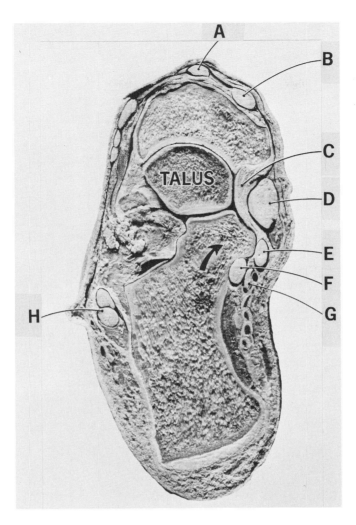

Fig. 2-6. Section through calcaneus, talar head, navicular and sustentaculum tali (arrow), A. extensor hallucis longus, B. tibiales anterior, C. deltoid ligament, D. tibialis posterior, E. flexor digitorum longus, F. flexor hallucis longus, G. plantar nerve, H. peroneus longus

which is constricted inferiorly, laterally and superiorly—is roughened by ligamentuous attachments and vascular foramina. It deviates medially about 15 to 20 degrees in the adult and is the most vulnerable area of the bone.

The rounded head has continuous articular facets for the navicular anteriorly, the spring ligament inferiorly, and the sustentaculum tali postero-inferiorly. The talus has no muscular attachments so that its connections to adjacent structures is by articular capsule and synovial membrane only. As the blood vessels must utilize these fascial structures to reach the talus, trauma associated with capsular tears may be complicated by avascular necrosis of the talus.

A bony tubercle projects backwards from the body of the talus. When prominent, it presents a vertical groove on its medial side for the tendon of the flexor hallucis longus. Occasionally this tubercle may fail to unite with the talus when it forms an accessory bone, the os trigonum. The talus forms the dome or keystone of the medial longitudinal arch.

The shafts of the five metatarsals are concave on their plantar aspect. The first metatarsal has a short thick shaft and a large head. The inferior surface of the head

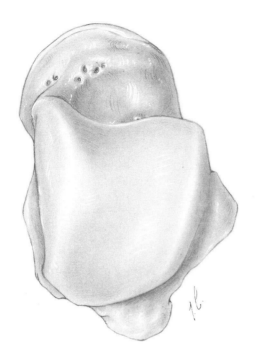

Fig. 2-7. Superior aspect of talus, note convergence of sides of trochlear surface in a posterior direction and vascular foramina on neck

is grooved by the medial and lateral sesamoids contained in the tendon of the flexor hallucis brevis (Fig. 2-8). The second metatarsal is the longest and has a slender shaft, most noticeable in the distal third which is also a site of fatigue fractures.

From a functional aspect the anatomy of the foot must also include the anatomy of the leg. The tibia outlines the antromedial aspect of the leg and conveys the body weight to the foot. It forms a strut between the lower femur and the dome of the talus. It is palpable subcutaneously from the medial condyle and tibial tuberosity down to and including the medial malleolus. The proximal end of the tibia is expanded to form the medial and lateral condyles. There are two slightly concave articular facets (medial and lateral tibial plateaus) for articulation with the femur. These surmount the tibial condyles. The thinnest part of the tibial shaft and the commonest site for fractures is at the junction of the middle and distal thirds.

On the lateral side, the slender fibula is buried in muscle except in its distal quarter where it comes subcutaneously to form the lateral malleolus. This projects about 1 to

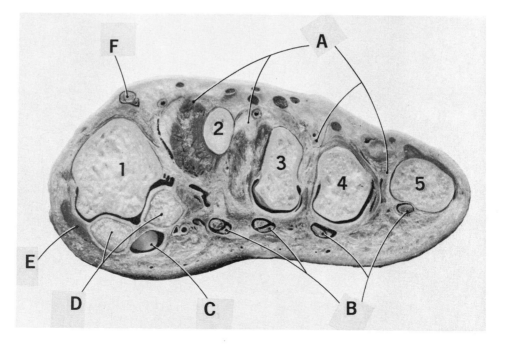

Fig. 2-8. Transverse section through the metatarsophalangeal joints. 1, 3, 4, 5 heads of corresponding metatarsals, 2 shaft of second metatarsal, A. dorsal interossei, B. digital flexors, C. flexor hallucis longus, D. sesamoids, E. abductor hallucis

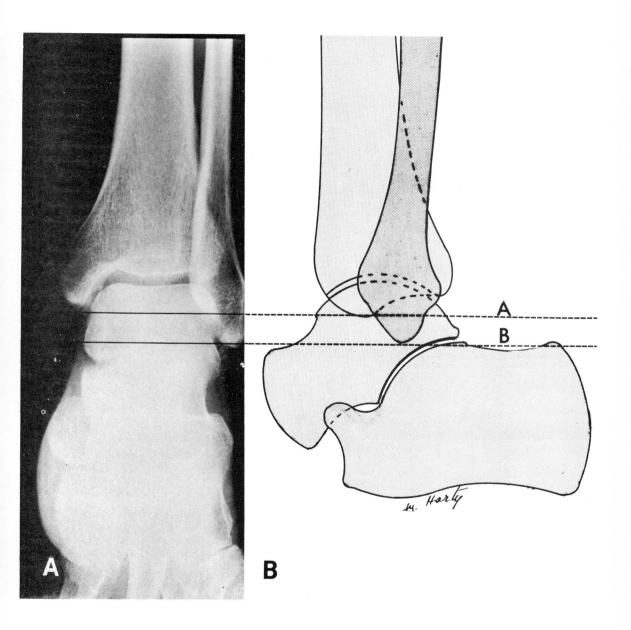

Fig. 2-9. Ankle joint to show the relationship of, A. the medial to, B. lateral malleolus

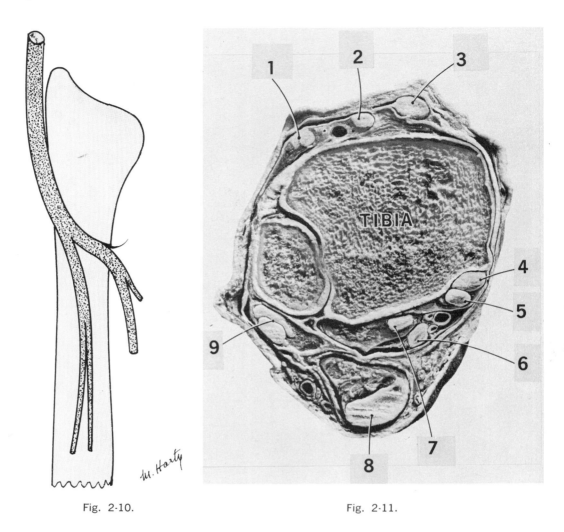

Fig. 2-10.   Fig. 2-11.

Fig. 2-10.   The common peroneal nerve crossing the neck of the right fibula

Fig. 2-11.   Transverse section through the inferior tibiofibular joint. 1. extensor digitorum longus, 2. extensor hallucis longus, 3. tibialis anterior, 4. tibialis posterior, 5. flexor digitorum longus, 6. tibial nerve, 7. flexor hallucis longus, 8. tendo calcaneus, 9. peronei

2 cm. distally and posteriorly to the medial malleolus. It is an accurate and constant bony landmark on the lateral aspect of the ankle joint (Fig. 2-9). Proximally the head is felt on the posterolateral aspect of the knee joint. The common peroneal nerve is palpable and vulnerable as it crosses on the neck of the fibula about 2 to 3 cm. distal to the head (Fig. 2-10).

The interosseous membrane joins the tibia and the fibula and has a hiatus at its proximal end. This allows the anterior tibial vessels to reach the extensor compartment of the leg by passing in close proximity to

the neck of the fibula rather than the tibia. At the distal end, the interosseous membrane thickens considerably to form the inferior tibiofibular joint, the only fibrous joint in the human body other than in the skull. This joint is further reinforced by the anterior and posterior tibiofibular ligaments. It is not a plane joint. The convex fibula fits into a corresponding concavity on the lateral side of the tibia (Fig. 2-11). For this reason, in a normal anteroposterior x-ray picture the tibial shadow overlaps that of the fibula. During extension (dorsal flexion) of the foot the wider anterior end of

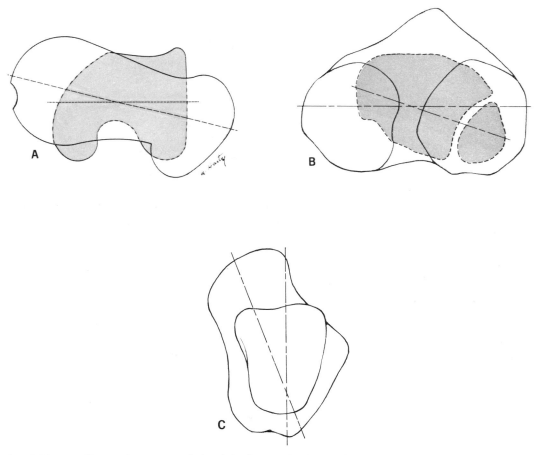

Fig. 2-12.   A. The torsion angle of the right femur, B. the torsion angle of the right tibia, C. the angle of medial deviation in the neck of the right talus (see text)

the talar dome forces the malleoli apart. They are brought together in flexion (plantar flexion) by the elastic fibers in the inferior tibiofibular ligament. The stability of the ankle joint mortice is reinforced by the overlapping of the medial and lateral malleoli, the wedging of the talus during extension, and the extra length of the posterior articular margin of the tibia which prevents posterior displacement of the foot.

Normal foot alignment is influenced by a number of variable factors such as the extent of the torsion angle in the femur and the tibia, as well as the medial deviation of the neck of the talus. The torsion or anteversion angle of the femur is that angle formed by the axis of the knee joint (parallel to the posterior surface of the condyles) and the axis of the femoral neck (Fig. 2-12A). It ranges from 35 degrees anterior (anteversion) to 25 degrees posterior with an average figure of 15 degrees anteversion. In the tibia the axis of the ankle joint is always laterally rotated in relation to that of the knee joint. The angle ranges from 9 to 40 degrees with a mean reading of 15 degrees (Fig. 2-12B). The neck of the talus is directed medially in relation to the axis of the ankle joint. This deviation measures 15 to 20 degrees in the adult (Fig. 2-12C). These three variable components, which come under genetic influences, play a major role in the alignment of the nonpathologic foot.

LIGAMENTS AND JOINTS

In the foot, needless to say, as in any other synovial joint, a fibrous capsule attaches adjacent articular margins. On the dorsum of the foot most of the ligaments derive their names from the adjoining bones which they connect. On the plantar aspect many of the ligaments get a strong reinforcement from the overlying fibrous tissues and some have acquired specific names.

Ankle Joint

The capsular ligament surrounds the ankle joint but it is strengthened on the medial and lateral sides to form the medial (deltoid) ligament and lateral ligament respectively.

The deltoid or the medial ligament of the ankle joint is made up of a strong concentration of fibrous tissue firmly attached to the tip and adjoining margins of the medial malleolus. Distally it splits indistinctly into

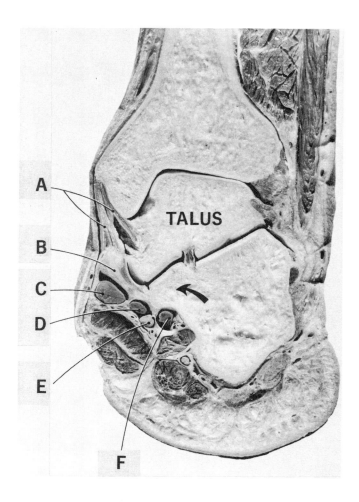

Fig. 2-13. Photograph of coronal section through the right ankle, A. deltoid ligament, deep and superficial parts, B. spring ligament, C. tibialis posterior, D. flexor digitorum longus. E. plantar nerve, F. flexor hallucis longus. Sustentaculum tali—arrowed

a deep and a superficial lamina. The deeper layer is attached by two condensations to the medial side of the neck and the medial aspect of the body of the talus (Fig. 2-13). The fibers of this deeper component, directed laterally and distally, maintain the talus in close contact with the medial malleolus. The superficial layer has a continuous attachment to the navicular tuberosity (tibionavicular), to the medial edge of the plantar calcaneonavicular (spring) ligament, to the sustentaculum tali (tibiocalcaneal), and to the posteromedial aspect of the talus. The strong deltoid ligament contributes not alone to the stability of the ankle joint but by its more superficial expansion to the stability of the subtalar joint. The ligament is covered and grooved medially by the tendon of the tibialis posterior which, in turn, is covered by the flexor retinaculum or lacinate ligament.

The so-called lateral ligament of the ankle joint is made up of three separate components (Fig. 2-14). The calcaneofibular, which may be cord-like or a flat band, passes distally and backwards to the calcaneus. It is an important stabilizer on the lateral side and counteracts inversion forces at the ankle joint. This is one of the ligaments which, under strain, may detach a flake of bone from its area of attachment rather than tear through the parent ligament (Fig. 2-15A & B). The anterior talofibular ligament passes anteriorly and medially to the neck of the talus. The posterior talofibular is a strong ligament directed almost horizontally from the malleolar fossa of the fibula to the posterior tubercle of the talus (Fig. 2-16). (The firm attachment of the lateral malleolus to the tarsal bones is emphasized in distal fibula fractures when this lateral malleolus stays with the foot rather than with the leg.) The transverse tibiofibular ligament extends from the posterior articular margin of the distal tibia (sometimes called the third or posterior malleolus) to the superior surface of the malleolar fossa. It occupies the bevelled posterolateral corner of the trochlea tali during ankle flexion.

Sinus Tarsi and Tarsal Canal

The funnel shaped orifice of the sinus tarsi is found anterior to the lateral malleolus. It is continued deeply as the tarsal canal between the groove under the neck of the talus and the corresponding sulcus on the calcaneus. The interosseous talocalcaneal ligament forms a strong connection in the tarsal canal and sinus. It is embedded in fat and often takes the form of a fibrous band with a marked condensation at the lateral and medial ends. The lateral margin may interdigitate with the attachment of the inferior extensor retinaculum (cruciate crural ligament) and is adjacent to the origin and belly of the extensor digitorum brevis which arises from the beak of the calcaneus. This bony prominence also gives origin to the bifurcate ligament, which is a short, condensed, conjoint, segment of the calcaneocuboid and calcaneonavicular capsule (Fig. 2-14 and 18).

Plantar Ligaments and Fascia

The plantar calcaneonavicular (spring) ligament is a short, powerful, fibrocartilaginous, structure which gains a very firm attachment to the inferior surface of the navicular and the anterior margin of the sustentaculum tali (Fig. 2-13 and 17). Superiorly, it forms the inferior synovial capsule of the talocalcaneaonavicular joint and inferiorly, the sheath of the tibialis posterior tendon.

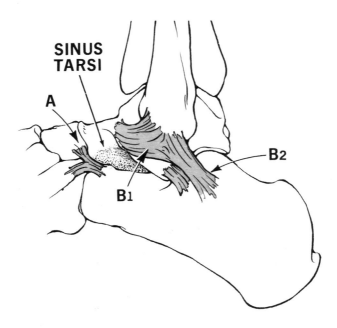

Fig. 2-14.   A. Bifurcate ligament of left foot, B. 1. talofibular and B. 2 calcaneofibular parts of lateral ligament

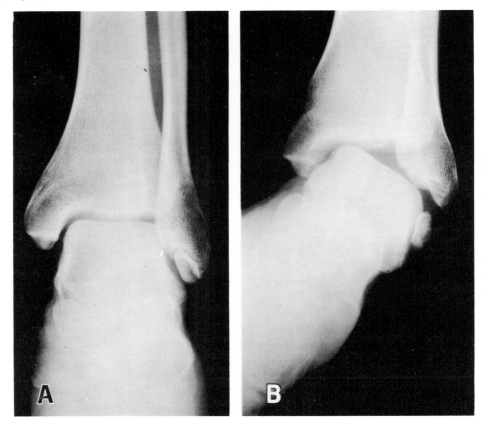

Fig. 2-15.   A. Detached proximal bony attachment of the calcaneofibular ligament, B. foot inverted in figure 15 A.

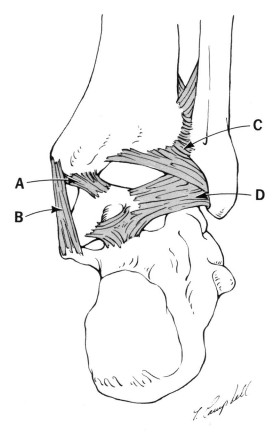

Fig. 2-16.   Right deltoid ligament, A. deep and B. superficial part, C. transverse tibiofibular ligament, D. posterior talofibular ligament

The distal surface of the talus articulates with the calcaneus and the navicular. The talocalcaneonavicular may be classified as a ball-and-socket joint, but unlike other joints of that variety, the socket moves around the ball and is not rigid. In fact, the malleable socket is exposed to constant change and deformities, some of which may reach the pathological stages. The talocalcaneal joint lies obliquely behind the sinus tarsi (Fig. 2-18).

The capsular ligaments are reinforced by the talocalcaneal ligaments in the sinus tarsi, by the spring ligament between the sustentaculum tali and the navicular, and by the bifurcate ligament between the lateral calcaneus, the cuboid and the navicular. The plantar calcaneocuboid (short plantar) and the long plantar ligaments reinforce the lateral longitudinal arch. The deeper short plantar ligament passes from the anterior tubercle of the calcaneus to the posterior groove on the cuboid and forms the inferior capsule of the calcaneocuboid joint (Fig. 2-19). The more superficial, long, plantar ligament has an extensive attachment on the plantar surface of the calcaneus. Its deeper fibers stretch to the ridge on the cuboid, and the more superficial ones pass over the tendon of the peroneus longus to the base of the lateral three or four metatarsals. The plantar intermetatarsal ligament forms a continuous band of transverse fibers which maintain the transverse arch outline of the metatarsal bases. (The short thick part between the medial (cuneiform and the base of the second metatarsal was known as Lisfranc's ligament.)

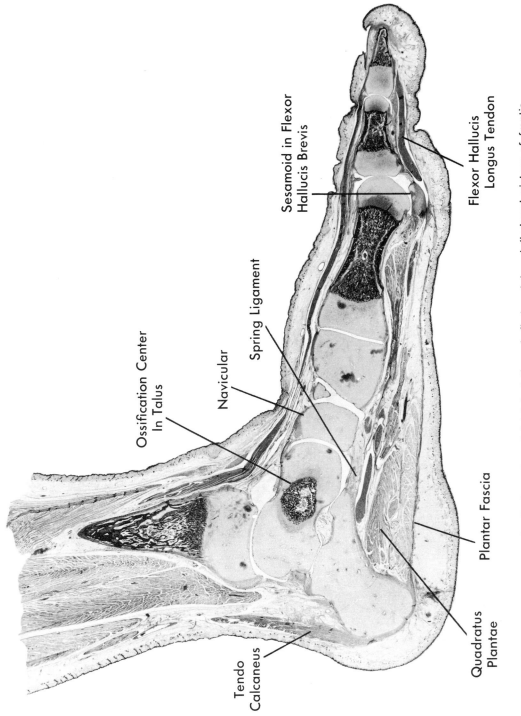

Ossification Center In Talus

Navicular

Spring Ligament

Sesamoid in Flexor Hallucis Brevis

Flexor Hallucis Longus Tendon

Plantar Fascia

Quadratus Plantae

Tendo Calcaneus

Fig. 2-17. Longitudinal section of fetal foot through first metatarsal (indexed picture of frontis-piece)

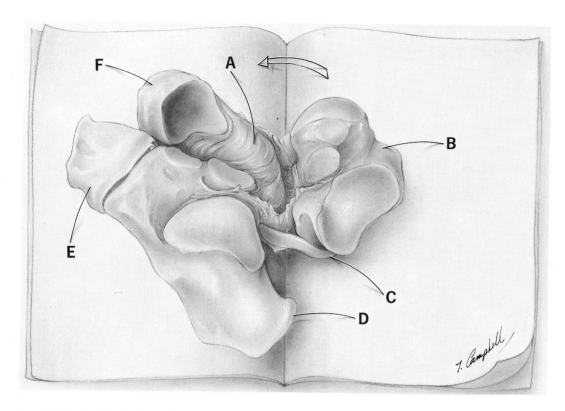

Fig. 2-18. Left talocalcaneal and talocalcaneonavicular joints opened to display, A. deltoid ligament, B. inferior facets of inverted talus, C. flexor hallucis longus tendon, D. calcaneus, E. cuboid, F. navicular

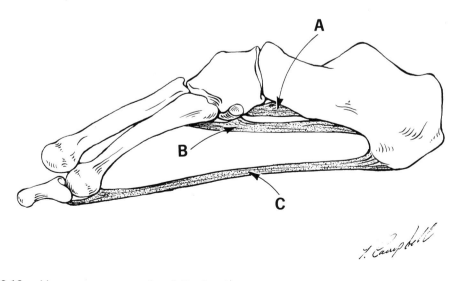

Fig. 2-19. Ligamentous supports of the longitudinal arch, A. short plantar ligament, B. long plantar ligament, C. plantar fascia

Metatarsophalangeal Toe Joints

The convex metatarsal heads fits into the concave facet on the proximal phalanx at the metatarsal phalangeal joints. The capsule is formed by the medial and lateral collateral ligaments, dorsally by an expansion of the extensor tendon, and on the plantar aspect by a strong thick fibrous plantar ligament (glenoid ligament of Cruveilhier) (Fig. 2-8). This is attached firmly to the base of the phalanx but loosely to the metatarsal. The plantar surface is fused with the transverse metatarsal ligament and grooved for the passage of the flexor tendons. The medial and lateral sesamoids in the tendon of the flexor hallucis brevis are embedded in the plantar ligament (Fig. 2-8).

The interphalangeal joint of the toes are of the hinge variety. The proximal bone is divided by a shallow groove into two small condyles with corresponding concavities on the distal bone. While each has collateral and plantar ligaments, an expansion from the extensor tendons forms the dorsal ligament.

MUSCLES AND FASCIA

The extrinsic foot muscles have their origin proximal to the ankle joint. They are the extensor group anteriorly and the peronei laterally. Both groups are innervated by the branches from the common peroneal nerve. The flexors situated behind the interosseous membrane are innervated by the tibial nerve. The muscles are covered by strong deep fascia which blends with the periosteum on the subcutaneous surfaces of the tibia and lateral malleolus. In the lower leg this deep fascia thickens to form the superior extensor retinaculum (transverse crural ligament) and the inferior extensor retinaculum (cruciate crural ligament). It then continues as the deep fascia on the dorsum of the foot (Fig. 2-20). The fascia dorsalis pedis is a thin membraneous layer which blends with the plantar aponeurosis at the sides while anteriorly it ensheathes the tendons on the dorsum of the foot and toes.

The distal margin of the popliteal fossa is formed by the medial and the lateral heads of the gastrocnemius, each of which arises from the femur. The soleus (originating from the proximal tibia and fibula) joins the tendon of gastrocnemius to reach the calcaneus as the tendo calcaneus. The plantaris, a diminutive muscle in man, arises from the lateral femoral condyle. The long slender tendon crosses medially

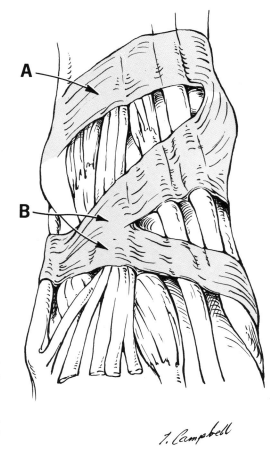

Fig. 2-20. A. Superior and, B. inferior extensor retinacula of right ankle

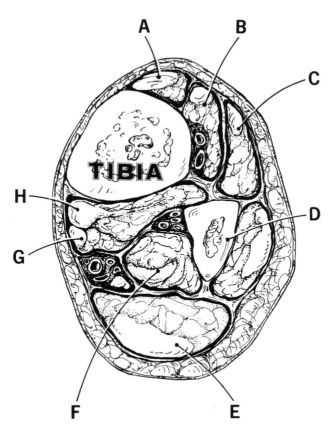

Fig. 2-21. Transverse section through the distal leg to show the proximity of the extensor hallucis longus tendon to the tibia. A. tibialis anterior, B. extensor hallucis longus, C. extensor digitorum longus, D. fibula, E. tendocalcaneus, F. flexor hallucis longus, G. flexor digitorum longus, H. tibialis posterior

between the soleus and gastrocnemius to reach the medial margin of the tendocalcaneus and continues into the calcaneus. These three muscles (triceps surae) are innervated by branches of the tibial nerve which sends superficial and deep branches to the soleus. The superficial innervation always passes between the lateral head of gastrocnemius and plantaris muscle, except when the plantaris is absent.

In the distal third of the leg the tendon of the extensor hallucis longus passes close to the periosteum of the tibia (Fig. 2-21). For this reason, following fractures of the distal tibia, extension of the great toe is one of the movements that is slower to return.

At the ankle region the long tendons, ves-

sels, and nerves have acquired a constant relationship to the bony points and are retained in position by the overlying fascial condensations (Fig. 2-11). The tendon of the tibialis posterior produces a shallow groove on the back of the medial malleolus, as does the peroneus brevis on the back of the lateral malleolus.

The attachment of tendons to bone is often more extensive than that shown in the anatomical illustrations. True, the area indicated has the principal insertion, reinforced by the penetrating Sharpey fibers through the bone cortex, but the tendon margin also blends firmly with the surrounding periosteum. This additional anchorage must be detached when mobilizing the tendons for transplanting.

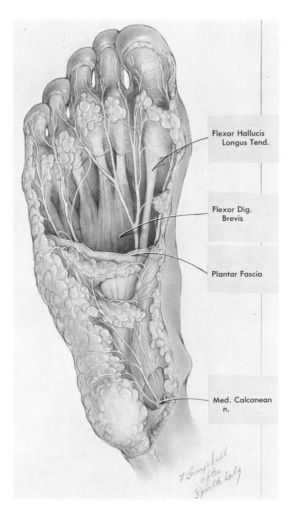

Fig. 2-22. Sole of right foot. Note subcutaneous fat lobules and plantar digital nerves

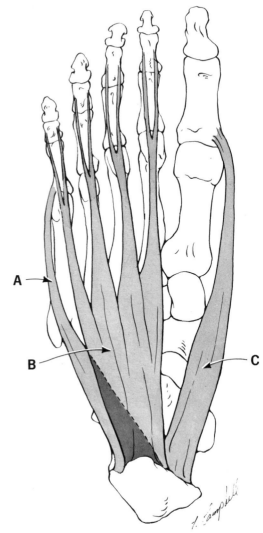

Fig. 2-23. Muscles of the first layer. A. abductor digiti minimi, B. flexor digitorum brevis, C. abductor hallucis

The fascia on the sole of the foot, or plantar aponeurosis, is a strong layer of white fibrous tissue. It is divided into a thick central part bounded by a medial and lateral portion. The central part is attached to the medial tubercle of the calcaneus. It spreads distally and divides near the metatarsal heads into five processes which straddle the flexor tendons, one for each toe. A superficial layer gains attachment to the deep skin fold between the toes and the sole. The deeper layer becomes continuous with the fibrous flexor sheath on the proximal phalanges, and it sends septa to the deep transverse ligament of the sole.

The plantar aponeurosis is firmly attached to the skin of the sole by numerous inelastic fibrous septa which enclose the fat lobules. On its deep aspect it gives origin to the flexor digitorum brevis. The weaker medial and lateral sections cover the abductor hallucis and abductor digiti minimi respectively (Fig. 2-17 and 22).

The muscles in the sole of the foot are divided into four layers. The first (subcutaneous) layer consists of the flexor digitorum brevis, the abductor hallucis, and the abductor digiti minimi (Fig. 2-23). The flexor digitorum brevis arises from the medial tubercle of the calcaneus and the

the lateral four toes. The abductor hallucis arises from the medial tubercle of the calcaneus and is inserted in the medial side of the base of the proximal phalanx of the great toe in common with the medial head of the flexor hallucis brevis. The abductor digiti minimi arises from the medial and lateral tubercle of the calcaneus and is inserted into the base of the proximal phalanx of the little toe. (The movements of abduction and adduction of the toes are poorly developed in man.) These three muscles together with the strong plantar aponeurosis form the principal tie beams of the medial and lateral longitudinal arches.

The second layer is made up of a tendon group and a muscle group (Fig. 2-24). The tendons are those of the flexor hallucis longus and the flexor digitorum longus which go to the lateral four toes. The quadratus plantae (flexor accessorius) has a bipennate origin from the calcaneus. The medial head, covering the margin of the long plantar ligament, is large and fleshly and may occasionally cause confusion in operative exposures. The four lumbrical muscles arise from the tendons of the flexor digitorum longus. They are inserted into the dorsal expansion of the extensor tendons of the lateral four toes, with a few fibers attached to the medial capsule of the metatarsophalangeal joint. The lumbrical tendons pass on the plantar side of the transverse metatarsal ligament, but the tendons of the interossei pass on its dorsal side. The foot lumbricals, although often poorly differentiated, extend the proximal interphalangeal joint and aid in flexion of the metatarsophalangeal joint of the lateral four toes. They counteract the tendency to claw toes.

The muscles of the third layer are the flexor hallucis brevis, the flexor digiti minimi and the oblique and transverse heads of the adductor hallucis (Fig. 2-25). The flexor hallucis brevis has a diffuse fibrous origin from the plantar tarsometatarsal ligaments and cuboid. At the head of the first metatarsal it splits into medial and lateral tendons which are inserted into the corresponding sides of the proximal phalanx of the big toe. Each tendon develops a sesamoid bone under the metatarsal head. The tibial (medial) tendon and sesamoid are

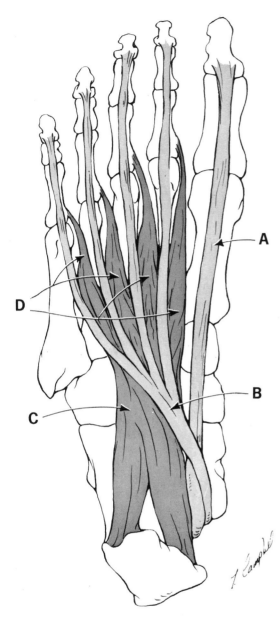

Fig. 2-24. Muscles of the second layer. A. tendon of flexor hallucis longus, B. tendon of flexor digitorum longus, C. quadratus plantae, D. lumbricals

plantar aponeurosis. It divides into four slender tendons which are inserted into the middle phalanges of the lateral four toes, having been previously perforated by the long flexor tendons. It is the prime flexor of the proximal interphalangeal joint of

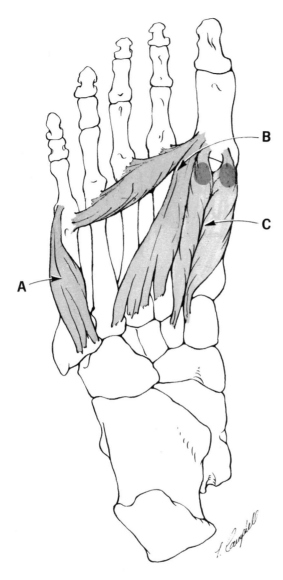

Fig. 2-25. Muscles of the third layer. A. flexor digiti minimi, B. adductor hallucis, C. flexor hallucis brevis

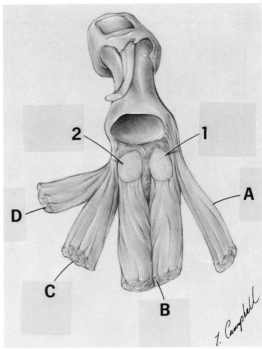

Fig. 2-26. The composite tendon of the flexor hallucis brevis. 1. medial sesamoid, 2. lateral sesamoid, A. abductor hallucis, B. flexor hallucis brevis, C. oblique head and, D. transverse head of adductor hallucis

jointed by the insertion of the abductor hallucis. The oblique and transverse heads of the adductor hallucis join the lateral or fibular tendon (Fig. 2-26). The diminutive transverse head of the adductor hallucis arises from the plantar capsule (plantar pad) of the four lateral metatarsophalangeal joints and from the transverse tarsal ligament. It crosses to the lateral tendon

of the flexor hallucis brevis on the deep side of the digital flexors and lumbrical tendons. The fleshy oblique head arises from the bases of the second, third and fourth metatarsals and the fascial sheath of the peroneus longus. It crosses obliquely under the concavity of the second, third and fourth metatarsal shafts to join the lateral tendon of the flexor hallucis brevis. The adductor hallucis reinforces the transverse tarsal ligament to counteract splaying of the forefoot. The flexor digiti minimi arises from the fifth metatarsal base and the sheath of the peroneus longus tendon. It is inserted into the base of the proximal phalanx of the little toe in common with the abductor digiti minimi.

The fourth layer consists of three plantar and four dorsal interosseus muscles together with the tendons of the peroneus longus and tibialis posterior. The three plantar interossei arising from the corre-

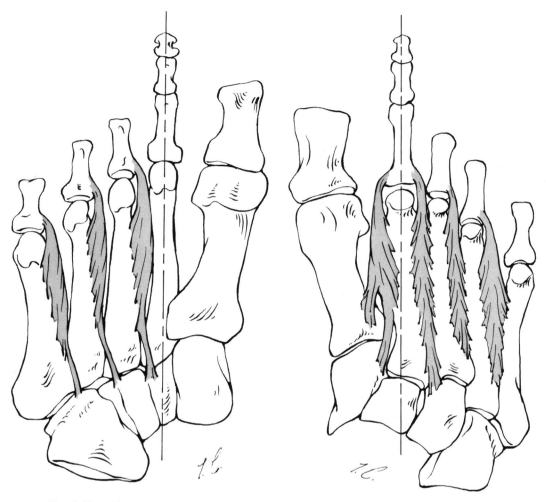

Fig. 2-27.   The plantar interossei   Fig. 2-28.   The dorsal interossei

sponding metatarsal shafts are unipennate and adduct the three lateral toes at the metatarsophalangeal joints (Fig. 2-27). The four dorsal interossei are bipennate and abduct the second, third and fourth toes from an axis through the second ray (Fig. 2-28). The interossei tendons are inserted into the bases of the proximal phalanges as illustrated with fibrous connections to the dorsal digital expansion.

The tendon of the peroneus longus passes through the groove on the cuboid in a medial direction to the lateral side of the first metatarsal base and medial cuneiform (Fig. 2-29). This insertion corresponds to the insertion of the tibialis anterior on the medial side of these two bones. The major insertion of the tibialis pos-

terior is into the medial aspect of the navicular tuberosity. In addition it attaches by fibrous expansion to all the other tarsal bones (except the talus) and to the bases of the second, third and fourth metatarsals.

The human plantar arches are maintained by:

1. the intrinsic shape and close interlocking of the foot bones. The posterior prolongation of the calcaneus enhances the support provided by the plantar fascia, the muscles of the first layer, the quadratus plantae and the long plantar ligament.

2. the strong plantar ligaments and fascia.

3. the postural tone and active contractions of the intrinsic and extrinsic foot muscles.

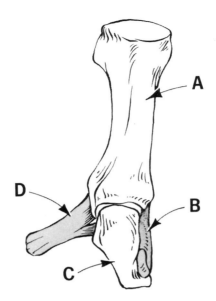

Fig. 2-29. A. First left metatarsal, B. tibialis anterior tendon, C. medial cuneiform, D. peroneus longus tendon

INNERVATION

The embryonic segmental distribution of the cutaneous nerves is maintained in the leg and foot. The preaxial or cephalic border is indicated by the long saphenous vein and the adjacent skin is innervated by segmental nerves, lumbar 3 and 4. The post axial border is indicated by the distal part of the short saphenous vein and is innervated by sacral segments 1 and 2. These segments overlap to a considerable extent and often show minor variations which may be exaggerated by prefixation or postfixation of the lumbosacral plexus in the spinal cord.

The sensory and motor innervation of the leg and foot is by sciatic nerve derivatives, Lumbar 4, 5, Sacral 1, 2 (except on the anteromedial aspect which gets its cutaneous nerve supply from the saphenous branch of the femoral, Lumbar 2 and 3). The saphenous nerve is distributed to the skin over the subcutaneous surface of the tibia and commonly reaches the medial side of the first metatarsophalangeal joint (Fig. 2-30). The common peroneal branch of the sciatic enters the leg behind the fibular head. It winds anteriorly on the neck of the fibula deep to the origin of the pero-

neus longus (Fig. 2-10). The superficial peroneal (musculocutaneous) branch stays in the peroneal compartment where it supplies the peroneus longus and brevis. It pierces the deep fascia at the lower third of the leg to split into medial and intermediate dorsal cutaneous nerves (Fig. 2-30). The medial branch crosses in front of the ankle joint to the medial side of the great toe and the adjacent margins of the second and third toes. It gives a communicating twig to the deep peroneal nerve in the first interdigital cleft. The intermediate dorsal cutaneous branches pass anterior to the lateral malleolus and fan out to reach the third and fourth interdigital spaces. During inversion one or more of these cutaneous branches are often visible.

The deep branch of the common peroneal nerve pierces the anterior peroneal septum to gain the extensor compartment of the leg. Here it is distributed to the extensor muscles of the ankle and toes and terminates as the dorsal digital nerve to the adjacent sides of the great and second toes (Fig. 2-30). The lateral margin of the foot gets its sensory nerve supply from the sural nerve (Sacral 1 and 2). Pos-

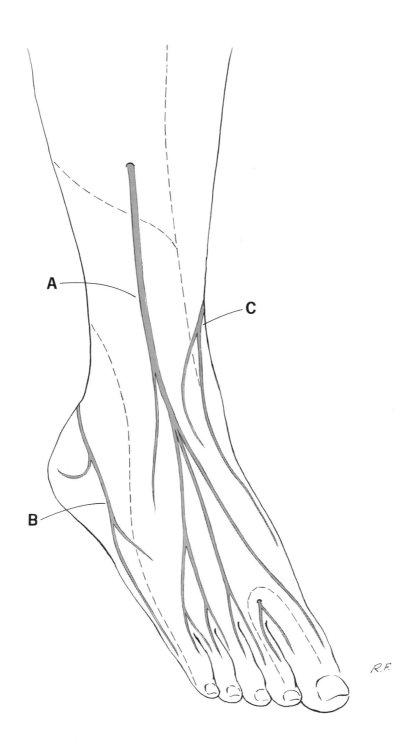

Fig. 2-30. Sensory innervation of dorsum of foot, A. dorsal cutaneous nerves from superficial peroneal, B. sural nerve, C. saphenous nerve. The terminal cutaneous branches of the deep peroneal nerve supply the first interdigital cleft.

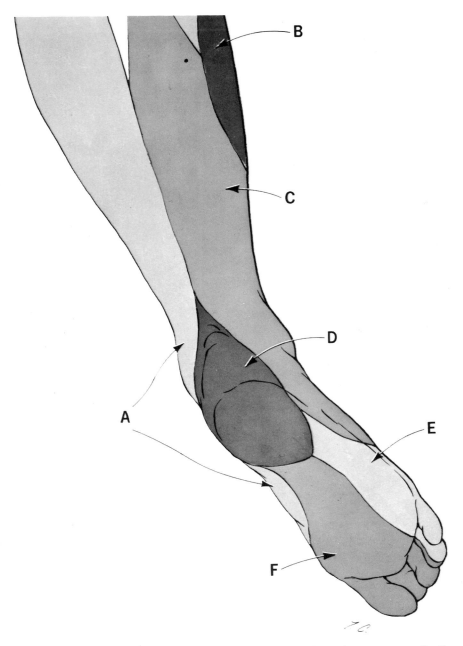

Fig. 2-31.   Sensory innervation of the right calf and sole. A. saphenous nerve (L. 3 and 4), B. superficial peroneal, C. sural (S. 1 and 2), D. tibial, E. lateral plantar, F. medial plantar

teriorly the medial calf is innervated by the saphenous (Lumbar 3 and 4). The lateral calf gets its nerve supply from the sural and peroneal communicating nerves (Sacral 1 and 2) (Fig. 2-31).

In the popliteal fossa the tibial branch of the sciatic nerve is placed superficial to the popliteal vein and artery. The sural

nerve pierces the deep fascia about the midcalf. In the subcutaneous tissue it passes downwards, gets a communication from the common peroneal nerve and then swings laterally to the outer margin of the foot and heel. At the soleal line the tibial nerve pierces the arched fibrous origin of the soleus to reach the intermuscular space between that muscle and the tibialis posterior. The adjacent superficial and deep calf muscles are innervated by this nerve. The medial calcaneal branch of the tibial nerve pierces the flexor retinaculum and is distributed to the skin on the medial, plantar and posterior aspect of the heel. This contributes the principal cutaneous innervation of the heel (Fig. 2-22).

The tibial nerve ends deep to the flexor retinaculum by dividing into medial and lateral plantar branches. The larger medial plantar nerve (Lumbar 4 and 5) has a limited motor but an extensive sensory distribution. It supplies the abductor hallucis, the flexor hallucis brevis, the flexor digitorum brevis and the first lumbrical. The cutaneous branches pass through the plantar fascia to supply the medial three-and-one-half digits and the corresponding skin of the sole — backwards to the level of the midtarsal joint (Fig. 2-31). It also sends interdigital twigs dorsally to innervate the area of the nail beds of the medial three toes. The smaller lateral plantar nerve (Sacral 1 and 2) passes laterally between the flexor digitorum brevis and quadratus plantae (Fig. 2-17) to the

region of the fifth metatarsal base where it divides into superficial and deep branches. The superficial branches supply the flexor digiti minimi, the interossei in the fourth intermetatarsal space, and the skin of the lateral one-and-one-half digits with a corresponding area of sole (Fig. 2-22 and 31). The deep branch moves into the space between the third and fourth layers to supply the remaining muscles of the foot.

John Hilton's comments on articular innervation are as germane today as they were when he made them a century ago. He said in 1863, "The same trunks of nerves, whose branches supply the group of muscles moving a joint, furnish also a distribution of nerves to the skin over the insertion of the same muscles, and (what at this moment more especially merits our attention) the interior of the joint receives its nerves from the same source. This implies an accurate and consentaneous physiological harmony in these various cooperating structures." The joint capsule and periosteum are morphologically similar. They have a rich nerve supply and are very sensitive to physical trauma, especially to stretch stimuli.

BLOOD VESSELS

The popliteal artery lies directly on the femur, the posterior knee-joint capsule, and the popliteus muscle. It is deep to the popliteal vein and tibial nerve. At the inferior border of the popliteus muscle the artery divides into an anterior and posterior tibial branch. Distal to the knee (and as at the elbow), venae comitantes flank the larger arteries. These form a valved plexus embedded in the periarterial fascia and, as in the valved lymphatic trunks, the contents derive a forward impetus from the adjacent arterial impulse.

The anterior tibial, the smaller branch of the popliteal artery, passes close to the fibular neck to gain the extensor compartment of the leg (Fig. 2-32). It descends on the interosseous membrane medial to the deep branch of the common peroneal nerve, between the tibialis anterior and the extensors which arise from the fibula. In the lower leg, it moves onto the tibia and crosses the center of the anterior capsule

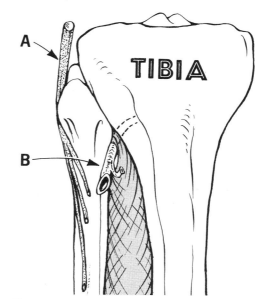

Fig. 2-32.   Proximal end of right fibula to show, A. the common peroneal nerve and, B. the anterior tibial artery (interosseous membrane-stippled)

of the ankle joint to become the dorsalis pedis artery.

On the dorsum of the foot the dorsalis pedis artery commonly lies between the tendon of the extensor hallucis longus on the medial side and the tendons of the extensor digitorum longus laterally. It terminates at the proximal end of the first intermetatarsal space by division into the deep plantar and first dorsal metatarsal branches. This arterial pattern often shows considerable variation. The anterior tibial artery may end about the midleg level, when the dorsalis pedis will be a branch of the peroneal artery. Occasionally the dorsalis pedis may be absent or it may be large enough to replace the lateral plantar vessel.

In the region of the ankle joint the lateral and medial malleolar arteries pass behind the long extensor tendons to reach the lateral and medial malleolus respectively. They join other articular branches to form the articular vascular circle or circulus articuli vasculosus of William Hunter (1743). This rich anastomosis which is characteristic of all synovial joints is situated immediately under the synovial membrane at the margin of the articular cartilage. Through the bony vascular foramina it also contributes an adequate blood supply to the adjacent bones.

The posterior tibial artery passes deep to the soleal origin and accompanies the tibial nerve and venae comitantes to the level of the medial malleolus. These structures lie posterior to the tibialis posterior, the flexor digitorum longus and lower tibia. They are deep to the soleus and the tendo calcaneus. The principal neurovascular bundle to the skin of the heel, the medial calcaneal branches, passes almost vertically downwards from the medial side (Fig. 2-22). Horizontal incisions in this area may jeopardize the nutrition of the heel flap. About one inch below the bifurcation of the popliteal artery the posterior tibial gives off the peroneal artery. It follows a course close to the fibula and ends by dividing into lateral calcaneal and perforating branches.

The posterior tibial artery ends deep to the flexor retinaculum by dividing into the medial and lateral plantar vessels. The larger lateral plantar artery accompanies the lateral plantar nerve and its deep branches. Under the second metatarsal shaft the vessel anastomoses with the deep plantar branch of the dorsalis pedis artery to complete the plantar arch. The plantar digital vessels come from this plantar arch. The more diminutive dorsal digital arteries are branches of the arcuate branch of the dorsalis pedis artery. The smaller medial plantar artery passes forward between the abductor hallucis and flexor digitorum brevis, both of which it supplies. It sends small terminal branches with the digital twigs of the medial plantar nerve.

The veins of the lower limb are divided into a superficial and a deep group. The superficial group consists of the great (long) and small (short) saphenous systems which lie in the subcutaneous tissue. The deep veins accompany the arteries and are under the deep fascia. Both venous systems are provided with numerous valves.

The great saphenous vein drains the medial marginal of the dorsal venous plexus. It passes proximally anterior to the medial malleolus and then onto the medial side of the leg, generally on the posterior side of the saphenous nerve. The small saphenous vein drains the lateral margin of the foot and the lateral side of the dorsal venous arch. It continues behind the lateral malleolus into the calf and pierces the deep fascia in the roof of the popliteal fossa to join the popliteal vein. The great and small saphenous venous systems communicate freely with each other and with the deep system of veins.

The deep veins of the lower extremity accompany the arterial tree and its branches. The deep plantar venous arch drains the digital blood into the medial and lateral plantar vessels. The venae comitantes around the peroneal, the anterior and the posterior tibial arteries unite at the proximal border of the interosseous membrane to form the popliteal vein. Many valved communicating or perforating veins join the superficial and deep systems through the deep fascia. They allow blood to pass from the superficial to the deep groups, but not vice versa under normal conditions. A constant communication is found at the termination of the great and small saphenous veins, at the fossa ovalis, and the popliteal fossa. Communications are also present proximal and distal to joints, such as the ankle, knee and transverse tarsal. Additional perforating veins are often noticed on the course of the great and small saphenous veins passing through the deep fascia of the calf and by the intermuscular septa to the venae comitantes of the posterior tibial artery.

LYMPHATIC VESSELS

Avascular structures, such as the epidermis, nails, hair and hyaline cartilage are devoid of lymphatic vessels. The lymphatic dermal plexus of the digits drains onto the dorsal aspect of the foot as in the hand. The lymphatic vessels follow the course of the great and small saphenous veins to the inguinal and pcpliteal lymph nodes, respectively. A few lymph nodes are situated closs to the popliteal vessels and occasionally at the proximal end of the interosseous membrane.

SKIN

The skin is made up of a felted, flexible elastic corium or dermis covered by an avascular and insensitive epidermis or cuticle. The dermis, which is developed from mesoderm, consists of a superficial, highly sensitive, vascular, papillary layer. The deeper reticular layer of strong interlacing bands of fibrous and elastic tissue covers the subcutaneous area. Careful scrutiny shows that the sensitive dermal papillae are actually dermal ridges which fit into reciprocal furrows on the deep aspect of the epidermis. The superficial corneal (horney) layer of the epidermis (ectodermal) includes a clear stratum lucidum and superficial keratinized layer of desquamating cells. Under conditions of excessive moisture the soft keratin of the epidermis becomes swollen and macerated as typically seen between the fourth and fifth toes, a relatively enclosed area which allows very little evaporation. Skin thickness ranges from 0.5 mm (as in the eyelid) to 4 to 5 mm in the sole of the foot. The thick skin of the digits and sole has a rich innervation, and although it is covered by 3 to 4 mm of epidermis, it is still very sensitive. The plantar skin is firmly bound to the plantar aponeurosis by fibrous septa which envelope the fat lobules. This fibrofatty layer acts as a buffer for protection of the deeper structures (Fig. 2-22).

Until recently the correct position and direction for skin incisions has been one of the more neglected aspects of surgery. Diagrams of Langer's lines have been reproduced for many years and have been suggested as the most appropriate direction for surgical exposures. Incisions parallel to the natural crease or wrinkle lines are recommended for better healing and cosmetic results. The crease or wrinkle lines, which are attached by fibrous septa to the deep fascia, are always directed at right angles to the pull of the underlying muscles or tendon, e.g., the palmar and digital creases. Holmstrand et al. have shown that most of the collagenous fibers in the dermis lie parallel to the wrinkle lines and, furthermore, that the new collagenous fibers of scar tissue invariably parallel the scar irrespective of the direction of the crease lines. Incisions made parallel to the wrinkle creases heal with their collagenous fibers in line with those in the normal dermis and produce a better cosmetic result. Undoubtedly other factors such as the site and size of the pathological lesion, the direction of the neurovascular bundle, the prominence of the underlying bone, and the problems of skin pressure also influence the type of skin incisions selected and must receive serious consideration.

SURFACE ANATOMY

In the foot accurate anatomical knowledge is a prerequisite to correct diagnosis. The visible and palpable bony prominences form the most constant and accurate landmarks in surface anatomy.

On the medial side (Fig. 2-33) the palpable bony points are:

1. the medial malleolus
2. the navicular tuberosity, most prominent on inversion

3. the base, shaft, and head of the first metatarsal
4. the phalanges of the great toe
5. the head and neck of talus, most obvious on eversion
6. the sustentaculum tali of the calcaneus

The posterior margin of the navicular indicates the medial end of the midtarsal joint. The tendo calcaneus is easily recognized as is the extensor hallucis longus

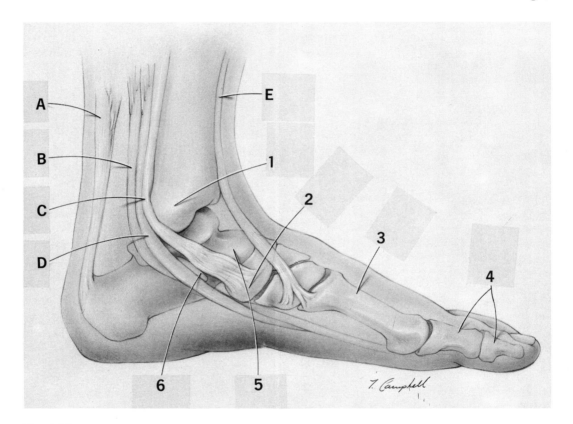

Fig. 2-33.   Medial aspects of left foot. 1. Medial malleolus, 2. Navicular tuberosity, 3. first metatarsal, 4. phalanges of great toe, 5. head of talus, 6. sustentaculum tali. A. tendocalcaneus, B. flexor hallucis longus, C. tibialis posterior, D. flexor digitorum longus, E. tibialis anterior.

tendon during extension of the great toe. Forced active inversion throws the tendons of the tibialis anterior and posterior into prominence. The sustentaculum tali, which is covered by the tendon of the flexor digitorium longus, forms the lower margin of the subtalar joint, and the principal neuro-

vascular bundle to the sole skirts its inferior border. The pulsations of the posterior tibial artery are felt about 2 cm. behind the medial malleolus.

On the lateral aspect (Fig. 2-34) the identifiable bony points are:

1. The lateral malleolus of the fibula

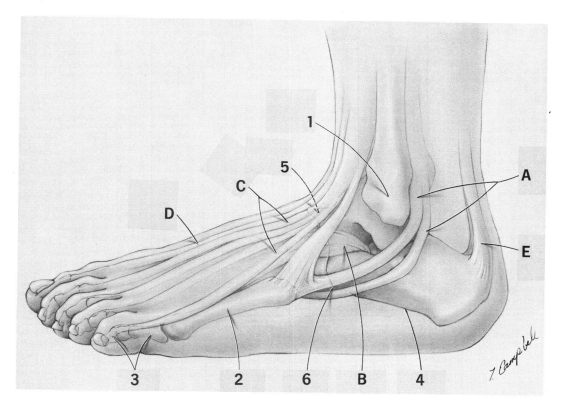

Fig. 2-34. Lateral aspect of left foot. 1. lateral malleolus, 2. fifth metatarsal, 3. phalanges, 4. calcaneus, A. peroneal tendons, B. belly of extensor digitorum brevis arising from inferior margin of sinus tarsi, C. tendons of extensor digitorum longus, D. tendon of extensor hallucis longus

2. The base, shaft, and head of the fifth metatarsal

3. The phalanges of the lateral toes

4. The calcaneus comprising the body, the peroneal tubercle (trochlear process) if present, projecting between the peroneal tendons and the inferior margin of the sinus tarsi, which gives origin to the palpable belly of the extensor digitorum brevis

5. The head and neck of the talus, more easily palpated during inversion and flexion.

6. The lateral end of the midtarsal joint is located midway between the lateral malleolus and the base of the fifth metatarsal and can be made more obvious by inversion and adduction of the foot.

The sinus tarsi is identified as a depression anterior to the lateral malleolus. It is an important landmark during surgical exposures of the subtalar joint from the lateral side. Having severed the attachments in the sinus tarsi, it is imperative to direct the posterior prolongation of the capsular incision *distally* and posteriorly to enter the posterior talocalcaneal joint. A posterior prolongation directed *proximally* invariably opens the ankle joint. The tendons of the peronei are palpable during eversion, passing from the posterior margin of the lateral malleolus in the direction of the base of the fifth metatarsal. The belly of the extensor digitorum brevis is easily recognized on the inferior margin of the sinus tarsi during active toe extension. Following tears of the lateral ankle ligament the depression of the sinus may be filled by a hematoma.

In addition to the items already mentioned on the dorsum of the foot, the tendons of the extensor digitorum longus are noticeable. Between these tendons and that of the extensor hallucis longus the pulsations in the dorsalis pedis artery are palpable. The dorsal venous plexus and the terminal branches of the superficial peroneal nerve may also be visible. The metatarso-phalangeal and interphalangeal joints are palpable between the plantar and dorsal aspects of the foot. On the sole the posterior tubercles of the calcaneus, the fifth metatarsal base, the tuberosity of the navicular and the sesamoids of the great toe are identifiable. The digital nerves can be occasionally and painfully rolled under the more lateral metatarsal heads.

GROWTH CHANGES

Even in fetal life the arched foot is a distinctive human characteristic, although it may be camouflaged by the subcutaneous baby fat according to some investigators.

Each tarsal bone is ossified from a single center, except the calcaneus which has an epiphysis at its posterior end. The primary centers for the calcaneus, the talus and the cuboid, appear at the sixth, seventh, and nine months respectively of fetal life. However in the navicular, which is a relatively large tarsal bone, the primary center does not appear until the third or fourth year. At birth the navicular is a flat plate of cartilage between the head of the talus and the cuneiforms, but in childhood the navicular shows a marked acceleration of growth rate compared to the other foot bones. Two directional changes occur in the talus during the growth period. In the adult the neck of the talus deviates medially 20 degrees or less from the antero-posterior direction of the trochlear surface. In the infant the axis of neck is directed medially 30 degrees or more (Fig. 2-35). In addition the neck of the talus undergoes a longitudinal rotation as seen in Figure 2-36. Some authorities maintain that the

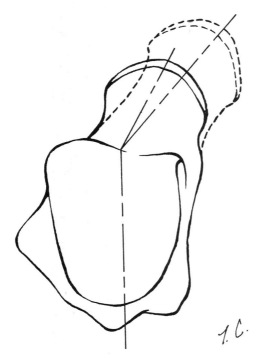

Fig. 2-35.

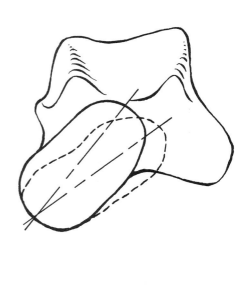

Fig. 2-36.

Fig. 2-35.   Left talus of adult (continuous outline) contrasted with the more angulated and longer neck of the fetal bone (broken outline).

Fig. 2-36.   Anterior view of left talus to show rotation of the head from the fetal (broken arrow) to adult life (continuous outline).

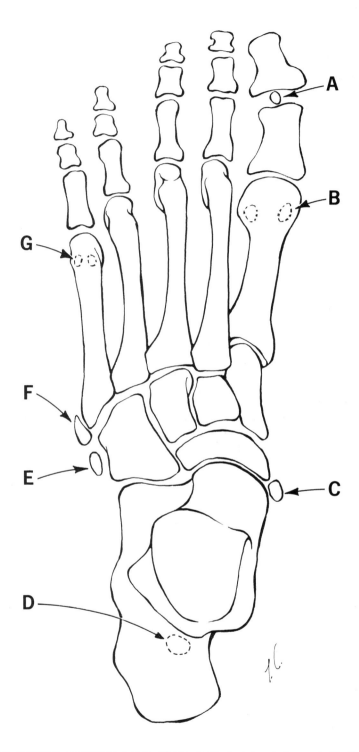

Fig. 2-37. The more common accessory bones of the foot. A. interphalangeal, B. flexor hallucis brevis, sesamoids, C. os tibiale externum, D. os trigonum, E. sesamoid in tendon of peroneus longus, F. ossicle at base of fifth metatarsal, G. sesamoids under head of fifth metatarsal

directional changes in the talus occur at the trochlear surface rather than in the neck.

The lateral deviation of the head and neck of the talus, together with the accelerated growth in thickness of the navicular, corrects the infantile adduction of the forefoot. The very active rate of growth in a large avascular cartilagenous mass and, later, in the ossification center, may be an etiological factor in the so-called osteochondritic changes of the navicular.

Anomalous ossifications, although rare, are found most commonly in the foot and may present diagnostic and medicolegal problems to the clinician. Ossification centers, which normally unite, may fail to do so and, more unusual, additional unions may occur between bone elements. The anomalies are so commonly bilateral, though not necessarily similar in size and shape, that when they come under consideration, a roentgenogram of the other foot should be available for comparison.

Perhaps the most dramatic and striking examples are the bony fusions seen in syndactylism and the additional bone formation of polydactylism. Rarely a bony bar may unite the calcaneus to the navicular, to the cuboid, or to the talus, or fusion may be found between the middle and distal phalanges of the toes.

Accessory foot bones are of two types.

The sesamoids which are typically embedded in a tendon and the true accessory bone (supernumerary ossicles) that may be either projections from a foot bone or separate ossicles. The sesamoids occur typically where the tendons are acutely angulated or subject to pressure. Under the first metatarsal head the medial and lateral sesamoids of the flexor hallucis brevis are constantly found. Whereas the medial bone may consist of two, three, or even four bone areas (multipartite sesamoids), the lateral sesamoid rarely divides and then only into two parts. Occasionally sesamoids are found in the tendon of the peroneus longus or under the heads of the lateral metatarsals.

The ossification centers for the accessory bones of the foot appear between the seventh and tenth years and attain full size at the age of twenty. The commoner accessory bones are the os trigonum at the posterior margin of the talus, the os tibiale externum (although at the medial side of the foot), or accessory navicular, placed on the medial side of the navicular. A separate bony nodule is found at the base of the fifth metatarsal. Two ossification centers which fail to unite may produce a bifid medial cuneiform or bifid navicular. The more common accessory bones of the foot are shown in Figure 2-37.

REFERENCES

Barnett, C. H., Davies, D. V., MacConaill, M. A.: *Synovial Joints*, Springfield, Charles C Thomas, 1961.

Fick, R.: *Handbuch der Anatomie und Mechanik der Golenke*, Vol. III, Jena, G. Fischer, 1911.

Gardner, E. *et al.*: *Anatomy*, 2nd Ed., Philadelphia, W. B. Saunders Co., 1963

Grant, J. C. B.: *Atlas of Anatomy*, 5th Ed., Baltimore, The Williams & Wilkins Co., 1962.

Gray, H.: *Anatomy of the Human Body*, 28th Ed., Philadelphia, Lea & Febiger, 1966.

Harty, M.: The Position of the Foot in Walking, Lancet 2, 275, 1953.

Hilton, J.: *Rest and Pain*, London, Bell and Daldy,

1863.

Holmstrand, K. *et al.*: The Ultrastructure of Collagen in Skin, Scar and Keloid, Plast. & Reconst. Surg., 27:597, 1961.

Humphry, G. M.: *The Human Foot and the Human Hand*, London, MacMillan & Co., 1861.

Hunter, W.: Philos. Trans. of Royal Society, *42*: 470, 514-521, 1743.

Inkster, R. G. *et al.*: The Anatomy of the Locomotor System. London, Oxford University Press, 1956.

Wood, Jones, F.: *Structure and Function As Seen in the Foot*. Baltimore, The Williams & Wilkins Co., 1944.

═ 3 ═

Definitions of the Normal

and of the Abnormal Foot

In this chapter we will begin to deal with movements and ranges of motion. The terms to be used will be defined and the ranges of motion will be listed in accordance with the recommended standards of joint motion recorded in the monograph *Method of Measuring and Recording* pub-lished by the American Academy of Or-thopaedic Surgeons in 1965. Furthermore, without a good working knowledge of the normal movements of the foot, one cannot evaluate the abnormal properly. Nor can one define motions of the foot without in-cluding the motions of the ankle joint.

DEFINITIONS

Extension (*dorsiflexion*) is a term used to describe the range of motion which takes place through the foot and the ankle joint when the foot is brought in an upward direction toward the leg. The average range of normal active extension varies with age. In the child, adolescent, young adult, and in the athletic adult the range of active extension of the foot and ankle is, on the average, 30 degrees from the neutral right angle position with the knee flexed at an angle of 90 degrees. In the middle-aged average adult the range of active extension is from 10 to 20 degrees. Furthermore, the preponderant part of this movement takes place through the ankle and only a very slight portion takes place through the tarsal joints (Fig. 3-1).

Passively the range of extension varies. "Relative Passive Extension" of the ankle from the neutral right angle position is 25 to 30 degrees in children and young adults. However, by *locking* the tarsal joints, so that the only motion is that which takes place through the ankle joint (called "True Passive Extension"), the range is limited to only 10 to 15 degrees in the child and from 0 to a maximum of 5 degrees in the adult. In order to lock the tarsal joints, one must invert the foot to a maximum amount. It is important to lock the tarsal joints at all times when testing for passive extension of the ankle because this will give the true range of motion of the ankle joint. It will

55

THE ANKLE

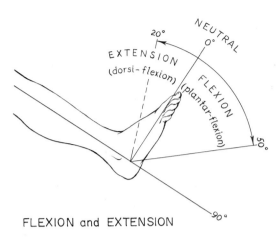

FLEXION and EXTENSION

Fig. 3-1. Range of active extension (dorsi-flexion) and flexion (plantar flexion) of the foot and ankle. **These motions should be tested with the knee extended.**

also yield information needed regarding the contracture of the calf muscle structures which it is so important to elicit in certain abnormal conditions, as well as in various deformities of the foot.

Contracture of the calf muscle group or of the tendo achillis, loss of extension of the ankle joint, etc., can be demonstrated only by locking the subtalar joint. Note the difference in the apparent range of motion when the same foot is extended with the subtalar joints unlocked (Fig. 3-2A) and in the true range of passive extension when the subtalar joint is locked (Fig. 3-2B).

Since the ankle is a modified hinge joint, its primary motions are flexion and extension. There is a minimal degree of lateral movement when the ankle is in a position of *flexion* (plantar flexion). The range of flexion of the ankle and foot is 50 degrees from the right angle position (Fig. 3-1). All eversion and inversion movements

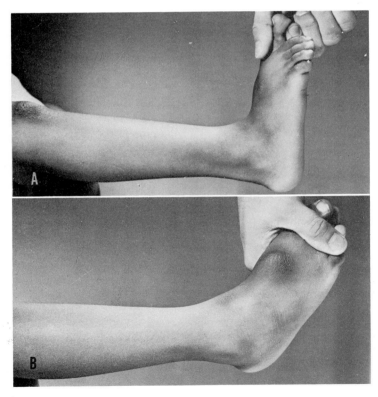

Fig. 3-2A. **Relative Passive Extension.** Note that the foot extends to an angle of 35 degrees when the tarsal joints are unlocked.

Fig. 3-2B. **True Passive Extension.** Same foot with tarsal joints locked. Extension is absent due to contracture of the calf muscle group. Locking of the tarsal joints is performed by maximum inversion of the midfoot and forefoot.

HIND PART of the FOOT

A
ZERO STARTING
POSITION

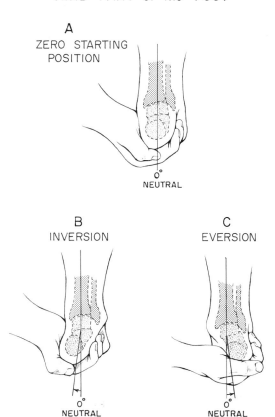

0°
NEUTRAL

B
INVERSION

C
EVERSION

0°
NEUTRAL

0°
NEUTRAL

Fig. 3-3.   Hind Part of the Foot.
A.   Neutral position of heel in relation to
the tibia.
B.   Passive Inversion: Motion takes place
through the talocalcaneal joint. The average
range of motion is 5 degrees.
C.   Passive Eversion: Motion takes place
through the talocalcaneal joint. The average
range of motion is 5 degrees.

FORE PART of the FOOT

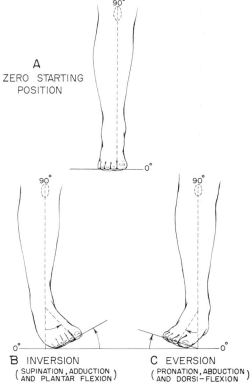

90°

A
ZERO STARTING
POSITION

0°

90°

90°

0°

0°

B   INVERSION
(SUPINATION, ADDUCTION)
(AND PLANTAR FLEXION)

C   EVERSION
(PRONATION, ABDUCTION)
(AND DORSI-FLEXION)

Fig. 3-4.   Active Inversion and Eversion Motion.
A.   Zero starting position: The foot is aligned
with the tibia in the long axis from the knee to
the ankle with the axis extending between the
first and second toes, and more specifically,
between the first and second metatarsal heads.
B.   Active Inversion: The forepart of the foot
turns medially. It includes supination, adduction,
and a slight amount of flexion (plantar flexion).
Average range of motion is 30 degrees.
C.   Active Eversion: The forepart of the foot
turns outwardly or laterally. It includes pronation, abduction, and extension (dorsi-flexion).
Average range of motion is 15 to 20 degrees.

*which are mistakenly attributed to the
ankle take place through the subtalar joint.*
If any such movement occurs through the
ankle joint per se, it should be considered
abnormal.

In measuring the movements of the foot,
one must differentiate those dealing with
the hind part of the foot, or more specifically, the subtalar joint, and those dealing
with the forepart of the foot consisting of
the mid-tarsal and the tarsometatarsal
joints. However, major emphasis must be

given primarily to the former, since there
is only a trace of motion in the tarsometatarsal joints actively and passively —
an amount so slight that it is difficult to
measure.

There is practically no active motion of
the hind part of the foot; therefore, only
the passive movements will be considered.
In the zero starting position the heel is
aligned with the midline of the tibia (Fig.
3-3A). To produce *inversion* (Fig. 3-3B)
the heel is grasped firmly in the cup of the

examiner's hand and is turned inwardly. The average range of motion is 5 degrees (slightly more in a child). When measuring *eversion,* which is also 5 degrees on the average, the heel is turned in the outward direction (Fig. 3-3C). There is also a certain amount of forward motion of the subtalar joint. This is minimal and difficult to measure but it is important to keep it in mind. At the same time, loss of the movements of the hind foot, as in a triple arthrodesis, leaves the foot quite stiff despite the fact that there may be some compensatory increase in the movements of the forepart of the foot.

In evaluating the motions of the forepart of the foot (more commonly called the forefoot), the zero starting position is designated as the position in which the foot is aligned with the tibia in the long axis from the knee to the ankle and the axis extending between the first and second toes (Fig. 3-4A). *Active inversion* is that movement in which the forefoot turns medially. It includes supination, adduction and a slight amount of flexion (plantar flexion). This motion averages approximately 30 degrees (Fig. 3-4B). In *active eversion* the foot is directed laterally with the sole of the foot facing in that direction. This motion includes pronation, abduction, and extension and its range measures 15 to 20 degrees (Fig. 3-4C).

The *passive inversion* and *eversion* movements (Fig. 3-5A and B) are informative. They should always be checked by the examiner since they give considerable clinical information that may not be derived from the active movements. The heel must be held by one hand of the examiner, while the other hand turns the foot inward. The amount of motion passively is only slightly greater than the active range of motion but the clinical "feel" of the foot, that is, how the foot feels in the examiner's hand, is highly informative. This also applies to passive eversion when the foot is carried outwardly in the same manner.

Passive adduction and abduction (Fig. 3-5C) motions are procured by moving the forepart of the foot in an inward and an outward direction, respectively, with one hand while the heel is held with the other, through the same axis. There are 20 de-

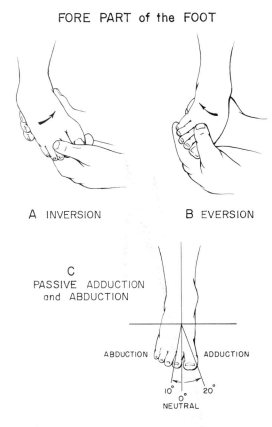

FORE PART of the FOOT

A INVERSION   B EVERSION

C
PASSIVE ADDUCTION
and ABDUCTION

ABDUCTION   ADDUCTION

10°   20°
0°
NEUTRAL

Fig. 3-5. Passive Inversion, Eversion, Adduction, and Abduction Motion.
  A. Passive Inversion: Testing the passive range of motion of the foot is as important as the active range of motion since this portion of the evaluation of the tarsal and ankle motion can be imformative.
  B. Passive Eversion: — Note position of hands in testing for both passive inversion and eversion.
  C. Passive adduction and abduction determine the range of motion of the forepart of the foot. This motion must take place in the plane of the sole of the foot.

grees of passive adduction and 10 degrees of passive abduction in the average normal foot. This motion must take place in the plane of the sole of the foot. Usually, one uses the opposite normal foot to measure some of these passive movements since it is seldom that both feet are involved. When both feet are affected, it is possible only to state that the active movements of eversion, inversion, adduction and abduction are mildly, moderately, or severely

THE GREAT TOE

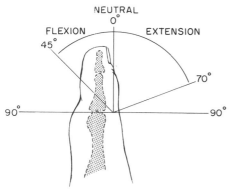

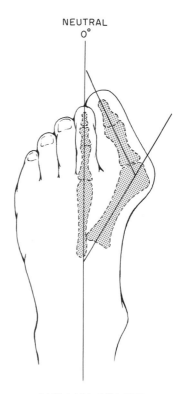

A   METATARSOPHALANGEAL JOINT

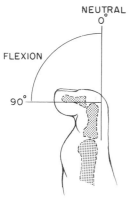

B   INTERPHALANGEAL JOINT

HALLUX VALGUS

Fig. 3-6. Motion of the Great Toe Joints.
A.   Metatarsophalangeal   Joint   Range   of
Motion:
In the zero starting position, the two phalanges are in line with the first metatarsal in the
lateral view. There are 45 degrees of **passive**
flexion and 70 degrees of **passive** extension on
the average at the first matatarso-phalangeal
joint.
B.   Interphalangeal Joint Range of Motion:
At the inter-phalangeal joint of the great toe,
there are 90 degrees of **passive** flexion and 35
degrees of **active** flexion on the average. There
is no active extension and only a trace of passive extension in the adult.

Fig. 3-7. Hallux Valgus. Hallux Valgus deformity and method of measuring same by bisecting the second metatarsal, the first metatarsal and the phalanges of the great toe. The
angle of the deformity is the angle between the
phalanges and the first metatarsal. The amount
of abduction of the first metatarsal is measured
as the angle between this structure and the line
bisecting the second metatarsal.

limited, since it is difficult to measure these
movements in degrees.
    When measuring the passive motion of
the great toe, the zero starting position is

that in which the great toe is in line
with the first metatarsal bone (Fig. 3-6A).
Flexion, an average of 45 degrees, is present in the first metatarsophalangeal joint,
and the range of extension in this same
articulation is 60 to 70 degrees (Fig. 3-6A).
In the interphalangeal joint of the first digit
there is no extension and 35 degrees of
active flexion (Fig. 3-6B). Should a de-

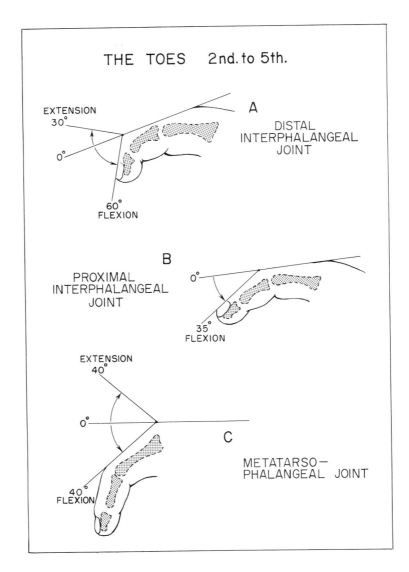

Fig. 3-8.   Range of Motion of 2nd to 5th Toes. A. The range of motion of the distal interphalangeal joint of each toe is 30 degrees of extension and 60 degrees of flexion, B. The proximal interphalangeal joint demonstrates on the average 35 degrees of flexion and no extension. C. The metatarso-phalangeal joint has a range of 40 degrees of extension and 40 degrees of flexion, on the average.

formity of the great toe be present, it may be measured by bisecting the first metatarsal and the bones of the great toe as in hallux valgus (Fig. 3-7).

The remaining digits have flexion motion of the metatarsophalangeal, proximal interphalangeal and distal interphalangeal joints as indicated (Fig. 3-8A and B), but only the metatarsophalangeal joints demonstrate any extension (Fig. 3-8C). Abduction and adduction of the digits (toe spread) are measured in relation to the second toe (Fig. 3-9).

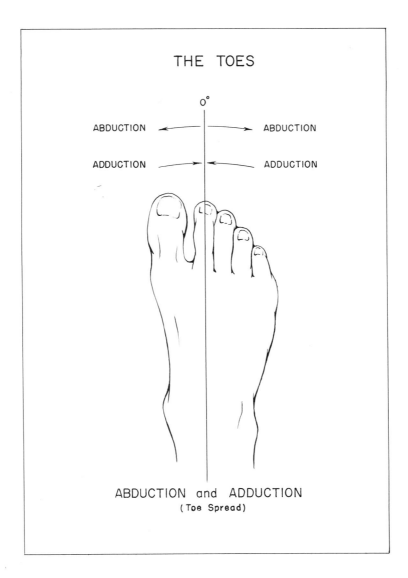

Fig. 3-9. Adduction and abduction movments of the toes are measured in relation to the second toe. This motion is passive in type.

THE COMMON DEFORMITIES

The deformities of the foot can involve either one or several joints and their surrounding soft tissues. Some of these deformities are acquired, but most are congenital. Only the more common ones will be defined in order to provide an easy, quick reference source.

Hallux Valgus. The deformity here involves the great toe at the level of the metatarsophalangeal joint (Fig. 3-10). In this deformity there is lateral deviation or adduction of the toe in relationship to the first metatarsal shaft and head. If, as in some instances, in addition to the valgus

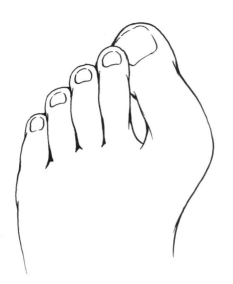

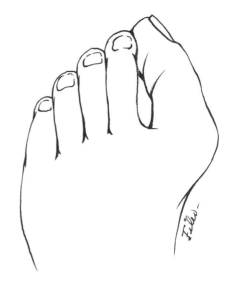

Hallux valgus

H.V. with metatarsus varus primus

Fig. 3-10. Hallux Valgus. The deformity consists of adduction of the great toe in relation
to the metatarsal shaft and head.

Fig. 3-11. Metatarsus Varus Primus. This is a
hallux valgus deformity with rotation of the
metatarsal producing a rotational deformity of
the toe as well. It is usually an hereditary type
of hallux valgus deformity.

deformity, the toe is rotated inwardly, in other words toward the great toe of the opposite foot, the condition is designated as hallux valgus with metatarsus varus primus (Fig. 3-11). This defect is due to the medial rotation of the first metatarsal shaft superimposed on the valgus deformity.

Hallux Varus. This connotes a medial deviation or abduction of the great toe in relation to the first metatarsal shaft. It is almost invariably a congenital deviation, frequently found in association with a varus deformity of the forefoot (Fig. 3-12).

Hallux Rigidus. This condition produces rather a marked or a complete limitation of extension and/or of flexion of the great toe at the first metatarsophalangeal joint. This is an acquired deformity and is associated with osteoarthrosis of the first metatarsophalangeal joint.

Cock-up Deformity. This is a condition in which there is flexion of the interphalangeal joint and extension at the metatarsophalangeal joint (Fig. 3-13). It is due primarily to muscle imbalance between the great toe flexors and the great toe extensors. It generally stems from a weakness of the extensor hallucis longus which permits overactivity of the flexor hallucis longus.

Hammer Toe. In this deformity there is usually involvement of either the proximal or distal interphalangeal joint. The defect consists of a flexion contracture of either of these two articulations (Fig. 3-14). Frequently a painful corn (clavus) or a callus will overlie the bony prominence. The capsule of the plantar surface of the involved joint is usually contracted.

Metatarsus Varus (Fig. 3-15). This deformity consists of medial deviation of the

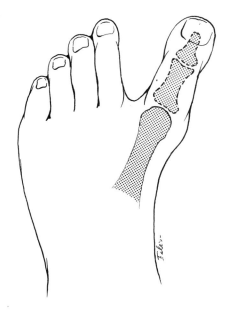

Hallux varus

Fig. 3-12. Hallux Varus. This is an abduction deformity of the great toe and is usually associated with a metatarsus varus or a varus deformity of the forefoot.

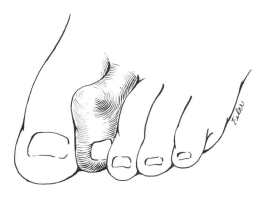

Hammer toe

Fig. 3-14. Hammer Toe. This deformity may involve either of the interphalangeal joints of the toe. The capsule on the plantar surface of the involved joint is usually contracted.

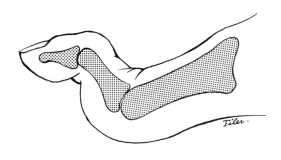

Cock-up deformity Great toe

Fig. 3-13. Cock-up Deformity. This deformity involves primarily the great toe with flexion of the inter-phalangeal joint and extension of the metatarso-phalangeal articulation due, usually, to muscle imbalance.

metatarsals and occasionally of the first row of tarsal bones. Although initially the deformity is one involving the soft tissue structures, if allowed to persist, it can extend to bony structures as well, if the basic condition remains unchecked. It can occur as either a congenital or an acquired malformation.

Pes Planus (Pronated Foot). This term refers to the presence of a flatfoot (Fig. 3-16). In this instance there are varying degrees of the flatfoot condition. The severe form of flatfoot, which is almost invariably of congenital origin, is indicated by the term *calcaneovalgus* (Fig. 3-17) since the heel is in a laterally deviated position due to a congenital or hereditary disturbance in the relative positioning of the os calcis, the talus, and the navicular bones.

Pes Cavus (Fig. 3-18). This term is used to designate the type of foot characterized by a higher than normal longitudinal arch. The deformity can be either hereditary or acquired. It may or may not be accompanied by flexion deformities of the toes. When such deformities are present in ad-

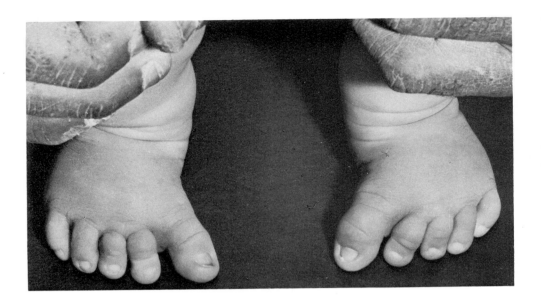

Fig. 3-15. Metatarsus Varus. This deformity can be either congenital or acquired and consists of medial deviation of the metatarsals and of the great toe.

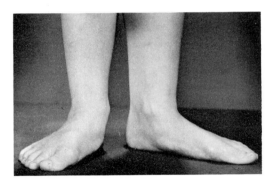 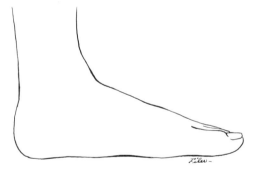

Fig. 3-16. Pes Planus—(Flat or Pronated Foot). The longitudinal arch of the foot is depressed or absent in the standing position.

dition to the cavus, the syndrome is called a *clawfoot deformity*.

Talipes Calcaneus (Fig. 3-19). As in calcaneovalgus, this defect also reflects a malposition of the os calcis in relation to the talus, but in this deformity the os calcis is in the neutral position in the postero-anterior relationship. In the lateral position the posterior half of the os calcis is displaced forward so that the calcaneal tuber-osity is situated directly under the superior articular surface of the os calcis. Clinically, the patient's foot is fore-shortened in the standing position and it does not rest on the plantar aspect of the heel pad but on the posterior portion of it. This is an acquired deformity.

Talipes Equinus (Fig. 3-20). This term denotes an irregularity of the foot in which the entire foot is held in a position of

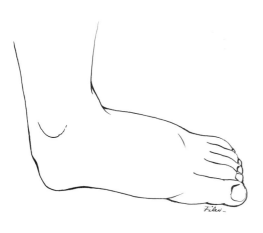

Calcaneo valgus

Fig. 3-17.   Calcaneo-Valgus Foot.
In this deformity, the foot presents no longitudinal arch. There is a valgus position of the rear foot in relation to the forefoot. The normal weight bearing axis falls on the medial side of the first toe. This deformity is either congenital, as in the plantar-flexed talus (or in the congenital rigid flat foot) or acquired as in patients with muscle imbalance due to poliomyelitis or cerebral palsy. In the latter two conditions, the tendo achillis is almost invariably contracted.

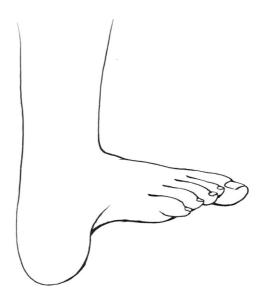

Talipes calcaneus

Fig. 3-19.   Talipes Calcaneus.
Malposition of the os calcis in relation to the talus is the cause of this deformity and is found in patients with muscle imbalance due, almost always, to post-poliomyelitic involvement.

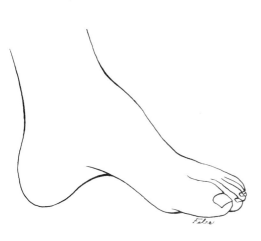

Pes cavus

Fig. 3-18.   Pes Cavus.
This deformity produces a foot which presents a higher than normal arch and may or may not be accompanied by flexion (cock-up) deformities of the toes. When the latter abnormality is found concurrent with the former, the foot is designated as a clawfoot.

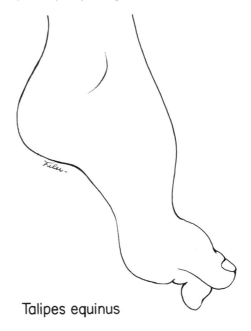

Talipes equinus

Fig. 3-20.   Talipes Equinus. The contracture of the Triceps Surae muscles (calf muscle group) causes the foot to assume a position of acute flexion. As the term indicates, the foot is held in a position similar to a horse's hoof.

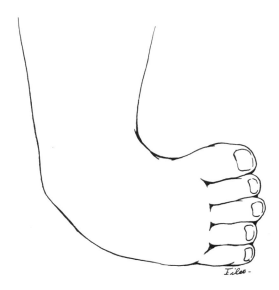

Talipes equino–cavo–varus

Fig. 3-21. Talipes Equino-Cavo-Varus (Clubfoot).
This foot malformation involves three deforming components: equinus, cavus, and varus. It is primarily a soft tissue contracture with varying degrees of involvement of the bony components in the severe cases. It is a congenital deformity with hereditary predisposition in a certain percentage of cases.

flexion in relation to the leg. The term "equinus" is used to denote that the foot is held in a position similar to a horse's hoof.

Talipes Equino-Cavo-Varus (Clubfoot) (Fig. 3-21). This is a malformation of the foot involving three different components as the term indicates. It is a congenital deformity with certain hereditary tendencies. It involves the ankle, the tarsal, and the metatarsal regions of the foot. It is primarily a soft tissue contracture with varying degrees of involvement of the bony components in the severe cases, but little or none in the slightly-deformed foot.

BIBLIOGRAPHY

Method of Measuring and Recording. Chicago, American Academy of Orthopaedic Surgeons, 1965.

=4=

The Normal Foot—Its Development and Care

Without the knowledge of the appearance of the normal foot, the various pathological conditions which are found from infancy to adulthood cannot be discussed.

Therefore, what is considered the normal foot will first be presented in progressive stages; from infancy to the ultimate development of the mature adult foot.

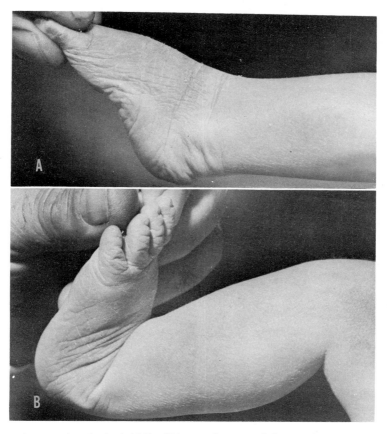

Fig. 4-1A. Normal appearing foot at birth. Skin on dorsum of foot and anterior aspect of ankle not tight. Range of passive flexion is 45 degrees.

Fig. 4-1B. Range of **relative passive extension** (dorsiflexion with subtalar joints not locked) in new born foot is 45 degrees.

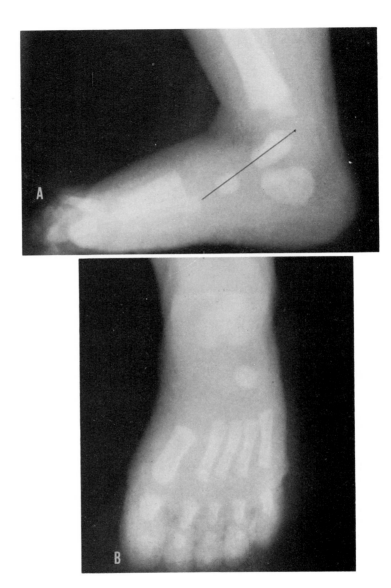

Fig. 4-2A. Talo-calcaneal relationship in the normal newborn foot at rest. The line bisecting the talus passes through the upper one-third of the cuboid and plantar to the first metatarsal.

Fig. 4-2B. Bones visible at birth: os calcis, talus, cuboid, all five metatarsals, all phalanges except for the distal two of the fifth toe.

At birth, the foot usually lies rotated somewhat externally because of the position of the neonate's lower extremities. In relation to the leg, the foot occupies a position that is at either the neutral right angle, or possibly at 15 degrees of extension and slight eversion.

When the infant's extremity is picked up for an examination of the foot, there is an immediate, perceptible withdrawal movement with the toes fanning out slightly and the foot extending another 10 to 15 degrees. A test of the movements will reveal the following: 1) Flexion is unrestricted

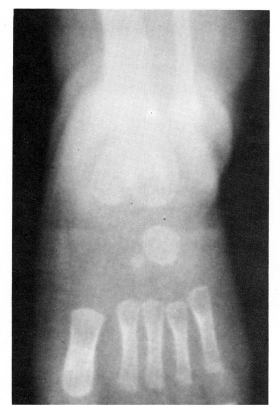

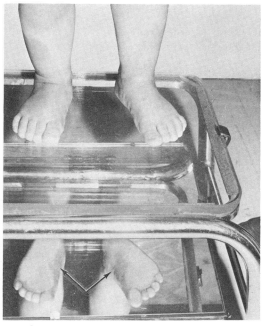

Fig. 4-4. Appearance of normal foot at one year of age. The child has been walking for one month. Note only beginning evidence of slight arching of the foot in the reflector mirror.

Fig. 4-3. At three and one-half months, the lateral cuneiform makes its appearance roentgenographically.

and the range from the right angle position is between 45 to 55 degrees (Fig. 4-1A). 2) Extension (dorsiflexion) with the subtalar joint locked is 10 to 15 degrees. Upon *relative* passive extension there is a maximum of 45 degrees of motion (Fig. 4-1B). Roentgenographically (Fig. 4-2A) the talocalcaneal relationship in the lateral nonweight bearing view reveals the talus to be lying fully outlined, slightly angulated plantarly in relation to the os calcis but with each structure clearly outlined with no overlapping of the talus. Furthermore, a line bisecting the talus should, upon forward projection, pass through the dorsal portion of the cuboid. Any overlapping between the os calcis and the talus, particularly when the bisecting talar line extends below the level of the cuboid, should be considered as indicative of a valgus foot. The roentgenogram of the infant or baby foot must be taken in the true lateral non-

weight-bearing position with the knee flexed at 90 degrees and the foot relaxed. At birth the bones that are visible roentgenographically are: 1) the talus, 2) the os calcis, 3) the cuboid, 4) all of the metatarsals and the phalanges (Fig. 4-2B), except for the distal two phalanges of the fifth digit.

The lateral cuneiform first appears at the age of three months in the male and two-and-one-half months in the female. This is the only perceptible change in the normal foot and it is evident roentgenographically (Fig. 4-3).

During the first twelve months after birth there is clinically, no demonstrable longitudinal arch per se (Fig. 4-4). Only after the child has assumed the plantigrade position and the various forces of weight-bearing stresses are applied to the foot does the longitudinal arch, as such, begin to be apparent. Therefore, since the foot is in the formative stage of development during this period of life, selection of the proper type of shoe to be worn by the toddler is an important consideration. The shoe should have a firm leather sole and should fit the foot properly. How often has the physician, particularly the pediatrician, seen babies with their feet either crowded or, on the other hand, swimming in a flimsy shoe which serves only as a cover and gives the foot no support whatsoever? One might conceivably ask why the child should be fitted with a firm leather-soled shoe which fits the foot properly even though it is not bearing weight. In addition, the foot grows so rapidly that it may seem uneconomical to purchase well fitted shoes. However, one has but to observe a child's early activities to realize why such cautious measures are vital to the development and maintenance of normal healthy feet.

To begin with, the foot is very elastic and resilient during the early months of life. Only 50 per cent of the tarsal bones exhibit partial ossification during the first twelve months and, in reality, they are all only an orderly arrangement of cartilaginous masses. They are held together loosely by ligamentous and muscular structures which have not developed the strength and the elasticity required to hold the bones of the foot in proper alignment with one another. The foot is very flexible and the application of abnormal stresses can place an undue burden upon it. Thus, it is necessary that the foot be given the advantage of proper support from the very onset of weight bearing, which is usually three to four months of age. Even though the baby does not begin to take his first steps until the seventh or eighth month, usually by the sixth month he begins standing in his crib or his playpen. But even earlier, proud parents often demonstrate an infant's prowess to doting grandparents and other admirers by holding the baby's hands to support him as they encourage the youngster to try to stand on a hard, firm, unyielding surface such as a floor. Usually the child's feet are covered only with socks or with flimsy soft leather shoes. One should keep in mind the fact that *Homo sapiens* has assumed the biped position only during the past 1,000,000 years and the tendency to pronation is still a predominant factor. Greater awareness of this would prevent parents from encouraging the baby to stand until he is absolutely ready to do so spontaneously without any assistance.

Furthermore, ideally, a child should be barefoot and on a resilient surface while learning to walk so that the foot can be exercised by permitting the toes to grasp into a surface that gives to some degree. Nature did not intend for the child to take his first steps, or those taken during the first two or three years of life, on a hard, unyielding surface of the modern home, or the concrete driveway, and the paved sidewalk. Therefore, since the surfaces on which the child first learns to walk are unyielding, of necessity the feet must give. Thus, an abnormal strain is placed on the child's feet during the most critical formative period covering the first two or three years of life.

It is important for the pediatrician to examine an infant's feet thoroughly, noting any abnormality that may exist. He should also question the mother as to whether or not either she or her husband have or have not had painful pronated feet. There is no doubt that there is a strong hereditary predisposition to pronated feet, and even though only one of the parents may have such a pronation, the child is almost certain to have the same problem eventually, if the feet are not properly supported during the critical period. Whenever a pediatrician or orthopaedist sees a child with pronated feet, he has but to question the mother and he will find that there is, almost invariably, an hereditary or familial diathesis in each instance. Only occasionally will one find pronated feet in the child yet normal feet in both parents. Sometimes the parents feet appear normal, but close questioning will elicit the information that the parents had received earlier treatment for the condition but had forgotten this fact.

Mothers should be instructed in how to place the baby properly in his crib for his sleep. Most infants have a tendency to sleep in a prone position with their feet either tucked under them in almost the fetal position or they assume the frog position (Fig. 4-5A and B). Such positions will almost invariably lead to a deformity of the foot. The infant's or baby's sleeping position should be changed by placing (Fig. 4-5C) him on his side with a small rolled towel or blanket placed anteriorly to prevent him

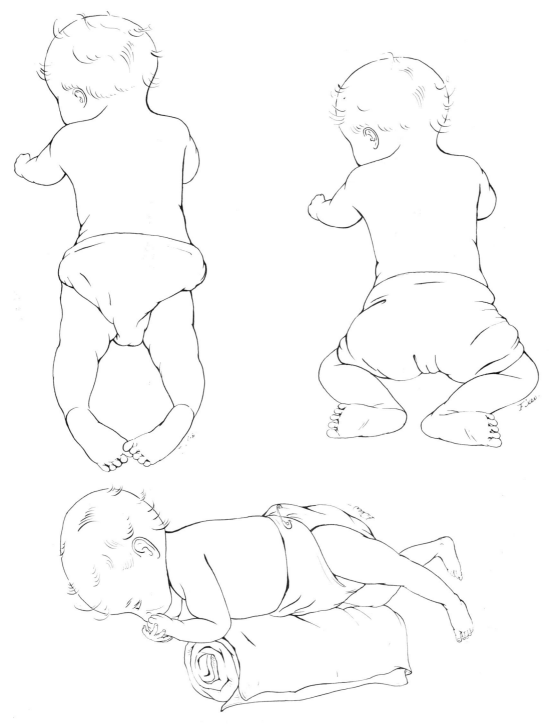

Fig. 4-5A. Child sleeping in the position which tends to produce internal tibial torsion and meta-tarsus varus.

B. Frog-like position of sleeping by the infant contributing to the development of external tibial torsion and valgus position of the feet.

C. Corrected position for the infant when sleeping. A small rolled blanket or large bath towel placed anterior to the abdomen will help to correct the improper sleeping position previously des-cribed.

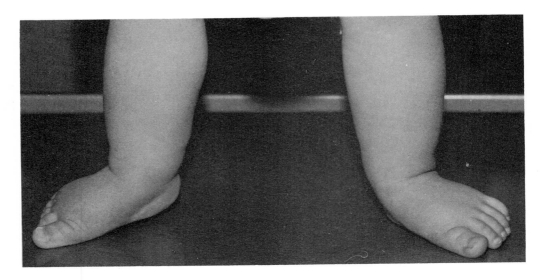

Fig. 4-6.   Broad standing stance assumed by child when first beginning to walk. Feet are placed wide apart in order to secure as broad a base of support as possible. Note that line of transmitted weight, if projected, would fall medial to the forefoot. Observe, also, apparent pronation of both feet. Age: eight and one half months.

from rolling over on his abdomen. Thus within a matter of two to four weeks, the deforming sleeping habits will have been eliminated.

When the child begins to take his first steps and for several months thereafter, his sense of equilibrium is not fully developed and is uncertain. Automatically, he places his feet wide apart to secure as broad a base of support as possible (Fig. 4-6). Furthermore, he will initially stand and toddle with one foot more externally rotated than the other, but almost invariably this external rotation corrects spontaneously as the child grows.

With the feet separated in order to maintain balance, the line of transmitted weight from the anterior superior iliac spine through the midpatella does not fall between the first and second toes but medial to the hallux. This places an undue strain on the foot, producing pronation. This, in turn, leads to flattening of the foot since the ligaments and the muscles fail to hold it in the proper position. The result of all this is a clumsy, springless, flatfooted gait. Progressively, as the child's sense of equilibrium develops, the feet are placed more closely together; the line of transmitted weight falls within the normal stance; the

foot comes into a better balanced position; the muscles and the ligaments function more efficiently as they tighten, thus maintaining the proper alignment of the tarsal bones into a compact arrangement. The superfluous fat, particularly on the medial side of the foot, disappears. The fulcrum forces, as previously described in Chapter 1, exert the necessary corrective effect on the foot, and the arch of the foot finally starts to take shape. This change, however, does not begin to take place before the sixteenth month (Fig. 4-7).

During this phase of development, the use of correct footwear is most important even if the foot appears to be perfectly normal. A high-top shoe should usually be worn during the first few months that the plantigrade position is assumed, but as soon as the child's foot can be fitted into an oxford-type or low-cut shoe, this step should be carried out. Furthermore, the mother should be informed that the shoe must be tied snugly in order to contain the foot properly. Very often a mother will ask her physician about the type of shoe she should purchase once the child is actively ambulatory. Many physicians, including some orthopaedists, have no specific criteria for making the proper selection. The

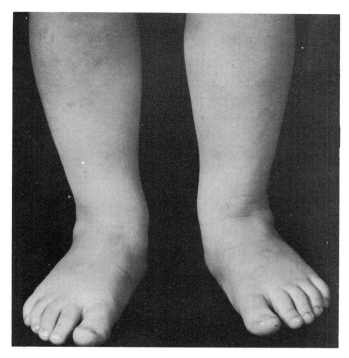

Fig. 4-7. The appearance of normal feet in a sixteen-month-old baby. Note closer stance. The ankles do not invert and the lower extremities, hence the feet, are not externally rotated. The line of transmitted weight is closer to the normal.

following detailed basic specifications will apply for all shoes, whether intended for children with normal feet or for those whose feet have a mild pronation.

1) The sole of the shoe should be firm, preferably a leather welt sole with a straight line construction on the medial edge, round tipped at the toe part to allow for the necessary freedom of the toes and wide enough through the metatarsal region to accommodate the child's short, plump foot (Fig. 4-8A).

2) The heel counter of the shoe should be narrow enough to hold the rear portion of the foot snugly and firmly and the counter should be high enough to cup around the posterior aspect of the rear foot just above the level of the ankle, and then curve down along the medial and lateral sides to clear the malleoli. If the oxford shoe can be slipped off the baby's foot after it has been laced snugly, the counter is not properly constructed and thus will not hold the child's heel. Occasionally the child will have a very narrow rear-foot and even the best of constructed shoes will not hold the

os calcis snugly. In such instances one can narrow the throat of the shoe by adding another set of eyelets just 1 cm. posterior to the top set, thus gaining some of the necessary support by the additional lacing. There should also be a medial elevation of the heel of at least 1/8 inch, preferably 3/16 inch (Fig. 4-8B), and a medial heel advance of 1/2 inch (Fig. 4-8A). The shoe should have a thin rubber heel of not more than 1/8 inch in thickness. This will not only give the child some stable traction during ambulation, but will also serve to indicate to the mother that the time has arrived for the application of a new set of rubber heels when the the rubber heel is worn down to the leather. (The shoes should not be permitted to become completely run down.) The application of the medial heel elevation and advance helps to invert the talocalcaneal area of the foot, lock the tarsal joints in the normal position, and support the foot properly.

3) The shank of the shoe should be rigid. Some orthopaedists recommend a flexible shank claiming it permits more flexibility of

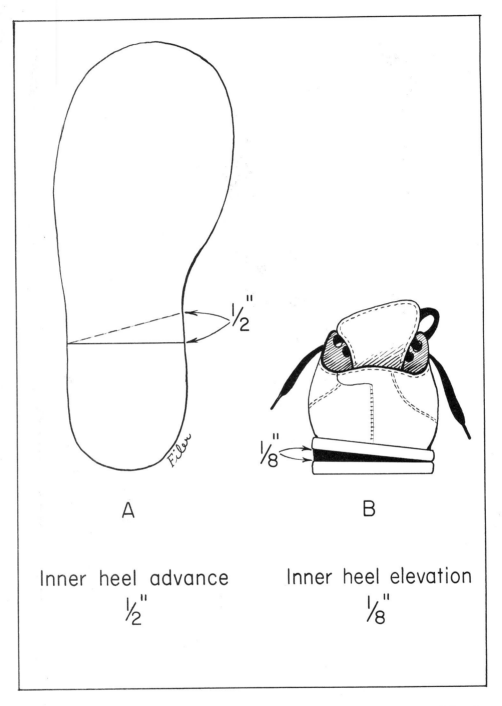

A

B

Inner heel advance
½"

Inner heel elevation
⅛"

Fig. 4-8. Type of shoe to be fitted on youngster's feet when first ambulatory and for the next three to four years even though feet and legs may be normal from the beginning.
A. Specifications: 1. straight line last; 2—welt sole; 3—rigid shank; 4—medial leading edge of heel half-inch longer than lateral leading edge—called: Inner Heel Advance; 5—Oxford type to be used as soon as child can be fitted in one.
B. Posterior view.—Note one-eighth inch medial heel wedge called: Inner Heel Elevation. This tends to raise medial edge of rear foot giving it the necessary support to maintain the os calcis under the talus.

the foot and, hence, freedom of the foot and toes; this in turn is conducive to better muscle and ligamentous development. We cannot agree with this premise. Many orthopaedists, including the author, who have a more than passing interest in foot problems, are of the opinion it is more necessary to maintain proper balance in growing feet than to attempt to stimulate muscle control. A flexible shoe will not hold the foot in a properly balanced position. Moreover, if the foot has a tendency to pronation, the shoe will break down rather than exert any corrective influence. There is no question that the muscles and ligaments play an important part in the function of the foot, but their function is dependent upon the integrity of the skeletal framework since the muscles will become fatigued and their effective function will be lost if the foot is unbalanced.

By and large, the present-day child no longer has the opportunity to play on the resilient surfaces of a lawn or in the fields but instead is constantly exposed at home and in the schools to hardwood floors which frequently cover a concrete slab. His activities are usually carried out on hard pavements. Under these conditions the foot obviously needs added support. Such additional protection can best be achieved by the use of a rigid shank in the shoe. Furthermore, it behooves the orthopaedist or the pediatrician, who, almost invariably, is the first to advise the mother regarding the child's footwear, to recommend the type of shoe to be worn and not permit the choice to be made by a shoe salesman who is generally not only inexperienced, but also seldom sincerely interested in the proper fitting of the child's feet.

At twenty-four months of age the child's foot should present a definite longitudinal arch in a standing position (Fig. 4-9). The heel should be in neutral position when viewed from the posterior aspect and the ankle should not invert. When the plantar surface is viewed in the reflecting mirror, there will be only little evidence of a longitudinal arch. However, this is due primarily to the characteristic adipose tissue which is still persistent on the medial plantar aspect of the baby foot. Roentgenographically (Fig. 4-10A), in addition to the os calcis,

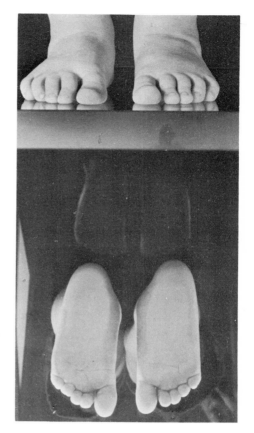

Fig. 4-9. Child's normal foot at twenty-four months of age. Heels are in neutral position, slight evidence of longitudinal arch when viewing plantar aspect of foot through reflector mirror. Medial aspect of foot demonstrates no inrolling.

talus, cuboid, and lateral cuneiform, the medial cuneiform and the phalangeal epiphysis of the first metatarsal will be demonstrable. In the lateral standing position (Fig. 4-10B) the talus is still angulated slightly plantarly in its relationship with the os calcis, and the line bisecting the talus projected distally now passes along the superior edge of the cuboid and almost touches the distal plantar edge of the first metatarsal.

Beginning at the age of twenty-four months any roentgenographic evaluation of the feet, particularly of the position of the tarsal and metatarsal bones during weight bearing, should be carried out with the subject in a standing position. To attempt to evaluate pronation and other static malpositions by studying films of non-weight-

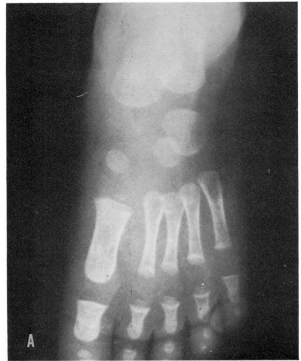

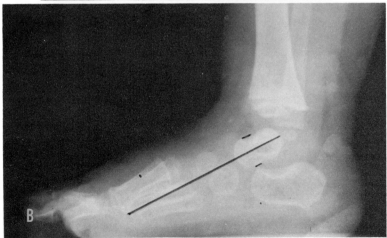

Fig. 4-10.   A.   Roentgenogram of foot at twenty-four months. In addition to the talus, os calcis, cuboid and lateral cuneiform, the medial cuneiform is now evident.

   B.   Lateral standing roentgenograms of normal foot at twenty-four months. Note that line bisecting the talus now passes along the superior edge of the cuneiform and practically touches the plantar surface of the distal tip of the first metatarsal.

bearing structures is useless. Lateral views taken at rest (Fig. 4-11A) cannot give an accurate evaluation of true talocalcaneal relationship as well as that of all of the tarsal bones; only standing roentgenograms will present the true picture (Fig. 4-11B). Note the difference in the appearance of the relationship of the tarsal bones. At rest, (Fig. 4-11A) the foot appears normal in this case, whereas in reality this youngster has a valgus foot while standing (Fig. 4-11B). Standing roentgenograms, both in the anteroposterior and lateral positions *must* be taken routinely in evaluating feet. However, in the final analysis, one must depend on both clinical evaluation as well

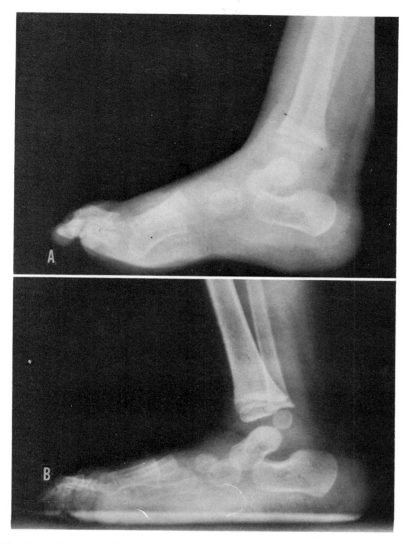

Fig. 4-11. The Importance of Standing Roentgenograms.
A.   Lateral of foot of twenty-four-month-old baby. At rest, the tarsal bones appear in essentially normal relation to each other.
B.   Observe the same foot upon standing. Note plantar flexion of the talus. Not only the child, but the mother and the maternal grandfather have valgus feet, symptomatic in the latter two.

as roentgenographic examination to make a diagnosis of pronation of the foot at this age, unless the malposition of the bones is very obvious.

At two-and-one-half years of age, the middle cuneiform bone can be visualized roentgenographically (Fig. 4-12). Between two-and-one-half and three years of age the youngster's physician (whether pediatrician or general practitioner) should evaluate both lower extremities carefully since this will be almost the last opportunity he will

have to detect any early deviations from the normal and apply minor corrective measures not requiring prolonged therapy. Both lower extremities of the child should be unclothed and his gait should be observed. Does he present a limp? Is he walking pigeon-toed or with both feet externally rotated? Does he present a genu valgus (knock knee) or a genu varus (bowleg) appearance? Normally the youngster's legs should be straight and he should be walking with each foot pointing directly forward with each step. A minimum intoeing of not more than 5 to 10 degrees, or a similar amount of outtoeing when walking, is considered to be within normal limits.

Next, the youngster should be placed on the examining table in a recumbent position. Both lower extremities should be checked for any discrepancy in length by measuring from the anterior superior iliac spine to the medial malleolus with the pelvis level. A difference of less than 1 cm. (3/8 inch) is considered to be within the normal limit of error. It is preferable to use a flexible steel tape measure since, concomitantly, one can observe whether the long axis non-weight-bearing line, extending from the anterior superior iliac spine to between the first and second metatarsal heads, bisects the patella. If it does not, then the lower extremities should be evaluated for possible lateral, medial, or rotational deviation from the normal. Muscle power evaluation should also be carried out routinely. The range of motion with the foot at rest, which automatically will include the ankle, should involve the following maneuvers:

Range of passive motion:

1)	Flexion (plantar flexion)	$50° \pm 5°$
2)	Extension (dorsiflexion)	
	relative:	
	tarsal joints unlocked	$30° \pm 5°$
	true:	
	tarsal joints locked	$10° \pm 5°$
3)	Eversion of foot	$10° \pm 5°$
4)	Inversion of foot	$10° \pm 5°$
5)	Adduction of forefoot	$20° \pm 5°$
6)	Abduction of forefoot	$15° \pm 5°$

With regard to flexion and extension of the metatarsophalangeal joints, the range is similar to that recorded in Chapter 3. Moreover, at rest the longitudinal arch should appear to have a normal conformation. The maximum arching should be located at the junction of the posterior one-third with the anterior two-thirds of the medial longitudinal arch. At this stage there is no evidence of the lateral portion of the longitudinal arch.

The youngster should then be seated on the examining table with both legs dependent over the edge of the examining table, the knees at right angle, with the patellae in the neutral anteroposterior position.

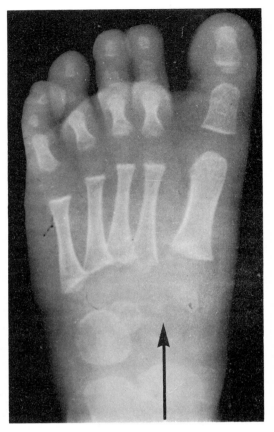

Fig. 4-12. At thirty months, the middle cuneiform makes its appearance.

When the child's feet hang in a relaxed attitude, the examiner will find both of them pointing slightly internally approximately 5 to 10 degrees. Any outward pointing of the toes beyond the neutral position, when the above posture is assumed, should be considered divergent from the normal. This also applies when the feet assume an internal rotary stance greater than 10 degrees.

The feet can best be evaluated as to position and weight distribution while in a standing position, preferably on a reflector stand (Fig. 4-13). The longitudinal arch is well developed. There is as yet no evidence of the lateral portion of the longitudinal arch. Both heels are in neutral position. The ankles do not invert. The navicular tubercle is not prominent. There is a slight prominence on the dorsolateral aspect of the foot just forward of the lateral malleolus which is within normal limits. It will progressively diminish and finally disappear by the time the normal foot has reached full growth. The toes are straight and relatively parallel to one another. As can be seen in the photograph the weight is evenly distributed. The legs are straight. With the knees touching, the medial malleoli are separated by not more than 3 cm. The patellae are in true anteroposterior position. This, then, is the normal foot and leg. This illustrates what is considered to be normal until the youngster is approximately ten years of age. At this time the lateral portion of the longitudinal arch will have developed, and the weight bearing will then be evenly distributed on the plantar aspect of the heel and the metatarsal region of the foot.

Only osseous changes will have occurred during this period and these are demonstrable only roentgenographically. At three years and eight months the tarsal navicular appears (Fig. 4-14). At approximately eight years of age the calcaneal apophysis makes its appearance (Fig. 4-15). Other changes evident by roentgenography are the appearance of the sesamoid bones under the first metatarsal head (Fig. 4-16) which become perceptible between the thirteenth and the

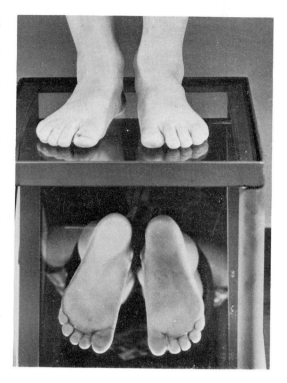

Fig. 4-13. Appearance of feet in standing position at three years of age. Note the presence of the longitudinal arch, medial portion of it, in the reflector stand. The baby adipose tissue on the medial side of the mid-foot has disappeared. Both heels are in neutral position and the ankles do not invert.

fourteenth year. (Maturation takes place earlier in the female.) The accompanying maturation chart (Chart 4-1) is based on a review of numerous articles and books. The most comprehensive compilation was by Drs. N. L. Hoerr, S. E. Pyle, and C. C. Francis from the Department of Anatomy, Western Reserve University School of Medicine.

After the age of sixteen in the male and fourteen in the female, all epiphyses have usually closed and the foot can be considered an adult foot. Its normal appearance is best described by illustrations (Fig. 4-17 A and B). In the anteroposterior view (A) the arch is visibly well developed and the malleolar prominences are in line with the axis of the foot. The navicular tubercle may or may not be slightly prominent. The toes are relatively parallel with one another.

CHART 4-1. MATURATION CHART OF THE BONES OF THE FOOT

Age of Appearance

Talus		
Os calcis		
Cuboid		
Metatarsals	1, 2, 3, 4, 5	At Birth
Proximal phalanges	1, 2, 3, 4, 5	
Middle phalanges	2, 3, 4	
Distal phalanges	1, 2, 3, 4	
Lateral cuneiform	3 mos. ♂	
	2.5 mos. ♀	
Distal phalanx—5th toe	6 mos. ♂	
	5 mos. ♀	
Middle phalanx—5th toe	7 mos. ♂	
	6 mos. ♀	
Medial cuneiform	24 mos. ♂	
	18 mos. ♀	
Middle cuneiform	30 mos. ♂	
	23 mos. ♀	
Navicular	3 yrs. 8 mos. ♂	
	2 yrs. 10 mos. ♀	
Calcaneal apophysis	8 yrs. ♂	
	6 yrs. 2 mos. ♀	
First metatarsal sesamoids	13 yrs. ♂	
	10 yrs. ♀	

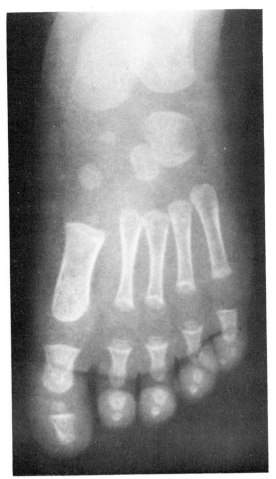

	Active	Passive	
Extension	20°	....Relative	....30°
		True	.... 0°- 5°
Flexion	50°	....	55°
Inversion of heel	0°	....	5°
Inversion of forefoot	10°	....	15°
Eversion of heel	0°	....	5°
Eversion of forefoot	10°	....	15°
Adduction	20°	....	20°-25°
Abduction	10°	....	10°-15°

Fig. 4-14. At three years and eight months, the tarsal navicular is evident roentgenographically.

The heel is in neutral position or in minimal valgus and the tendo Achillis stands out as a definite anatomical aligning landmark. There should be no bow-stringing of this structure. The medial view (B) demonstrates the normal appearance of the longitudinal arch; the highest point of the arch is located at the junction of the posterior one-third with the anterior two-thirds of the foot at the level of the navicular tubercle. In examining the foot at rest, the range of motion, both actively and passively, should be evaluated since excursion of the foot actively differs from the passive range of movement. Motions, on the average, are as follows:

An analysis of the motion of the metatarsophalangeal and the interphalangeal joints is given in the previous chapter. It is also necessary to keep in mind that as the individual ages, or as he becomes more sedentary in his mode of living, the extremes of the various ranges of motion will diminish by 5 or 10 degrees. Arterial pulsations in the feet should be tested as well as venous return.

It is also interesting to note that, although the epiphyses are closed by the end of the fourteenth year, the foot, in the female, will continue to increase in size under one particular circumstance: during and following pregnancy. Almost invariably, following gestation, the female foot increases in both its length and its width. Although this is a common observation, thus far there is no valid explanation for this tendency.

As can be seen, the normal foot is therefore a rather complex mechanism containing 26 bones with their multiple, as well as single, articulating surfaces; innumerable ligamentous structures; 17 tendons from muscles arising in the leg, and 10 small muscles and 3 small muscle groups arising in the foot itself. It is small wonder, then, that we are faced with so many medical problems arising in this structure. This is particularly so in view of how the feet are abused in the present day and age by failure to exercise them properly and by covering them with footwear (especially in the case of the adult female) which is physiologically and functionally incorrect and often even crippling.

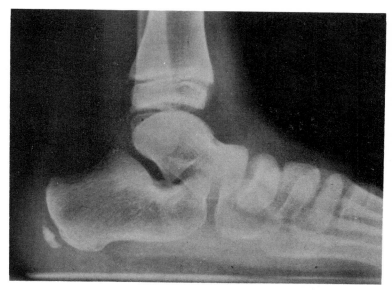

Fig. 4-15. At approximately eight years of age, in the male, the calcaneal apophysis makes its appearance.

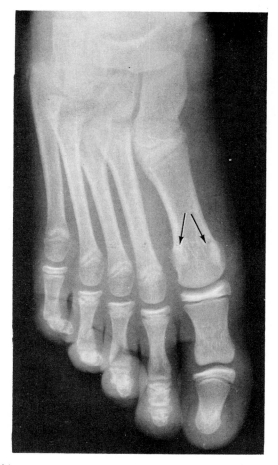

Fig. 4-16. The sesamoids appear under the first metatarsal head between the ages of thirteen and fourteen years in the male.

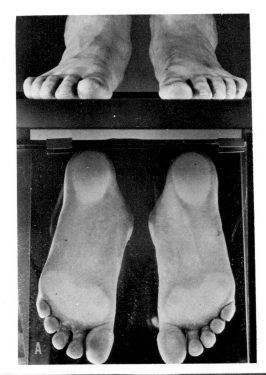

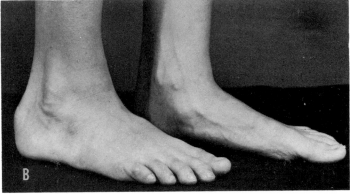

Fig. 4-17A.   Anteroposterior view of sixteen-year-old foot. Observe that the entire longitudinal arch is now developed. The weight is borne evenly on the heels-and the metatarsal region of the foot. The navicular tubercles are slightly prominent.

17B.   In the medial view of the rear foot, standing, note the longitudinal arch. In the lateral view of the foot in the foreground, observe that all of the toes are straight and parallel to one another. Further, from this same aspect, one cannot see the lateral portion of the longitudinal arch which is visible from the plantar reflected view.

BIBLIOGRAPHY

ANDERSON, M., BLAIS, M., AND GREEN, W. T.: Growth of the Normal Foot During Childhood and Adolescence. Amer. J. Phys. Anthrop. *14*:287, 1956.

HAUSER, E. D. W.: *Diseases of the Foot.* Philadelphia, W. B. Saunders Co., 1950.

HOERR, N. L., PYLE, S. E., AND FRANCIS, C. C.: *Radiographic Atlas of Skeletal Development of the Foot and Ankle.* Springfield, Charles C Thomas, 1962.

HUBAY, CHARLES A.: Sesamoid Bones of the Hands and Feet. Amer. J. Roentgen Radium Ther. *61*:493, 1949.

JONES, F. W.: *Structure and Function as Seen in the Foot.* Baltimore, The Williams & Wilkins Co., 1944.

LEWIN, P.: *The Foot and Ankle.* 4th Ed., Philadelphia, Lea & Febiger, 1959.

MORTON, D. J.: *The Human Foot.* New York, Columbia University Press, 1935.

= 5 =

Problems of the Foot from Birth

to the Stage of Ambulation

This chapter covers foot problems (except clubfoot and other major abnormalities) from birth to the time of ambulation which is usually between ten and fourteen months of age.

From birth on, the normal foot changes a number of its characteristics as it grows to full maturity. What may be considered normal at one stage of its growth may be considered abnormal during another phase of development. Therefore one cannot rely on the same type of examination at all times. It is essential for the physician to recognize not only the obvious deformities present in a newborn's foot, but also minor deviations from the normal. He should institute therapy equally soon in both situations if the growing and maturing youngster is to be spared some of the static foot deformities frequently encountered clinically. It is not sufficient for the obstetrician, pediatrician or general practitioner to observe the infant's feet casually during the initial examination and to note that the foot is not obviously deformed in appearance. Nor should the first evaluation be limited to the foot alone but should include the entire lower extremity. This is necessary because, however minimal the mal-position and mal-appearance of the foot may be, it is not necessarily due to deformity in this structure per se, but may be due to some minor abnormal deviation in the femur, the tibia or the ankle. Any defect in one of these structures can be reflected in an apparent deformity of the foot.

In the newborn, the normal foot when examined appears to be slightly internally rotated. The heel is in neutral position in relation to the ankle. On flexion (plantar flexion) there are 50 degrees of motion from the neutral position. The skin does not appear tight on the anterior aspect of the ankle and the midtarsal region of the foot (Fig. 5-1A). There are 45 degrees of relative passive extension (dorsiflexion) from the neutral right angled position and upon extension the foot tends to evert slightly (Fig. 5-1B). Furthermore, the foot can be everted and inverted passively from the neutral position between 20 to 30 degrees in each direction. To all intents and purposes this is considered a normal appearing foot at birth even if, at a later date, such a

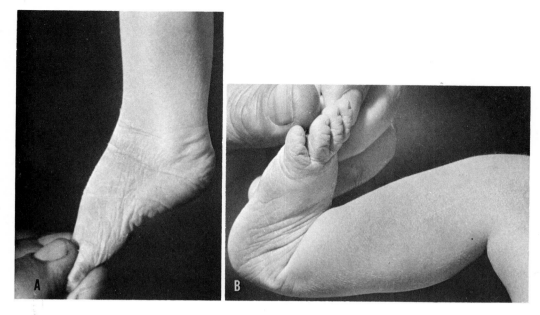

Fig. 5-1A. Normal newborn foot in flexion position. There are 50 degrees of motion and the skin does not appear tight on the dorsum of the foot and ankle.
1B. On passive extension, the foot demonstrates 45 degrees of motion.

foot should present a pronated appearance upon bearing weight. On roentgen examination, the following bones are visible (Fig. 5-2): the talus, the os calcis, the cuboid, all of the metatarsals and all of the phalanges except for the distal two phalanges of the fifth toe. As the foot matures, other tarsal bones and apophyses gradually appear.

When the foot presents the slightest variation from the normal, the examiner should devote the necessary time evaluating any minor abnormality or difference, not limiting the examination to the foot alone, but also checking the entire lower extremity.

The hip joint should be evaluated not only to determine the presence of any possible dislocation or subluxation, but with regard to the range of internal and external rotation. If the range of internal rotation is greater than 90 degrees, it is essential to realize that such an infant has an internal femoral torsion which, if left uncorrected, will later result in a pigeon-toed gait. Rarely, if ever, does one find an external femoral torsion. The normal range of internal femoral rotation averages 75 degrees. The therapy for this internal femoral torsion consists of nothing more than the application of several diapers, rather than a single one, so that the lower extremities can be kept in a position of abduction at the hip joints for several months. The mother can apply this corrective measure easily, and when correction has been achieved (usually within three to six months), this method of diapering can be discontinued. Furthermore, once corrected, the defect will not recur.

If, on the other hand, the femoral component is found to be normal, then the tibia should be evaluated. Again, the knee in the newborn or the infant should be held in the straight anterolateral position, and the foot should be slightly externally rotated from the neutral position by not more than 10 degrees. The tip of the medial malleolus should be located slightly forward in relation to the tip of the lateral malleolus. Here again, one may find an internal or external tibial torsion as a cause for what may appear to be either an inward or an outward mal-position of the foot.

If the tibia, on examination, should be internally rotated, the ankle and foot will present the following positional differences: the medial malleolus will be located much further posterior than the lateral malleolus,

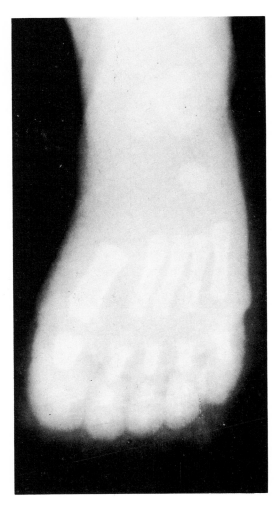

Fig. 5-2. Visible bones at birth are: talus, os calcis, cuboid, all of the metatarsals, and all of the phalanges except for the distal two in the fifth toe.

and if the torsion should be extreme, as for example an internal tibial torsion of 90 degrees, the lateral malleolus will be found to be in an almost anterior position and the medial counterpart in an almost posterior one. Consequently the foot is held in a position of adduction and slight varus. There is a common error that is made by the examining physicians. He is apt to observe the apparent mal-position of the foot and advise the parents that the infant has a deformity of the foot. He may even attempt to treat it when, in reality, the deformity is in the tibia.

Frequently there is a combination of minor deviations from the normal wherein the infant presents a mild internal tibial

torsion, along with a minimal or mild forefoot varus with medial divergence of the great toe. Again in this instance, the foot may be treated with corrective shoes while the torsion will be overlooked. As a result the child will have a pigeon-toed gait when he begins to ambulate, and the physician will be at a loss to understand this outcome, while the parents will naturally be highly dissatisfied.

If such an abnormality is noted in a child, a careful history should be obtained from the mother. If it is a first-born child, the parents should be questioned as to whether or not either of them ever walked pigeon-toed, since there is a definite hereditary tendency to certain minor deviations of the foot and leg, just as there are other skeletal or facial tendencies that are hereditary. If the mother has had other children, she should be questioned as to whether or not any of them have had a bowlegged appearance or a pigeon-toed gait, and whether or not these children outgrew such defects.

If the case history reveals a definite hereditary trait, and if the deformity in the siblings failed to correct itself without orthopaedic treatment, then the infant is in need of definite corrective therapy. If, on the other hand, the deviation from the normal is minimal and the family history indicates spontaneous recovery, then the infant needs nothing more than periodic observation. Such medical supervision is *particularly* important during the first six months after the child starts to walk and the gait pattern becomes established. This is so because in some instances, an apparently improving situation will suddenly worsen when the child begins to walk.

In some infants the foot and leg abnormality will appear to be disappearing satisfactorily with no treatment and the physician will tend to dismiss the problem. However, the mother will suddenly appear with the child (now between eighteen and twenty-four months of age) and demand to know why the youngster is walking pigeon-toed or is bowlegged when she had been advised that the problem had been corrected. It is therefore wise for the physician to refrain from categorically telling the parents that the infant or the child

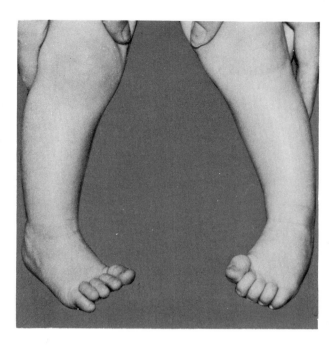

Fig. 5-3. Mild internal tibial torsion which was easily overlooked and the youngster treated for minimal forefoot varus instead.

will outgrow this mild deformity. The possibility that this may and can be permanently corrected should be indicated to the parents, but they should not be assured that it "will happen" spontaneously.

What, then, is the therapy for a mild degree of internal (Fig. 5-3) or external tibial torsion or a corresponding femoral torsion with no foot deformity. It is nothing more than careful observation particularly when the child begins to walk. In addition, the baby's sleeping habits should be investigated. If the baby or infant is an abdominal sleeper, the position of the lower extremities should be checked since sleeping throughout the night in a frog position will undoubtedly contribute to the development of external femoral or tibial torsion and a valgus position of the feet (Fig. 5-4). Conversely, sleeping with the lower extremities internally rotated will lead to the development of internal rotation of the tibia and a varus deformity of each forefoot (Fig. 5-5). Should either of these situations be found, they should be corrected by placing the infant on his side (Fig. 5-6) with a large rolled bath towel anteriorly to prevent the baby from rolling over onto his abdomen. Within one or two weeks the

infant's postural sleeping habits will have changed so that this deforming factor will have been eliminated. If the torsion corrects itself spontaneously, well and good. Should it fail to do so and the baby acquires a pigeon-toed stance at the age of twelve months, then treatment is indicated. Usually with this degree of torsion there is mild forefoot varus as well, so that both components require correction. Treatment consists of the application of neutral surgical open-toed shoes with a Dennis-Browne bar (Fig. 5-7). At the beginning the shoes should be placed at the neutral position on the bar since the infant's feet will not tolerate greater correction. The mother should be advised that the shoes are to be kept on constantly, except during bathing, for one hour in the afternoon, and for another hour before the infant is given his last feeding. The mother should be instructed to massage the feet gently for two or three minutes each time the shoes are removed and to watch for possible irritation of the heels. She should also be advised of the necessity of properly fitted socks. Wrinkled socks lead to irritation of the skin. The infant should be reexamined one week after the initial application of

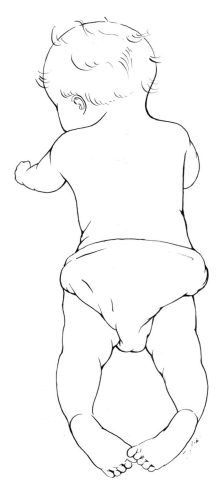

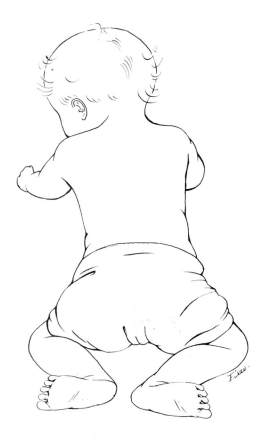

Fig. 5-4. Frog-like sleeping position leading in many instances to external femoral, but more frequently tibial torsion and valgus feet.

Fig. 5-5. Abnormal sleeping position leading to the development of internal torsion of the tibia or femur with varus foot deformity and therefore apparent bow-legs and pigeon toes.

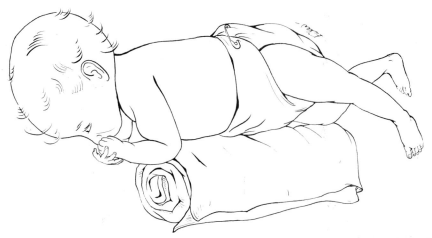

Fig. 5-6. Corrected sleeping posture by placing infant on his side with rolled blanket or bath towel anteriorly to prevent him from rolling on his abdomen and subsequently assuming previously described deforming sleeping positions.

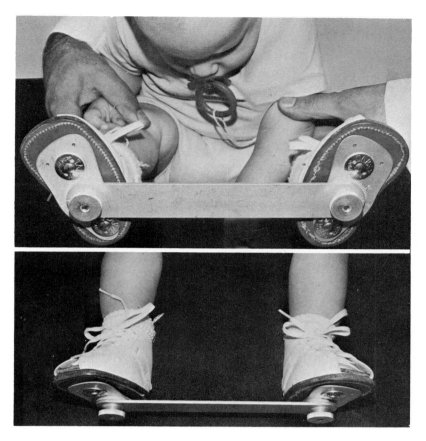

Fig. 5-7. Dennis-Browne bar with tarso-pronator (out-toeing) shoes externally rotated to correct internal tibial torsion and mild forefoot varus.

the shoes and at that time, if the tolerance to them and to the bar has been satisfactory, the shoes should be externally rotated to an angle of 45 degrees at the maximum. At *no* time is it necessary to place the shoes in a position of 90 degrees external rotation to correct this mild type of deformity. If one should do so, the result quite frequently will be a corrected tibia with a valgus foot. The same type of therapy in reverse should be applied if the infant displays an external tibial torsion of any consequence, whether or not the deformity is accompanied by a mild valgus position of each foot.

If, on the other hand, the infant should display an internal or external tibial torsion of more than 35 degrees, a more definite form of treatment is indicated. Snug, long, leg casts should be applied with a sufficient amount of sheet wadding (or similar substitute) which will protect the soft tissues but will not be so bulky as to cause the cast to lose its purchase. The cast should extend from the mid-thigh to the tips of the toes with the knee flexed about 90 degrees and the foot held in the neutral right angle position, but no attempt should be made to position the foot in neutral in relation to the long axis of the lower extremity. Twenty-four to forty-eight hours later the cast should be cut circumferentially at the junction of the middle and the lower third of the leg (Fig. 5-8) and the distal end of the cast should be *gently* externally or internally rotated, as the indications may be, up to the point of resistance. The cast should be wrapped with crepe paper to permit further derotation without the need of changing it on each occasion, and one roll of extra fast setting plaster of paris should be applied to close the defect. One week later the derotation should be repeated until the foot, and automatically therefore the ankle, are rotated into the

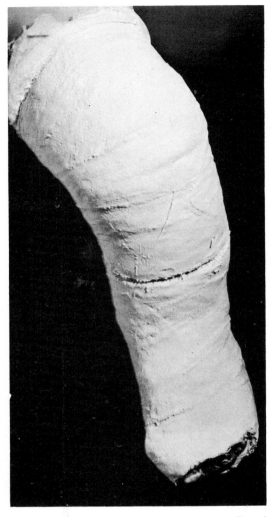

Fig. 5-8. Long leg cast applied with knee flexed at 90 degrees, the foot at neutral right angle position, and location of circular cut in cast just above ankle to correct internal tibial torsion.

neutral position in relation to the long axis of the lower extremity.

Should it become necessary to change the cast during the process of correction, the cast should again be applied with the foot held lightly at a right-angled position. No attempt should be made to gain correction. If this should be attempted, it would result in either a valgus or varus deformity of the foot without any effect on the tibia and fibula. Once the neutral position has been reached (that in which the long axis bisects the patella and falls between the first and the second toes) cast immobilization and control should be maintained for at least three months. Cast changes should be done as often as is necessary to accommodate the growth of the infant's lower extremity. After removal of the cast or casts, the Dennis-Browne bar should be used at night, but only until the age of eighteen months since the deformity could recur until that time.

At birth and during early infancy, the more commonly found congenital and/or hereditary malformations of the foot are pes adductus (metatarsus varus), prehensile tendency of the great toe (hallux varus), overlapping toes, congenital flatfoot (talipes calcaneovalgus) and congenital clubfoot (talipes equinocavovarus) or any single component of it. The talipes equinocavovarus deformity and the flatfoot, and their myriad problems will be discussed in separate chapters, but the other deviations will be presented in this section.

PES ADDUCTUS, WITH OR WITHOUT HALLUX VARUS

The two forms should be considered simultaneously since the therapy is essentially the same for both, varying only in degree. Many physicians frequently dismiss this imperfection as being of no consequence, believing that the infant will outgrow it. This is not so at all. Others may advise the mother that the condition should be watched, recommending therapy in six months if the deformity does not correct itself. This attitude is also wrong. The

sooner therapy is instituted after the infant is a week old, the easier and more rapid, as well as successful, will the correction be.

In a mild case of pes adductus or hallux varus, the mother should receive specific instructions as to the care of this abnormality. These instructions consist of nothing more than gentle manipulation of the foot for ten minutes four times daily in a direction opposite to that of the defect. Not only should the mother be told what to do,

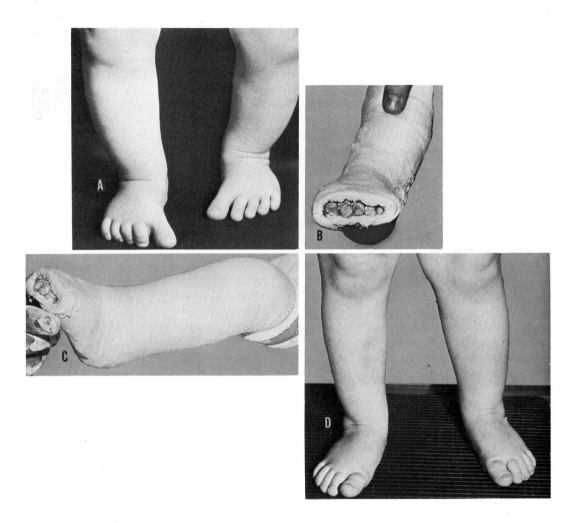

Fig. 5-9A. Moderate pes adductus. Note varus of forefoot and abduction of great toe from the second digit.

B. Foot portion of cast applied. Note molding of cast about the toes with application of pressure over the cuboid laterally and the first metatarsal head medially.

C. Completed cast extending above knee. D. Corrected feet—six months later.

but the procedure should be demonstrated to her repeatedly until it is understood. The manipulation consists of holding the heel firmly in one hand with the thumb exerting pressure on the cuboid and with the other hand gently stretching the forefoot in the direction opposite to that of the deformity. The foot should be held in this stretched position for ten seconds; it should be released for an equal amount of time and the entire exercise then repeated. If this exercise is performed carefully and conscientiously by the mother for the prescribed period, no other treatment is necessary.

However, such exercises are ineffectual in the moderately deformed foot (Fig. 5-9A) that is, one that upon stretching in the opposite direction reaches only to the neutral position. In this instance, the mode of therapy can consist of either the application of clubfoot shoes with a Dennis-Browne bar or the utilization of corrective casts. When the former regimen is prescribed, the use of the shoes, the length of time of application and the position are the same as in the correction of a mild internal tibial torsion: namely, neutral position of the shoes on the bar when starting this form of therapy, followed by an increasing external rotational position of the shoes on the bar to a 45 degree angle. Once the deformity has been corrected, the Dennis-Browne bar need be applied only at night, but the shoes should be worn constantly. This regimen should be maintained until the child has become ambulatory and for three months thereafter. If the correction is maintained, then the child is given a regular type Oxford or low-cut shoe with an outer sole elevation of 3/16 of an inch. This type of corrective shoe is worn for at least one year. If there is no recurrence, no further therapy is needed except for semiannual check-ups for the next three years.

An alternate form of therapy is the use of corrective casts. In our opinion this is by far the preferable method for the correction of the moderate forefoot adduction, although there are ardent exponents of the previously described method. With a cast, one uses a positive form of therapy. Nothing is left to chance or to the whim of the mother who may feel sorry for the infant and leave the shoes off for two hours instead of one "because the baby was fussing". It is true that the application of a cast takes more time than the fitting of a pair of shoes and a bar, but if the orthopaedist is to treat deformities of the feet conscientiously as well as carefully, time should not be considered—only perfection— if possible, and perfection is the correction of a deformed foot that can be achieved solely by the devotion of time, patience and the meticulous application of plaster of paris casts. An ideal example of such an orthopaedist is Dr. J. Hiram Kite of the Shriners Hospital for Crippled Children in Atlanta, Georgia. Because of his dedication, perseverance and preciseness, he has revolutionized the care and correction of the equinocavovarus foot.

The cast is applied from the mid-thigh to the toes with the knee at a 90 degree flexion position, while the foot is held at a right angle flexion position. The use of a short leg cast in an infant is almost invariably valueless because it will slip off, either partially or completely, no matter how well it may be applied initially. One must apply the cast in sections and it must be properly molded. In order to carry this out it is necessary to apply the Webril or the sheet wadding carefully and snugly, since this is the foundation of a well-fitted cast. The sheet wadding to be used for an infant should be not more than 3 inches wide (preferably only 2 inches in width). Prior to application of the cast, the skin should be sprayed with tincture of benzoine compound or one of the other skin adherents. The sheet wadding should be applied snugly and without wrinkles. Small tears can be made in it to make it lie flat on the foot and leg. As it is rolled on, it should not be folded on itself. One should have no fear of applying it too tightly because standard sheet wadding tears easily. The first section of the cast is the most important since it will be applied to the foot. It is preferable, whenever possible, for the surgeon to hold the foot while the plaster assistant applies the cast. For the average orthopaedist this may be a rather difficult problem to solve when he first establishes his practice, but it can be accomplished by stimulating interest and applying patience in teaching the office nurse or the attendant in charge of the plaster room at the hospital how to apply the plaster of paris.

The cast is applied from the tips of the toes up to and including the ankle. The foot is then held with one hand molding the plaster around the heel and the calcaneocuboid joint while the other hand applies firm pressure on the medial side of the cast over the region of the first metatarsal head (Fig. 5-9B). It is preferable to use extra-fast-setting plaster of paris bandages. After the cast has set, the anterior portion over the ankle should be trimmed to permit the extension of the foot to the neutral position. The cast should then be completed up to the mid-thigh with the knee flexed (Fig. 5-9C). The toes should not be crowded together but should lie flat and parallel to one another. Again, this can be accomplished only by the meticulous application and molding of the cast.

The cast should be changed weekly or wedged until the forefoot deformity is not only corrected, but is slightly overcorrected. The method of testing for adequate correction is to check the position the foot

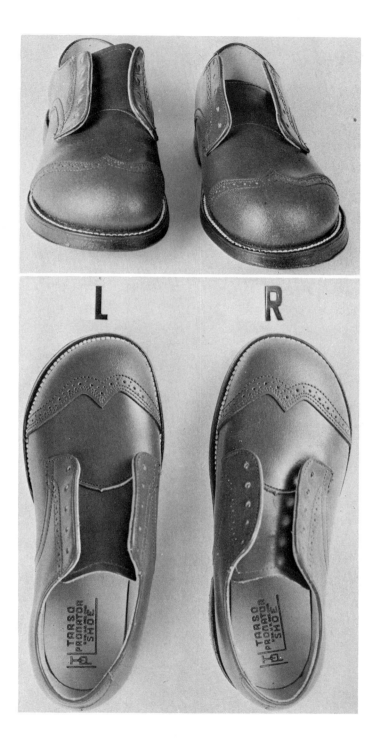

Fig. 5-10. Front and top views of the tarso-pronator shoe. It can be used to correct either a mild hallux varus (adductus) or a pigeon-toed gait due to poor walking habits.

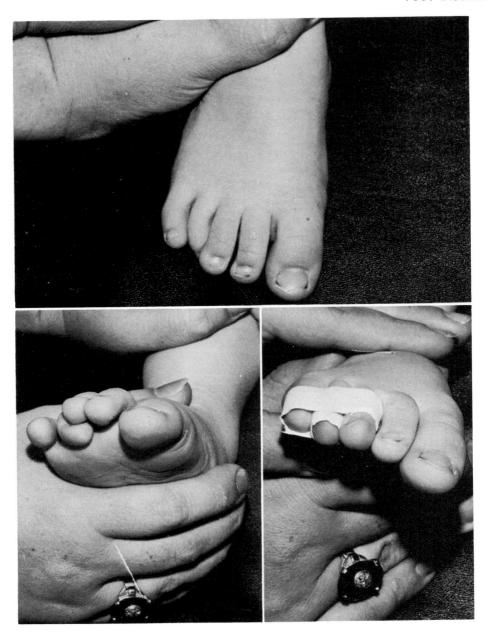

Fig. 5-11. A and B. Varus deformity of the fourth toe.
   C. Method of correction by taping to adjacent toes. (see diagram).

assumes when the leg and foot are permitted to hang over the edge of the plaster table. If the forefoot is minimally adducted or even in neutral position, it is
incompletely corrected. It should hang in
a slightly abducted position.

Once correction has been achieved by
weekly cast changes or wedgings, if one
prefers, a retaining cast should be applied

for a six- to eight-week period with the cast
being changed at least every three to three
and one-half weeks. Following this, the
mother should be instructed in the method
of massage and exercise of the child's foot.
This regimen is the same as in the mild
form of pes adductus (Fig. 5-9D). I prefer
also to prescribe a clubfoot shoe for the
corrected foot. The shoe should be worn

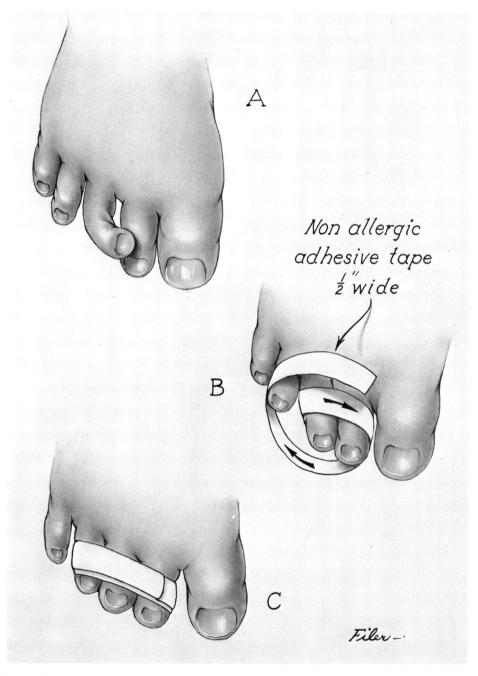

A

Non allergic adhesive tape ½" wide

B

C

Filer—

Fig. 5-12. Diagrammatic sketch of taping. Note direction of application of the tape to hold the deformed digit in corrected position.

constantly throughout the entire twenty-four-hour period, except during bathing and exercising. The parents should be told of the possibility of a slight recurrence when the infant begins walking and they should be apprised of the possibility of addi-

tional casting should there be a recurrence.

If no relapse occurs when the biped position is assumed, no further corrective shoes are necessary. On the other hand, any slight recurrence calls for re-casting or re-correcting, and out-toeing (tarso-pronator) shoes (Fig. 5-10) should be worn for at least twelve to eighteen months following removal of the casts. The same regimen is applied in the correction of the moderately severe pes adductus (metatarsus varus). In this last type, clubfoot shoes with a Dennis-Browne bar have no place in the initial corrective phase of therapy.

VARUS OR VALGUS DEFORMITIES OF THE TOES (OVERLAPPING TOES)

The valgus or varus deformity, as well as overlapping of one toe on another (Fig. 5-11A and B), warrants early recognition but treatment is not indicated until the infant is at least six months of age since prior to this time the toe is too small to manage. The treatment consists of the strapping of the deformed toe between the adjoining two toes in such a manner as to splint it between the two normal ones. This is best carried out with the use of half inch wide non-allergenic adhesive tape since it does not irritate the skin. The tape should be reapplied daily after the baby's bath. Correction usually requires from three to six months. The tape is first applied to the deformed toe with the digit held out straight. It is then brought over the dorsum of the involved toe to the dorsum of the medial adjoining toe, around the plantar surface of the latter to the lateral adjoining toe on the plantar aspect, around the lateral side of this digit to the dorsum, and across again over to the dorsum of the medial normal digit (Fig. 5-11C). Thus the deformed toe is held in a corrected position. The mother should be carefully instructed (Fig. 5-12) as to the proper application of the tape and the orthopaedist should request the mother to tape the toes in his presence, thus making certain that she understands precisely how to apply the tape. The baby's toes should be inspected regularly once a month until correction has occurred. In the case of varus deformity of the fifth toe, the deformed toe obviously can be taped only to the fourth toe and correction requires considerably longer time.

BIBLIOGRAPHY

FLIEGEL, O.: Bemerkungen zum angeborenen Pes adductus. Wien klin Wsch, 66:616. 1954.
Congenital Pes Adductus. Bull Hosp. Joint Dis. 16:65 (April) 1965.
FRIEDMAN, B.: Foot Problems in Infants and Children. Rotational Deviations of Lower Extremities. J. Pediat. 46:573 (May) 1955.
HERZMARK, M.D.: Flat Feet in Children. An Ounce of Prevention. Med. Times. (Feb.) 1963.
KITE, J. H.: Treatment of Flatfeet in Children. Med. Ann. Dist. Columbia 21:316 (June) 1952.
The Treatment of Flat feet in Small Children. Post-Grad. Med. 15:75 (Jan.) 1954.
Torsion of the Legs in Small Children, J. Med. Assoc. Georgia, (Dec.) 1954.
Flat Feet and Lateral Rotation of Legs in Young Children. J. Internat. Coll. Surg. 25:77 (Jan.) 1956.

Torsional Deformities of the Lower Extremities, West Virginia. Med. J. 57:92 (Mar.) 1961.
LLOYD-ROBERTS, G. C.: Orthopaedic Problems in Childhood. The Practitioner, 193:634 (Nov.) 1964.
MARGO, E.: Metatarsus Varus in Static Feet. Southern Med. J. 48:724 (July) 1955.
STAMM, T. T.: Foot Health and the General Practitioner. Common Defects and Deformities of the Foot. Med. Press, 30, (Nov.) 1955.
SWANSON, A. B., GREENE, P. W. AND ALLIS, H. D.: Rotational Deformities of the Lower Extremity in Children and Their Clinical Significance. Clinc. Orthop. 27:157, 1963.
ZACHARIAE, L.: The Grice Operation for Paralytic Flat Feet in Children. Acta. Orthop. Scand. 33:80, 1963.

= 6 =

The Pronated Foot in Infancy and Childhood

The appearance of the normal foot was described in Chapter 4. As indicated in Chapter 5, there is a definite hereditary predisposition to flat feet. In this chapter the emphasis is placed on the importance of early recognition and immediate corrective treatment to prevent many of the static deformities resulting from lack of or from

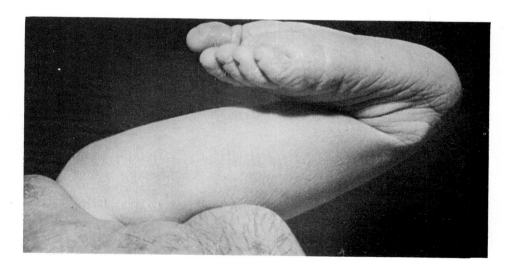

Fig. 6-1.   Congenital Calcaneo-Valgus at Birth.
   Note the acute extension position of foot in relation to the leg. The heel is in a valgus position as is the foot in relation to the ankle and leg. **With immediate institution of therapy, a good result can be achieved in most instances.**

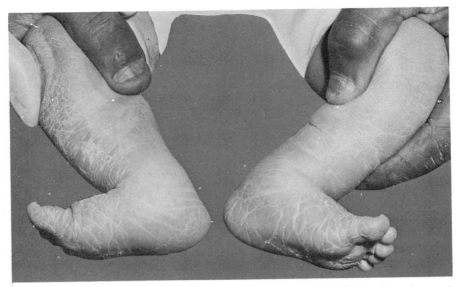

Fig. 6-2.   Bilateral calcaneo-valgus feet five days after birth. Although they have begun to assume a more normal appearance, still on passive extension the feet will touch the anterior aspect of each leg. This is the type of feet which are so often disregarded with the remark, "They don't look too bad. We'll watch them." Fig. 6-6 is the roentgenogram of these feet taken at the same time. Note the almost vertical tali.

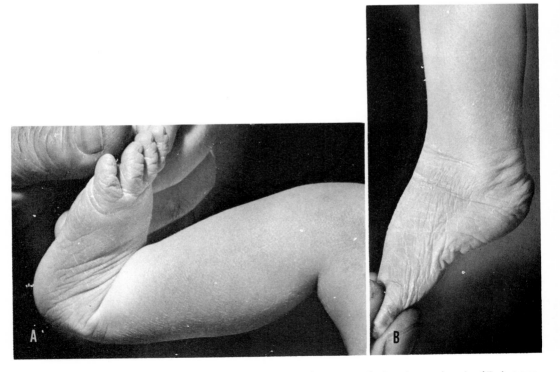

Fig. 6-3.   A.   Relative passive extension of the normal newborn foot only reaches to 45 degrees. Even with force, the foot cannot extend any further. Note position of heel in relation to ankle as compared to Figure 6-1.
    B.   Range of passive flexion in the normal newborn foot is 50 degrees. Note that skin on anterior aspect of ankle and dorsum of foot does not appear tight and the anterior transverse creases are not stretched.

insufficient therapy, deformities that necessitate prolonged periods of care. Furthermore, early treatment can prevent the need for later surgical intervention which is frequently required in the case of inadequately treated symptomatic feet.

CALCANEOVALGUS FOOT

The type of flatfoot deformity found at birth is known as the calcaneovalgus foot (Fig. 6-1). It can be unilateral or bilateral. Study the illustration carefully. As can be seen, the foot lies in acute extension and slight valgus. The dorsal surface of the foot is in contact with the anterior surface of the lower leg. Figure 6-2 demonstrates a moderately severe deformity on clinical examination. There are varying degrees of the same malformation. Early recognition even of a mild deviation is of paramount importance. Careful clinical and roentgenographic evaluation is necessary for the immediate institution of proper therapy.

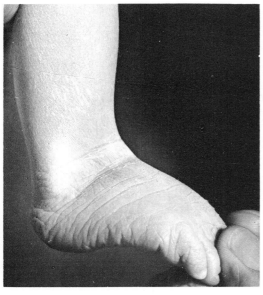

Fig. 6-4. This is the side view of the foot illustrated in Figure 6-1. Note that flexion is limited to the neutral position and the skin on the anterior aspect of the ankle and the dorsum of the foot is quite taut. In fact it stands out as a tight band. The skin is blanched over the band whereas, the surrounding skin is pink. The creases are stretched. Although there are various gradations of this deformity, depending on the severity of the contracture of the soft tissues, the end result is invariably a plantar flexed talus.

Examination of the normal newborn foot shows that relative passive extension is limited to an angle of 45 degrees (Fig. 6-3A) and passive flexion to an angle of 50 degrees (Fig. 6-3B). To all intents and purposes, in the calcaneovalgus type, extension is practically absent at birth and flexion is limited to the neutral position with the anterior soft tissue structures appearing tight and preventing further flexion of the foot (Fig. 6-4). If the deformity is of a lesser degree, the feet will present the appearance illustrated in Figure 6-2. In the lesser deformity, the examiner will find that he can extend both feet passively with little, if any, force so that they touch the anterior tibial cutaneous surface. Furthermore, flexion will be limited to at least half of the normal range, if not more, and the soft tissue structures will be contracted.

On roentgenographic examination definite malalignment of the visible tarsal bones will be found. In the lateral roentgenogram of the normal foot at rest, the line bisecting the talus traverses through the upper half of the cuboid (Fig. 6-5A). There is no overlap between the talus and os calcis. In a calcaneovalgus foot, in the same projection, the talus is plantar-flexed and the line bisecting the talus (Fig. 6-5B) extends below the plantar surface of the cuboid. In addition there is overlapping between the head of the talus and the anterior superior edge of the os calcis. (See arrow). The roentgenograms of the feet illustrated in Figure 6-2 demonstrate even greater talocalcaneal malposition with the right foot presenting an almost vertical talus and the left a lesser talar malalignment (Fig. 6-6).

Treatment. Correction of such a deformity should begin with the obstetrician's, pediatrician's, and general practitioner's recognition of this malposed foot at the time of birth and the subsequent request for an orthopaedic evaluation and initiation of therapy within a few days after birth. *It is just as important to institute corrective treatment in this type of tarsal malposition as it is in clubfeet!*

Following clinical and roentgenographic

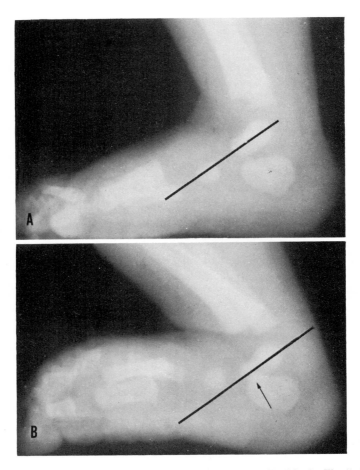

Fig. 6-5A.   Radiograph of Normal Foot at Birth (In the Lateral Position). The talus is so posi-tioned that a line bisecting it will bisect the lateral cuneiform or pass through the dorsal half of this bone. Its position in relation to the os calcis is a slightly plantar flexed one but there is no overlap of one bone upon the other. Each osseous component is well delineated. The positioning of the foot is described in the text.

  B.   Roentgenogram of newborn foot illustrated in Figure 6-1. Note that the line bisecting the talus falls plantar to the cuboid. There is overlapping of the talus on the os calcis anteriorly. Arrow points to area of overlap. This is a calcaneo-valgus foot which, **if recognized early and immediate therapy instituted, can be corrected.**

evaluation, the plan of orthopaedic man-agement consists of the application of cor-rective casts. These are applied from the level of the knee joint to the tips of the toes with the foot held in a complete equi-nus position, but *no varus*. The skin should be sprayed with tincture of benzoin or one of the other skin adherents. Webril is pref-erable to sheet wadding since it can be applied more smoothly and more snugly as a covering prior to application of the cast. Before the cast has had an opportunity to harden, the foot is molded under the longi-tudinal arch (Fig. 6-7) to a maximum de-gree just distal to the talus. The cast should

be well molded around the heel. A lateral roentgenogram should be taken after the cast has hardened to determine the align-ment of the talus in relation to the os calcis. If the position is not within the prescribed normal, as indicated in Figure 6-5A, the cast should be removed the following day, the foot remanipulated without a cast so that the orthopaedist can directly observe the amount of tension applied to the soft tissues in order to secure maximum correc-tion. Next, a new cast, again firmly molded under the midtarsal region and the heel, should be applied. Check roentgenograms should then be procured. Usually, either

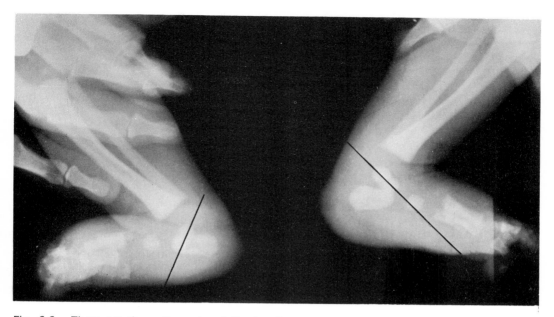

Fig. 6-6. These are the radiographs of the feet illustrated in Figure 6-2. Note position of tali in relation to the os calcis. The right talus is practically vertical although clinically the feet do not appear so malaligned. Immediate institution of corrective casts is necessary.

with the first or at most the second cast application, realignment is achieved. Occasionally, in the vertical talus type deformity, several cast changes on consecutive days may be necessary to achieve the desired correction, but it can be usually accomplished. In the vertical talus deformity, if one is unsuccessful in securing adequate correction initially, the heel and foot should be placed in varus along with the equinus position, since in such a deformity the talocalcaneal malposition is not only in the vertical rotational position but also in the lateral one. The care of the vertical talus type foot from birth to adolescence is discussed in detail in the next chapter since this is a different clinical entity from the plantar flexed talus.

Once correction is secured, the foot is kept in the equinus position for at least four weeks, although the cast is changed weekly to accommodate for growth. No attempt should be made to correct the equinus prior to this time. At the end of this period, the cast should be removed and roentgenograms should be procured in the anteroposterior as well as the lateral views (Fig. 6-8). This illustration represents the corrected position of the talus shown in Figure 6-5B. The foot should be permitted

to seek its own level of extension (dorsiflexion) without manipulation and a new cast applied, care being taken to mold the cast properly under the longitudinal arch of the foot. The cast is changed every two weeks until the neutral right angle position is achieved *without* forcible manipulation, but simply by holding the foot gently from the toes and permitting the weight of the leg to bring about the gradual correction of the equinus position. Once this position is reached, the foot is maintained in the corrective cast for a period of at least three months. Any temptation to remove it sooner than this will result in loss of the correction.

By this time the infant will be approximately six months of age. The baby is then fitted with a pair of hard-soled, steel-shank, straight-last shoes with a rubber cookie inserted in the shoe to fit under the longitudinal arch of the foot. The shoes are not removed at any time except when the infant is bathed. The parents are advised to strictly discourage the baby from standing even if they hold him by his hands. The child should be permitted to begin standing only when he wishes to do so spontaneously without parental support. The baby should be seen at least once a month

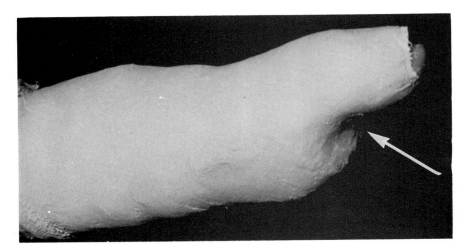

Fig. 6-7. Corrective cast. Observe position of foot in complete equinus and molding of cast on the medio-plantar aspect at level of the talarnavicular and navicular cuneiform joints. This molding extends across the entire plantar aspect of the foot but more pronounced on the plantar medial aspect. Cast extends to the tips of the toes and toes **must** be lined up parallel to one another and all five digital tips should be visible.

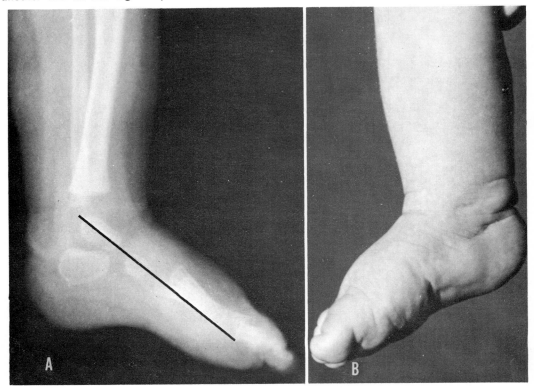

Fig. 6-8. A. Lateral roentgenogram of same foot illustrated in Figure 6-5B after application of corrective casts for eight weeks. Note talo-calcaneal relation, there is no overlap. Note also that line bisecting the talus traverses the upper half of the cuboid and touches the plantar edge of the first metatarsal. Although the position of the osseous components is normal, the foot will continue to be casted in an overcorrected position. (Refer to text).

B. Clinical appearance of same foot after two months of corrective casts. Compare this with Figure 6-1. Note the longitudinal arch of the foot.

The roentgenogram in Figure 6-8A was unfortunately reversed when printed by the photographer thus causing it to appear as though it were the opposite foot.

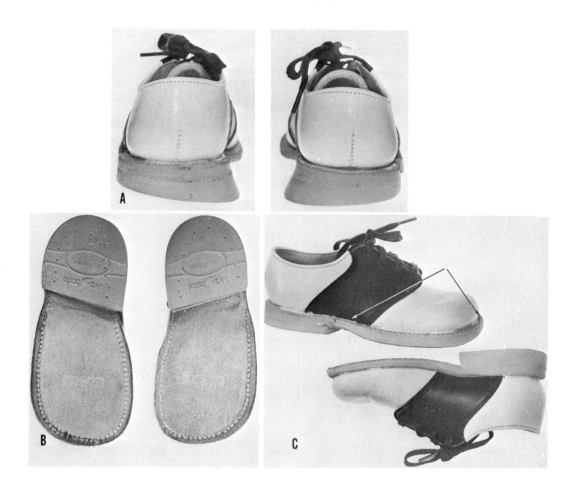

Fig. 6-9A.   Posterior view of shoes to illustrate inner heel elevation and flare. The elevation places the rear foot in inversion and thus helps to maintain locked position of os calcis and talus. Inner heel elevation may vary from $\frac{1}{8}$ to $\frac{1}{4}$ inch. Less than $\frac{1}{8}$ inch is useless and more than $\frac{1}{4}$ inch is not well tolerated by the patient. The flare, usually $\frac{1}{4}$ inch, broadens the size of the heel and is synergistic with the inner heel elevation.

B.   Plantar aspect of shoes demonstrating inner heel advance. This varies from $\frac{3}{8}$ to $\frac{3}{4}$ inch. Its action is to reinforce the effect of the elevation and flare to the plantar aspect of the talo-navicular joint and, if needed, to the navicular-cuneiform joint.

C.   Outer sole elevation is used for a twofold effect. First, to invert the forefoot while the rearfoot is everted. Second, to balance the shoe so that the eversion forces of the heel will not cause the youngster to run the shoes over on the lateral aspect. It may vary from $\frac{1}{8}$ to $\frac{1}{4}$ inch and extends from the midline anteriorly (see arrow) to the junction of the posterior $\frac{1}{3}$ with the anterior $\frac{2}{3}$ of the shoe on the lateral aspect. It is tapered from a thin edge medially with the maximum width along the lateral edge of the sole. The sole should be split and the wedge inserted, cemented, and sewn in.

D.   Rubber cookie inserted in the shoe on the medial side. There are various graduated sizes. The size to be installed in the shoe depends upon the child's foot size. The anterior tip of the cookie should be at the level of the medial outflare of the shoe, and it should extend posteriorly so that the posterior tip is located at a spot perpendicular to the tip of the medial malleolus (observe arrows).

E.   Observe how feet are held in properly supported position. The ankles do not invert. The laces should be drawn snugly at each eyelet.

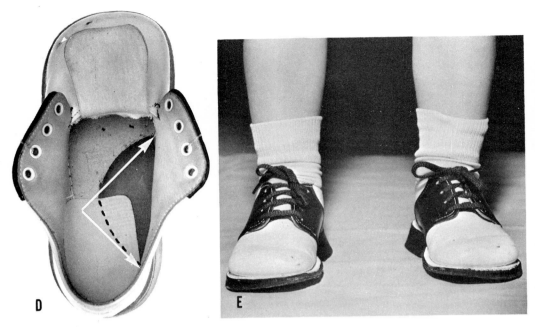

Fig. 6-9.   See page 103 for Figs. 6-9 D and E.

and the parents should be instructed to bring the child in as soon as he begins to pull himself up to a standing position. At that time a corrective heel is added to the shoe. This is of the Thomas type consisting of an inner heel elevation of 1/8 inch, an inner heel flare of 1/4 inch, and an inner heel advance of 3/8 inch. In addition to this, x-rays of the standing child's feet should be procured for the first time in order to determine whether or not the talus is maintaining its proper relation to the os calcis and to the other tarsal bones.

The parents should be warned that occasionally one series of casts will be insufficient and that a second series may be necessary should the original correction be lost. If another series of casts is required, one should start from the beginning with the feet again in the full equinus position. Instructions of this phase of correction will be given later in this chapter.

If the standing roentgenograms taken at this time demonstrate normal talocalcaneal alignment, the corrective shoes are kept on constantly until the child is sixteen months of age. If the foot or feet on clinical examination appear to be within normal limits at this time, and the roentgenograms taken with the child standing again demonstrate normal talocalcaneal alignment, the child is fitted with oxford (low-cut) straight-last shoes, again with the application not only of a corrective heel and rubber cookie, but also an outer sole elevation of 1/16 inch. The shoes can now be removed at night, but no weight bearing is permitted without the corrective shoes until twenty-four months of age. At that time, the correction in the shoes is changed to an inner heel elevation of 3/16 inch, inner heel flare 1/4 inch (Fig. 6-9A), inner heel advance 1/2 inch (Fig. 6-9B), outer sole elevation 1/16 inch (Fig. 6-9C). A rubber cookie of proper size (Fig. 6-9D) is installed inside the shoe. The youngster is then kept in this type of corrective shoes until the age of six (Fig. 6-9E). When the youngster is six years old, a final evaluation of the feet should be carried out both clinically and roentgenographically. No further correction is needed if all findings are normal.

This same regimen is carried out even if the infant is first brought in for care up to the age of six months, but the period of immobilization and correction in casts will be much longer and will usually require at least one year's treatment in corrective casts. However, there is a difference in one step and that is the application of walking casts after the proper correction has been procured and the foot has been brought up to the neutral position without loss of correction.

This same principle of therapy can be applied up to the age of twenty-four months, but with certain variations of the technique. In a child six months or older who has had no therapy, what will be the appearance of the feet? At rest the feet will present little if any longitudinal arch. Relative passive extension will still be over the normal 30 to 45 degrees. True passive extension with the tarsal joints locked will be greater than 10 degrees. In other words, the foot will present greater flexibility than normal. In a standing position the heels will be in valgus, the medial border of the foot will be quite prominent and the entire foot will "rock inwardly" as though the youngster were bearing his weight on the medial surface of the navicular. There will appear to be, and in truth there is, a valgus deviation of the rear foot in relation to the forefoot (Fig. 6-10). Is it any wonder that such a child is slow in walking? Still, the baby whose feet are illustrated in Figure 6-10 had been regularly checked by a physician. The physician had advised the mother that the child was slightly retarded and therefore was slow in walking. One wonders if the child's shoes and socks were even removed during any of the regular bi-monthly physical evaluations.

The initial cast or casts for the correction are applied in the same manner until proper alignment is secured between the os calcis and the talus. By this time, in some cases of vertical talus such correction may be almost impossible. An attempt should be made to correct the malalignment but the parents should be warned of the great probability of failure.

Once the proper alignment has been achieved, then *very gradual* dorsal wedging of the cast is carried out weekly along with lateral roentgenograms as indicated to make certain that there is no loss of the normal talocalcaneal position. This correction may take as long as eight to twelve weeks, if not longer. If it is necessary to change the cast between wedgings, either because of softening or due to the wear and tear imposed upon the cast by the baby's crawling, the cast should be reapplied in the complete equinus position; on the first wedging it can be brought up to its previous position. On subsequent weeks the foot is gradually wedged to neutral. Once the neutral position has been reached and the foot appears to be within normal limits, clinically as well as roentgenographically, walking casts are applied. Here again, certain steps must be followed.

The application of a walking cast must be carried out in two stages. Any tendency to hurry, to be slipshod, or to take short cuts will only lead to loss of correction. One *must* be patient and meticulous. First the foot portion of the cast is applied snug-

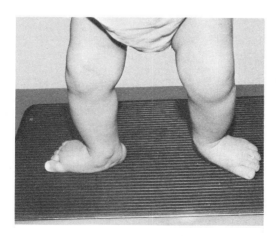

Fig. 6-10. Unexamined, untreated, unrecognized calcaneo-valgus feet at age of fourteen months. Mother concerned why child had not begun to walk as yet. At this age, if the child does not have vertical tali, intensive cast therapy and support, as described, will frequently produce a good result.

ly over well-fitted Webril with the foot in the equinus position. The cast should extend from the tips of the toes to just above the ankle joint. It is then molded not only on the plantar aspect to mold the longitudinal arch, but also around the heel so that the cast will grasp the heel and hold it in position when the foot is dorsiflexed. After the cast has hardened, its anterior portion is cut out in an elliptical fashion from its edge above the ankle joint down to the level of the talonavicular joint anteriorly. The foot is then slowly extended to bring it up into the neutral position and with minimal varus of the heel. The cast is then extended up to the knee. A lateral roentgenogram should be procured to check the position of the talus in relation to the os calcis. If this proves satisfactory, a walking heel is applied. Such corrective immobilization is maintained for *at least* six months and in some instances even longer. If at the end of this period of immobilization,

from the support laterally and run the shoe over on the outer aspect. With Whitman plates the lateral heel flange holds the tarsal region of the foot in the desired position.

It is realized that a number of orthopaedists will be critical of the use of a steel arch-support on the basis that it is unyielding and does not permit the ligamentous and the musculo-tendinous structures to receive sufficient exercise so as to strengthen the foot structures and thus support the bony components. This premise may apply to the normal foot, or to the mildly flat foot, but not to a calcaneovalgus foot. The latter is, or was, to begin with, a structurally unsound foot with regard to the osseous elements. Furthermore, the ligamentous structures were, and still are, stretched and non-supporting. As indicated in the first chapter, the ligaments and muscles act as stays when the bones of the foot are in proper anatomical alignment. Any strain placed on the ligaments because

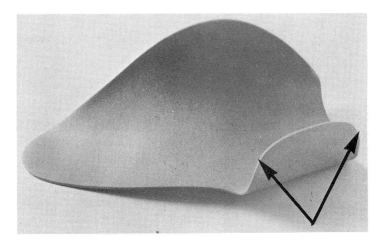

Fig. 6-11.   Whitman arch support manufactured from monel steel. Note lateral flange to grip tarsal region of foot and hold it in proper position. The use of a heel cup is optional. The author prefers not to use it.

lateral standing roentgenograms reveal normal alignment of the talus, the child is fitted with previously prepared Whitman steel plates which have been manufactured according to the size and shape of the child's feet (Fig. 6-11). The use of the leather, leather and steel, or rubber ordinary arch supports is contraindicated since the foot will have a tendency to slide away

of improper alignment and locking of the tarsal bones will place such a strain on these ligamentous structures and they will stretch. Therefore, in an abnormal foot such as the calcaneovalgus type, radical measures are necessary to gain the result desired. We agree that this type of arch support is a crutch, but it is a crutch that this type of foot requires for several years.

After the child has been fitted with the already described style of shoe with the arch support properly placed in it, the parents are given specific instructions. Initially and until advised otherwise by the orthopaedist, the shoes are to be removed only for bathing. The child *may not* run barefoot or in house slippers around the house or on the concrete play area. *In other words, the shoes and arch supports are to be worn constantly.* The child should be reexamined in one month to make certain that the foot is maintaining itself in the corrected position. If the roentgenograms, as well as the clinical evaluation, reveal any loss of correction, the child's feet should be recast for a period of at least another three months. If the correction is maintained, then the youngster is placed on a regular three-month follow-up basis. The arch supports usually require changing on an annual basis, but if the child's feet should grow at a more than usually rapid rate, then the arch supports are changed earlier.

How does one tell when new plates are needed? The distal leading edge of the Whitman plate fits under the first metatarsal head. When this edge of the support is proximal to the plantar prominence of the first metatarsal, the child is in need of new arch supports. The length of time that the youngster is maintained in Whitman steel arch supports will depend largely on the clinical judgment of the orthopaedist. As a form of a yardstick — for each year of delay in correcting such feet, one adds two additional years of corrective support. Thus a youngster whose initial casting was started at one year of age will wear arch supports until the age of eight. Furthermore, one will not discard all correction when one discontinues the use of the arch supports. Appropriate sized rubber cookies should be placed in the shoes and an inner heel elevation of 1/4 inch, and inner heel flare of 1/4 inch should be added to each heel. If, after wearing such shoes for six months, the foot position is maintained, the heel correction is discontinued, and six months later the rubber cookie is discarded. In other words, children with flat feet due to plantar flexed tali should continue under orthopaedic supervision up to the age of ten to twelve years at a minimum.

One word of caution: every foot does not turn out to be perfectly corrected no matter how diligently one may try. In most instances, however, the results will be worth the effort.

THE PRONATED FOOT AT SIXTEEN MONTHS

As mentioned in previous chapters, the infant does not present a true longitudinal arch of the foot at birth nor will he demonstrate one under ordinary circumstances until he is approximately eighteen months of age (plus or minus three months). What then of the youngster who is first seen between the ages of eighteen to twenty-four months having been referred by the physician because of pronated feet (Fig. 6-12 A and B), which, furthermore, are not of the calcaneovalgus type?

Incidence. Although it would be difficult to obtain a reliable estimate of the percentage of children who have faulty foot balance, there is no doubt that between 40 and 45 per cent of the children brought to a pediatric clinic have pronated feet though they are asymptomatic. This lack of symptomatology is one reason why many children with faulty foot stance do not receive early therapy. Furthermore, there is a certain percentage of physicians, fortunately diminishing in number, whose attitude is "let the foot grow as it wishes as long as it isn't deformed or symptomatic. Many people have pronated feet which are symptom free."

Etiology. The predisposing causes of pronated feet in children are several. The most common one is hereditary predisposition (familial diathesis). In addition to heredity, there are such causes as external tibial torsion, internal torsion, either femoral or tibial, genu valgus, congenital shortening of the first metatarsal, hypermobile first metatarsal, and metatarsus varus primus. The presence of an accessory scaphoid (os tibiale externum) has been given as a cause for pronated feet, but this idea is not en-

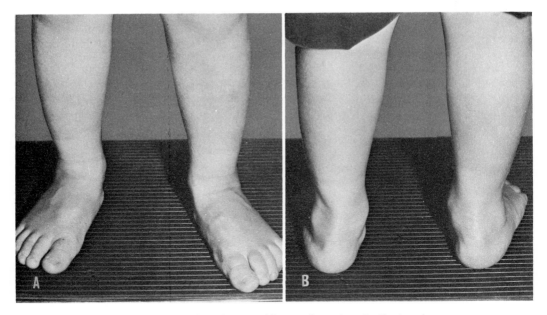

Fig. 6-12.   Pronated Feet.   A.   There is no evidence of any longitudinal arch.
B.   Note bow-stringing of tendo Achillis and mild valgus position of both heels.

tirely correct. I have seen a number of feet with an accessory scaphoid which on cursory examination appeared pronated but which, upon careful evaluation, had a normal longitudinal arch.

Deficiency in the strength of some of the musculature in the foot and/or leg, either actual or relative, can produce a pronated foot. Causes of actual muscle imbalance leading to flatfoot deformity are acute anterior poliomyelitis and cerebral palsy. Other deficiencies also producing a similar type of foot are those associated with endocrine imbalances of the pituitary and/or the thyroid type with or without obesity. Diseases due to vitamin deficiencies, such as rickets and scurvy, can also be considered as causative agents.

The more frequent causes will be discussed in greater detail when therapy will be considered. Moreover, there are other factors which produce symptomatic pronated feet but these occur in the adolescent and in the adult group. They will be discussed in the chapters dealing with the adolescent and with the adult foot.

Symptomatology. The complaints associated with pronated feet in children up to the age of four or five are almost in-variably negligible. Children of this age (from two to five years) will not complain of pain in the feet per se. Their symptomatology is usually indirect. The parents will observe any one or several of the following symptoms: They will state that the child tends to be clumsy; to fall frequently; is unable to keep up in play or in running with the youngsters of his own age; walks with one foot externally rotated; limps on one or both feet; walks with a pigeon-toed or an out-toeing gait; is knock-kneed or bowlegged; asks to be carried frequently; awakens from his sleep complaining of pain in both legs. At times the mother will bring in the youngster stating that she is just unable to put her finger on it, but that something is wrong with the child's feet or legs and that he doesn't walk "right". On other occasions the reason for the office visit is that the child is running over the heels and soles of the shoes either inwardly or outwardly. Often the mother will bring in the child for evaluation stating, "I've always had trouble with my feet and I want you to check Johnnie's feet and correct them even if the child has no complaints now. I can remember that my feet didn't begin to bother me until I was in

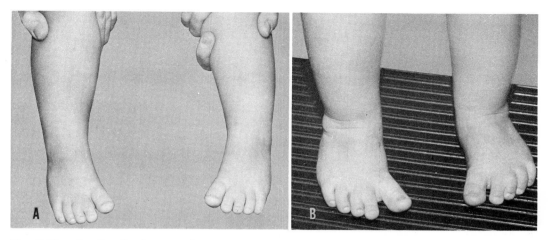

Fig. 6-13.   A.   Practically normal appearance of foot when the youngster is non-weight bearing.
   B.   Notice obvious bilateral metatarsus varus which had been missed since the child had not been examined in a standing position.

my late teens and the boy's feet are like mine."

Whatever the complaints may be, one word of advice: *Do not treat them lightly.* Even if the child has completely asymptomatic pronated feet, treat them. There are some physicians who will disagree with this blanket statement, but this statement is made as a result of thirty years' experience and observation. If the physician permits a child with pronated feet to go on untreated, eventually when the latter will have grown to adulthood, disability will result either in the lower extremities or in the low back. Whether minor or major, these difficulties can be definitely attributed to pronated feet. Contrary to the belief of some orthopaedists that only the flattening foot is symptomatic, it is our firm conviction that a flat foot exposed to the uses and abuses of modern living, will inevitably become symptomatic.

Examination. Physical evaluation should not be limited to the feet alone. Both lower extremities should be evaluated. The range of motion of both hips should be checked and particular attention should be directed to rotatory movement. Knee motion and any varus or valgus deformity should be determined. Torsion of the tibia, whether internal or external, should be recorded. The feet should be examined in the standing position as well as at rest and preferably on a reflector mirror stand. Thus one

can observe the plantar as well as the dorsal, the medial, and the lateral aspects of both feet. The heels should be evaluated since any valgus position of the heels with bow-stringing of the tendo achillis will be indicative not only of pronation, but probably also of a contracted calf muscle. A careful and complete neurological check is necessary. One will be surprised how often he may find a minimal muscular spasticity of both lower extremities associated with apparent pronation of the feet and accompanied by slight stumbling on the part of the patient. Muscle power examination and leg length evaluation should also be carried out. Anterioposterior and lateral standing roentgenograms of both feet should be procured.

The importance of examination of the feet in a standing position cannot be stressed adequately. If one does not examine the child's feet and both lower extremities in an erect position, the remaining evaluation is practically useless. The same applies to standing roentgenograms. Figure 6-13 A serves as an excellent example. This child had been examined by another orthopaedist with the youngster being held on the mother's lap. He reassured the parents that the child's feet were perfectly normal and no therapy was indicated. Subsequently she reported to our office since the child still had a pigeon-toed gait. When the child was made to stand, it was obvious that she had a bilateral hallux-metatarsus varus (Fig. 6-13B) and was definitely in need of therapy. Still this little girl might have been permitted to go along with this deformity if the mother had accepted the first medical verdict.

Therapeutic Regimen. The plan of treatment cannot be exactly the same in all pronated feet since, quite often, there are other lower extremity problems associated with the main one. Each patient presents his own individual problem. If, let us say, a two-year-old child, on examination, presents bilateral third degree pes planus only (Fig. 6-14A and B) and the standing roentgenograms do not demonstrate any deformity or malposition of the tarsal bones, the plan of therapy is as follows: Corrective shoes should be ordered as described in Chapter 4 and a prescription incorporated in the shoes consisting of:

Inner heel elevation . . . . 3/16 inch
Inner heel flare . . . . 1/4 inch
Inner heel advance . . . . 1/2 inch
Outer sole elevation . . . . 1/8 inch
Rubber cookie of appropriate size
Rubber heels

The mother should be instructed that the child is to wear the shoes from the first waking moment until placed in bed at night. He should not go barefoot and should not be permitted to walk in house slippers. Often the mother will ask if little "Susie" may not wear patent leather slippers on Sunday because the corrective shoes "are not pretty". This answer should be a firm and unequivocal, "No". The orthopaedist must be firm and should leave no doubt in the parents' minds that there can be any exception to the therapeutic routine. Another question which will often be raised is whether or not the wearing of tennis shoes during the summer months is acceptable. Again the reply should be in the negative. If the orthopaedist wishes to achieve good results with the use of corrective shoes, he must not only prescribe the necessary corrective shoes, but must establish such good rapport with the parents, especially the mother, that they will follow his directions to the letter.

Having prescribed the shoes and the correction, the child should next be seen within four weeks in order to make certain that

the shoes are well fitted and that the prescription has been installed according to the physician's specifications. The child should stand with his shoes on his feet in order to have the fit checked. The fit of the shoe around the heel counter should be carefully examined since, in some instances, it will be found that the child's heels are too narrow. Should such a situation present itself, then an extra pair of eyelets should be added 1.5 cm. posterior to the top set. This addition will help to narrow the throat of the shoe and will improve the fit around the rear of the child's foot. Furthermore, the mother should be instructed to lace the shoes snugly and to apply a double knot that will not slip. It is useless to prescribe corrective shoes if they are not laced snugly so as to support the foot properly. The mother should also be advised to buy a new pair of shoes with the same prescription when the child either outgrows or wears out the first pair.

She should, additionally, check the wear of the rubber heels at least once a week and as soon as the heel is worn down almost to the overlying leather prescription, the rubber heels should be replaced to prevent them from becoming completely run down. The child should not be permitted to run about with uncorrected shoes while such repairs are carried out. The orthopaedist should have made prior arrangements with the shoe repairman to whom the prescription work is sent to be certain that such repairs can be carried out while the youngster and the mother are waiting at the shop.

Parents frequently ask "How long will the child be required to wear such shoes?" The answer should be a qualified one. To a great extent the outcome will depend on the manner in which the feet will respond to the correction and also how faithfully the mother follows given instructions. For the average type of pronated feet, corrective shoes will be required for *at least* four years. In some, less time will be needed. Furthermore, the youngster should be placed on a regular follow-up routine. He should be reexamined at least once every six months. In order to make certain that the child will be brought in every six months, a card should be sent to the par-

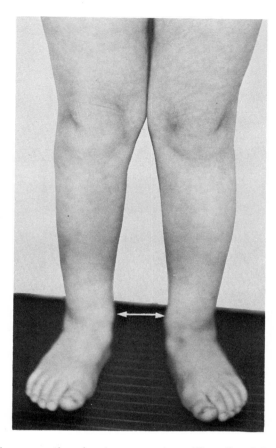

Fig. 6-14.   Intermalleolar separation due to genu valgus. When the distance is less than 10 cm., the genu valgus can be gradually overcome with the use of orthopaedic corrective shoes. When the intermalleolar distance is over 10 cm., genu valgus braces are almost invariably required to effect the desired correction.

ents reminding them that the child is due for such a reevaluation. Nor will the prescription remain the same during this entire period. As the foot grows, the size of the rubber cookie will change. Also after the age of four the heel correction should be increased to:

Inner heel elevation	1/4 inch
Inner heel flare	1/4 inch
Inner heel advance	3/4 inch
Outer sole elevation	1/8 inch

If, let us say, the foot has eventually developed into a normal one by the age of six, will all correction be discarded? No, it will not. The outer sole elevation and the inner heel advance will be discontinued. The inner heel elevation will be cut down to 3/16 inch and the inner heel flare will remain at 1/4 inch. The size rubber cookie to be installed will depend on the size of the foot. At the end of another six

months, if the foot has not lost any of its correction, the heel correction will be completely discarded and only the rubber cookie will be retained in the shoe. The youngster will now be permitted to wear "gym shoes" during the play period after school, and on Sundays and other dress occasions little girls will be permitted to wear party shoes. If at the end of the next six-month period the feet still appear normal, all corrections are discarded and the patient is discharged.

We realize that this regimen sounds didactic but any attempts to short cut this period of therapy will assuredly result in an unsatisfactory correction.

If, in addition to pronated feet, the child has a genu valgus, the course of therapy will remain essentially unchanged unless the valgus deformity is severe. Many children with pronated feet will also demon-

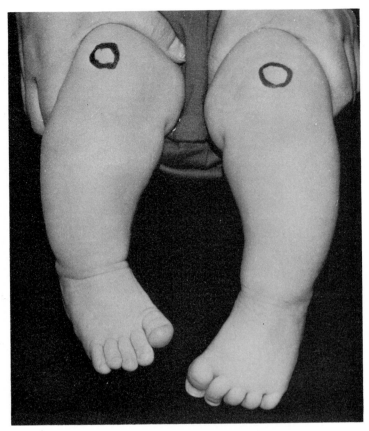

Fig. 6-15. Mild internal tibial torsion which is found only when the knees are held in a true antero-posterior direction. The bowing of the legs is an apparent one due to the torsion.

strate some genu valgus. This is measured by having the child stand barefooted with both lower extremities exposed from the level of the hips distally, with the knees in an anteroposterior direction and in contact with one another (Fig. 6-14). The distance between the medial malleoli should be measured and recorded. If it is not more than 10 cm., the same shoe correction that has been prescribed for the pronated feet can be used and the same regimen followed. Gradually the genu valgus deformity will correct as the feet do. On the other hand, if the separation is over 10 cm., the use of corrective shoes is insufficient to correct the knee condition. Furthermore, standing x-rays of both knees should be procured in the anteroposterior position on 14 x 17 films with the knees centered on the plate to make certain that there is no lateral proximal epiphyseal tibial dysplasia (Blount's disease).

When there is severe genu valgus, the therapy recommended is the application of genu valgus braces as well as corrective shoes. These braces and shoes are worn around the clock until complete correction has been achieved. Following correction, the braces are to be applied during the child's sleeping periods for at least six additional months. The valgus will be corrected much sooner than the pronated feet so that the corrective shoes are to be continued until the pronation deformity is also corrected although the braces can be discarded.

At times, one will see a child whose mother will complain that he walks pigeon-toed or appears bowlegged, or that he walks with his feet held in an out-toeing position. The pigeon-toed or bowlegged gait is due to internal torsion either femoral or tibial, and the out-toeing is due to external tibial torsion. Therapy will depend

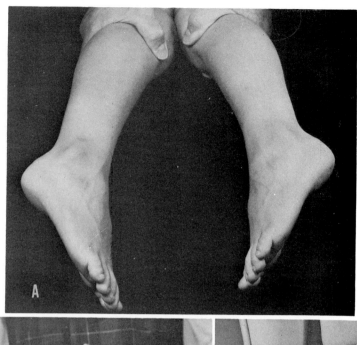

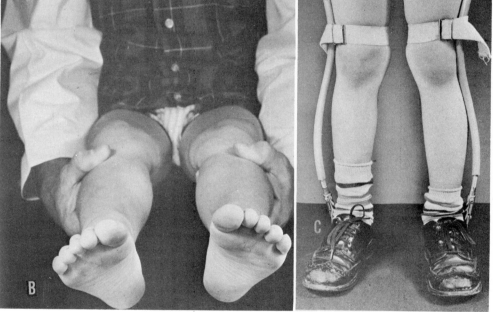

Fig. 6-16A.   There is an excessive amount of internal rotation of the feet of over 90 degrees due to internal femoral torsion.

   B.   Note limitation of external rotation of the feet due to the internal femoral torsion.

   C.   Observe position of feet with the application of twisters to hold both lower extremities externally rotated when the youngster is standing or walking.

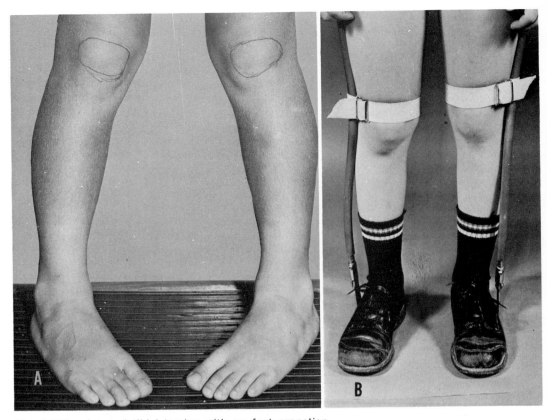

Fig. 6-17A.   Internal tibial torsion with no foot pronation.
   B.   Correction of pigeon-toed gait as a result of the application of the twisters.

upon the child's age and the severity of the torsion.

If the internal tibial torsion is mild (Fig. 6-15), the use at night of a Dennis-Browne bar applied to the shoes is indicated. The examiner will observe that when the baby is standing, there will also be present a mild or moderate hallux varus and at times a minimal metatarsus varus. The feet will be pronated as well. During his waking hours the baby will be required to wear corrective shoes which must serve a two-fold purpose: first, to correct the pronation of the feet, and secondly, to maintain the great toe in the corrected position. A straight-last shoe is required with the following correction:

Inner heel elevation . . . . 3/16 inch
Inner heel flare . . . . 1/4 inch
Inner heel advance . . . . 1/2 inch
Outer sole elevation . . . . 1/4 inch
Rubber cookie according to required size
Rubber heel

There is a question that is likely to be asked: if the outer sole elevation is greater than the inner heel raise, will not the former offset the latter and thus aggravate the pronation? Fortunately, it will not have such a nullifying effect. At first the night Dennis-Browne bar is placed in neutral position and the shoes gradually rotated until the feet are held in a 60 degree position of external rotation. There is no question that the bar will most definitely contribute to further pronation of the feet, but one must temporize for the few months that are necessary for the torsion to be corrected. Following correction the bar is not discontinued, but the shoes are rotated toward neutral so that there will be only a 10 degree external rotation of each shoe. Since the varus of the great toe will require several months longer to correct, the shoe prescription remains unchanged, usually for nine months. At the end of this period, if the leg and foot are well cor-

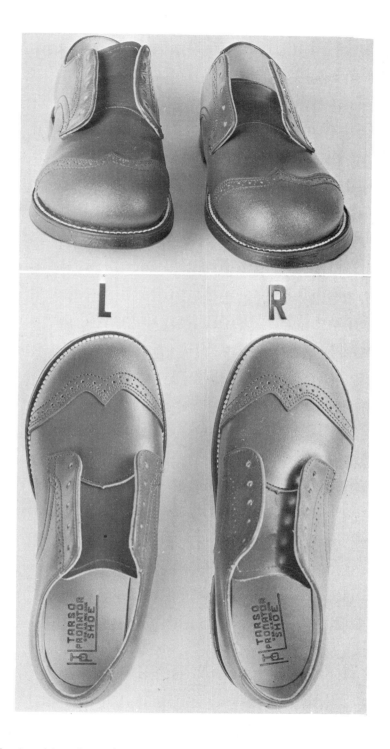

Fig. 6-18.   Front and top views of the tarso-pronator shoe. It can be used to correct either a mild hallux varus (adductus) or a pigeon-toed gait due to poor walking habits.

rected, the outer sole elevation is reduced to 3/16 inch. Corrective shoes are then maintained as for the pronated feet and with, of course, the routine follow-up regimen.

Occasionally the orthopaedist will find that the pigeon-toed gait is due not to internal tibial torsion, but to internal femoral torsion. How is this determined? If the youngster on examination does not demonstrate any internal tibial torsion, one will find that upon internal rotation of the hip or thigh the feet will assume a position of more than 90 degrees of internal rotation (Fig. 6-16A). One will also find that on external rotation there will be definite limitation of motion (Fig. 6-16B). Foot pronation almost invariably accompanies internal femoral torsion. In such instances a Dennis-Browne bar is useless. The youngster should be fitted with twisters (Fig. 6-16C) which are to be worn day and

night along with the corrective shoes. Since there is no varus deformity of the great toe, the shoe correction worn with the twisters is the usual:

Inner heel elevation . . . . 3/16 inch
Inner heel flare . . . . 1/4 inch
Inner heel advance . . . . 1/2 inch
Outer sole elevation . . . . 1/8 inch
Rubber cookie according to size
Rubber heel

The twister is adjusted to force the youngster to walk with the feet held in 10 to 15 degrees of external rotation. The brace should be adjusted by the orthopaedist. The patient should be re-examined at least once every eight to twelve weeks to check the brace as well as to evaluate the child's progress. The twisters should be worn constantly until the lower extremities can be passively externally rotated to 90 degrees. This may require the use of twisters for twenty-four months.

Subsequently, the twisters are to be worn

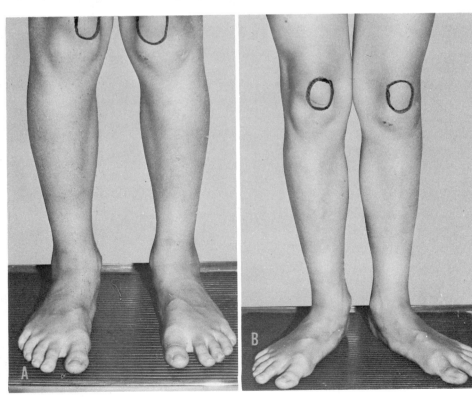

Fig. 6-19A.   Apparent normal appearance of feet when placed parallel with one another. Note position of patellae which is obvious enough to warrant more than a cursory evaluation of the feet.

B.   With knees properly placed in the antero-posterior position, the external tibial torsion is obvious. This torsion, in turn, places an abnormal stress and strain on the feet leading to symptomatic pronation.

at night for at least another six to twelve months since there is a tendency for the femoral torsion to recur if the corrective force is discontinued too early. The corrective shoes are continued until the feet demonstrate a normal longitudinal arch. Internal tibial torsion without foot pronation is occasionally encountered (Fig. 6-17A). In such a situation, twisters alone (Fig. 6-17B) will correct this problem.

Occasionally, one will be faced with a problem of a youngster who walks pigeon-toed but who upon examination does not present any apparent cause for this abnormality. Such a condition is due to bad walking habits, and the use of tarso-pronator shoes (Fig. 6-18) will help to overcome this gait. The shoes must be worn for at least eighteen months and then gradually discarded.

The older the youngster is when his foot condition is diagnosed, the longer will be the necessary period of correction. After the age of six or seven, correction of even a mild tibial torsion, that is, 15 to 20 degrees, will require the use of twisters for at least three to four years. If the torsion is greater in amount, the only recourse is surgical intervention by the performance of a derotation osteotomy of the tibia and fibula.

External tibial torsion is not as frequent as the internal type. One finds that this entity will also tend either to aggravate and increase the amount of pronation of the feet or produce such a pronation. Usually the condition is not recognized, or no attention is paid to it until the youngster is five or six years of age when he complains of pain in his feet or his legs. On initial examination, the feet will appear to be within normal limits. (Fig. 6-19A). However, on careful evaluation it will be found that the boy walks and stands ordinarily with both feet externally rotated. This stance, of course, places an abnormal strain on the feet causing them to pronate. (Fig. 6-19B). In addition to the application of twisters, Whitman plates should also be prescribed. This therapy may sound a bit stringent. However, it is necessary if one wishes to avoid surgery since the orthopaedist does not have the advantage of the time element which he has with a two- or three-year-old youngster.

What of the use of foot exercises such as picking up marbles or other objects with the toes, spreading the toes, walking along a sloped surface, to build up the longitudinal arch? The author feels that such therapy is as useless in the development of the longitudinal arch of the foot as manipulation of the cervical spine is in the curing of an upper respiratory infection. Such measures may be an excellent mental cathartic for the mother since it gives her something to be done and she feels that she is contributing to the improvement of the youngster's feet. In reality they are of no help. However, they do not cause any harm, and if the parents should request a series of exercises to strengthen the child's feet, and if the attending physician is disposed to prescribe, then he can do so with the knowledge that they will not do any good, but on the other hand, they will do no harm.

BIBLIOGRAPHY

BLOUNT, W. P.: Tibia Vara: Osteochondrosis Deformans Tibiae. J. Bone Jt. Surg. 19:1 (Jan.) 1937.

BONNET, WILLIAM L., BAKER, WILLIAM L., AND BAKER, D. R.: Diagnosis of Pes Planus by X-Ray. Radiology, 46:36 (Jan.) 1946.

DICKSON, FRANK D., AND DIVELEY, REX L.: Functional Disorders of the Foot. 3rd Ed. Philadelphia, J. B. Lippincott Company, 1939.

FLIEGEL, O.: Bemerkungen zum angeborenen Pes adductus. Wien klin Wschr, 66:616, 1954.

FRIEDMAN, B.: Foot Problems in Infants and Children. Rotational Deviations of Lower Extremities. J. Pediat. 46:573 (May) 1955.

HERZMARK, M. D.: Flat Feet in Children. An Ounce of Prevention. Med. Times (Feb.) 1963.

HOWORTH, M. BECKETT: A Textbook of Orthopaedics, Philadelphia, W. B. Saunders Co., 1952.

KIDNER, F. C.: The Pre-Hallux (Accessory Scaphoid) in its Relation to Flat Foot. J. Bone Jt. Surg. 11:831 (Oct.) 1929.

KITE, J. H.: Treatment of Flatfeet in Children. Med. Ann. Dist. Columbia, 21:316, 1952.
The Treatment of Flatfeet in Small Children. Postgrad. Med. 15:75 (Jan.) 1954.
Torsion of the Legs in Small Children. J. Med. Assoc. Georgia (Dec.) 1954.
Flatfeet and Lateral Rotation of Legs in Young

Children. J. Internat. Coll. Surg., *25*:77 (Jan.) 1956.

Torsional Deformities of the Lower Extremities, West Virginia Med. J., *57*:92 (Mar.) 1961.

LEWIN, PHILIP: *The Foot and Ankle,* 4th Ed., Philadelphia, Lea & Febiger, 1959.

LLOYD-ROBERTS, G. C.: Orthopaedic Problems in Childhood. The Practitioner, *193*:634 (Nov.) 1964.

MARGO, E.: Metatarsus Varus in Static Feet. Southern Med. J. *48*:724 (July) 1955.

STAMM, T. T.: Foot Health and the General Practitioner. Common Defects and Deformities of the Foot. Med. Press, *30* (Nov.) 1955.

SWANSON, A. B., GREENE, P. W., AND ALLIS, H. D.: Rotational Deformities of the Lower Extremity in Children and Their Clinical Significance. Clin. Orthop. *27*:157, 1963.

ZACHARIAE, L.: The Grice Operation for Paralytic Flat Feet in Children. Acta. Orthop. Scand., *33*:80, 1963.

= 7 =

Static Foot Problems

in the Pre-Adolescent and Adolescent Stages

Although the causes of static foot problems remain essentially unchanged throughout childhood, in children from eight to sixteen years of age the types of therapy for the pronated foot differ as compared to treatment for the child below the age of eight. However, from the standpoint of maturity of the foot, and thus any plan of therapy, a different set of standards must be used.

According to Drs. Hoerr, Pyle, and Francis, the human foot is considered to be fully mature by the age of eighteen in the male, and fifteen years and three months in the female. Thus the adolescent stage for the foot should not be regarded as extending beyond the age of sixteen in the male and fourteen in the female. Although this axiom may sound somewhat arbitrary, experience has proved that any corrective surgery for flatfeet after the above ages is not as successful either cosmetically, symptomatically, or functionally. The remaining articular surfaces of the foot do not have an opportunity to adjust to their new positions if corrective surgery is performed after the foot is physiologically mature. One can cor-

rect such pronated feet after the adolescent stage if the feet are very flexible on examination, but the orthopaedist should advise the patient of the likelihood of achieving at best only a good result cosmetically, and a fair to good result symptomatically.

If a child has been under proper and well-supervised therapy for his feet during infancy and childhood, he has a 75 to 85 per cent chance of reaching adolescence with a well-corrected, normally functioning pair of feet. One must realize, however, that in spite of careful conscientious therapy and supervision, approximately 15 per cent of the youngsters treated (and most often they are the ones with the plantar flexed tali or the severely relaxed flatfeet) will not respond to conservative treatment. This lack of response to treatment in infancy and early childhood is serious since such feet respond even less to conservative therapy during pre-adolescence. It is a still more grave problem if such a patient is brought to the orthopaedist for initial therapy during the adolescent stage.

Conservative therapy should, however, be prescribed for the majority of youngsters up to the age of twelve. When a child with severe pronation of both feet is first brought in for treatment between the ages of eight and ten, the parents should be advised that there is a bare possibility of securing the correction desired by conservative means, but that should such treatment fail, surgery may be necessary to achieve the desired result. Some parents, either because of ignorance or poor advice, will discontinue or neglect the recommended therapy. In some instances, where surgery is the only alternative whereby such feet can be corrected and the parents are so advised, they will disregard such recommendations and seek the services of another orthopaedist or even a chiropodist who will assure them that since the feet are asymptomatic, conservative therapy alone is needed. It is impossible to overemphasize the seriousness of the responsibility of the physician who dismisses the problem of foot imbalance in the adolescent as being of no consequence. It often results in a lost opportunity to correct the feet and the physician consulted will thus condemn the individual to a future of discomfort and limitation of physical activity.

Undoubtedly, some orthopaedists will criticize the recommendations which will be listed for the therapy of certain problems of the adolescent foot as being too radical. However, these recommendations and conclusions are based on sufficient follow-up study that they can be substantiated and with a sufficient number of end results. While the mildly pronated feet do not require surgery, a totally pronated foot which has not responded at all to conservative therapy warrants corrective surgery even if relatively asymptomatic. The ideal time for such surgery is usually, *but not always*, between the ages of twelve and fourteen. These criteria will be enumerated in more detail further on in this chapter.

Types of Static Foot Imbalance. There are essentially two basic types of imbalanced feet in the adolescent: *a*) the flat or planovalgus foot, and *b*) the cavus or high-arched foot. There are various degrees of involvement in each of these types as well as a variety of combinations. This multiplicity can be attributed to the disturbance in articular alignment of the various tarsal joints. For example, a planovalgus foot may be due to malalignment of the talocalcaneal joint (plantar-flexed talus), a sag of the talonavicular joint, or of the naviculocuneiform joints, or a combination of all three. It can also be due to congenital or acquired defects of the first metatarsal, short tendo Achillis, as well as torsional deformities of the tibia. Equally, the cavus foot can be congenital in origin, or it can be caused by plantar soft tissue contracture, acquired muscle imbalance, or such hereditary problems as Friedreich's ataxia.

THE NORMAL FOOT

Before discussing the recognition and treatment of the pronated foot, it would be best to consider both the clinical and the roentgenographic findings of the normal foot in the adolescent. Certain basic criteria, particularly from the roentgenographic standpoint, must be established, since this knowledge will aid in the diagnosis and the establishment of the proper therapeutic regimen later on. Furthermore, treatment should not be prescribed for a pronated foot until a complete clinical and roentgenographic evaluation has been carried out. One will often see youngsters whose feet may appear to be not too severely involved clinically. The subjective findings may be moderate. Yet the roentgenographic findings may reveal definite mal-relation of the tarsal components of the longitudinal arch.

Physical examination should begin with the patient's legs hanging over the edge of the examining table and with the knees at right-angle position and with the feet dangling. In such a position both feet will assume complete flexion and 5 to 10 degrees of external rotation. The range of active and passive motion has already been described in Chapter 4 which should be read thoroughly prior to this chapter. One test of motion, however, will be reviewed since it is an important evaluating sign.

This is the range of relative passive and true passive extension. The average range of relative passive extension in this age group is 45 degrees plus or minus 5 degrees. This involves motion of the tarsal joints as well as of the ankle joint. True passive extension, on the other hand, permits motion to take place only through the ankle joint. Motion of the tarsal joints is eliminated by locking them. This is accomplished by inverting the foot forcibly to the maximum amount and then extending it to the maximum. The range of true passive extension in the normal foot is the neutral right-angle position or possibly *at most* 10 degrees of extension—never more. If the foot does not come up to the neutral right-angle position with the tarsal joints locked, this indicates the presence of a contracted calf muscle (short tendo achillis). In a standing position with the feet parallel, the heels are in neutral position and the feet and ankles do not roll in (Fig. 7-1A). There is no prominence of the navicular tubercle and no ankle inversion. The longitudinal arch is normal in appearance and upon examination of the plantar aspect of the foot on the reflector stand, the weight is seen distributed on the heel and the metatarsal area (Fig. 7-1A). The conformity of the longitudinal arch is clearly visible. Posterior and medial views are not illustrated since the clinical appearance of the normal foot has been discussed previously.

The roentgenograms should be taken in the standing position with full weight bearing on both feet. A specific procedure should be established with the radiologic technologist and should not be varied. In the anteroposterior view the *talonavicular angle* in the normal foot may vary from a minimum of 60 degrees to a maximum of 80 degrees (Fig. 7-1B). This is determined by drawing a line along the edge of the medial and lateral borders of the neck of the talus. These lines—a and a'—are parallel or almost parallel to one another (Fig. 7-1B). The distance between these two lines is measured and the midpoint located and a line is drawn between a and a', but parallel with them—line b—which bisects the

neck and the head of the talus. A third line —line c—is drawn parallel to the body of the navicular. The angle formed by the two lines is called the dorsal *talonavicular angle*. This angle will vary, as mentioned previously, from 60 to 80 degrees.

In the lateral standing position (Fig. 7-1C) again certain landmarks are located and lines drawn. First, the dorsal and plantar edges of the neck of the talus—d—are drawn. Next, the superior and inferior edges of the proximal articular surface of the navicular—e—are marked. Following this a line—f—is drawn extending from the previously located superior to the inferior edges of the navicular. The distance between these two points is measured and bisected. A line at right angles to f is then drawn bisecting the navicular. It will be observed that it runs parallel with the trabeculae of this osseous structure. Next, the distal articular surface of the medial cuneiform is located and a line—g—is drawn. The superior and inferior edges of the distal articular surfaces of the medial cuneiform are located on line g, the distance between the two points is measured, and a line is drawn at right angles to line g, both distally and proximally. Distally, the line when projected should either touch the plantar portion of the first metatarsal head or at most bisect it. Proximally, it should meet the navicular bisecting line to form a straight line or a slight angle dorsally (Fig. 7-1D). Proximally at the talonavicular joint the line from the navicular extending posteriorly should bisect the talus equidistant between point d as a straight line. Any plantar angulation at either the talonavicular or naviculocuneiform joint is to be considered abnormal. These, then, are the criteria for a normal foot both clinically and roentgenographically. It is important that these criteria be well understood since inadequate knowledge of them will tend to mislead the physician in evaluating what is considered to be normal. Furthermore, one does not arrive at a diagnosis by the use of either a clinical or a roentgenographic evaluation, alone, but by the assessment of both.

THE PRONATED FOOT

There are various degrees of pronation, and for simplicity the United States Army standard nomenclature "pes planus, first degree, second degree, third degree" will be used to classify this static deformity. Neither the term "pes planus" nor that of "flatfoot" are exact from a scientific standpoint; but clinically, they best describe this type of abnormality. Edmonson, in *Campbell's Operative Orthopaedics*, classifies pes planus "by whether the arch is relatively too flexible or too rigid and by whether the peroneal muscles are spastic or normal." His three principal types are: (1) the flex-ible type with normal peroneals, (2) the rigid type with normal peroneals, and (3) the rigid type with spastic peroneals (peroneal spastic flatfoot). What we classify as the rigid type of flatfoot, which is congenital in origin, he classifies as "rocker-bottom foot." The treatment of pronated feet, whether symptomatic or not, will be presented progressively, *i.e.;* the symptomatology, the degree of pronation, the cause, the age of the patient, the treatment particularly as it relates to the patient's age, the results that can be expected, and how they can be achieved.

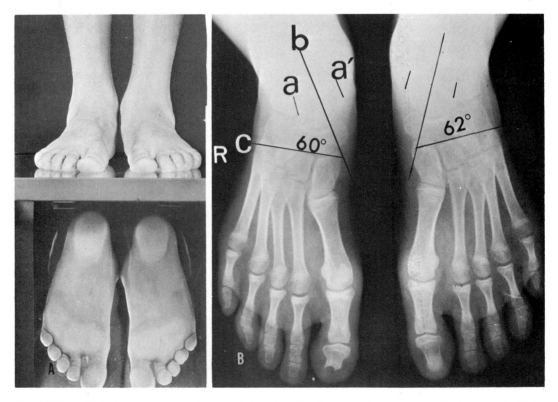

Fig. 7-1A. Clinical appearance of normal feet in standing position on the reflector stand. Note that in the reflection, the weight is borne on the heel and the metatarso-phalangeal area. The longitudinal arch, both the medial and the lateral portion, is well delineated.

B.   Standing antero-posterior roentgenograms. Normal **anterior talo-navicular angle** varies from a minimum of 60 degrees to a maximum of 85 degrees. Refer to text for its determination.

Pes Planus — First and Second Degree

Symptoms. The symptomatology in the adolescent does not necessarily bear any specific relation to the severity of the pro-nation. In many instances the feet may be *completely* pronated but asymptomatic, particularly up to the age of twelve. On the

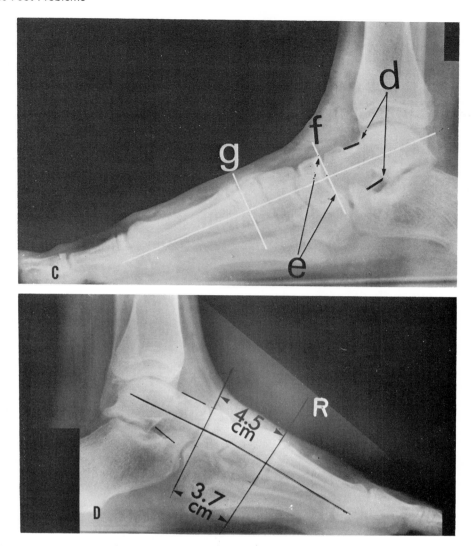

Fig. 7-1.   Continued.
   C.   Lateral standing view of the feet illustrated in Figures A and B above. Note that line bisecting talus also bisects navicular and cuneiform bones parallel to the trabeculae of these osseous structures. It extends to plantar surface of the first metatarsal. Such a straight line is considered the lower limits of normal. Refer to text for its determination.
   D.   Lateral standing roentgenogram of another foot demonstrating slight dorsal angulation at the talo-navicular joint. From a roentgenographic standpoint this is the appearance of a normal foot. It is found in 80 to 85 per cent of the clinically normal feet.

other hand, there are youngsters whose subjective symptoms are so disabling that they can hardly walk without some type of support. Even with the use of corrective shoes or arch supports, some are still incompletely relieved of their complaints. particularly in the planovalgus type foot (Fig. 7-2 A and B). The most common subjective findings appear after a day's activity. They usually are fatigue, or pain and soreness along the medial plantar aspect of both feet with or without radiating discomfort to the legs and/or the knees. With other children the only complaint may be leg ache. In other instances, even though the youngster does not admit to any discomfort, the parents may have noticed that he is unable to keep up with his playmates when he participates in any athletic activities. He walks clumsily. He does not have any "spring" to his walk and he walks "flatfootedly." The parents are dismayed because he runs down a pair of new shoes within two or three weeks and breaks down the inner counter of the shoes. Parents have presented themselves at the office—particularly a father who has been a thwarted athlete—stating, "My son walks and runs like a duck with his feet turned out." The youngster is not at fault. The father does not realize that the boy has inherited the paternal pattern of feet.

Causes. The causes of pronation will be presented in the order of their progressive importance to the development of the pronated foot.

Contracture of the calf muscle, more commonly known as short tendo achillis, will cause a foot to go into mild pronation. In this situation, since the calf muscle structures are tight, the tendo achillis throws the heel into slight valgus because of the bow-stringing effect of the tendon due to contracture. This produces an eversion of the talocalcaneal joint with stretching of the medial calcaneal ligaments and, hence, mild pronation. This is best recognized by placing the knee in the neutral zero position, locking the tarsal joints, and passively extending the foot via the ankle joint. If the calf muscle structures are tight, the foot will not reach the neutral right angle position (Fig. 7-3).

Dudley J. Morton in his book, *The Human Foot,* in 1935 popularized three concepts as being the causes of all static evils of the foot. These were: shortening of the first metatarsal, hypermobility of the first metatarsal segment, and posteriorly displaced sesamoids. Not only did he attribute foot pronation directly to either or all of these three factors, but also the development of hammer toes, claw toes, metatarsalgia, etc. To quote, "Of the three types of structural defects identified in these studies, hypermobility of the first metatarsal seg-

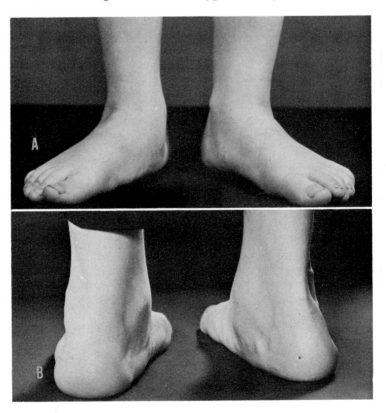

Fig. 7-2A. Plano-valgus foot or Pes Planus, third degree. Note the absence of the longitudinal arch particularly of the right foot with inrolling of the ankles. The feet are held in the typical stance this youngster uses when standing or walking.

B. Posterior view. Observe that the tendo achillis is bowed due to the valgus position of both heels even when the feet are rotated to the midline. The longitudinal arch is absent.

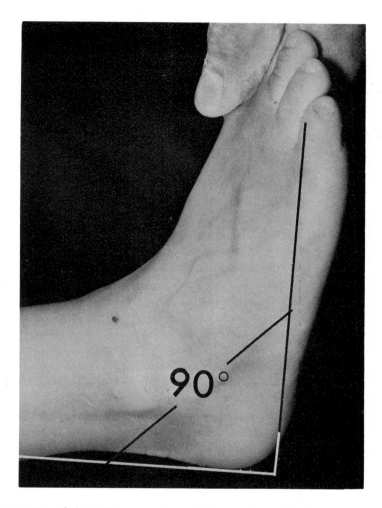

Fig. 7-3.   Contracture of the calf muscle group. (Short tendo achillis).
Note 15 degree limitation of extension of the foot when the tarsal joints are locked and extension can take place through the ankle joint only (true passive extension). Normally there are at least 5 degrees of true passive extension in the adolescent.

ment (this refers to the first metatarsal and medial cuneiform bones) is responsible for the widest range of foot trouble."

We will not take up any more of the reader's time to delineate all of the dire consequences which according to Morton developed because of hypermobility of the first metatarsal, etc. Suffice it to say that at that time, and for some years thereafter, orthopaedists accepted these statements as gospel. In our opinion these conclusions of Morton are unsound. The presence of any one of these three factors, or all of them put together, does not produce pronation of the foot, inflammatory reactions, neuritic mani-

festations, sluggishness in the vascular circulation, etc., in the adolescent as he reaches adulthood. Upon examination of the feet illustrated in the photographs (Fig. 7-4A) the reader will agree that the first metatarsal is short bilaterally. However, there is no evidence of widening of the second metatarsal shaft. The talonavicular angle is within normal limits. Furthermore, in the lateral standing roentgenograms of both feet (Fig. 7-4B) there is no evidence of any pronation of either foot. In our opinion, a short first metatarsal is contributory to the production of foot strain or, at most, a mild first degree pronation

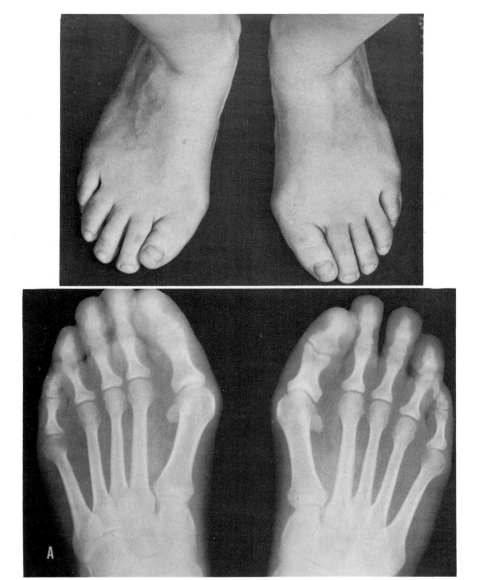

Fig. 7-4A. Short First Metatarsal Shaft. Anteroposterior standing views demonstrating short first metatarsal with hallux valgus bilaterally in a fourteen year old female. There is no widening of the second metatarsal which, according to Morton, occurs whenever there is shortening of the first metatarsal.

similar to the type associated with calf muscle contracture, but certainly nothing more.

External tibial torsion is commonly regarded as a cause of foot pronation since the youngster walks with the feet externally rotated. This places an abnormal strain on the medial aspect of the foot, causing the foot to roll in. This, in turn, frequently produces some degree of pes planus (Fig. 7-5A). With the knees in an anteroposterior position one can observe that the feet are "turned out." The line of weight bearing falls medial to the great toe. The feet roll in. Upon examination of the plantar aspect of the feet on the reflector stand (Fig. 7-5B), it is evident that the lateral one-third of the longitudinal arch on the right foot and the lateral one-half on the left are absent.

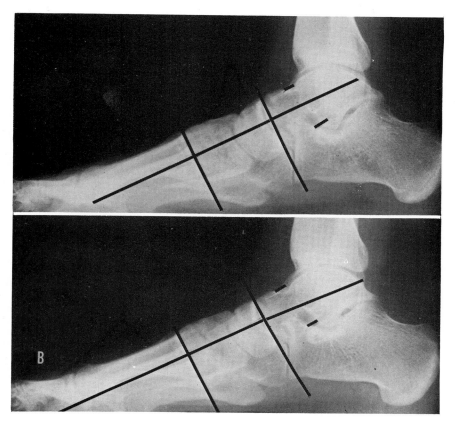

Fig. 7-4.   Continued.
   B.   Lateral standing views of the feet illustrated in previous figure. There is no roentgenographic evidence of pronation of either foot due to the short first metatarsals, which is frequently found with such shortening according to Morton.

Sagging of the naviculocuneiform joint or of the talonavicular joint, diminution of the anterior talonavicular angle, or a plantar-flexed talus are the most common causes of moderately-severe pronated feet. The presence of a talonavicular bar in most instances is accompanied by foot pronation. If the situation is a mild or minimal one, second degree pronation (Fig. 7-6A and B) will result. Any deviation more significant than mild results in third degree pronation as illustrated in Fig. 7-2A and B). What is the reason for the development of a naviculocuneiform sag, a plantar-flexed talus, etc.? Heredity plays the most prominent role. Occasionally, this deformity is produced by muscle imbalance such as that following poliomyelitis, or that due to cerebral palsy wherein the peroneal group of muscles is over-active.

What of the vertical talus, better known as the plantar-flexed talus? Fortunately this cause of foot pronation is relatively infrequent. I have yet to see flat feet due to vertical tali which have not had some attempt at correction prior to adolescence. However, if the treatment has been inadequate, such feet indeed present a most difficult problem when seen in an eight- to ten-year-old youngster. The feet are symptomatic. The patient has a "heel gait," *i.e.*, he does not come up on his toes in order to propel himself. In fact, if one watches such a patient ambulate barefooted, the examiner will observe that the youngster does not use the distal one-third of the foot when completing a stride.

Treatment. In considering the treatment of the pronated foot, it is necessary to consider the different causes individually

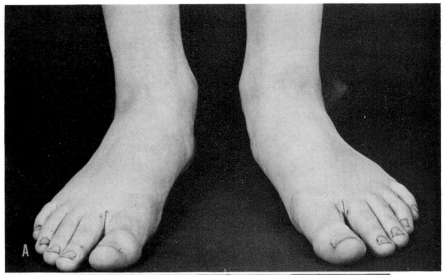

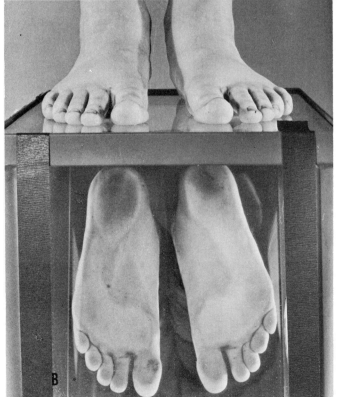

Fig. 7-5.   Pes Planus, Second degree.

A.   In the front standing position note that the ankles roll in slightly and that the navicular tubercles are only slightly prominent. In the ordinary standing position of a patient with this type of feet there is slight external rotation of the feet. The longitudinal arch is depressed although present bilaterally.

B.   On the reflector mirror note the appearance of the plantar aspect of both feet. The lateral portion of the longitudinal arch is absent bilaterally.

and, in addition, at various age levels. When treatment is instituted early in adolescence, certain pronated feet will respond to conservative therapy, whereas certain types will require surgical therapy in order to achieve correction.

Let us, therefore, begin with the patient, who following complete clinical examination as well as roentgenographic evaluation presents normal feet from an X-ray standpoint, but clinically has a first or a mild second degree pronation. The only positive finding is a 10 to 15 degree loss of true passive extension (Fig. 7-3). The regimen recommended applies from age eight to fourteen. A corrective heel should be prescribed with an inner heel elevation of 3/16 inch, inner heel flare 1/4 inch, inner heel advance 1/2 inch, a rubber cookie of appropriate size, and a rubber heel. The shoe should have ties with a minimum of four eyelets on each side of the shoe. It should have a steel shank and a firm leather or composition sole. In addition, calf-stretching exercises should be prescribed. The parents and the patient should be instructed that the exercises are to be performed at least twice daily (when the youngster has arrived home from school and at bedtime). The exercises should first be demonstrated to the patient and to the parent or parents. The patient should then be asked to perform the exercises in the presence of the examiner to make certain that they are being carried out correctly.

The exercises are as follows: A length of 3-inch muslin, 5 feet long, is doubled on itself and a loop is made around the forefoot with the loop on the medial side of the foot (Fig. 7-7) so as to lock the tarsal joints. With the knee in the neutral position a firm pull is applied to the muslin for a slow count of ten. The count should be carried on the one-thousand-and-one, one-thousand-and-two, one-thousand-and-three basis. The patient will feel a definite pulling discomfort along the lateral and posterior aspect of the leg up to the knee. The pull is relaxed for a similar count of ten, and then repeated. Initially this is performed for ten times. An additional time is added every other day until the exercise is performed twenty-five times on each occasion. Thus gradually over a period of a month to six weeks, if the exercise is carried out conscientiously, stretching of the calf muscle or muscles will have taken place. Once the patient has gained 5 degrees of true passive extension, the exercise is continued at the rate of twenty-five times once daily for at least another three months. It may then be discontinued, but the shoe correction is maintained until the age of fourteen in the female and sixteen in the male. The patient should be placed on a regular follow-up re-examination every six months. In the greater majority of such patients the pronation will be corrected. The same regimen is prescribed if the patient is twelve years of age or over when he is first brought in for medical attention. He is usually brought to the doctor because of a mild foot and leg pain. The parents should be taken aside and advised that although the exercises will correct the contracture and eliminate the symptoms, the pronation will remain unchanged since it is now too late to overcome the tarsal ligamentous relaxation which has taken place. Occasionally, the pronation will correct even this late, but it is the exception to the rule. The question of inserting the heel correction and the rubber cookie in the so-called casual or slipper type shoe may be brought up. The answer should be in the negative, but it should be explained why to the patient and the parents. With the average adolescent, if a reasonable explanation is given, the desired cooperation invariably ensues. When the epiphyses have closed, then all heel correction is discontinued, but the rubber cookie remains in the shoe as long as the patient feels the need for it.

Lengthening of the tendo achillis as a procedure to correct pronated feet due to contracted calf muscles has been recommended by others in the past. We have not found the need for this operation if the exercises are carried out faithfully. It has been found necessary to perform a lengthening of the tendo achillis as part of a flatfoot plasty procedure, but not as the principal operation to correct foot pronation. This operation (tendo achillis lengthening) is mentioned, but not recommended.

The next cause presented as a contributing factor to foot pronation is the short first metatarsal. In the adolescent this entity, per se, has not been the cause of foot pronation. It is an incidental finding roentgenographically in association with a splay foot or a hallus valgus deformity (Fig. 7-4 A and B). It is mentioned at this time so that the reader may be conscious of its occasional appearance. If there is a mild foot pronation, but the lateral standing radiographs are normal in appearance, the therapy consists of the wearing of a corrective shoe similar to that used in the contracted calf-muscle-type foot. If there is a definite splay foot or hallux valgus deformity, then that should be cared for accordingly. The reader is referred to Chapter 13 for further information.

If the pronation is due to external tibial torsion, both problems must be attacked simultaneously. If on roentgenographic examination both feet are found to be within normal limits, and if the torsion is less than 25 degrees, then conservative therapy is recommended. This consists of the use of twisters along with Whitman plates. This therapy will give good results up to the age of ten in the female and twelve in the male. The parents should be informed that the youngster still has a substantial growth

period ahead, that the twisters and the supports may very well correct both problems. The twisters are so adjusted as to cause the patient to walk slightly pigeon-toed. They are worn throughout the child's waking hours. Usually by the time the youngster has reached his fourteenth birthday, both the torsion and the pronation will have been corrected.

If the torsion is over 25 degrees, or if the patient is a female more than ten or a male more than twelve years old, derotation osteotomy of the tibia and fibula is recommended. The site of the osteotomy is left to the operator's choice. I prefer to osteotomize both the tibia and fibula at a point 4 cm. below the level of the tibial tubercle. After the osteotomy is completed, the distal fragments should be externally rotated 5 degrees in this last mentioned deformity. Correction should never be beyond neutral, in fact, 5 degrees of external rotation is preferable. It is not within the scope of this book to describe the technique of the osteotomy. It is delineated in all of the recent orthopaedic texts. The same therapy applies to youngsters who present themselves with internal tibial torsion.

Pes Planus — Third Degree (Planovalgus)

We now arrive at the crux of the subject, the planovalgus or third degree pronated foot and its problems: in other words, the flexible completely flatfoot.

There are three common causes of the flexible flatfoot. In the order of their frequency, they are: (1) the naviculocuneiform sag, (2) the dorsal talonavicular sag, and (3) the plantar flexed talus.

1. The Naviculocuneiform Sag. In this type of completely pronated foot, the subjective symptoms can be totally absent or at most the patient will complain of some fatigue or pain in the feet or the legs. Occasionally the patient will complain of knee pain. On physical examination one will find the typical pronated foot with complete absence of the longitudinal arch when standing, prominence of the navicular tubercle, slight or mild valgus position of the heel and inversion of the ankle. There may or may not be shortening of the tendo achillis. In the standing roentgenograph of

the foot one will find that there is a definite sag of the naviculocuneiform (Fig. 7-6).

If the patient is between the ages of seven and nine when treatment is initiated, the use of corrective shoes is useless. A more positive corrective force is needed— the Whitman steel plate (Fig. 7-7). These supports should be individually tailored to the patient's feet. It is necessary to have available the services of a good bracemaker to manufacture these plates. Otherwise, if they are not constructed to fit each individual foot properly, they will be painful and the patient will not wear them. A properly-constructed, properly-fitted Whitman, steel, arch support can be placed into the shoe and the young patient will complain of discomfort for a day or two but will have no pain in the foot. Once he is accustomed to them, he should not even be actually conscious of the presence of the arch supports in his shoes. These should be worn throughout the patient's waking hours

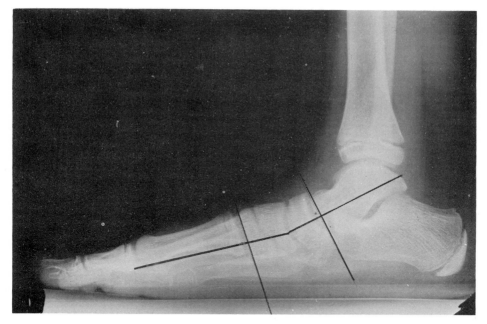

Fig. 7-6.   Lateral standing roentgenogram of a flexible flatfoot. Note sag of the naviculo-cuneiform joint.

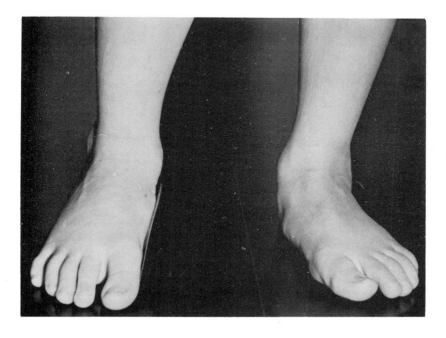

Fig. 7-7.   Moderately pronated foot held in a corrected position by a Whitman steel arch support. Note difference in position between right foot and unsupported left foot.

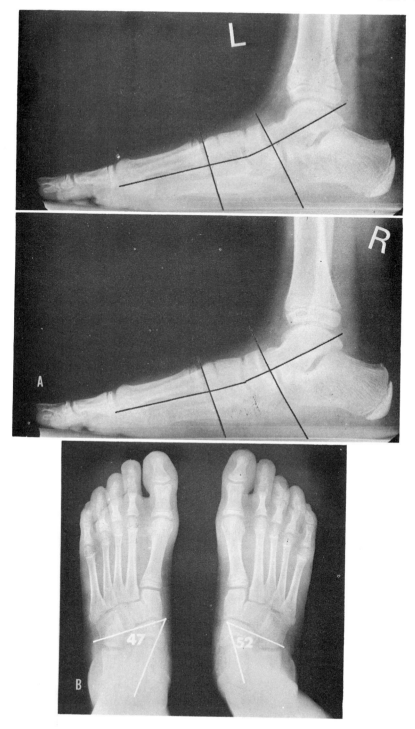

Fig. 7-8. A and A'.   Lateral standing roentgenograms of feet of an eight-year-old white female presenting a bilateral naviculo-cuneiform sag. Clinically she presented bilateral pes planus, third degree.

B.   Standing anteroposterior views reveal that the **anterior talo-navicular angle** is below normal bilaterally.

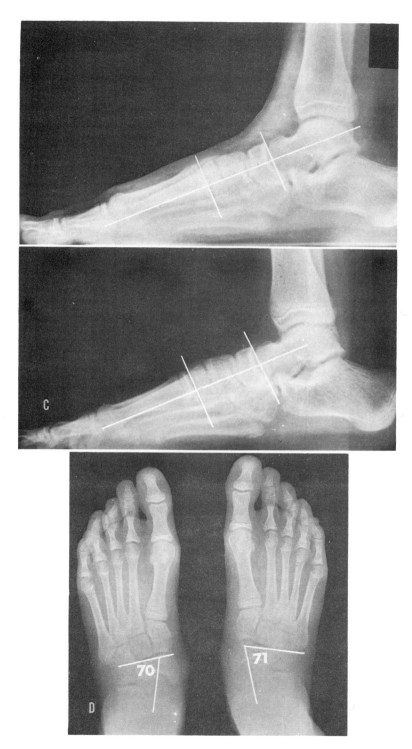

Fig. 7-8. Continued. C and C'. Lateral standing views of same feet four years later. Whitman plates had been prescribed for both feet and had been worn for four years.

D. Standing anteroposterior views four years later. Anterior talo-navicular angle is now within normal limits.

in all of his shoes. After the initial fitting, the patient should be re-examined in one month to make certain that there are no abnormal pressures. It is true that with these supports the patient will develop calluses over the navicular tubercle and along the edge of the lateral flange of the support. The parents should be reassured that these calluses will disappear spontaneously once the supports are discontinued. The patient should then be placed on regular six-month follow-up care. The supports require replacing usually every twelve months unless there should be a sudden spurt of growth.

The following case report is from my files. An eight-year-old white female was brought in by her parents. The mother stated that the youngster had had prominent bones on both the inner and outer aspects of her feet since birth, but that these prominences had increased in size. The feet were asymptomatic. On clinical examination the feet were completely pronated. The flexibility of each foot was normal; the muscle power and the range of motion of each foot were within normal limits. Both heels were in valgus position when standing. This disclosed one of the bony prominences about which the mother complained. In addition, on the medial aspect of the foot the navicular tubercle was quite prominent, which, of course, was due to the pronation. On roentgenographic examination in the lateral view, there was a sag of the naviculocuneiform joint bilaterally (Fig. 7-8A). In the anteroposterior view the dorsal talonavicular angle was appreciably below the normal limits (Fig. 7-8B).

Treatment in the above case consisted of the prescription of monel Whitman plates. The parents were advised that with the constant use of these arch supports, there was approximately a 75 per cent chance of achieving correction. If, on the other hand, the feet did not respond by the time the youngster was twelve, or at the most thirteen years of age, surgery would have to be considered. The child wore the arch supports faithfully. The parents were cooperative. She was seen every six months on a routine check-up visit and the arch supports were changed as the feet grew in size. No foot exercises were prescribed.

Four years later, on routine examination, the feet were normal in appearance. Roentgenographically, the lateral views demonstrated no naviculocuneiform sag (Fig. 7-8C) and the talonavicular angle was within normal limits bilaterally (Fig. 7-8D). The youngster was advised to discard the arch supports gradually over a period of six months. When last seen her feet were normal in appearance and asymptomatic (Fig. 7-8E).

Nevertheless, all patients with pronated feet due to the naviculocuneiform sag do not respond in this manner. The preference for the use of the Whitman plates was presented in the previous chapter. However, a few of the remarks will be repeated for emphasis. The Whitman type plate is preferred because of the lateral flange which does not permit the foot to slide off the medial portion of the arch support. There are many orthopaedists who feel that any steel arch support is a crutch, and that its rigidity impairs the function of the foot and does not aid in the correction of the foot in any manner. The Whitman plate, in our opinion, is considered a brace for a flatfoot. It certainly does not inhibit the flexibility of the adolescent foot and it holds the latter in the desired position.

When the patient has been treated with corrective Whitman plates for four to six years and the feet are unimproved by the age of twelve, either roentgenographically or clinically, or both, surgery is recommended irrespective of whether they are or are not symptomatic. If the youngster is first brought in for treatment at the age of twelve, Whitman plates are prescribed, but the parents are shown the roentgenograms and the problem must be discussed thoroughly with them. They should be advised that there is little possibility that the feet will respond to the Whitman plates as the sole therapeutic measure. However, they should also be informed that such a procedure should and will be attempted. On the other hand, when the patient reaches his thirteenth birthday, if the feet are not normal both roentgenographically and clinically, surgical procedure will be necessary. At the time when surgical procedure is recommended, the parents frequently seek the services of another orthopaedist or a chiropodist who will supply them with the answers that they wish to hear. The parents may, on the other hand, express a desire to continue the use of arch supports until the patient can decide for himself whether or not to undergo surgical correction. *The ideal period for surgical correction of flatfeet is between ten and fourteen years of age.* After fourteen the end results may be satisfactory, but seldom excellent. The reason for this diminution in the rate of excellent results is that after the age of fourteen, the foot has reached maturity and the surgeon cannot achieve the desired correction. There is little time left for the articular surfaces to grow and adjust to their newly-corrected position. In an occasional case, one can operate after the age of fourteen, providing the foot demonstrates the same range of motion and flexibility that a twelve-year-old foot has. However, this is a rare instance. These specifications may appear to be restrictive and didactic, but they are sound. Following them will lead to results that will please patients and generally, but not always, to normal appearing feet. Disregarding these criteria can leave a large percentage of your patients unhappy.

The Operation. There are a number of operative procedures which have been described for the correction of this type of flatfoot. In *Campbell's Operative Orthopaedics* one can find a minimum of eight different procedures for correction of the flexible flatfoot. This number in itself is indicative of the fact that apparently no one particular operation has been completely satisfactory. The operative procedure about to be described for the correction of the flatfoot *due to naviculocuneiform sag* is no more than a modification of the Miller and the Young procedures. This operation has proved most effective in my experience. It is not recommended before the age of ten in females and twelve in males. When it has been performed at an earlier age, as the foot has grown, there has been a development of a slight varus distal to the naviculocuneiform arthrodesis. *The procedures about to be described should be used only in the foot completely pronated due to the naviculocuneiform sag.*

Under tourniquet control a slightly curved incision is made along the medial aspect of the foot from the level of the posterior edge of the medial malleolus to 1 cm. distal to the first metatarsocuneiform joint (Fig. 7-9A). The operator must give himself adequate room for this procedure. The skin and subcutaneous tissues are raised and reflected back 1.5 cm. both dorsally and plantarly. A longitudinal incision is then made along the plantar-medial surface to expose and reflect the small muscles of the foot on the plantar surface to the level of the lateral edge of the navicular and the medial cuneiform bones, as well as the talar head. The tibialis anterior and the tibialis posterior tendons are identified. The sheath of the tibialis anterior tendon is split from a point just distal to the anterior cruciate ligament to the medial aspect of the cuneiform. The tendon is raised and severed. Similarly, the posterior tibial tendon sheath is incised from the level of its insertion in the navicular tubercle to the distal edge of the laciniate ligament. The tendon is detached from the navicular tubercle. An identifying suture of number 2 chromic catgut is attached to the ends of each of these tendons with the suture ends at least 10 cm. long. The tendons are permitted to retract.

The next two incisions are extremely important and must be carefully planned and executed (Fig. 7-9B). The first incision is made on the medial aspect of the foot. The capsular and ligamentous structures are incised down to the underlying bones. The incision begins at the distal articular surface of the cuneiform and extends proximally to a point 1 cm. below the level of the tip of the medial malleolus along the medial edge of the talocalcaneal joint. It ends at the sustentaculum tali. The second incision is made parallel to the first, but on the plantar medial aspect approximately 1.5 cm. apart. When the second incision reaches the area of the last proximal 2 cm., the dissection must be carried out carefully since the flexor hallucis longus tendon lies directly in the line of the incision, and so does the tibial nerve which is posterior and inferior to this tendon. These structures must be identified and retracted and the incision completed to the level of the sustentaculum tali. Distally the two incisions

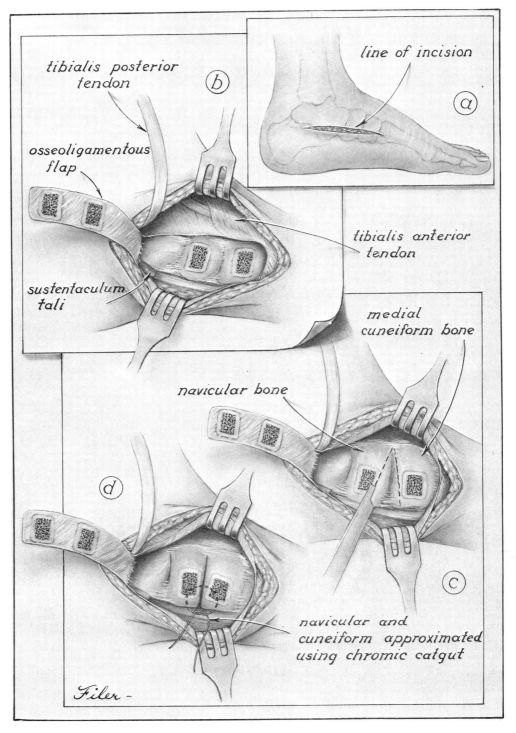

Fig. 7-9A. Line of incision extends from level just posterior to the medial malleous distally to the first metatarsal cuneiform joint.

B. Diagramatic sketch of the osseoligamentous flap developed to include a thin sliver of cortex of the plantar medial surface of the medial cuneiform and the navicular tuburcle extending proximally to the sustenaculum tali.

C. Diagramatic sketch of removal of wedge of bone from the apposing surfaces of the navicular and medial cuneiform bones.

Fig. 7-9. D. Raw surfaces approximated using number 2 chromic cat—gut suture.

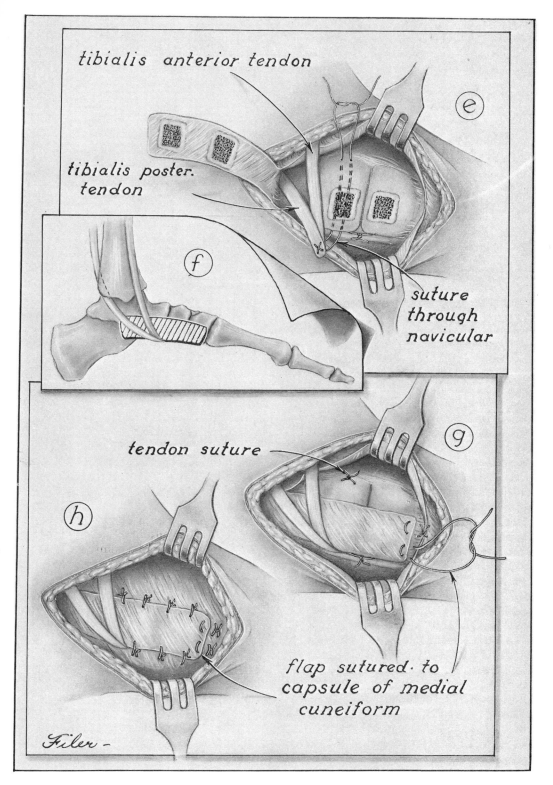

Fig. 7-9. Continued.
E. Tibialis anterior and tibialis posterior tendons transposed to the plantar surface of the navi-cular.
F. Diagramatic sketch of osseoligamentous flap and tendons. READ DETAILED DESCRIPTION OF PROCEDURE IN THE TEXT.
G. Mattress sutures re-attaching shortened osseoligamentous flap to the metatarsal cuneiform capsule.
H. Sutures to indicate complete re-attachment of flap.

are joined by a transverse incision just proximal to the first metatarsocuneiform joint.

With a *thin sharp osteotome* an osteoligamentous flap of tissue 1.5 cm. wide is raised (Fig. 7-9C) containing as thin a layer as possible of the cortex of the medial surface of the cuneiform, as well as a thin layer of the cortex of the navicular tubercle. The surgeon must bear in mind that the ligamentous structures over these two bony segments are quite thin and care must be exercised in raising this flap over the cuneiform and the navicular. Proximal to the latter bone, the flap is quite substantial. As it is lifted back to the sustentaculum tali, the medial surface of the head and neck of the talus is exposed as well as the medial talocalcaneal joint edge. The osteo-ligamentous flap is then wrapped in a moist sponge and retracted proximally. The capsular-ligamentous covering over the navicular and the medial cuneiform bones (both dorsally and plantarly) is then reflected carefully, particularly on the plantar surface, to expose the dorsal and plantar surfaces of the medial cuneiform and of the navicular.

Next a small wedge of bone ⅛ inch in thickness is removed along with the entire articular surface of the medial cuneiform, the base of the wedge being properly located on the plantar surface. Therefore, care must be taken as to the proper positioning of the foot prior to removal of the wedge (Fig. 7-9D). A thin, *sharp* osteotome is mandatory. If the ordinary type of osteotome is used, no matter how careful the surgeon may be, almost invariably a larger wedge than desired is removed making closure of the defect difficult and at times leading to overcorrection of the naviculocuneiform joint. The articular cartilage is then removed from the distal surface of the navicular exposing the underlying cortex. The foot is pronated and plantar flexed at the naviculocuneiform joint to make certain that the foot is adequately corrected and that there is good contact between the two raw bone surfaces. If adequate correction is achieved then a large heavy tenaculum is used to form a suture hole through the navicular beginning at the level of the plantar edge of the proximal

articular surface, the opening coming out at the distal surface 1.5 cm. lateral to the medial cortical edge of the navicular (Fig. 7-9E).

A similar hole is prepared in the cuneiform beginning at the distal articular edge and progressing proximally and dorsally. Care must be exercised in preparing this suture opening to ensure adequate cortex in both bones so that the suture does not tear out when it is passed through and tied. A number 2 double chromic catgut suture is passed through the cuneiform and then through the navicular. The foot is held in the desired corrected position by the surgeon while the assistant pulls the suture tightly and ties it in order to approximate the raw edges. Under no circumstances should the assistant be permitted to hold the foot in the corrected position (particularly during his first few scrubs) since he will have no true concept of the correction desired. This is the surgeon's responsibility.

Having achieved the desired correction, the next step is to drill a second hole in the navicular close to its *lateral* edge in order to prepare for the new insertions of the tibialis anterior and posterior tendons. The plantar surface of the navicular should be completely denuded of soft tissues. The drill hole is made only large enough to accommodate a large, heavy, cutting-edge needle and the suture. No attempt is made to pass the tendons into the substance of the navicular. The drill point is left *in situ* while a number 2 chromic catgut suture is passed in a figure 8 style through both tendons similar to that used in tendon repairs. The two suture ends of adequate length, at least 10 cm., are threaded into one needle. As the drill is removed, the needle follows and emerges on the dorsal surface of the navicular. The suture ends are clamped with a hemostat and the tendons and the suture are temporarily retracted proximally.

The previously prepared osteo-ligamentous flap is now pulled taut with the use of two Kocher hemostats to cover the cuneiform and navicular bones. The flap should now have a bow string effect since an arch has been constructed on the plantar medial aspect of the midfoot. With the flap in this position a number 0 chromic suture on a cutting needle as fine as possible is passed through the capsule of the metatarsocune-iform joint on the dorsal-medial edge and thence through the flap at a slightly proximal level. The same procedure is carried out at the plantar edge (Fig. 7-9F). Both sutures are tied with the foot held in the corrected position. The redundant portion of the flap is severed. The metatarsocune-iform joint is not disturbed. Two or three more sutures are placed to anchor the distal end of the flap to the adjoining capsular structures. If the procedure has been carried out according to directions, the portion of the navicular which was resected and incorporated in the flap will overly the naviculocuneiform joint plantar medially, and the flap will assume the function of a plantar medial osteo-ligamentous sling. Several additional sutures are taken both along the dorso-medial and plantar medial edges to reattach the flap to the adjoining ligaments and to shorten automatically the osteo-ligamentous sling even more. Following this, the two tendons are pulled over the flap to the plantar surface of the navicular. As the suture is pulled to bring the tendons to the new area of insertion, it will be observed that the foot and heel will go into slight varus. The suture is tied on the dorsum of the foot by passing each end separately through ligamentous tissue. Additional sutures of number 0 chromic are then placed from the tibialis anterior and posterior tendons to the underlying osteo-ligamentous flap.

Prior to closing the subcutaneous and cutaneous layers the surgeon may carry out one of two maneuvers: he may release the tourniquet and spend another fifteen to twenty minutes, controlling the bleeding or he may insert a Snyder hemovac unit to aspirate the blood. The point of exit of the unit should be as far away from the incision as possible. Wall suction should be applied immediately even if the tourniquet has not been released. Careful closure of the sub-cutaneous tissues is performed. The skin layer is closed with a subcuticular wire suture. If there is evidence of a short tendo achillis prior to surgery on the foot, lengthening of the tendon is first performed. One can use either the White type of tendon lengthening procedure or the Hauser tech-

nique. In the former the tendo achillis is exposed through a 4-inch posteromedial incision beginning at the level of the insertion of the tendon in the os calcis and extending proximally. The anterior two-thirds of the tendon is divided at the level of the insertion. While moderate force is applied, the medial two-thirds of the tendon is divided 3 inches proximal to the site of the initial partial tenotomy. Extension of the foot accomplishes the desired amount of lengthening. In the Hauser procedure the only difference is that after the tendon sheath has been opened, the medial two-thirds of the tendon is tenotomized at the level of its insertion and the posterior two-thirds is tenotomized 3 inches above the distal partial tenotomy. The foot is then extended and the desired length is procured.

The application of the postoperative cast is of paramount importance since immobilization in overcorrection is undesirable. On the other hand, the cast should be applied snugly and should be well molded. Too much sheet wadding is undesirable since the dressing and, automatically, the cast become too bulky. In addition, within a week the sheet wadding becomes padded and the cast is too loose. With the loosening of the cast, loss of correction can ensue. Furthermore, it is not wise to plan to remove the cast in two weeks to reapply a new, more snugly fitting one. Occasionally this may be necessary. If a change is required, it should be carried out under general anesthesia.

The cast is applied in sections. First, using 4-inch wide rolls of extra-fast plaster of paris, the cast is wrapped snugly around the midfoot, hindfoot and lower one-third of the leg. This is done with the foot held in neutral right angle position at the ankle joint and with minimal varus of the heel. One small helpful hint: hold the foot gently by the toes with the knee flexed at 90 degrees. Begin the plaster roll from the outside toward the inside so that it can be wrapped firmly around the newly constructed longitudinal arch. Also snug the cast up around the heel to maintain a minimal varus position. After the application of one roll, the plaster is molded snugly and firmly under the longitudinal arch and around the heel. The tourniquet is then released if the operator has inserted a hemovac unit.

After this portion of the cast has set, the remaining portion of the foot is wrapped in plaster of paris. Before doing so, the forefoot must be brought down to maximum pronation and the cast applied to the tips of the toes and again molded on the plantar medial surface (Fig. 7-9G). The remainder of the leg is then incorporated in the cast up to the level of the tibial tubercle. The toe portion of the cast is trimmed so that the tips of all five toes are visible. The cast should then be reinforced with a plaster of paris splint extending from the tips of the toes to the proximal edge. Two more rolls of plaster of paris are used to finish the cast. The circulation is observed at the tips of the toes. The operator should make certain that there is good capillary response.

As the surgeon becomes more adept he can correct both feet at one session (within two hours' tourniquet time, if not less). However, for at least the first few times, one should correct one foot only and one week later the other foot.

Postoperative Care. The foot should be elevated on at least two pillows. Ice bags are maintained constantly for forty-eight hours on the dorsal and plantar surface of the cast. The hemovac unit is removed on the third postoperative day. The patient will experience a good deal of pain during the first forty-eight hours and sedation should be liberal. Postoperative roentgenograms in the anteroposterior and true lateral positions are usually procured on the first postoperative day to ascertain the position of the naviculocuneiform joint. In the lateral radiograph the sag should be absent and the landmark lines, when drawn, should demonstrate normal alignment of the tarsal bones. If the desired correction has not been achieved, the foot should be remanipulated under general anesthesia within the first forty-eight hours after surgery to gain the necessary correction and position of the naviculocuneiform surfaces. On the fifth postoperative day the patient is permitted to get out of bed and go about in a wheelchair. One week later correction of the other foot is carried out by the same surgeon unless there are two operating teams available both of whom are equally experienced in this procedure. Immobilization of the feet is maintained for a minimum of eight weeks.

When the casts are removed, much to the dismay of the patient's parents, the feet will appear in a varus position. The parents should be warned of this in advance, as well as be reassured that when the casts are removed, the feet will be in this position only temporarily.

Roentgenograms are taken upon removal of the casts to ascertain the fusion of the medial naviculocuneiform joint. Occasionally, the fusion may appear weak, but this is of no immediate consequence. The patient is fitted with a new pair of shoes of the rigid shanked, Oxford, tie-type and permitted to become ambulatory on crutches under supervision. At first the youngster will walk on the lateral aspect of both feet. The parents should be reassured that this position will correct itself gradually and spontaneously. The youngster is encouraged to walk as much as he can as soon as the discomfort becomes minimal. The more he is ambulatory, the sooner he will discard his crutches. At the end of two or three weeks, at most, the crutches are discarded. The child must be carefully instructed to use the heel-toe gait. The patient will walk with a clumsy, stiff-footed gait for a period of at least eight weeks. Jumping, running, in fact, all athletic activities, except swimming (but no diving) are totally restricted for six months. At the end of the six-month period all restrictions are lifted (Fig. 7-10, A, B, C and D). Three months after surgery the patient can begin wearing any type shoe he or she desires.

The "Don'ts" of the Operation. Do not use staples to maintain the naviculocuneiform correction. In each instance when they were used, it was subsequently necessary to remove them. Do not hesitate to split the cast and the underlying sheet wadding to relieve any pressure or circulatory impairment, but do *not* remove the foot from the posterior two-thirds of the cast. Do not panic, if, unfortunately, either a superficial or deep infection should develop. At the slightest suspicion of infection, cut a window in the cast, making it of adequate size to expose the entire incision and

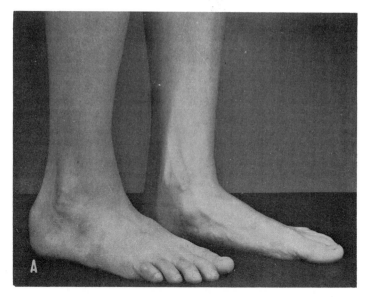

Fig. 7-10A.   Pre-operative appearance of the feet. (See pages 142, 143 and 144.)

treat the local infection parenterally with a broad spectrum antibiotic. Above all, do not remove the entire cast.

Do not attempt to correct both feet at the same time until you have mastered the technique. This is not a simple procedure nor is this a procedure to be attempted for the first time by a neophyte orthopaedic surgeon without the assistance of an experienced orthopaedist. On the initial attempt the average operating time will be one-and-one-half to two hours. Do not insert any type of arch support in the shoes postoperatively. Do not permit the youngster to walk in the preoperative flatfooted manner. Demonstrate both to the patient and the parents the proper method of heel-toe walking. If you do not take the time to do this, a patient will occasionally develop peroneal spasm with loss of some of the correction. This will necessitate remanipulation of the feet under anesthesia and re-immobilization in walking casts for an additional six weeks.

Do not discharge the patient too soon no matter how excellent the result appears. Following removal of the casts, the patient should be reexamined weekly for at least one month. He should then be evaluated monthly for six months and then placed on a tri-monthly check-up visit for one year. If at the end of eighteen months following

surgery, he is asymptomatic and the feet are well corrected, and he is able to participate in all types of activities, he may be discharged. Occasionally, a pseudoarthrosis of the naviculocuneiform joint may result. If the foot is asymptomatic, disregard the pseudoarthrosis. If it is painful, repair will be necessary.

In conjunction with this procedure, there is a question which probably arises in the minds of some readers. "Why transfer both the tibialis posterior and the tibialis anterior tendons to the plantar surface of the navicular?" First, as to the tibialis posterior. In 90 per cent of the feet on which I have performed surgery, approximately 200 thus far, the tendon was abnormally inserted to the medial aspect of the navicular tubercle rather than to the inferomedial surface. Thus, with this abnormality present, according to Edmondson "the normal support of the longitudinal arch by the posterior tibial muscle is lost." By transferring the tendon to the plantar aspect of the tarsal navicular it helps to reinforce the action of the osteo-ligamentous sling as well as to continue its function of inversion. "But why transplant the tibialis anterior as well?" The answer to this is not difficult. One of the functions of the tibialis anterior is that of supinator of the forefoot. When supination of the forefoot takes place, pronation of the

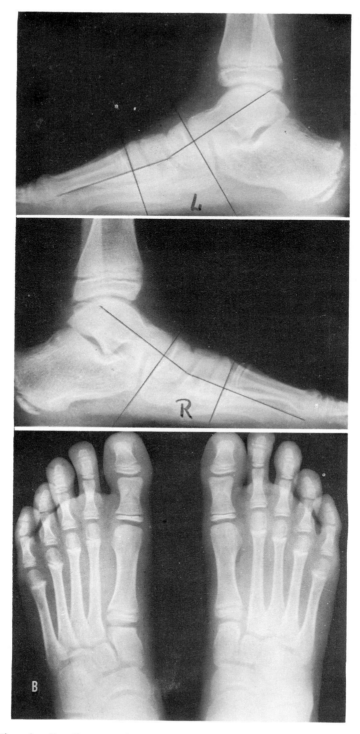

Fig. 7-10. Continued. B. Pre-operative roentgenograms of the same feet in the anteroposterior and lateral standing views. Note naviculo-cuneiform sag.

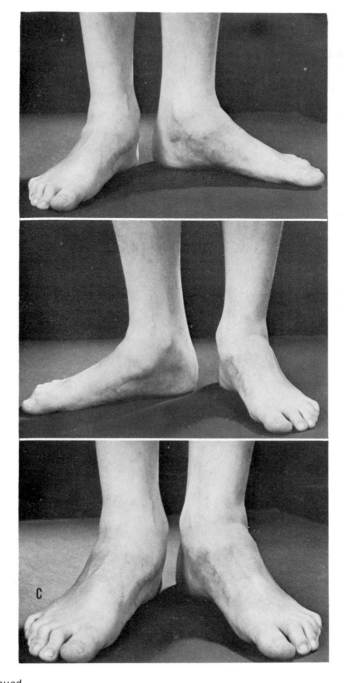

Fig. 7-10.   Continued.
   C.   Postoperative appearance of same feet one year following surgery.

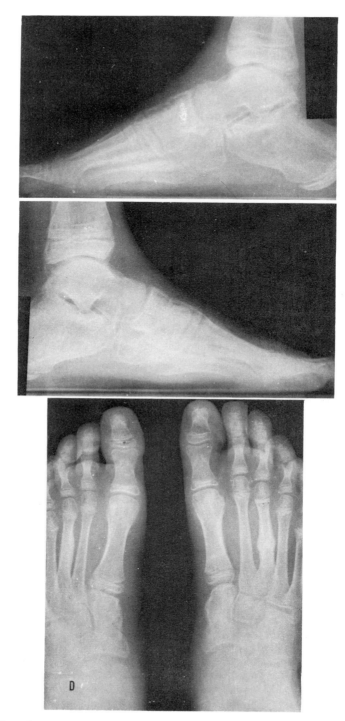

Fig. 7-10. Continued.
    D. Postoperative standing roentgenograms of the same feet one year following surgery.

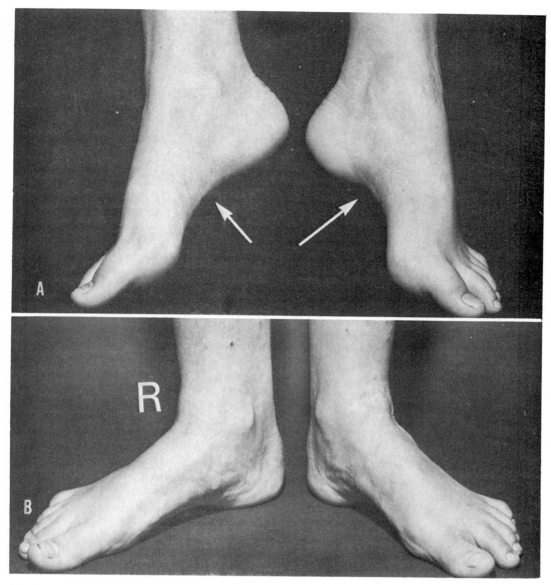

Fig. 7-11A.   Note cavus deformity of the left foot which developed over a period of six years following laceration of tibialis anterior tendon.
   B.   Standing views of same foot.

foot develops. A good example regarding this function was most evident when a nine-year-old girl was brought into the office because of a cavus deformity of her left foot (Fig. 7-11 A and B). The only positive subjective finding was that the patient had suffered a laceration over the anteromedial aspect of the left ankle at the age of three. The only positive objective finding was the absence of tibialis anterior muscle function. Apparently, this tendon had been lacerated at the time of injury. The defect went unrecognized, and therefore, remained unrepaired with the resulting development of a cavus foot deformity.

2. Dorsal Talonavicular Sag. In this type of pronated foot there are certain findings evident both clinically and roentgenographically which are not present in the previously described type of foot. On physical examination one usually finds that there is limitation of true passive extension due to contracture of the tendo achillis. In a standing position the foot presents only a second degree pronation. When the foot is viewed on the reflector stand, there is evidence of a longitudinal arch. The main deforming appearance, however, is the marked inversion of the ankle, producing an appearance of complete pronation. When viewed from the rear, both heels present a marked valgus with bow stringing of the tendo achillis. On examination of the standing roentgenograms there is marked diminution in the dorsal talonavicular angle. In the lateral view, there may be a mild or minimal sag at both the talonavicular and naviculocuneiform joints, indicative of a minimal generalized ligamentous relaxation.

Treatment of this type of foot is again conservative up to the prescribed age of ten in the female and twelve in the male. This entails the use of the Whitman type plate, but with the medial flange of the plate elevated slightly higher in order to attempt to correct the ankle inversion and the heel valgus. In addition, calf stretching exercises are prescribed. If conservative means fail to correct the problem (and, again, in approximately 25 to 30 per cent of the patients, failure will occur), or if it is too late to begin conservative therapy, surgical intervention is indicated. The procedure of choice is the classical Grice operation.

The Operation. For the sake of clarity, the procedure will be described verbatim: "A short curvilinear incision is made on the lateral aspect of the foot directly over the subastragalar joint. The incision is carried down through the skin and subcutaneous tissues to expose the cruciate ligament overlying the joint. This ligament is split in the direction of its fibers and the sinus tarsi is dissected free of adipose tissue and ligamentous structures. In most instances in order to get better exposure, the short toe extensors have been displaced from the calcaneus and reflected forward. With this exposure, the relationship of the calcaneus to the astragalus can be readily seen and the mechanism of the deformity can be clearly demonstrated. If the foot is placed into equinus, the calcaneus can usually be replaced beneath the astragalus by inverting the foot. . . . . An osteotome or blunt periosteal elevator is inserted in the sinus tarsi as a block to demonstrate the stability which might be obtained with the graft. This is also done to determine the size of the grafts and the optimum position in which they may be placed. . . . . The sinus tarsi is prepared for the graft by the removal of the thin layer of the cortical bone from the under surface of the astragalus and the superior aspect of the calcaneus."

Instead of procuring the graft from the tibia, it is procured from the fibula. A second incision is made over the lateral aspect of the leg directly overlying the fibula approximately 10 cm. proximal to the tip of the lateral malleolus. The fibula is exposed subperiosteally between the peroneal and the flexor digitorium longus muscles and the entire fibula is removed for a distance of 3 or 4 cm. This depends, of course, upon the size of the foot, and the size of the graft required. Almost invariably, as long as the periosteum is maintained, the defect will fill in with new bone within a matter of six to nine months. Even when the defect in the fibula has persisted, none of the patients have complained of any symptomatology referable to the absence of a section of the fibula. One must exert some care in the dissection to prevent injury to the superficial peroneal nerve during the exposure of the fibula. The fibular graft is then split in two, thus forming two grafts.

The Grice procedure continues: "The grafts are cut to size and are trapezoid in shape. The corners of the broad base are removed with a rongeur so that the graft will countersink into the cancellous bone and prevent lateral displacement (Fig. 7-12). The grafts are placed in the sinus tarsi with the foot held in the slightly overcorrected position and then as the foot is everted, the grafts are locked in the desired position. The tension on the graft should favor healing. . . . . The foot is usually very stable after the insertion of the graft and in many instances the planus deformity can be corrected at operation.

Lengthening of the tendo achillis may or may not be necessary. The decision to lengthen it should be made preoperatively by testing the passive range of extension with the subtalar joint locked. If it is obvious that the tendon is tight and the foot cannot be brought up to the neutral position, then lengthening of it should be carried out prior to performance of the Grice procedure. (In a certain number of instances it will be found that such lengthening is unnecessary.) Following this a plaster cast is applied extending from the tips of the toes to the knee with the foot in neutral right angle position and with the cast well molded under the heel and around the ankle. The cast should also be well molded under the newly formed longitudinal arch with the forepart of the foot pronated slightly above the normal to accentuate the arch. Weight bearing is permitted between eight to ten weeks with the use of crutches depending upon when the roentgenograms reveal that union of the fibular graft has taken place between the talus and the os calcis. The postoperative care is similar to that previously described for the naviculo-cuneiform sag type of foot.

Occasionally one may find a patient in whom despite early, adequate, conservative therapy, the foot still everts due to medial sag of the talonavicular joint. One such patient was seen at the age of nineteen months. Standing roentgenograms revealed mildly plantar flexed tali (Fig. 7-13A.) The feet were first placed in corrective casts for nine months, followed by the use of Whitman plates. When this child reached ten years of age, his feet revealed a good longitudinal arch in a standing position, but there was marked inversion of the ankles. The heels were in neutral position (Fig. 7-13B.) Standing roentgenograms revealed normal appearing feet in the lateral view, but diminution of the dorsal talonavicular angle in the anteroposterior view (Fig. 7-13C). Subjectively the patient stated that his feet tired easily and ached after a day's activity. The procedure recommended for this type of foot is transposition of the tibialis anterior to the plantar surface of the navicular. The end result is quite satisfactory (Fig. 7-13D).

3. Plantar-Flexed Talus (Vertical Talus). Plantar flexion of the talus, as previously

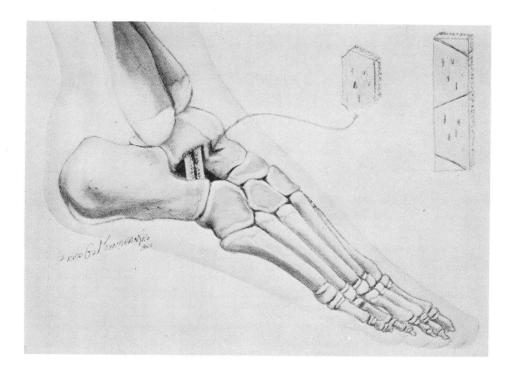

Fig. 7-12.   The Grice procedure. Grice, D. S.: Courtesy of J. Bone & Joint Surg.

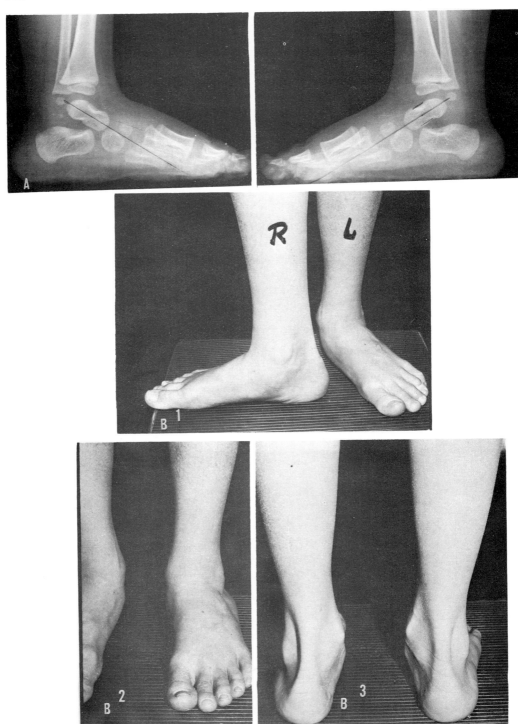

Fig. 7-13A.   Roentgenograms of both feet standing at age nineteen months presenting mild bilateral plantar felxed tali. Patient brought in because of severe pronation of feet clinically.

   B-1.   Standing photograph of the same feet at eleven years of age. Note normal appearance of longitudinal arch of the right foot but apparent pronation of the left foot due to in-rolling of the rear portion of the foot. The feet are symptomatic and patient tires easily. B-2.   Note valgus appearance of the left heel in the front view and apparent pronation of both feet due to the in-rolling. B-3. Rear view of same feet. The medial aspect is prominent and there is slight valgus of the heels.

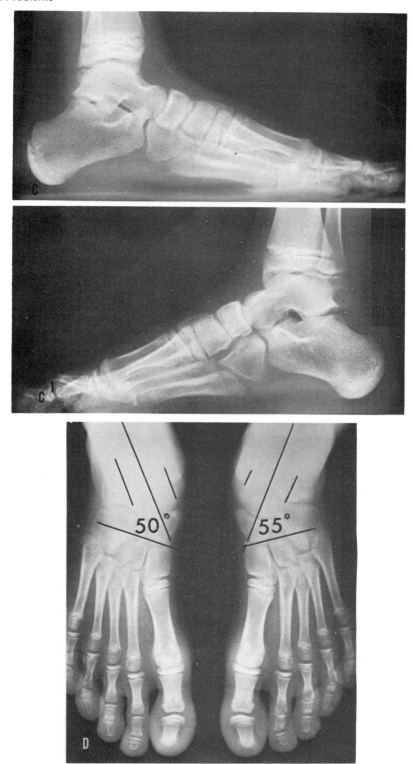

Fig. 7-13. Continued. C. Lateral roentgenograms reveal normal appearing longitudinal arch in each foot substantiating clinical findings.

D. Anteroposterior view of both feet standing demonstrating diminution of the dorsal talonavicular angle which accounts for the clinical appearance of in-rolling of the rear portion of the foot.

pointed out, is the plantar malposition of the talus in relation to the os calcis found in the calcaneovalgus foot at birth. When such a malposition is found as the cause of the planovalgus type of foot in the pre-adolescent or the adolescent stage, it is due either to inadequate or ineffectual treatment, to failure to recognize and treat it, or the deformity did not respond to adequate treatment as is the case in 50% of such feet. The subsequent therapeutic regimen will depend not only upon the patient's age and clinical evaluation of the feet, but also upon severity of the plantar flexion of the talus as seen by roentgenography.

Careful clinical as well as roentgenographic evaluation of the feet is of utmost importance. If a mild *congenital rigid flatfoot* is wrongly diagnosed as a severe plantar flexed talus type deformity, it can lead to incorrect treatment and ultimately to poor results. There are, however, specific clinical and roentgenographic findings which differentiate the one type of foot from the other.

In the planovalgus type of foot due to a plantar flexed talus, the foot is flexible. Upon examination at a position of rest, the rear foot can be inverted passively by the examiner, and the forefoot pronated so that the foot is corrected into an almost normal appearance. Furthermore, with the patient standing, the foot should be flexible enough so that the valgus of the rear foot, and, therefore, automatically the inversion, can be corrected passively and the forefoot pronated. The patient should then be able to hold this position by contracting the tibialis posterior and flexor hallucis longus muscles. Standing roentgenograms in the anteroposterior and lateral views (with the foot held in this corrected position) should demonstrate satisfactory reposition of the talus in relation to the os calcis and an increase in the dorsal talonavicular angle to within the normal range of 60 to 70 degrees. If both clinically and roentgenographically it can be seen that the foot cannot be passively and/or actively corrected to the near-normal position from the planovalgus one, the condition is due to dislocation of the talonavicular articulation and the resultant fixed deformity is due to a congenital, rigid, flatfoot.

The type of treatment chosen will depend upon the patient's age as well as the severity of the plantar flexion. For example, an eight-year-old male was referred to me because of moderately symptomatic third degree flatfeet (Fig. 7-14A). On roentgenographic examination the talus was bilaterally plantar-flexed in the lateral views (Fig. 7-14 B and B'). In the anteroposterior views the dorsal talonavicular angle was within the lower limits of normal on the right and below normal on the left (Fig. 7-14C). Since the feet appeared flexible on examination and the patient was only eight years of age, Whitman plates were prescribed. The parents were advised that the prognosis, at best, was only fair, but that conservative therapy would first be attempted. They were told that while the boy's feet would remain asymptomatic with the use of arch supports, this did not necessarily indicate that the feet would be corrected. They were also apprised of the need to obtain roentgenograms annually. If by the age of twelve, there would be no appreciable improvement seen either clinically or roentgenographically, surgical procedure would then be considered.

Occasionally, with the use of Whitman plates, moderate correction has been achieved by the age of twelve. In such a patient a fairly satisfactorily appearing and functioning pair of feet can be obtained by the continued use of arch supports until full growth is reached.

On the other hand, if the plantar flexion is moderate to severe, and the dorsal talonavicular angle is less than 45 degrees, or if the patient is first treated after the age of ten, surgical procedure is indicated. It is a waste of time and effort to attempt to treat such feet by conservative means if either of the above criteria are fulfilled.

The operation recommended for the naviculocuneiform sag-type of foot *is not recommended* for the plantar-flexed or vertical talus.

The Operation. The operation for the plantar-flexed talus, planovalgus type of foot is the Grice procedure with transplantation of the tibialis anterior and posterior tendons and with or without lengthening of the Achilles tendon. The decision to

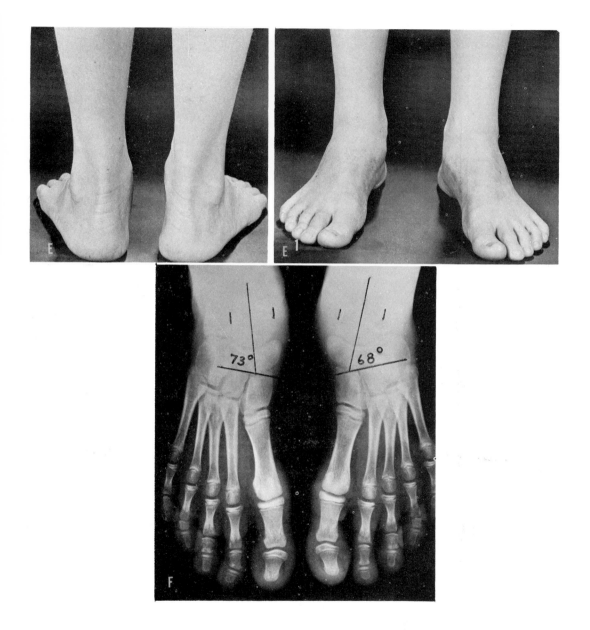

Fig. 7-13. Continued. E. Appearance of the same feet nine months following transposition of the tibialis anterior to the plantar aspect of the tarsal navicular. The feet are asymptomatic.

F. Standing roentgenograms of the same feet in the anteroposterior view The dorsal talonavicular angle is within normal limits.

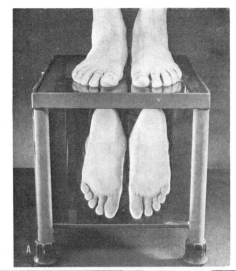

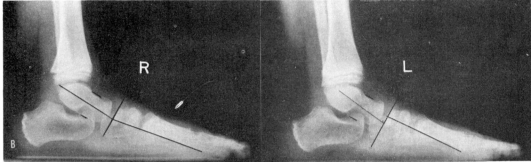

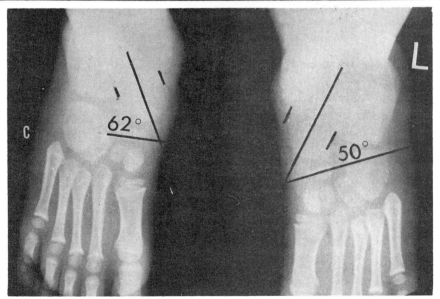

Fig. 7-14A.   Pes planus third degree due to mildly plantar flexed tali. Note almost complete absence of the longitudinal arch when observing plantar surface reflection in mirror.
  B. & B'.   Mild plantar flexion of talus bilaterally in lateral standing views.
  C.   Anterior talo-navicular angle at lower limits of normal on the right and below normal on the left. Standing anteroposterior views.

lengthen this tendon must be made prior to surgery. If true passive extension is limited on the preoperative examination, then lengthening is indicated. This procedure should be performed first. The type of tendon-lengthening procedure chosen is up to the discretion of the surgeon.

We prefer the Hibbs double L reverse method (Fig. 7-15). In this procedure the Achilles tendon is exposed either through a transverse or posteromedial incision beginning from the level of the insertion of the tendo achillis into the os calcis and extending proximally for 8 cm. The tendon sheath is split and the tendon is delivered from the sheath at this level. The first cut in the tendon begins from the lateral edge of the tendon just above its insertion into the os calcis and extends transversely across three-quarters of the tendon width (a to a'). A second transverse incision is carried out from the medial edge, extending three-quarters of the width across the tendon (b to b'). A longitudinal incision from a' to c and from b' to d is carried out parallel to the medial and lateral edges of the tendon, respectively, and to within 1 cm. of the transverse cuts. Upon extension of the foot the desired length is achieved. The tendon sheath is loosely closed and the skin incision is closed with a continuous subcuticular wire suture.

If tendon lengthening is not indicated, the Grice procedure is first performed as described ealier in this chapter. Frequently, capsulotomy of the dorsal talonavicular capsule is necessary in order to permit reposition of the talus on the os calcis. Then, through a medial incision beginning just proximal to the navicular tubercle and extending distally to the level of the metatarsocuneiform joint, the tibialis anterior is exposed and detached at the plantar medial aspect of the foot. The tendon sheath is split to the level of the inferior edge of the anterior cruciate ligament. The plantar aspect of the navicular is denuded of soft tissues and a drill hole is made dorsoplantarly in the middle portion of the navicular just distal to the proximal cortical surface. The tibialis anterior tendon, having had a No. 2 chromic suture passed through its end in a figure 8 fashion, is then transferred to the plantar aspect of the navicular by passing the suture through the drill hole and through the capsular structures and tying it. The tendon should be placed in position under physiologic tension. An additional one or two sutures of Number 00 chromic are passed through the edge of the tibialis anterior to the tibialis posterior tendon as the former crosses over the latter just posterior to the navicular tubercle. After all incisions have been closed, a cast is applied as in the Grice procedure, followed by a period of immobilization as in the latter technique.

Postoperative Care. The postoperative care differs from that described previously. Upon removal of the cast at eight to ten weeks, a plaster mold of each foot is made and Whitman steel arch supports are manufactured from the molds. Weight bearing is not permitted until the steel arch supports are fitted to the feet and inserted in the shoes. Oxford, lace-type shoes with a steel shank should be used. Weight bearing is first initiated with the use of crutches. The patient must be instructed as to the manner of walking he must employ. He must not be permitted to fall back into his old preoperative method of ambulation. He must be instructed to walk in the heel-toe method with the toes pointing directly ahead. He must learn to come up on his toes with each step. The crutches should be discarded only after the patient has learned the proper method of walking. The arch supports are worn for at least nine to twelve months. Athletic activities, even running or jumping, are not permitted until six months after surgery. Here again, the parents should be informed prior to surgery that the youngster will not resume the normal method of walking as soon as the casts are removed, and that a prolonged period of convalescence and of instruction will be necessary.

Finally, one word of advice. This procedure is not for neophytes. This type of foot is difficult to correct and if one is not well versed in foot surgery, he should not attempt to correct such feet without the aid and advice of an experienced orthopaedic surgeon.

4. Mild Cavus Feet. Occasionally the orthopaedist will have the opportunity to examine and treat a mild cavus foot which may or may not be symptomatic. Frequently, the parent will state that he has difficulty in purchasing shoes for a son or daughter because of the exceptionally "high arch." Occasionally the patient will complain that if he stands for a long period of time, or if he walks for a long distance, "the bottom of the foot hurts and the pain goes up into the back." On the other hand, the patient may complain of having difficulty finding comfortable shoes because none of them "helps to fill the arch part of the foot."

On examination the only positive finding will be the presence of a mild cavus deformity. Some orthopaedists tend to dismiss this finding and advise the parents that the boy or girl will probably outgrow the symptoms. This is far from correct. Upon procurement of a careful history one will find that this type of foot is hereditary and that there is a definite familial diathesis. There is no evidence to indicate any muscle imbalance of the feet such as is found in Friedreich's ataxia, etc. The type of cavus foot deformity which occurs with these last mentioned disease entities is described in Chapter 17. In the mild cavus foot the toes are not claw-like; the patient simply has a high longitudinal arch.

The treatment of this problem is usually conservative since with properly fitted rubber cookies to fill in the space in the shoe and with the prescription of a shoe not requiring lacing, the patient can in most instances be made comfortable. Occasionally, it is necessary to consider resection of a portion of the plantar fascia. Should such an operative procedure be required, the Steindler technique should be considered. This procedure is as follows: A longitudinal incision is made along the medial aspect of the foot beginning at the level of the os calcis and extending forward for 8 cm. After dividing the skin and the underlying subcutaneous tissues, the lower or plantar aspect of the plantar fascia is dissected free

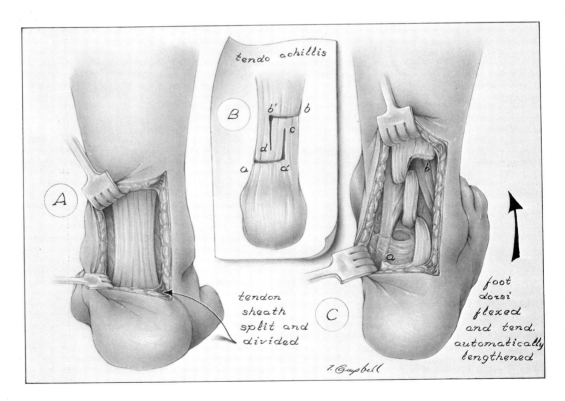

Fig. 7-15. Hibbs Method of tendo achillis Lengthening.
A. Exposure of tendon through lateral incision. B. Diagrammatic sketch of incisions. C. Tendon lengthened, but continuity maintained.

from the subcutaneous layer through its entire width. The fascia is then incised transversely close to its origin into the lower surface of the os calcis. The muscles covered by the plantar fascia are as follows, as one goes from medial to lateral: the abductor of the big toe, the short flexors of the toes, and the abductor of the fifth toe. These muscles are stripped off the periosteum of the os calcis with periosteal elevator. In addition to this, the long plantar ligament, which extends between the os calcis and the cuboid, is also stripped off. This ligament is often contracted and if not severed or stripped, it produces a cavus deformity of the outer border of the foot. By keeping close to the bone in stripping, one is at a safe distance from the plantar vessels and nerves. The procedure should be performed under tourniquet ischemia and a Shantz pressure dressing is applied postoperatively.

This procedure should be considered only as a last resort. It is a procedure whereby one can merely overcome a soft-tissue contracture of the foot. One must not expect too much from it in so far as correction of the appearance of the foot is concerned. It simply relieves the tension on the plantar soft-tissue structures.

BIBLIOGRAPHY

BUTTE, F. L.: Navicula-Cuneiform Arthrodesis for Flat Feet, J. Bone Jt. Surg. *19*:496 (April) 1937.

EDMONDSOM, S. A.: *In Campbell's Operative Orthopaedics,* 4th Ed. Vol. II, St. Louis, C. V. Mosby Company.

GRICE, D. S.: An Extra-Articular Arthrodesis of the Sub-Astragalar Joint for Correction of Paralytic Flat Feet in Children. J. Bone Jt. Surg. 34A:927 1952.

HAUSER, E. D. W.: *Diseases of the Foot.* Philadelphia, W. B. Saunders Co., 1950.

HOERR, N. L., PYLE, S. E. AND FRANCIS, C. C.: *Radiographic Atlas of Skeletal Development of the Foot and Ankle.* Springfield, Charles C Thomas, 1962.

HOKE, M.: An Operation for the Correction of Extremely Relaxed Flat Feet. J. Bone Jt. Surg. *13*:773. 1931.

HOWORTH, M. BECKETT: *A Textbook of Orthopaedics.* Philadelphia, W. B. Saunders Co., 1952.

MILLER, O. L.: A Plastic Flat Foot Operation. J. Bone Jt. Surg. *9*:84. 1927.

MORTON, D. J.: *The Human Foot.* New York, Columbia University Press. 1936.

STEINDLER, ARTHUR: *Orthopaedic Operations,* Springfield, Charles C Thomas, 1940.

YOUNG, C. AND CHARLES, S.: Operative Treatment of Pes Planus. Surg. Gyn. Obstet. *68*:1099. 1939.

=8=

Congenital Rigid Flatfoot

(Congenital Convex Pes Valgus)

During the past forty years several terms have been suggested by various authors, primarily in Europe, to describe the congenital rigid flatfoot. Nové-Josserand in 1923 chose to designate this deformity as "Pied Plat Congénital". Rocher and Pouyanne, in 1934, recommended the term "Vertically Oriented Talus". In 1939, after an extensive review of the world's medical literature pertaining to this subject, Lamey and Weissman suggested the term "Congenital Convex Pes Valgus". In fact, their article was the first to be reported in the English literature. Osmond-Clarke described his experiences with this type of deformed foot in 1956 and termed it "Congenital Vertical Talus".

Although each of these descriptive terms adequately expresses the problem to the orthopaedist, the term *congenital rigid flatfoot* conveys more completely to the medical profession, as a whole, the clinical as well as the pathological picture. Furthermore, the possibility of earlier recognition of this deformity is heightened by the use of this more figurative appellation. We strongly advise that this suggested, more descriptive term be used for this type of flatfoot deformity.

Some of the readers may wonder why an entire chapter is devoted to a condition which is reportedly rare and for which so little can be done. A review of the published literature (over 150 articles) reveals that this malformation of the foot occurs with sufficient frequency to warrant devoting more than the few lines written about this subject in the average orthopaedic textbook. Moreover, recognition of this deformity by those who first examine the infant would lead to the establishment of early corrective therapy and before the bony malalignment had become fixed. As in the management of the clubfoot, early correction could result in the achievement of a certain percentage of nearly normal feet. Those that failed to respond to conservative therapy could then undergo surgical correction. Unfortunately, one gains the impression from the current literature that surgical procedure is the only form of therapy. In the severely deformed congenital rigid flatfoot, surgical procedure is undoubtedly the only form of treatment. But, on the other hand, a fair portion of such feet do not present extreme deformity and do respond to conservative measures if these are instituted immediately after birth. It is my considered opinion that early recognition and treatment would obviate the necessity of surgical intervention in a fair number of such patients. Certainly even if the foot were rigidly fixed at birth, as does occur in the severe cases, repeated gentle manipulation and casting would do no harm.

Certainly the last words have not been written about this deformity and its management. Much more investigation needs to be done. Only the surface has been scratched so far. It is becoming more and more apparent that this deformity (even of a mild degree) should not be treated lightly or passed over by the physician simply because the youngster does not complain of painful feet. It is equally derelict to recommend that the infant be merely observed for a year or more to determine what the outcome may be of the deformity during the child's development, rather than to treat the condition with early definitive measures.

ETIOLOGY

The severe form of the congenital rigid flatfoot fortunately does not occur too frequently, but if one were to include in the same group all the congenital flat feet, such as the tali that are plantar flexed, or that are vertical but not rigidly fixed, one would find that 1.5 to 2.5 per cent of all newborn infants present a flatfoot deformity. There is no question that there is a strong hereditary factor in the plantar-flexed talus-type of flatfoot. On the other hand, the role of heredity, at best, is only questionable in the congenital rigid flatfoot. According to Lamey and Weissman the hereditary occurrence of the congenital convex pes valgus has been reported in the literature in mother and son, father and son, two brothers, and in identical twins. On the other hand, one gains the impression that it occurs more frequently in conjunction with congenital deformities such as congenital dislocation of the hip, clubfoot deformity, vertebral synostosis, microcephaly, arthrogryposis, prematurity, and cerebral agenesis. We have observed the presence of severe plantar-flexed tali in every ambulatory mongoloid child that has been referred for foot correction. In two children afflicted with mongolism there was an associated congenital rigid flatfoot deformity. Böhm's studies in the development of the human foot in the embryo throw some light on this problem. He states that there are constant changes in the position of the bones of the foot in relation to the leg during the first four months of fetal life, particularly during the latter half of the second month and the entire third month. During the second month of intrauterine life, the leg and the foot are in the same axis. At the end of the second month and the early part of the third, there occurs supination of the foot in relation to the leg. Concurrently the os calcis rotates under the talus but both are in the vertical (equinus) position. As adduction and supination of the foot develop during the midportion of the third month, equinus diminishes. By the end of the third month, the foot assumes a position of pronation in relation to the leg with slight, if any, equinus. Therefore, the malformation of the foot, according to Böhm, is an arrest of the normal evolution of the tarsal region of the foot during this period of development. He does not offer any explanation as to the cause of this arrest.

Many explanations have been given by various investigators according to Drs. Lamey and Weissman. Some of these suggested causes are spinal cord lesions, spina bifida occulta, abnormal insertion of the tibialis anterior, and overaction of the peroneal muscles, to list a few. None of the explanations are tenable. Craig feels quite strongly that this foot deformity is as much a congenital lesion as the clubfoot. Hern-

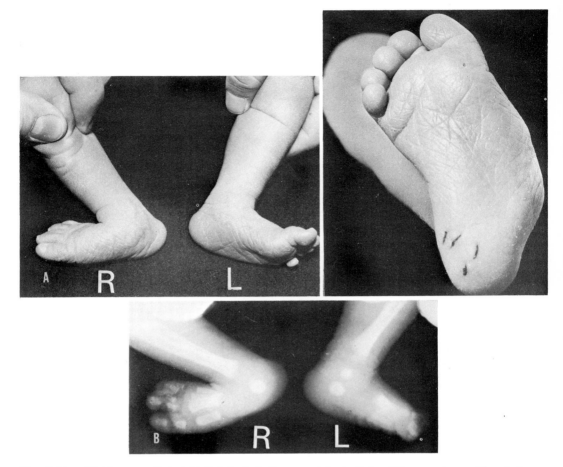

Fig. 8-1A. Right congenital rigid flat foot. Left normal foot. Note difference in **position between the two feet. Close-up** of same foot reveals valgus of forefoot in relation to rear foot. The heel is in neutral position. The deformity is a dorsolateral dislocation of the navicular on the talus.

B.   Roentgenographic appearance of same feet. Note normal relation of os calcis to talus in the left foot. On the right, note overlap of talus on os calcis with valgus position of forefoot in relation to rear foot.

don likens the dislocation of the talonavicular joint to that of the congenital dislocations of the hip joint. In their reported series of congenital rigid flatfoot deformities which they termed "Congenital Vertical Talus", Lloyd-Roberts and Spence observed that in the improperly corrected clubfoot leading to the development of a rocker bottom type deformity, both the clinical and the roentgenographic appearance were similar to that of the congenital convex pes valgus.

An opportunity was presented to us to study the possibility of any muscular dysfunction as an underlying cause of this type of deformity. The patient was a new-born female who presented a right congenital rigid flatfoot and a clinically normal left foot (Fig. 8-1A). Careful clinical evaluation failed to reveal any congenital, neurological, neuromuscular, or hereditary factors which could be considered as the cause of the deformity. Electromyographic studies failed to reveal any muscular abnormality in either lower extremity.

In the final analysis, one can only conclude that this is a congenital type deformity which on rare occasions demonstrates an hereditary pattern and that, in some instances, it occurs in association with other congenital birth defects or endocrine disturbances.

CLINICAL AND ROENTGENOGRAPHIC MANIFESTATIONS

In attempting to describe the clinical and roentgenographic appearance of this deformity, one single description does not suffice for all ages. In the newborn or in the infant prior to ambulation, the conformation of the foot, as well as the roentgenographic picture (Fig. 8-1 A and B), varies somewhat from that seen after the child has once become ambulatory (Fig. 8-2). Furthermore, the picture changes even more if the foot is seen during adulthood (Fig. 8-3). The same applies as far as treatment is concerned.

In the newborn or during infancy there is some similarity between the congenital calcaneovalgus foot and the congenital con-

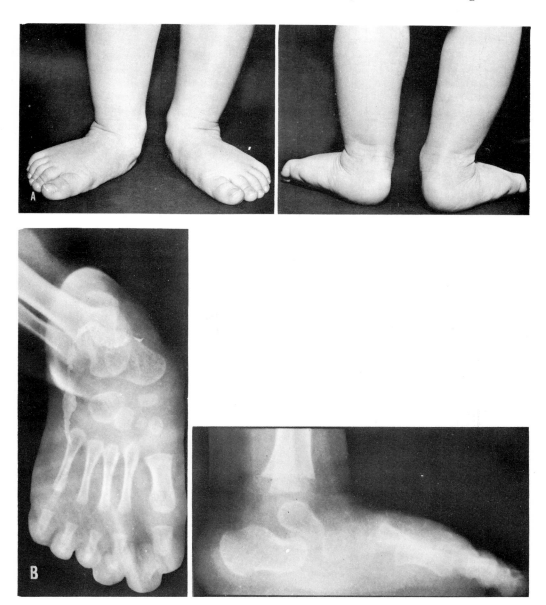

Fig. 8-2A.   Clinical appearance of congenital rigid flat feet in a child of sixteen months.

B.   Standing roentgenograms anteroposterior and lateral. Note malposition of the talus in relation to the os calsis with dislocation of the talonavicular joint.

vex pes valgus, but there are certain important differences which aid in the differential diagnosis between the two. However, in the newborn there is a certain so-called "grey area" where it is difficult to distinguish between the severe plantar-flexed talus and the mildly-deformed congenital rigid flatfoot.

The congenital calcaneovalgus foot presents the following characteristic features at birth:

1) The foot is in a position of extension and valgus with the dorsal surface frequently touching the anterolateral surface of the lower leg (Fig. 8-4A).

2) The Achilles tendon is not tight even in complete extension.

3) The heel is in valgus when the foot is extended.

4) Upon flexion of the foot the anterior soft tissue structures are contracted and, therefore, tight so that it is difficult, if not impossible, to flex the foot beyond the neutral position (Fig. 8-4B).

5) The plantar surface of the foot is flat, but the foot is flexible and can be arched on manipulation.

6) The head of the talus is palpable and points plantarly and medially, but can be repositioned.

In the congenital rigid flatfoot (congenital convex pes valgus) the distinctive features in the infant are as follows:

1) There is a valgus relationship of the rear portion of the foot with the forepart of the foot due to abduction of the latter at the mediotarsal joints (Fig. 8-4C).

2) The heel is not in valgus (Fig. 8-4C).

3) The heel is tilted downward in flexion.

4) The foot is in mild extension only and if the examiner attempts to extend the foot completely, he produces a convexity of the plantar surface of the foot (rocker-bottom deformity).

5) The foot cannot be easily inverted upon manipulation.

6) The head of the talus is palpable as a medioplantar prominence, but it cannot be easily reduced as in the calcaneovalgus foot. One gets the impression that there is a bony obstruction preventing inversion of the anterior one-half of the foot.

In the newborn, one is unable to differentiate roentgenographically between the two types of foot deformities. After the onset of weight bearing, there is only one roentgenographic feature which may help to differentiate between the congenital calcaneovalgus foot and the congenital convex pes valgus. In the former the talus is more frequently plantar flexed than it is vertical. In the latter, the talus is invariably in the vertical position. Since the navicular is not demonstrable at birth, the dislocation of the talonavicular joint, which is present in the congenital rigid flatfoot, is not evident. These two deformities can be confused

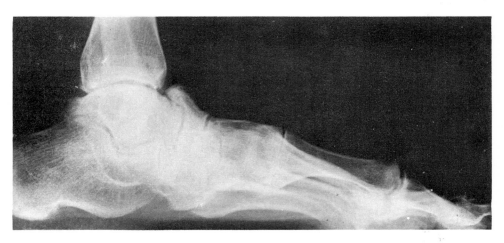

Fig. 8-3. Standing roentgenogram of congenital rigid flat foot in an adult. Note absence of the head of the talus with extensive changes in the talo-navicular and calcaneo-cuboid joints. Clinically this foot was symptomatic for years but recently the patient's feet are no longer painful. This is in all probability due to total loss of tarsal motion.

during infancy, particularly if the congenital convex pes valgus deformity is a mild one.

In a child past the age of one year, the differentiation between the two types of feet is clearcut both clinically and roentgenographically. Herndon and Heyman in 1963 listed eight differential points. Some of these warrant reviewing. In the congenital convex pes valgus (Fig. 8-5A and B) they state that:

1) The head of the talus is displaced into a vertical position in relation to the os calcis.

2) There is posterior displacement of the os calcis in relation to the talus with lateral deviation of the anterior portion of the os calcis.

3) There is dysplasia of the head and neck of the talus and abnormal development, probably due to the malrelation between the talus and the os calcis.

4) There is a forefoot valgus in relation to the rear foot due to the medioplantar dislocation, as well as relative forward displacement of the talus in relation to the os calcis. The calcaneocuboid relationship remains essentially unchanged or, at most, subluxated only slightly dorsally. Coleman recently reported two cases of dislocation of the calcaneocuboid joint with the os calcis displaced posteriorly.

5) There is true dislocation of the talonavicular joint with the navicular resting on the neck of the talus. In a child over five years of age, there is not only wedging of the plantar portion of the navicular, but I have also found that the head of the talus is flattened to some extent in the dorsoplantar direction.

6) The os calcis is in slight equinus with extension of the forepart of the foot through the midtarsal region producing the convex deformity which is demonstrable clinically.

7) There is contracture of the extensor, peroneal, and calf muscles.

After two years of age, the deformity of the foot becomes even more fixed due to contracture of the extensor tendons and the dorsal and lateral capsular structures of the talonavicular joint.

Furthermore, because of the malposition of the talus and the dislocation of the talonavicular joint, the peroneus longus and the tibialis posterior tendons are malpositioned in relation to the axis of the foot. Thus, they act as extensors rather than flexors of the foot. Coleman also pointed out that because of the contracture of the extensor muscle group, a dynamic muscle imbalance exists in this type of foot. In his evaluation of twelve congenital rigid flatfeet, he observed that because of the fixed talocalcaneal subluxation, structural changes take place in both of these bones and because of these alterations, "there is a strong tendency following correction for the talus and calcaneus to revert to their abnormal position." In two of his cases he reported a complicating "extreme subluxation at the talocalcaneal joint." He classifies this type of deformity as a "Type II deformity" and the congenital rigid flatfoot without this type of calcaneocuboid subluxation as "Type I".

SYMPTOMATOLOGY

In the infant and the child there are no symptoms which can be attributed to this type, or for that matter, any type of foot deformity. We have observed, however, that the children affected by this type of a foot problem are somewhat delayed in becoming adept in coordinated ambulation. After the age of three a certain number of these youngsters complain of tiring easily. Others will express a sense of discomfort in the feet and legs. Among the teenagers and adults occasionally one may find a patient who apparently has no symptoms in spite of the malformed feet. But one wonders if this asymptomatology is only a relative one. It is our opinion that pronated feet, let alone severe deformities such as congenital rigid flatfeet, are almost invariably symptomatic, but the individual concerned does not realize this. He is accustomed to living with uncomfortable feet.

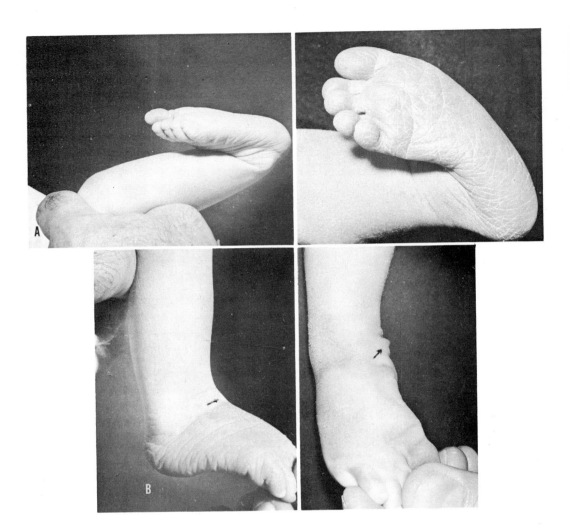

Fig. 8-4A. Congenital calcaneovalgus foot. A'. Congenital rigid flatfoot. Note the difference in appearance between the two. In a the foot is in a position of extension and valgus with the dorsal surface touching the anterolateral surface of the lower leg. The Achilles tendon is not tight and the heel is in valgus. In a' the deformity is between the rear foot and the mediotarsal region. There is valgus relation between the two. The heel is not in valgus and the tendo achillis is almost invariably tight.

B. Calcaneovalgus foot in extension. Note tight tissue structures on anterior portion of foot and ankle. B'. Congenital rigid flatfoot in flexion. Note redundancy of soft tissues on the dorsomedial aspect of the foot.

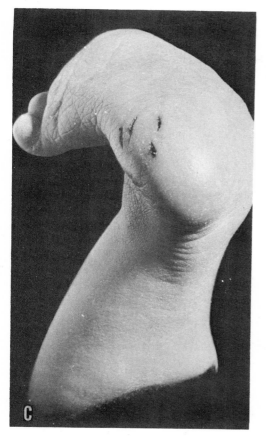

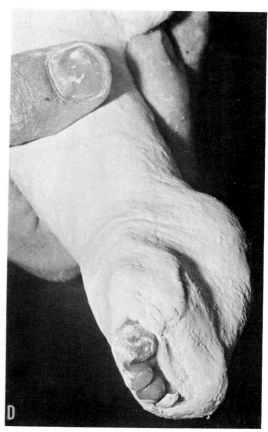

Fig. 8-4. Continued. C. Congenital rigid flatfoot. Note that the heel is in neutral position. Observe the valgus position of mid-and forefoot in relation to rear foot.

D. Initial, corrective cast applied in as much equinus, inversion, and adduction as can be tolerated.

TREATMENT

Most observers have advised that the treatment of choice in this type of foot deformity is, almost invariably, surgical intervention. In fact, they are extremely pessimistic about achieving any correction with the use of wedging casts. There is no question that in the severe congenital rigid flatfoot, correction with the use of casts may be well nigh impossible. However, in the newborn and in the infant up to six months of age, conservative therapy is definitely worth attempting. If it is successful, all well and good. If it is not, one has lost nothing but effort and some time. In my opinion, not to attempt to correct such a foot with plaster casts is indicative of a lack of knowledge of the problem. Furthermore, since at this stage it is often difficult to differentiate between the severe plantarflexed (vertical) talus-type of foot and the mildly deformed congenital rigid flatfoot (congenital convex pes valgus), plaster correction is most definitely indicated.

Figure 8-6 is an illustration of what appears to be a pair of congenital rigid flatfeet in a sixteen-month-old female. All outward appearances, as well as the roentgenographic findings, indicated this type of foot deformity. There is one clinical exception, the feet are flexible. Therefore, does not this child warrant a trial of conservative plaster correction, even for as long as one

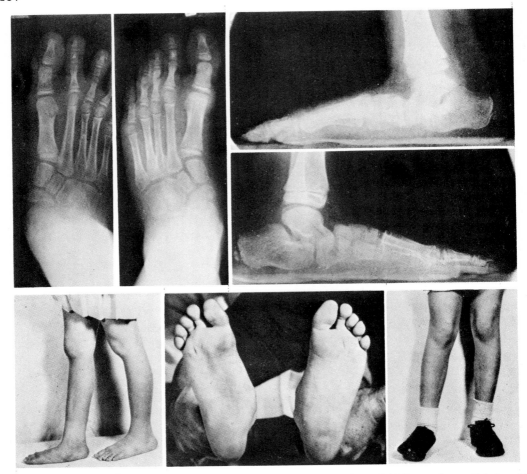

Fig. 8-5A.   Anteroposterior and lateral roentgenograms of both feet of M.F., made on October 17, 1959, when she was eight years old. The patient was first seen at nineteen months, on June 2, 1953, because of bilateral congenital valgus. Repeated manipulations at that time did not improve the deformity. Note the persistent equinus of the calcaneus, plantar convexity of the mid-tarsal region, vertical position of the talus, dorsal dislocation of the navicular which articulates with the superior aspect of the neck of the talus, and marked medial deviation of the talus with respect to the calcaneus.

B.   Both feet on October 17, 1959, show extreme valgus and prominence of the head of the talus in the region of the longitudinal arch. Note the manner in which the right shoe is worn. (Herndon and Heyman, courtesy of J. Bone & Joint Surg.)

year, before recommending surgical procedure?

One must realize that this type of foot, as well as the moderately severe to severe plantar-flexed talus-type of flatfoot, is very difficult to correct either conservatively or surgically. One must also recognize the fact that, similar to the clubfoot therapy, the earlier corrective treatment is instituted, the better chance one has of succeeding. If the child is first brought in for treatment after the age of six months, surgical correction is almost invariably the only meth-

od by which one can hope to obtain a satisfactory end-result in the congenital rigid flatfoot. But by this age, differentiation between the two types of feet is easily performed. If the rigidity of the foot is only slight, one should still carry out conservative management before progressing to surgical intervention. We feel that after a child is past six months of age and the foot is still rigidly fixed, the sooner surgical correction is attempted, the better are the chances of success.

In the newborn or the infant the therapeutic regimen should initially consist of cast correction. It is not only permissible, but absolutely necessary (even if the child should require surgery at a later date) to attempt plaster of paris correction first, since by gentle manipulation and plaster of paris wedging, one at least can stretch the extensor tendons to the point where it will be unnecessary to lengthen them at a later date. Thus, even though the correction of the talonavicular dislocation may not have been successful, at least stretching of the tendons will have occurred and thus the magnitude of the surgical corrective procedure diminished. It must be realized that the foot cannot be corrected to normal appearance within three or four wedging and cast applications. One must be patient, even more so than with clubfeet. The cast should be applied from midthigh to the tips of the toes, with the knee in 90 degrees flexion, and the foot in as much flexion (plantar flexion), adduction, and inversion as can be tolerated (Fig. 8-4D). The wedging is carried out in the same manner as

in the clubfoot cast except that, instead of wedging the foot laterally, one wedges the foot medially and plantarly to overcome the dislocation of the talonavicular joint, as well as the subluxation of the calcaneocuboid joint. Although it may appear difficult to reduce the talocalcaneal malposition, it can be done by grasping the heel in one hand and gently forcing it into the varus and equinus position and at the same time by lateral pressure against the head of the talus, realignment of the talocalcaneal malposition can be achieved. Having lined up this joint, the talonavicular dislocation can then be reduced gradually by gently manipulating the midfoot and the forefoot into a position of cavus and varus. One will be able to palpate the head of the talus easily and with this portion of the talus as a landmark, the remainder of the foot can be realigned around it. This correction should be carried out slowly every other day. With patience, one will frequently succeed in correcting and aligning the talus in proper position with the

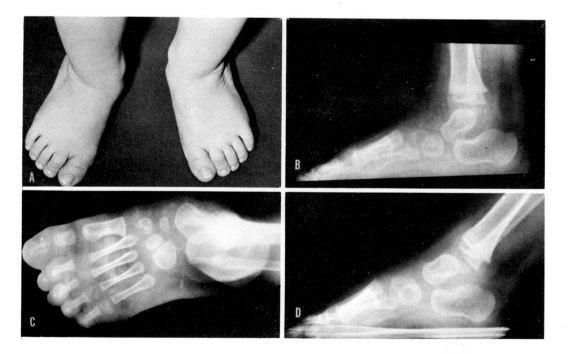

Fig. 8-6A.   Clinical appearance reveals what appears to be a pair of congenital rigid flat feet.

   B. Roentgenograms in the standing anteroposterior and C—lateral position also indicate this of foot. However, note standing roentgenogram Figure 8-6D.

   C.   The foot is flexible and normal talo-navicular and talo-calcaneal relationship established by placing the foot in the equinus position.

navicular and with the os calcis, even in the extremely rigid flatfoot deformity where there is marked contracture of the lateral soft tissue capsular and tendinous structures along with the dislocation. The result will be a nicely arched foot in an equinus position (Fig. 8-7). The foot should then be permitted to remain in this corrected equinocavovarus position for a period of at least six weeks.

The wedging cast that is next applied to correct the equinus should be a long leg-cast with 90 degrees flexion at the knee and with proper padding to protect the soft tissues on the anterior aspect of the foot and ankle. The heel and forefoot should be held in neutral position as far as varus is concerned but with maximum cavus and equinus. Once the bones of the foot are properly aligned, then dorsal anterior wedging is carried out to correct the equinus. If there is a question in the mind of the orthopaedist regarding the correction of the talonavicular dislocation, he should not attempt to correct the equinus deformity. Any attempt to do so will result in further dislocation of the talonavicular and the calcaneocuboid components. The complete corrective process cannot be accomplished in one or two weeks. Wedging should be carried out every third day and only a minimal amount, and the casts changed at least once weekly. It usually requires from four to six weeks of gentle and careful wedging of the foot to correct the equinus position and bring the foot up to the neutral right angle position. Once it has been accomplished, the feet should be kept in a corrective cast for at least three months, preferably for six. Prior to removal of the final plaster casts, a mold of the foot or feet should be made for the manufacture of Whitman steel arch supports. Such feet require constant supportive therapy and careful, conscientious follow-up supervision until full growth has been attained. This therapeutic regimen should be attempted in most, if not all, patients prior to the age of five months. After this period, if the deformity is a mild one, correction by the above described method can be attempted and sometimes accomplished, but after complete correction immobilization in the retention casts will be necessary for at least

nine to twelve months followed by the use of steel arch supports.

Although the technique of the cast application for the correction of this deformity is well known, its re-presentation may undoubtedly be of value to some readers.

Webril is the preferable material to use to cover the extremity prior to the application of the cast. The first portion of the cast should be applied from mid-thigh to lower leg with the knee flexed at 90 degrees. After the cast has hardened, the foot part of the cast is applied with the necessary pads to protect the skin at the area of wedging. The cast should be permitted to dry and then wedged. After the second wedging the cast should be changed. Prior to the application of a new cast, the foot should be gently massaged and manipulated in an attempt to stretch the dorsal structures of the foot. At the time that the cast is changed, roentgenograms should be procured to determine if there has been any correction of the talocalcaneal malposition, since the talonavicular dislocation cannot be visualized, although if the foot is carefully examined, the dislocation can be palpated. In the lateral view the talus should be almost parallel with the os calcis. In the anteroposterior view the talus should not be as medially deviated in relation to the os calcis as seen in the original roentgenograms. If the first series of wedgings does not demonstrate marked improvement, one should not be discouraged. The corrective process should be repeated until satisfactory alignment is achieved. As long as the wedging is carried out gently and slowly, no damage to the bony structures will result.

If the child is brought into the office after the age of one year, the use of corrective casts is of no value even in the mildly rigid congenital flatfoot.

If the corrective casts should fail to produce the desired results, then surgical intervention is the only alternative. Craig has corrected such feet as early as one year of age. Herndon and Heyman have reported surgical correction of two feet at eight to nine months of age. In our opinion the Grice procedure is most definitely contra-indicated in the congenital rigid flatfoot unless the patient is over five years of age.

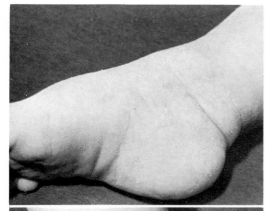

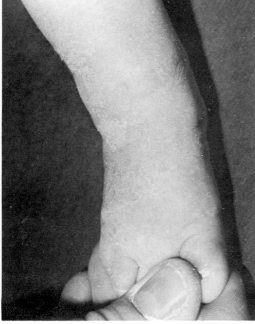

Fig. 8-7. Note appearance of same foot illustrated in Figure 8-1 and 4 a', b', c & d after gentle manipulation and cast correction over a period of six weeks.

Coleman recommends its use at an even earlier age. We believe this procedure can be used successfully in the plantar-flexed talus and the vertically displaced talus-type of flexible flatfoot deformity, since there is no dislocation of the talonavicular joint and the os calcis is not in an equinus position. In addition it is easy to reposition the talus on the os calcis. Any tendency to medial subluxation of the talus is prevented by placement of the grafts in the sinus tarsi to hold the talus in proper position,

reinforced by the transposition of the tibialis anterior to the plantar aspect of the navicular. Therefore, in the congenital calcaneovalgus foot or the vertical or near-vertical talus-type of flatfoot found in youngsters afflicted with cerebral palsy or some of the other neurological disorders, the Grice procedure gives excellent results. We have not found it successful for the achievement of satisfactory correction of the congenital convex pes valgus.

In the congenital rigid flatfoot, the procedure of choice is either Craig or the Herndon-Heyman operation. Both of these operations achieve the same result although the approach differs somewhat. In the Craig technique the following steps are carried out: A transverse dorsomedial incision is made at the level of the talonavicular joint beginning at the medial aspect of the foot and extending dorsally and laterally to the lateral edge of the common extensor group of tendons. Care must be taken not to sever the terminal sensory branches of the superficial peroneal nerve. The tibialis anterior and the extensor hallucis longus tendons are identified; their respective sheaths split, and the tendons lengthened by a Z-plasty. According to Craig, if the tibialis anterior tendon is not lengthened, a cavus deformity of the foot is produced. This has not been confirmed by other investigators including us. Craig further states that failure to lengthen the flexor hallucis longus tendon results in a cock-up deformity.

A second transverse curved incision is made at the level of the metatarsophalangeal joints from the second to the fifth toes with the arc of the curve in the proximal direction (Fig. 8-8).

Through the proximal incision (Fig. 8-9), the long extensor tendon of the fifth toe is sutured to that of the fourth toe and similarly the tendon of the third toe to that of the second. The fifth and third toe tendons are then divided distal to the suture. Through the distal curvilinear incision the tendon sheaths of the long toe extensors are split. The free ends of the third and fifth toe tendons are delivered into the lower incision. A number 00 chromic catgut suture is passed just distal to the cut end of each of these tendons and the suture of the fifth tendon is passed through the fourth tendon at the level of the lower incision. The suture is clamped with a hemostat, but not tied. The same procedure is carried out between the third toe extensor tendon and the second. The extensor tendons to the fourth and second toes are then sectioned just distal to the recently placed sutures. The ends of these two tendons are temporarily permitted to lie freely in the distal incision. The peroneus longus and brevis tendons are severed through a small lateral longitudinal incision just distal to the lateral malleolus.

Following this step the talonavicular joint is approached through the proximal incision. The capsule of this joint is divided both on the dorsal and the medial aspects exposing the appositional surfaces. The forefoot is flexed plantarly, adducted, and pronated, thus reducing the talonavicular dislocation. At times, it is necessary to slip a blunt dissector under the neck of the talus to lift the latter into proper position in relation to the os calcis and the navicular. Craig then advises the use of a stainless steel wire to maintain the talonavicular correction. I prefer to use a threaded Kirschner wire for this purpose. After reduction, the Kirschner wire is spun through the navicular and into the head, neck, and body of the talus. The wire is cut level with the skin and the latter is pulled over the cut end so that the wire can be palpated subcutaneously for removal at a later date. One will observe that the foot will assume a position of flexion when this reduction is effected except in the one- or two-year-old children.

The tendon ends of the distal incision are then approached and tied, i.e., the distal tendon end of the fifth to the proximal portion of the fourth, and the distal tendon end of the third to the proximal end of the second. It is important to remember that these tendons should be sutured to one another under careful physiological tension. Once this step has been carried out, the distal tendon ends of the second and fourth toes are sutured to the distal tendon ends of the third and the fifth toes. Any redundant tendon ends are then severed. The incisions are closed and a cast is applied with the foot in as much equinus as is

indicated. The cast extends from the toes to the knee.

Prior to the application of the cast, the foot should be extended carefully and gently to determine whether or not there is a contracture of the Achilles tendon as well as of the posterior capsular structures of the ankle. Should there be, then lengthening of the Achilles tendon and a posterior ankle capsulotomy are performed as a second-stage procedure eight weeks later. A plaster cast is then applied, extending from the tips of the toes to the mid-thigh as follows: With the use of extra-fast-setting plaster of paris the slipper cast is first applied from the tips of the toes to the level of the ankle with the foot in 20 degrees of equinus, varus of the heel, adduction of the mid-foot and pronation of the forefoot. After this portion has set, the cast is then extended to the mid-thigh with the knee in 20 degrees of flexion. Immobilization is maintained for eight weeks. At the end of this period of time, the cast is removed for the performance of a second stage procedure, if this is indicated. The second procedure is necessary if there is contracture of the Achilles tendon and the underlying posterior capsule of the tibiotalar joint. It consists of a posterior capsulotomy at the tibiotalar articulation, as well as lengthening of the Achilles tendon by one of the techniques mentioned. A plaster mold of the foot is made for the preparation of a Whitman steel or plastic arch support. A well-molded short leg-cast is then applied with the foot extended to the neutral position. Immobilization is maintained for another four weeks. The cast is then removed and the Kirschner wire is spun out through a small stab wound. The arch support is fitted to the foot. The support or supports are worn for at least one year (Fig. 8-10).

In the Herndon-Heyman procedure lateral and medial incisions are carried out (Fig. 8-11). The latter is a lazy S-type incision beginning below and behind the lateral malleolus at the level of the talocalcaneal joint, extending distally and dorsally to the level of the naviculocuneiform joint. The medial incision begins just below the tip of the medial malleolus and with a slight plantar curve

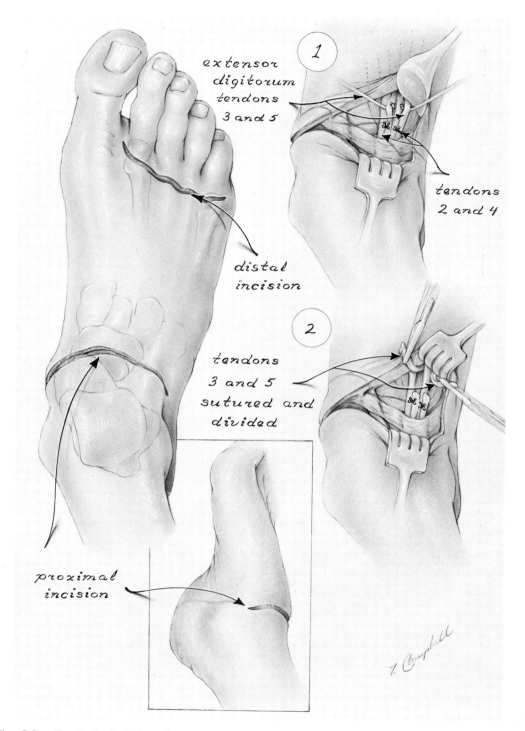

Fig. 8-8. The Craig technique for the correction of the congenital rigid flatfoot. Skin incisions on the dorsum of the foot: A transverse dorsomedial incision beginning at the medial aspect of the foot at the level of the talonavicular joint and extending dorsally and laterally to the lateral edge of the common extensor group of tendons.

Second transverse curved incision at the level of the metatarsophalangeal joints from the second to the fifth toes with the arc of the curve in the proximal direction. In addition to referring to the illustrations, the text must be carefully read should one wish to perform this procedure.

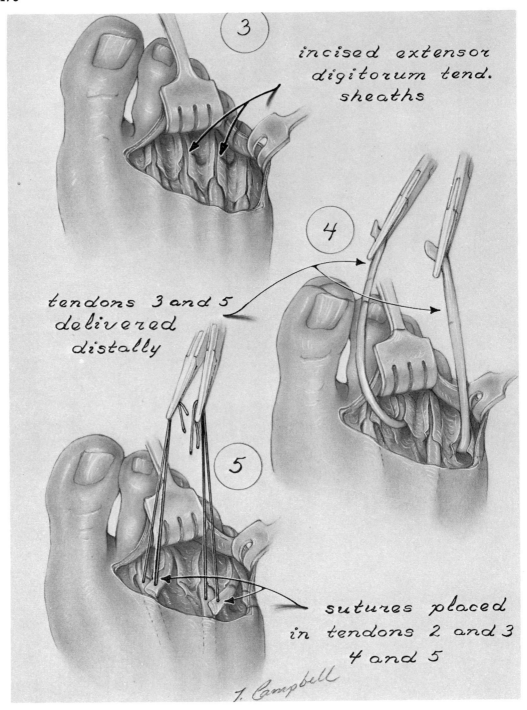

Fig. 8-9.   Craig Technique—Detail of Tendon Surgery.
    Step 1.   Through proximal incision extensor tendon five sutured to extensor tendon four. Extensor tendon three sutured to extensor tendon two.
    Step 2.   Extensor tendons five and three are divided distal to the suture.
    Step 3.   Through distal curved incision, split long toe extensor tendon sheaths.
    Step 4.   Deliver free ends of tendons five and three into the lower incision.
    Step 5.   Pass number 00 chromic suture through distal end of tendon five and through tendon four in the distal incision. Repeat procedure between tendons two and three. Clamp each suture with hemostat, cut tendons two and four below suture but do not tie.

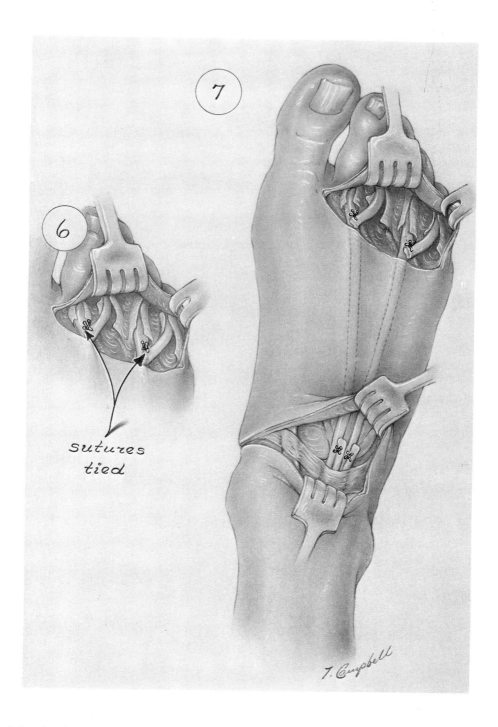

Fig. 8-9. Continued.

Step 6. After reduction of talonavicular joint and application of wires, tie tendon five to tendon four under physiologic tension and discard redundant portion of tendon. Carry out same procedure between tendons three and two.

Step 7. Suture free ends of tendons two and four in distal incision to tendons three and five.

extends distally to the level of the medial surface of the medial cuneiform. Through these two incisions both the medial and the lateral aspect of the talonavicular joint are exposed, as well as the lateral aspect of the talocalcaneal and calcaneocuboid articulations. The ligamentous and capsular structures of the talocalcaneal and talonavicular joints are completely sectioned, but with only enough dissection on the dorsal surface of the neck of the talus as is necessary to effect reduction of the talonavicular dislocation. The above two au-

thors believe that too extensive dissection of the dorsal capsular structures of the talus may lead to avascular necrosis of the talar head. Craig, on the other hand, is of the opinion that such necrosis occurs only when the sinus tarsi is dissected too extensively in addition to the other capsular structures.

After the necessary structures have been divided both medially and laterally, reduction of the dislocation is carried out by levering the head of the talus into the normal articular position with the navicular.

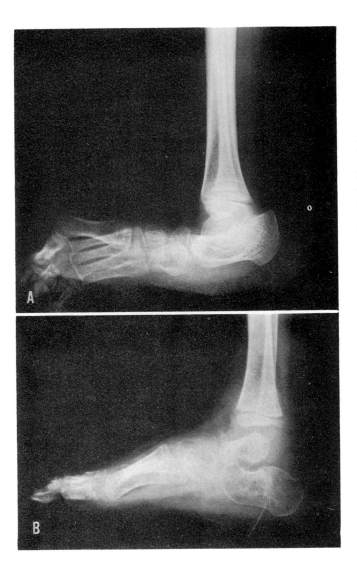

Fig. 8-10A.   Preoperative roentgenographic appearance of congenital rigid flatfoot.
   B.   Same foot after surgical correction by the Craig Procedure.

If at this time the dorsal and lateral tendons are found to be tight, lengthening is carried out of the long toe extensors as well as of the peroneals. Heyman and Herndon have not found it necessary to lengthen the tibialis anterior or the extensor hallucis longus.

Reduction of the joints is maintained by passing a Kirschner wire through the talonavicular as well as the talocalcaneal joints. Cast immobilization is maintained for six weeks. At the end of this time, posterior ankle capsulotomy and lengthening of the Achilles tendon are carried out, if the posterior capsule of the ankle and the Achilles tendon are contracted. The wires are removed four weeks later. A plaster walking cast is then worn for another six to eight weeks.

Osmond-Clarke has reported transplantation of the peroneus brevis into the neck of the talus to maintain reduction of the talonavicular dislocation after the soft tissue structures have been completely freed both medially and dorsally. His results have been satisfactory in the two cases he has reported.

Coleman recommends the performance of a Grice procedure through the usual lateral incision. Capsulotomy is carefully carried out around the talonavicular joint to reduce the dislocation through a dorso-medial incision. Tenotomy of the tibialis posterior is performed since this tendon is displaced anteriorly because of the malposition of the talus. Following reduction of the talonavicular joint, a Kirschner wire is passed through the medial cuneiform and the navicular and into the head and neck of the talus to maintain position. Following correction of the foot, the tendons on the dorsum of the foot are lengthened if they are contracted. The foot is immobilized for six weeks in a cast extending from the mid-thigh to the toes. This cast is well molded around the heel and the foot even if it is in the equinus position. The tibialis posterior tendon is sutured to the plantar aspect of the navicular in a manner similar to that employed in the Kidner procedure. At the end of six weeks the cast is removed. Tendo achillis lengthening and posterior ankle capsulotomy are also performed. Cast immobilization is maintained for another

six weeks. Upon removal of the cast the Kirschner wires are removed. One must realize, however, that arthrodesis of the talocalcaneal joint cannot be easily carried out before the age of three.

The results of operative correction, no matter which procedure one uses, are not always excellent. On the other hand, the function and the appearance of the feet are almost invariably appreciably improved. All of the investigators of this problem are in agreement that even if there is no pain, and in children this is frequently true, correction of the deformity is indicated. Even a moderate correction of the foot helps to improve the child's awkward gait and the unsightliness of the foot.

In the adult, and occasionally one may see such an individual, the foot must be carefully evaluated (Fig. 8-12). If it is asymptomatic in spite of the deformity, no treatment is indicated. If the patient's feet are symptomatic or if he wishes to have the feet corrected because of difficulty in shoe-fitting, or for other cosmetic reasons, the procedure of choice is a triple arthrodesis. The patient should be advised that although, both cosmetically and functionally, the feet may be improved to a certain extent, he must not expect too much. Symptomatically, the improvement will be appreciable. Functionally and cosmetically, the results will be fair, at best. At no time should the adult patient be advised that after such correction the result will be a normal or near-normal foot. In my opinion, in the adult surgical correction should not be recommended for cosmetic purposes as long as the feet are not disabling.

One word of caution should be added. Such a triple arthrodesis in a young or middle-aged adult is difficult. Occasionally, it is necessary to resect the entire head of the talus to effect reduction. Both a lateral sinus tarsi Kocher incision and a medial incision over the talonavicular joint are necessary in order to expose the bones properly for a triple arthrodesis. The orthopaedist should make certain that he will be able to close the lateral incision since the lateral soft tissues are so contracted that he may find closure quite difficult. A hemovac unit should invariably be used to aspirate the hematoma which almost al-

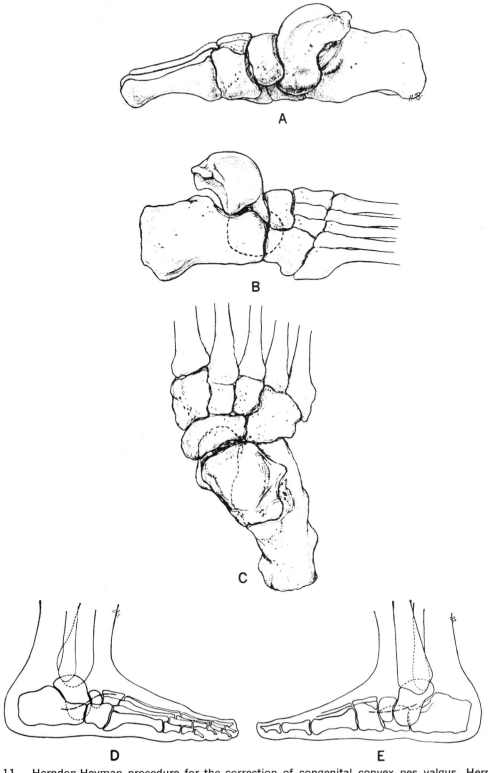

Fig. 8-11. Herndon-Heyman procedure for the correction of congenital convex pes valgus. Herndon-Hayman, courtesy of J. Bone & Joint Surg.

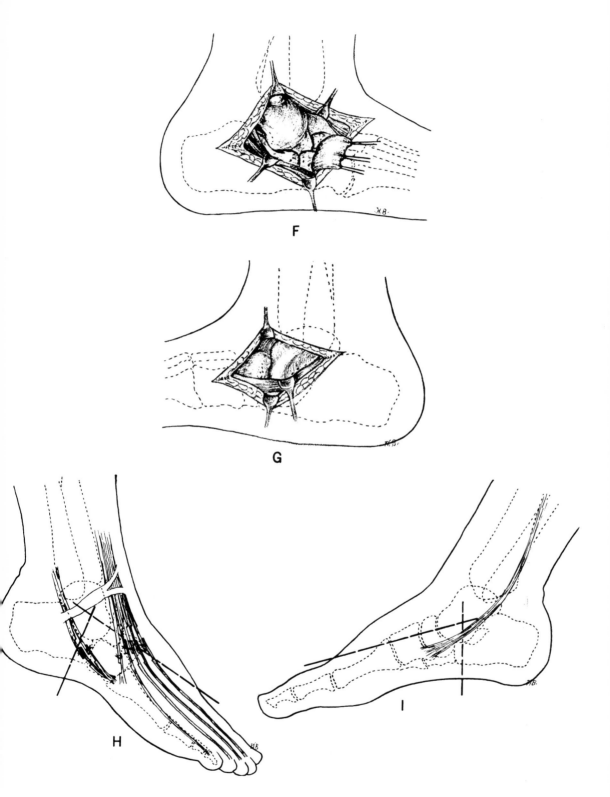

Fig. 8-11. Continued.

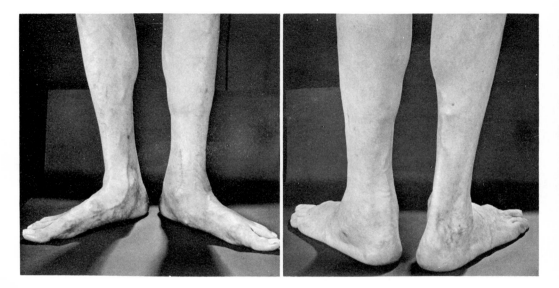

Fig. 8-12.   Adult congenital rigid flat feet asymptomatic at present. Roentgenograms of right foot illustrated in Figure 8-3.
    Feet were symptomatic for quite a number of years, but of late have been relatively comfortable.

ways results in an adult foot after a triple arthrodesis of such magnitude. Nor should such corrective surgery be attempted by a beginner without the assistance of an experienced surgeon.

BIBLIOGRAPHY

Böhm, M.: Der Fötal Fuss. Beitragzur Entstehung des Pes Planus, des Pes Valgus und des Pes Plano-Valgus. Ztschr. F. Orthop. Chir., LVII, 1932.

Coleman, Sherman S.: Personal Communication.

Craig, F. S.: Personal Communication.

Hark, F. W.: Rocker Foot Due to Congenital Subluxation of the Talus. J. Bone Jt. Surg. 32A: 334-350 (April) 1950.

Herndon, C. H.: Personal Communication.

Herndon, C. H. and Heyman, C. H.: Congenital Convex Pes Valgus. J. Bone Jt. Surg. 45A: 413-429 (March) 1963.

Heyman, C. H.: The Diagnosis and Treatment of Congenital Convex Pes Valgus or Vertical Talus. Instructional Course Lectures, The American Academy of Orthopaedic Surgeons, 16:117-126, 1959.

Kidner, F. C.: The Pre-Hallux Accessory Scaphoid in Its Relation to Flatfeet. J. Bone Jt. Surg. 11: 831, 1929.

Kidner, F. C.: The Pre-Hallux in Relation to Flatfeet. J.A.M.A., 101:1531, 1933.

Lamey, L. and Weissman, L.: J. Bone Jt. Surg. 21:79-91 (Jan.) 1939.

Lloyd-Robert, G. C. and Spence, A. J.: Congenital Vertical Talus, J. Bone Jt. Surg. 40A: 33-41 (Feb.) 1958.

Nové-Josserand: Formes Anatomiques du pied plat. Rev. d'Orthop. 10:117, 1923.

Osmond-Clarke, H.: Congenital Vertical Talus. J. Bone Jt. Surg. 38B:334-341, 1953.

Rocher, H. L. and Pouyanne, L.: Pied plat congenital par subluxation sous-astragalienne congenitale et orientation verticale de l'astragale. Bordeaux Chirl, 5:249, 1934.

Stone, K. H.: Congenital Vertical Talus: A New Operation. Procee. Roy. Soc. Med. 56:12 (Jan.) 1963.

=9=

The Normal and the Pronated Foot

in the Adult

There is no question but that the adult symptomatic pronated foot poses a problem which is still unresolved. This is evidenced by the plethora of so-called "orthopaedic shoes" from which the average individual is called upon to choose in his or her attempt to seek relief.

Furthermore, the problem will not be completely solved by any of the recommendations presented in this chapter. An attempt will be made, however, to present measures that have in my experience helped a fairly substantial number of people over the years.

First, a short discussion would not be amiss regarding the various supportive shoes that are on the market today. If one were to believe the claims of the advertisers about the merit of each particular shoe that is sold on the basis that it will solve all static foot problems, there would not be any need to write this chapter. I made a careful study and survey in the past and found that only 25 per cent of all adults suffering from static foot problems are relieved by purchasing and wearing this or that particular brand of "paedic"

shoe. Furthermore, the problem is more easily solved for the male patient than it is for the female. This, because "Dame Fashion" has decreed the type of shoes to be worn by the female which, under the best of circumstances, are unphysiologically constructed. Poorly-fitted or poorly-constructed shoes not only interfere with the function of the foot, but produce actual damage. One could unqualifiedly state that a large portion of the foot problems of the present day is due to faulty shoes. In fact, DuVries estimated that at present approximately 85 million people in the United States exhibit foot problems and that 90 per cent of these problems are caused by ill-fitting shoes.

First and foremost one should remember that the shoe should protect the foot, not disturb it. What, then is the proper type shoe? The properly-constructed shoe is one that is shaped like the human foot with a straight inner border, a rounded toe portion with sufficient room for the toes, and a well-fitted instep and heel. Its length should be such that the first metatarsophalangeal joint should be located at the point of the rounding in of the sole when the patient is in a standing position (Fig. 9-1). A steel shank should be built into the shoe to lend stability and reinforcement. The sole should be flat and firm. The Army shoe, which is built on what is known as the Munson last, is the type which best fits the requirements of a shoe built to conform to the shape of the foot. But, then, how many women would wear such a physiologically-shaped shoe in this modern age? None!

At the present time there is no single type of shoe which fits every foot. Nor is there a prescription shoe which is a "cure-all." Built-in arch supports, metatarsal pads, heel or sole wedges may be harmful, not only to a symptomatic foot, but also to an asymptomatic one. This is due to the fact that whatever type of support is built into the shoe, it is fitted to the size of the shoe and not according to the contour of the foot. It is the foot that is symptomatic and the support should be "tailored" to fit the foot. Nor should it be something that is taken off the shelf and placed into the shoe according to the shoe size.

The high-heeled type shoe which most women wear today was originally intended as a dress shoe and as such, it fulfilled its purpose quite satisfactorily. It was not intended, however, as the general utility foot cover which many women have made it. On the other hand, sandals and loafers are equally unsatisfactory unless one has a normal foot and is not required to stand or to walk for long periods of time on today's hard pavements and concrete floors. Both of these latter styles of shoes were intended to be used as "country shoes." Furthermore, when worn in the city, they tend to aggravate and render a weakly-constructed foot even more symptomatic.

The fitting of a shoe is most important. It is unfortunate that in the training of most orthopaedic residents, specific instruction is not given as to the proper fitting of shoes. Furthermore, the average shoe salesman today knows so little regarding the proper fitting of shoes that it is no wonder that so many people's feet are symptomatic. It is common practice among such salesmen that if, for example, a person requires a size 7 C and the size is unavailable in the

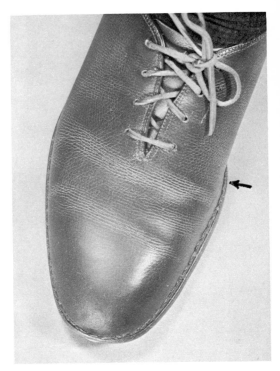

Fig. 9-1. Note arrow indicating level in the shoe where the first metatarsal joint should be located.

particular shoe style that the customer desires, to fit the purchaser in a 7½ B shoe on the basis that the fit is essentially the same. The average salesman today is interested in selling shoes and not in fitting them. Furthermore, sizes of shoes vary in that a size 7 of one brand might be a size 6½ of a different manufacturer and probably a size 7½ of a third brand.

There are certain basic principles which must be followed in fitting a shoe. First, the exact length and width should be decided with the individual standing. The shoe should be at least ⅜ of an inch, and preferably ½ of an inch, longer than the foot. The heel part of the shoe or heel cup should fit snugly around the heel of the foot, but not tightly. The first metatarsophalangeal joint should be located at the level of the change in the counter of the medial side of the sole. Ideally the instep of the shoe should fit the instep of the foot, but this is well nigh impossible to find in today's shoes. The shoe should be wide enough across the "ball" of the foot so that it will not feel tight but, on the other hand, it should not be loose. *The normal foot is so constructed that it is able to support itself.* It needs no external support. The shoes are only a protective covering against the outside elements. The normal foot no more needs support than the normal individual needs crutches, a hearing aid, or glasses. Support, as such, should be prescribed only when indicated and under orthopaedic supervision after careful evaluation of the particular foot problem.

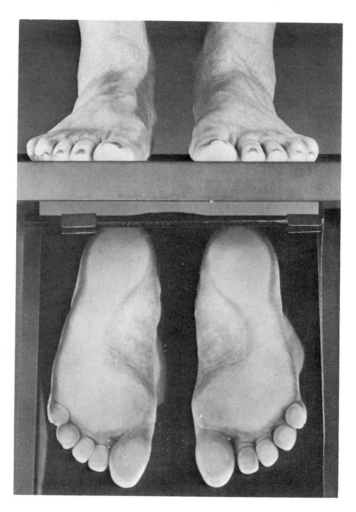

Fig. 9-2. Illustration of well-balanced adult foot. Note the normal conformation of **the medial** longitudinal arch. Although in the reflected image there is no evidence of the lateral **portion of the** longitudinal arch, the weight is evenly distributed on the plantar aspect of the foot. **The toes are** straight and relatively parallel to each other.

THE NORMAL ADULT FOOT

Appearance. The normal foot of an adult is best described by illustration (Fig. 9-2). In the standing position it is well-balanced in appearance in that there are no particularly outstanding bony prominences. There is a medial and a lateral portion of the longitudinal arch. The weight of the body is evenly distributed on the plantar aspect of the foot on the heel and the metatarsal region.

The toes are straight and lie parallel to one another. The heel is in neutral position and the contour of the heel cord (Achilles tendon) is in a straight line.

The ranges of motion of the adult ankle and foot have already been described and illustrated in Chapter 3. For the sake of clarity these will be relisted. One must keep in mind that with progressing age, there is a slight loss of motion in the various joints. The figures listed below represent the average ranges of motion.

ANKLE

EXTENSION (Dorsiflexion) 20° active motion
FLEXION (Plantar flexion) 50° active motion
TRUE PASSIVE EXTENSION 0 to 5°
  (Subtalar joint locked)
RELATIVE PASSIVE
  EXTENSION   25°
  (Subtalar joint
    unlocked)

FOOT

HINDPART
  (Subtalar joint)
INVERSION   5° passive motion
EVERSION   5° passive motion
FOREPART
  (Midtarsal joints)
INVERSION   30° active motion (includes supination, adduction, and flexion)
EVERSION   20° active motion (includes pronation, abduction, and extension)
                On passive manipulation of the forefoot (with the heel grasped firmly in the other hand) the range of motion is increased approximately five degrees.
ADDUCTION   20° passive motion
ABDUCTION   10° passive motion

Both the dorsalis pedis and the posterior tibial arterial pulsations should be palpable. Occasionally, particularly in the older individual, the dorsalis pedis pulsation will be absent. This absence, of itself, is not pathognomonic of any disease process as long as the posterior tibial pulse is strong and bounding.

Biomechanics. The biomechanics of the foot cannot be properly presented if the foot is considered as an isolated unit. After all, the foot is the link that transmits the forces of the body to the ground and, conversely, the ground reaction forces to the body in such a fashion as to provide constant adequate body stability. The foot, of necessity, therefore, acts as a flexible structure on some occasions and as a rigid lever on others. Furthermore, motion of the foot rarely, if ever, occurs in a single axis of rotation. It is a sequence of multiple coordinated movements through several axes. Therefore, in spite of the presentation of the various foot axes individually, one must keep in mind that they function as multiple units.

Manter in 1941 demonstrated that the axis of the subtalar joint passed from medial to lateral at an angle of 16 degrees to the longitudinal axis of the foot and 42 degrees to the vertical axis (Fig. 9-3). In addition Close and Inman proved that eversion of the joint occurs during the first 10 per cent of the walking cycle and then it goes progressively into inversion until the toe-off phase of the cycle. Wright and his co-workers substantiated these findings and also demonstrated that the amount of subtalar motion which takes place during the phases of the walking cycle varies with the angle of the ground, i.e., whether the individual is walking uphill, downhill, or on the level.

In the talonavicular joint there are two axes of rotation for the talar head: one for its long convex curvature and one for its short convex curvature. In the calcaneocuboid joint there are also two axes for the calcaneal surface. However, one is for its concave surface and one for its convex. From these observations, Elftmann in 1960 calculated the resultant axis and concluded

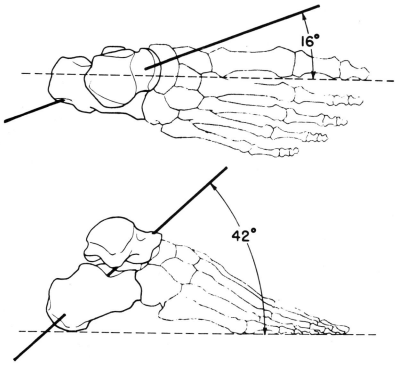

Fig. 9-3. Axis of subtalar joint. (Mann and Inman, courtesy of J. Bone & Joint Surg.)

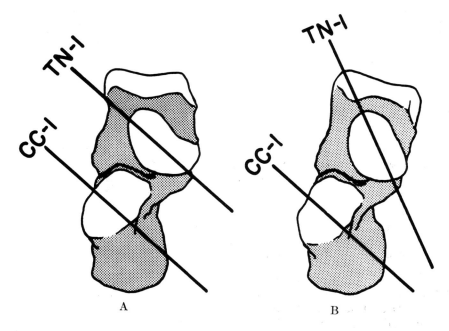

A

B

Fig. 9-4. Arrows represent resultant axes of rotation of the calcaneocuboid and talonavicular joints: A, pronated foot. When the resultant axes are parallel to each other, free motion of the talonavicular and calcaneocuboid joints is possible. B, supinated foot. When the resultant axes are divergent, motion is restricted in the transverse tarsal articulation since each individual joint has a different axis of rotation. (Mann and Inman, courtesy of J. Bone & Joint Surg.)

that these axes are parallel to each other in the flatfoot and divergent in the normal foot or in the inverted foot (Fig. 9-4). Since divergent axes provide greater stability, it is therefore obvious that the normal foot and/or the inverted flatfoot is more stable than the flatfoot per se. (There are additional axes in the foot that have been described by other investigators but are not as important in the understanding of the stability of the foot and therefore are not included in this discussion.) In addition to the position and relation of the talonavicular and talocalcaneal joints to one another, stability of the foot depends upon such active mechanisms as its intrinsic and extrinsic musculature as well as the passive mechanisms. These latter are the basic structural arches, their elastic ligamentous structures, and the plantar fascia.

Mann and Inman, in 1964, carried out electromyographic studies of the intrinsic muscles of the foot and demonstrated that these muscles act essentially as a single functional unit. Furthermore, the patterns of muscle activity proved to be different in the normal and the pronated foot only during level walking. The studies of these investigators also proved that the direction of the forces of the intrinsic muscles is, to all intents and purposes, parallel to the long axis and perpendicular to the transverse tarsal joints of the foot. They adduced that the activity of these muscles paralleled the progressive inversion of the subtalar joint and thus exerted considerable flexion on the forefoot. Hence these muscles are the principal stabilizers not only of the transverse tarsal joints, but also of the longitudinal arch.

Arches. The longitudinal arch consists of two components: the tibial or dynamic arch and the fibular or static supporting arch. The former consists of the talus, the portion of the os calcis supporting the talus, the navicular, the three cuneiforms and their corresponding rays. The latter consists of the os calcis, the cuboid, and the fourth and fifth rays.

In the standing position there is a transverse arch at the level of the tarsometatarsal joints. This gradually flattens out so that there is no arching of the foot at the metatarsophalangeal joints. In 1964 Schwartz et al. essentially substantiated my roentgenographic investigations which showed that there is no true metatarsal arch at the metatarsophalangeal joint level in the standing position. Schwartz demonstrated that all five metatarsal heads share in the weight bearing although there is some inequality as to the amount of the weight that is borne by each.

THE ADULT PRONATED FOOT

Pronation of the foot may be mild (first degree), moderate (second degree), or severe (third degree). At times, mildly pronated adult feet are more symptomatic than the completely flat ones. Frequently, it is the *pronating* foot that is symptomatic and not the pronated one. This symptomatology is usually due to poorly-fitted or poorly-constructed shoes.

Examination. It has been our experience that 85 per cent of the foot complaints in the young adult, as well as the older person, are due to problems of the forefoot. Therefore, the symptoms and therapy of the forefoot problems will be covered more fully in Chapter 19. They will be mentioned in this section when there is some close relation between the forefoot and the mid- and rearfoot complaints. In the adult a careful history should be procured to determine the location of the pain.

Subjectively, the patient will present a history which usually will have many, if not all, of the following complaints.

1. The feet feel somewhat stiff and sore when first arising in the morning. After taking several steps, the stiffness and soreness gradually disappear.

2. Usually by noontime or midafternoon at the latest, the feet again become painful, the greatest amount of discomfort being located along the medioplantar surface of the foot.

3. As the day progresses, the pain in the feet increases so that by nightfall it becomes quite severe.

4. With the increase of the symptomatology in the feet, the pain radiates to the back. (It is not common, but some patients will complain only of back pain which, on careful evaluation, proves to be due to foot pronation).

5. Frequently, the statement is made, "Doctor, when my feet hurt, I hurt all over."

6. The patient finds he has developed the habit of kicking off his shoes as soon as he gets home in order to experience some relief.

7. Some patients may complain of swelling of the feet and ankles after a day's activities particularly during the summer months.

8. In addition to the pain in the medioplantar and plantar aspect of the foot, some patients will also have pain under the second or third metatarsal heads with or without callus formation. The latter symptomatology is associated with an improper walking stance. It is found more frequently in females who wear high-heeled shoes constantly.

The objective examination should be a careful, methodical procedure. The following routine, with such modifications as one may wish to add, should be followed:

1. Observe the patient's walk with his shoes on. Does he come up on his toes with each step or does he use only the posterior three-fourths of the foot with each step? Are the heels of the shoes run down either on the lateral or the medial edge? Are the counters of the heels broken down? The examiner will frequently find that the older adults, particularly males, do not complete each step by coming up on the metatarsophalangeal portion of the feet and on the toes (the toe-off portion of the walking cycle). Also the patient with moderate-to-severe pronation quite frequently walks with the feet externally rotated more than 15 degrees. This type of gait causes the heel to wear down more rapidly along the lateral edge and the shoe to "run over toward the lateral aspect".

2. Following removal of the shoes and socks and trousers, the feet, legs, and knees, should be evaluated. Exposure of only the feet and ankles is insufficient. The patient should be asked to stand on the reflector stand in his accustomed position of standing. Do *not* suggest that he stand with his toes pointing directly ahead, with his feet parallel to one another, and with the knees touching. Let him assume his normal postural stance. The examiner should then observe if the patient presents any genu valgus of any consequence. More than 5 degrees in each lower extremity is above normal.

3. Is there any external tibial torsion (normal: less than 10 degrees for each leg)? An abnormal amount of external tibial torsion will place an undue strain on the foot and thus lead to pain and discomfort (Fig. 9-5A). For several years a twenty-two-year-old male had been complaining primarily of backache, as well as foot and leg pain. He had been treated with a lumbo-sacral support as well as corrective shoes but with no improvement. With the correction of his tibial torsion, his symptomatology referable to his back and both lower extremities subsided.

4. Is the navicular tubercle prominent, and if so, is it tender upon palpation? Prominence with associated tenderness of the navicular tubercle occurs with sufficient regularity in severe pronation to warrant careful evaluation.

5. In the standing position, is the foot pronated and, if so, how severely? In some patients one will find only a mild pronation, but accompanied by other findings, *e.g.*, external tibial torsion, contracted calf muscle, medial prominence of the rearfoot, etc., which lead to symptomatic feet.

6. Is the heel in valgus position, and is there an associated bow-stringing effect on the tendo achillis along with medial prominence of the rearfoot?

7. Are there severe varicosities present in the ankle and leg? One should realize that untreated varicose veins can cause foot and leg pain and can be very disabling.

8. Are there any deformities of the toes? Do they directly affect foot posture and contribute to the general symptomatology of the foot or are the symptoms due to the deformities only and completely localized, as in bunions?

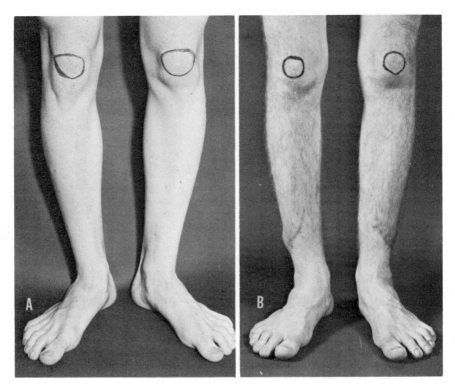

Fig. 9-5A.   Bilateral symptomatic feet, lower extremities, and back ache, due to external tibial torsion in an adult. Patient twenty-two-year-old male, photographs taken just prior to surgery.
   B.   Postoperative appearance nine months later. Patient is now asymptomatic. Such radical surgery should be considered only as a last resort after all conservative means have failed.

9. Observe the plantar aspect of the foot in the reflector. Are there any abnormal weight-bearing pressure areas with or without callus formation?

The feet should next be evaluated with the patient in a sitting position. One should have a foot stand on which to rest the leg in order to support the leg, ankle, and foot and also to free the examiner's hands so that he may examine the foot more easily.

1. Palpate the dorsalis pedis and the posterior tibial arteries on the dorsum of the foot and behind the medial malleolus respectively. No attempt will be made to describe the location of these pulsations specifically since this is knowledge that is gained while in medical school.

2. Determine the active and passive ranges of motion of the subtalar, tarsal, and metatarsophalangeal joints. There is only a trace of motion in the tarsometatarsal articulations. Limitation of inversion should be carefully evaluated since any restriction of this motion either unilaterally

or bilaterally is indicative of a pathologic condition in the subtalar region of the foot and is commonly known as "peroneal spasm". This condition will be discussed more fully in Chapter 19.

3. Inspect the plantar aspect of the foot to determine the location of callus formation or of any palpable masses. The evaluation of the plantar aponeurosis should be carefully performed to determine whether or not it is tight or shortened.

4. True passive extension should be tested since restriction of the foot in reaching the neutral position with the subtalar joints locked is indicative of a contracture of the triceps surae muscle group. Contracted calf muscles can and do produce pain in the feet and in the legs.

5. Should the navicular tubercle be prominent and painful, the examiner should palpate it to determine if the tubercle is movable as well as to evaluate the amount of tenderness present.

6. The presence of a bony prominence on

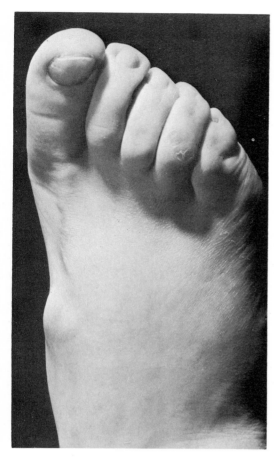

Fig. 9-6.   Dorsal Exostosis. Can occur at either tarso-metatarsal or naviculo-cuneiform joint.

the dorsum of the first tarsometatarsal joint or the talonavicular joint (Fig. 9-6) should be recorded. Also, whether it is or is not symptomatic. This prominence is an exostosis which develops at either of these two levels due to irritation produced by lacing the shoes too tightly or by other abnormal pressures. It can also represent a localized osteoarthritic process.

7. In spite of a negative history of any muscle weakness, muscle power of the four main groups of muscles should be checked. These are the invertor group consisting of the tibialis anterior and posterior, the evertors — namely, the peroneals, the extensors which comprise the long toe extensors and the tibialis posterior, and the flexor group consisting of the long toe flexors and the triceps surae.

8. Last, but not least, does the patient have diabetes or gout? The latter condition is discussed in detail in Chapter 16. Both of these systemic diseases can, at times, manifest themselves by the presence of pain in the feet. The examiner should always keep this possibility in mind, particularly in a patient whose feet are painful yet exhibit only minimal objective findings. The possibility of lead poisoning should also be kept in mind since pain in the feet and legs can be a precursor of this condition.

Following completion of the physical examination, standing roentgenograms of the foot or feet should be procured in the anteroposterior and lateral views, as well as an oblique view at rest. The salient points of the roentgenograms which should be evaluated are: 1) the relation of the various tarsal and metatarsal bones in the standing position; and 2) any pathologic changes and abnormalities which may aid in correlating the subjective with the objective findings.

At times, the examining physician may have a patient who may present minimal physical findings but who may still complain of markedly painful feet. In such situations a blood uric acid and blood sugar evaluation should be performed. I strongly advise that a blood uric acid examination be carried out routinely on all patients (male or female) who have a long-standing history of painful feet in spite of the use of various types of shoes, arch supports, or other external remedies. Gout, particularly the subclinical type, often manifests itself in the form of pain in the feet or in the low back area.

Treatment.   The therapeutic regimen to be prescribed will depend upon the correlation of the various subjective, objective and laboratory findings. Should the patient manifest any findings of a systemic disease, these should be evaluated and treated first before prescribing any corrective measures for the pronated feet. Varicosities should be treated either conservatively, with the use of supportive hose, or surgically in addition to treating the pronated feet.

External tibial torsion can, at times, produce foot, leg and back pain, although the feet may appear to be within normal limits on physical examination (Fig. 9-5A). This patient normally walked with his feet practically at a 50 degree angle in relation to his knees and with resulting foot pain due to the strain placed on his feet. On the other hand, when he attempted to walk with his feet in the normal position, he developed pain in his legs, knees, and low back, although his feet were comfortable. As a last resort, since all conservative measures had been exhausted, low derotation osteotomy of the tibia and high osteotomy of the fibula was performed bilaterally (September, 1964). Nine months after surgery, both of his lower extremities were asymptomatic (Fig. 9-5B). Such radical therapy should be performed *only as a last resort and only in a young adult who is still anxious to lead a vigorous active life.*

Absence of the dorsalis pedis pulsation in the presence of a normal posterior tibial pulsation is not necessarily an indication of circulatory disease in the foot. It does warrant, however, careful evaluation of the circulatory tree with at least a series of three oscillometric examinations at one-week intervals. If the readings are normal, the absence of the dorsalis pedis pulsations is of no great moment. One must not lose sight of the fact, however, that occasionally Buerger's disease (now more generally referred to as thromboangiitis obliterans or arteriosclerosis obliterans), as well as arteriosclerosis in the lower extremity, may first manifest itself as intermittent pain in the feet associated with activity.

At times in the adult female one will encounter the presence of pain in the feet and legs after a day's activity about the house. The patient will also state that she feels more comfortable in shoes with a heel of moderate height rather than in a low-heeled shoe. True passive extension is limited to between 10 and 15 degrees in such a patient due to contracture of the calf muscle group (triceps surae). Calf stretching exercises (as described in Chapter 7) will ameliorate this condition rapidly. Of course, if the feet are pronated, these should be treated as well.

In teenagers, prominent navicular tubercles with or without accessory scaphoids can be symptomatic and at times do require surgical intervention. In the adult, however, surgical extirpation is seldom, if ever, indicated. Almost invariably, the pain is due to pressure from the shoes on the tubercle. Fitting of a U-shaped pad in the inner side of the shoe to relieve the pressure on the tubercle usually renders the foot symptom free. Should this therapy fail to relieve the pain, excision of the accessory scaphoid, with or without the navicular tubercle, is indicated. The tibialis posterior tendon is transplanted to the plantar aspect of the navicular (Kidner procedure).

If the patient presents a symptomatic flat or pronated foot which is due to a musculoligamentous relaxation, a talonavicular or a naviculocuneiform sag, the treatment will depend upon the flexibility of the foot. This regimen of therapy does not apply to the so-called spastic peroneal flatfoot (talonavicular syndesmosis). This is a separate entity. It will be presented in detail in Chapter 19. The symptomatic pronated foot in the adult is at times a challenge, but it can also be an anathema.

If the foot can be inverted on passive manipulation or by adducting the rearfoot through the subtalar joint and pronating the forefoot, the tarsal and metatarsal bones can be realigned to form a normal-appearing longitudinal arch, an external support will be helpful. In such a patient a properly-fitted longitudinal arch support composed of rubber or cork and reinforced with spring steel stays (Fig. 9-7) will give appreciable relief. The arch support must be made to order. The insertion of an arch support in a patent's shoe on the basis of the shoe size is utterly useless. It is a waste of the patient's money, his efforts, and the physician's time. No two pair of feet are alike. In fact, no two feet are similar. Why then apply a pair of arch supports which are exactly alike and expect the patient to gain any relief from his symptoms?

The amount of elevation to be prescribed in the arch support will depend on the severity of the pronation and the flexibility of the foot. One should begin with a moderate amount of raise, usually 1/2 an inch. The patient should be advised that for the first twenty-four to forty-eight hours his symptomatology will be increased because of the realignment of the tarsal bones. After

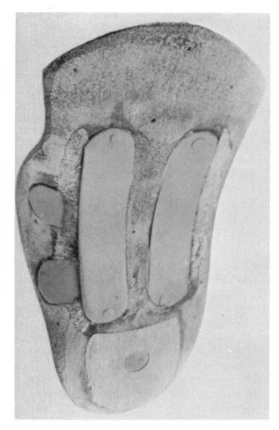

Fig. 9-7. Structural appearance of leather and cork longitudinal arch support with spring steel stays.

make it comfortable. The patient should be placed on a monthly follow-up basis for a period of three months. If by this time the feet are quite comfortable, the patient should be advised to return once a year in order to be refitted with a new pair of arch supports. Whenever new supports are ordered, a new imprint of the feet should be taken. The addition of a metatarsal support will depend upon whether the patient has metatarsalgia associated with the pain due to pronation. It frequently occurs concomitantly.

Are steel arch supports ever prescribed for an adult to support pronated feet? The answer is: practically never. Occasionally, one may see a patient complaining of painful feet which are absolutely flat. On examination there is some restriction of motion in all directions in the subtalar and midtarsal joints accompanied with pain. Blood uric acid test, sedimentation rate, and blood sugar test, as well as all other physical findings, are negative. Roentgenographically, the feet are pronated in the standing lateral view, but not due to malalignment of any one particular articulation. It is a general relaxation and pronation. There may or may not be minimal osteoarthritic changes demonstrable. In such a situation a plaster mold of the foot in a standing position is procured. When the positives are made on which the arch supports are to be constructed, the brace maker should be advised to raise the longitudinal arches not more than 1/8 of an inch. In other words, a steel brace is made simply to give the feet sufficient support to render them comfortable. Under no circumstances should one attempt to correct such feet to a normal contour. It is not only impossible, but such an attempt will render the feet even more symptomatic.

Daily contrast baths (wherein the feet are soaked alternately for thirty seconds first in fairly warm water up to the point of tolerance and then in cold water, for a period of ten minutes, followed by massage and manipulation of both feet by the patient) do help to relieve some of the soreness. This is particularly true after a hard day's activity. Salicylates are an effective adjuvant. However, these are at best only temporary measures of relief and do not

this period of time the pain will gradually subside until his feet become relatively comfortable. The patient should be advised that as his feet become totally asymptomatic, he will continue with the use of the initial arch supports prescribed for him. Should he experience moderate, but not complete, relief of his foot symptoms within a three-month period, then a new pair of arch supports with a higher elevation will be ordered for him and fitted in his shoes. The large majority of patients with this type of feet will experience practically complete relief. Minor adjustments of the supports may be necessary to make them more comfortable. At times, the support may press a trifle too much in one particular area of the foot. This will require a slight lowering of the arch support in that particular location; in fact, just enough to produce permanent results. Of course, if the patient is over-weight, and many of them are, this should be corrected to relieve the excessive pressure on the feet. Nor should the physician accept the flimsy excuse that "no matter how hard I try, I can't lose weight". Obesity is due to excessive caloric intake. If the patient is not interested enough in his own well-being to follow a prescribed diet, then the physician should not waste his time attempting to render the feet asymptomatic. Most patients will be cooperative providing the physician is firm in his attitude. In such circumstances, the patient should be referred to his own family physician or internist who should be requested to conduct a careful general physical evaluation and then place the patient on the limited caloric intake that will be required for the proper weight loss.

All manner of quackery has been practiced in the past on the unfortunate individuals who suffer from painful feet. And this is because few orthopaedists are interested sufficiently to take the time required to evaluate and prescribe for the adult afflicted with the problem of painful feet. If the patient is advised, after thorough examination, that the therapeutic regimen which will be prescribed for him will relieve most of his symptoms but will not cure him, he will be most cooperative. The physician must make a sincere effort to make the patient as comfortable as possible. In a certain number of these people, no matter what one tries in his attempt to relieve their disability, nothing helps. In such a situation an honest discussion of the problem with the patient will help the latter understand and, to some extent, accept his disability. As a desperation measure, walking casts may be applied with the feet in the corrected position and worn for six weeks. Should this treatment render the feet asymptomatic, fitted cork or rubber arch supports with spring steel stays should be then prescribed. Occasionally, this regimen dose gives effective relief.

Frequently, patients with symptomatic feet will present only a minimal amount of flattening of the longitudinal arch on examination. This type of a situation usually requires nothing more than a well-fitted steel shank shoe with a 1-1/4 inch heel to which is added a Thomas modification of an inner heel elevation of 3/16 of an inch and an inner heel flare of 1/4 of an inch. A rubber cookie commensurate with the length and width of the longitudinal arch may be inserted in the shoe as additional temporary support, although it is usually unnecessary.

One final reminder — order a blood uric acid test *routinely* in an adult with symptomatic feet in order to rule out the possibility of gout.

BIBLIOGRAPHY

CLOSE, J. R., AND INMAN, V. T.: The Action of the Subtalar Joint. The National Research Council, Series II, Issue 24, May, 1953.
DU VRIES, HENRI L.: *Surgery of the Foot*, 2nd Ed., St. Louis, C. V. Mosby Company. 1965, p. 45.
ELFTMANN, H.: The Transverse Tarsal Joint and Its Control. Clin. Orth. 16:41-46, 1960.
KIDNER, F. C.: The Prehallux (Accessory Scaphoid) in its Relation to Flatfeet. J. Bone Jt. Surg. 11:831, 1929.
KIDNER, F. C.: The Prehallux in Relation to Flatfeet. J.A.M.A., 101:1539, 1933.
MANN, R. A. AND INMAN, V. T.: Phasic Activity of Intrinsic Muscle of the Foot, J. Bone Jt. Surg. 46A:469, 1964.
MANTER, J. T.: Movements of the Subtalar and Transverse Tarsal Joints. Anat. Rec. 80:397, 1941.
SCHWARTZ, R. P., HEATH, A. L., MORTON, D. W., AND TOWNS, R. C.: A Quantitative Analysis of Recorded Variables in the Walking Patterns of "Normal" Adults. J. Bone Jt. Surg. 46A:324, 1964.
WRIGHT, D. G., DESAI, S. M. AND HENDERSON, H. W.: Action of the Subtalar and Ankle Joint Complex During the Stance Phase of Walking. J. Bone Jt. Surg. 46A:361, 1964.

= 10 =

The Clubfoot

SAWNIE R. GASTON, M.D.

ELEMENTS OF DEFORMITY

As one views the clubfoot in a newborn, there are certain features of the deformity which are clinically apparent. The heel is in equinus with the tuberosity of the os calcis pointing cephalad, forming a conspicuous prominence behind the ankle joint. The heel and forefoot are swung medially in inversion with supination of the forefoot. The forefoot is adducted, supinated and flexed on the hindfoot. The total picture is one of equinus of the entire foot with varus of the heel in relation to the leg and varus of the forefoot in relation to the heel. This position of equinovarus is fixed and rigid and cannot be manually altered on first examination. Occasionally one finds a severe metatarsus adductus foot which appears to simulate a clubfoot but which is easily differentiated and must be differentiated, since it bears an entirely different prognosis in terms of length of treatment and end-result. The severe metatarsus adductus foot differs from the true clubfoot in one simple aspect: There is no fixed varus or fixed equinus of the heel. The heel can be manually placed in valgus and the foot easily extended (dorsiflexed) to normal. Regardless of how severe the forefoot adduction and supination may be, as long as the heel is supple, it is not a true clubfoot (Fig. 10-1).

Equinus

Clubfoot equinus occurs at both the ankle joint and the subtalar joint. It is extremely important in terms of correction to appreciate this fact. Anteroposterior and lateral roentgenograms of the untreated clubfoot in the newborn will show that the talus is in equinus in relation to the tibia and that the calcaneus is in equinus in relation to the talus. Correction of tibiotalar equinus can be brought about by extending (dorsiflexing) the foot over a period of time. Correction of the talocalcaneal equinus cannot be corrected by extending the foot until the varus position of the calcaneus beneath the talus is corrected.

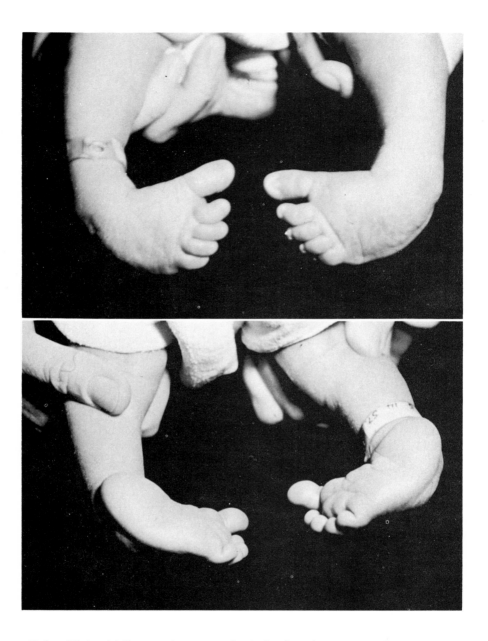

Figure 10-1. Bilateral talipes equinovarus prior to treatment.

Varus

Clubfoot varus occurs at the subtalar joint, the midtarsal joint and the tarsometatarsal joints. Heel varus is due to the relationship of calcaneus to talus at the subtalar joint. The anterior part of the calcaneus is tilted downward and rolled under the head of the talus and fixed in this position. This is apparent in the anteroposterior x-ray view of the clubfoot. This view shows that, whereas normally the long axis of the talus heads in the direction of the first metatarsal ray and the long axis of the calcaneus heads in the direction of the fourth and fifth metatarsal rays, in the clubfoot the axes of talus and calcaneus are superimposed and both are directed toward the lateral border of the foot.

The navicular, at the midtarsal joint, is displaced medially on the talar head. This relationship is obscured by the absence of the ossification center of the navicular on radiologic examination of the infant foot, but the axis of the first metatarsal to talus runs through the cartilaginous navicular and the projection of this axis of first metatarsal to talus interpolates the medially displaced position of the navicular. This observation is confirmed when one operates on a fixed varus-foot and finds that the medial articular portion of navicular is uncovered by the more laterally placed head of talus and that the navicular is partially dislocated medialward on the head of talus.

The other major element of varus is at the tarsometatarsal joints with adduction of the metatarsal shafts on the cuneiforms and cuboid through their capsuloligamentous structures. Furthermore, there may be actual bowing of the metatarsal shafts in varus which contributes to the deformity. It is unusual to see bowing of the metatarsals in a simple metatarsus adductus foot.

Etiology

Various theories involving genetic, environmental and anatomic factors have been advanced to explain the etiology of the clubfoot. Wynne-Davis concludes from her studies that the basis of the clubfoot does not fit into a purely genetic or purely environmental category. She found no recognizable pattern of inheritance to indicate a dominant, recessive, or sex-linked gene as the responsible factor. She suggests that the cause of clubfoot is partly genetic and partly environmental due to a factor acting on the fetus in utero. It is not known whether basic anatomic anomalies in the developing fetus are a cause of the clubfoot or a sequel to it.

In two studies by Wynne-Davis and Stewart the incidence of clubfoot deformity was found to be 1 in 1,000 births, and if one child in a family had the deformity, the chances of a second child being born with the same anomaly was increased to 1 in 35. The incidence of clubfoot is twice as high in males as in females.

Treatment

Only the relatively uncomplicated form of this congenital anomaly will be discussed. Patients with meningomyelocele and other neurogenic disorders, as well as those with arthrogryposis multiplex congenita, are omitted since these are extremely complicated cases to manage. Nevertheless despite this fact, these cases must not be abandoned. Treatment should be instituted at birth and persistently followed as in the less complex types. Correction will be achieved at a much slower rate, operative intervention is almost always necessary and the end-result must be evaluated with respect to the entire disorder.

Although the etiology of clubfoot is unknown, the problems inherent in its treatment constitute a familiar experience. The outstanding problems are the unpredictable response of the individual foot to correction, the necessity and difficulty of maintaining correction, and the potential for recurrence of the deformity even under diligent supervision. In my opinion no single solution for this problem is known other than a standardized method of treatment, vigilantly pursued and, ideally, *under the personal direction of the same physician from start to finish.* The proposed program of treatment is basically not new but what is fundamental and of paramount importance in order to insure uniformly good results is comprehension of the proper choice and administration of the various methods available.

THE PROPOSITION

Complete rapport between family and doctor is essential to the successful treatment of the clubfoot deformity. One must begin with explaining the defect to the parents and reassuring them that with their complete cooperation a nearly normal foot will result. It is also important to make clear that a clubfoot is not an inherited or inheritable deformity in the strict Mendelian sense. It has been shown by Stewart in certain ethnic groups that inheritance may be a factor. Moreover, if one sibling has a clubfoot, there is a greater than normal tendency for a subsequent sibling to have it also. Contrary to these published observations, not more than one child in the same family has had this deformity in the large series of children treated for this condition over a period of fifteen years by me at the New York Orthopaedic Hospital.

In the case of a child with unilateral clubfoot, it should be pointed out to the parents that, no matter how successful the correction may be, there are two unalterable sequelae beyond correction. One is that the circumference of the calf of the afflicted limb will be smaller than the opposite normal calf and the foot will be smaller than the opposite normal foot. These are minor defects in the overall picture and most parents accept them as unalterable.

It is also important to explain to the parents that correction is easily obtained in certain feet yet in other instances it is difficult to achieve even with the same methods. It can also be pointed out that in an infant with bilateral clubfeet one foot may prove to be more resistant to correction than the other although both are treated simultaneously by the same method to the same degree.

Once assured that a correction can be achieved by non-operative, or a combination of non-operative and operative means, the parents are generally willing to accept the essential need for their cooperation as a requisite to successful treatment. They must be told of the importance of not missing any arranged visits or discontinuing treatment and observation for *a minimum of seven years*. It is necessary and, in the long run, much easier on everyone if from the beginning the patients are aware of the duration of the proposed treatment. With the clinic patient, the language barrier or the level of understanding may require the cooperative vigilance of a Social Service Department to keep in touch with these patients and assist in their regular clinic visits. With this same group, the expense of the treatment is an important factor and the cost of equipment, such as shoes and splints, can be kept at a minimum or largely eliminated by developing a pool of discarded shoes and splints which can be loaned or given to these families with low income. This approach has worked most successfully in the clubfoot clinic of the New York Orthopaedic Hospital and does much to promote good will, cooperation and continuity of care.

The doctor's awareness of his responsibility in the treatment of the clubfoot is as important as indoctrination of the family. The methods which will be described require the doctor's insistence on weekly attendance for a minimum of four months from the initiation of treatment, possibly longer. Once a correction is obtained, it is essential to see the patient at least every three months until he is six years or more of age in order to detect any tendency toward recurrence of the deformity and alter the treatment according to the circumstances.

It has been our experience that few patients under such a conscientious program require operative treatment for persistent heel-varus. By and large, the clubfoot that gives us the greatest problem is one in which treatment was given early only to have the family leave the country or go to another city where treatment was discontinued due either to family circumstances, medical indifference or poor advice. Following such an experience, there is invariably a fixed deformity.

It is important to adopt a standard method of treatment with a regular progression and continuity of treatment along a well-thought-out plan with any alterations in the treatment made on specific clinical and roentgenographic criteria. Each step must be methodically pursued until the foot is ready for the next step. Surgery should not be undertaken without careful considera-tion of its indications and contraindications and its place in the treatment plan for the particular foot.

SEQUENCE OF CORRECTION

There are three basic elements of deformity in the clubfoot. They are forefoot varus, heel varus and equinus. The sequential correction of these three elements is of major importance. Equinus cannot be corrected until the varus is corrected because calcaneal equinus and varus beneath the talus at the subtalar joint are a concomitant deformity. The anterior part of the calcaneus, which is in equinus and varus beneath the talar head, cannot be brought out of equinus until it is brought out of varus. In simple terms: The anterior part of the calcaneus must be brought to a normal lateral position in relation to the head of talus before the calcaneus can be extended (dorsiflexed) in relation to the talus. This can best be illustrated by Figure 10-2. A and B can be studied simultaneously since A is a lateral view and B an anteroposterior view of an uncorrected clubfoot. A shows the calcaneus in flexion beneath the talus. B shows the axes of talus and calcaneus superimposed in the anteroposterior view. C and D can be studied simultaneously as they are the lateral and anteroposterior views of the corrected foot. C shows the more normal relationship in extension of the calcaneus in relation to the talus, and D shows the divergence of axes of talus and calcaneus, indicating a full correction of heel varus with the anterior portion of the calcaneus lateral to the anterior talus.

The achievement of this correction of the hindfoot deformity is the crux of the treatment of the clubfoot whether the correction is obtained by non-operative or operative means. As long as the calcaneus is in equinovarus in relation to the talus, the deformity will persist. Once this relationship is restored to normal by increasing the divergence of axes of talus and calcaneus as described, heel varus will be corrected and an element of equinus will be corrected. Further correction of equinus will require stretching of the calf or lengthening of the tendo achillis, as well as stretching or op-erative division of the contracted posterior capsule and ligaments of the talotibial and talocalcaneal joints. Further correction of forefoot adduction will require continued treatment with plaster, splint or surgical tarsometatarsal capsular and ligamentous release.

With this concept of correction as a guide, the forefoot and heel varus are simultaneously corrected by the application of a below-the-knee plaster cast over webril (or some similar rolled-on dressing) to protect the skin and bony prominences. We have not found it necessary to carry the plaster above the knee. As the plaster is hardening, the forefoot and heel are gently molded out of the varus position without using undue force and without causing the patient any discomfort. *There is no place for force in the correction of a clubfoot.* A fracture of the low shaft of tibia and fibula produced by forceful manipulation of a clubfoot in a newborn has been seen by the author. Unfortunately, the equinovarus deformity was corrected at the level of fracture. The foot deformity remained unaltered. This example is cited to emphasize that force is undesirable and can be harmful.

Treatment is started approximately two weeks after birth when the mother and child have been discharged from the hospital. It is well to commence on an outpatient basis, although if one wishes, plaster correction can be started while the infant is still in the nursery.

Removal of the plaster cast in the office by means of an electric saw is frightening to a child and such a practice spoils what might otherwise be a calm and quiet relationship between the doctor and patient. For this reason, the end of the plaster bandage is rolled back on itself a few turns, leaving a vertical ridge on the surface of the cast which can be marked along an edge. This will indicate the direction for lifting up the end of the plaster and un-

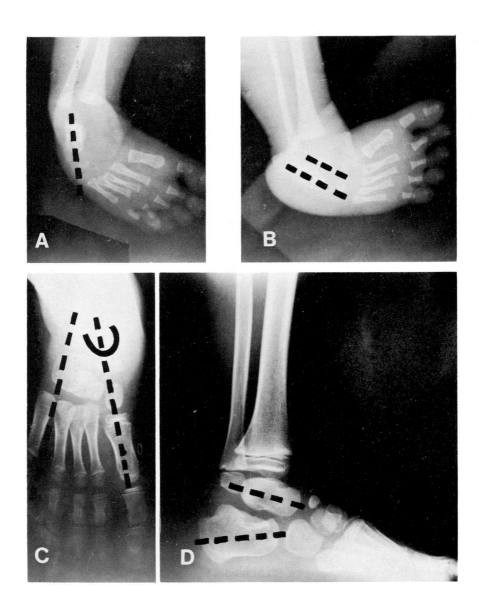

Figure 10-2.   Unilateral clubfoot before and after treatment.
   A.   Longitudinal axes of talus and calcaneus are superimposed and directed toward lateral border of foot.
   B.   Talus is in equinus beneath tibia and calcaneus is in equinus beneath talus.
   C.   Normal divergence of longitudinal axes of talus and calcaneus shows a full correction of varus.
   D.   Talus is in optimum dorsiflexion beneath tibia and calcaneus is in dorsiflexion beneath talus showing full correction of equinus.

winding the plaster bandage (Fig. 10-3). The mother is instructed to soak the plaster in warm water for approximately one-half hour the night before the next planned application of plaster. Thus when the plaster is soft, the mother can unwind it and remove it. This provides the child the privilege of a full bath and leaves the skin unencumbered overnight prior to the application of the next plaster.

Kite's method of wedging casts to correct the cavovarus deformity will also achieve the same result. The choice of the method of correction is left to the discretion of the individual orthopaedist.

Each week a new plaster is applied with further stretching of the forefoot and heel varus to a position of corrected valgus. It has been our experience that in about six weeks the foot is plantigrade enough to

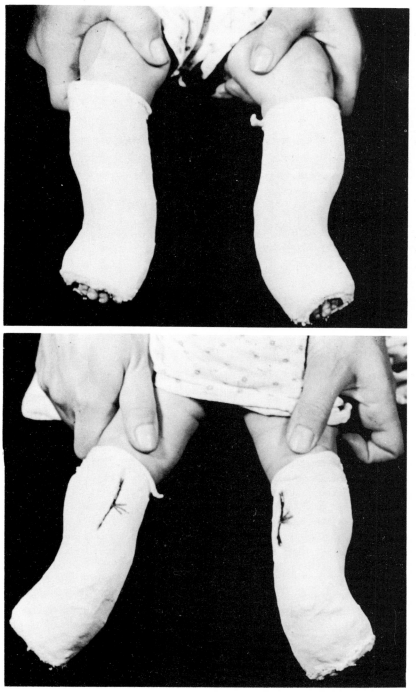

Figure 10-3.   Plaster cast correction of the varus deformity. The markings are a guide for the home removal of the plasters the day before each reapplication of the plaster casts.

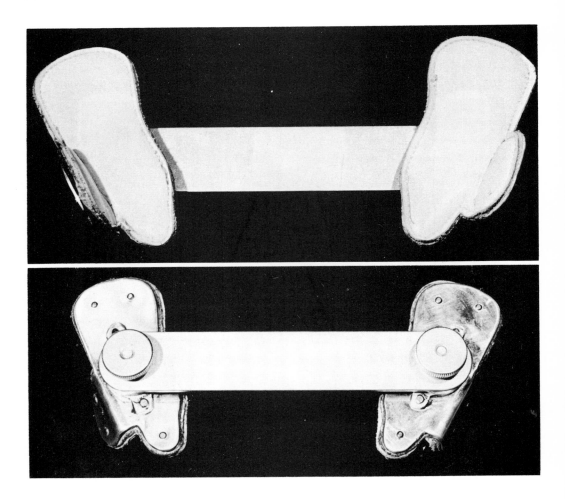

Figure 10-4.   Rubber or plastic covered foot plates and cross-bar used for the strapped-on kicking splint. The proper position of foot plates to bar and bend of the bar are illustrated in Figures 10-5 and 10-6.

permit a change from plaster correction to a strapped-on, crossbar kicking splint. The kicking splint is favored because it is a dynamic splint and the child assists in the correction of the deformity by the constant movement of his legs and feet attached to the splint. This method furthers the correction of varus and starts the correction of equinus.

Figure 10-4 shows the rubber-covered metal foot-plates of the strapped-on kicking splint and the crossbar. The lateral flange of the foot-plate is placed against the lateral aspect of the foot at approximately the calcaneocuboid articulation. It should be bent away from the plate so that the flange does not press into the lateral side of the foot and cause a pressure sore as the foot

goes into increasingly more valgus. The method of strapping the foot to the foot-plate is one of individual choice and is not important as long as the foot remains attached to the foot-plate until the next visit which should be a week later.

Correction is achieved by external rotation of the foot-plates on the bar and by a bend at the midpoint of the bar (apex distal) to produce an additional valgus influence on the treated foot. This midpoint bend is modified when treating a unilateral clubfoot to avoid ligamentous overstretching of the normal foot (Fig. 10-5). As the foot-plate is gradually externally rotated on the bar, it will be found that the varus and equinus will further correct in direct proportion to the degree of external rotation of the foot-plate to the bar. The circulation of the foot is the determining factor in how much the foot-plate can be externally rotated at any one time. As the foot is externally rotated, it will be observed that the toes become cyanotic if external rotation is excessive. One should apply the foot-plates and fasten them to the crossbar with a slight degree of external rotation of the plates to the bar. This child's foot is ob-

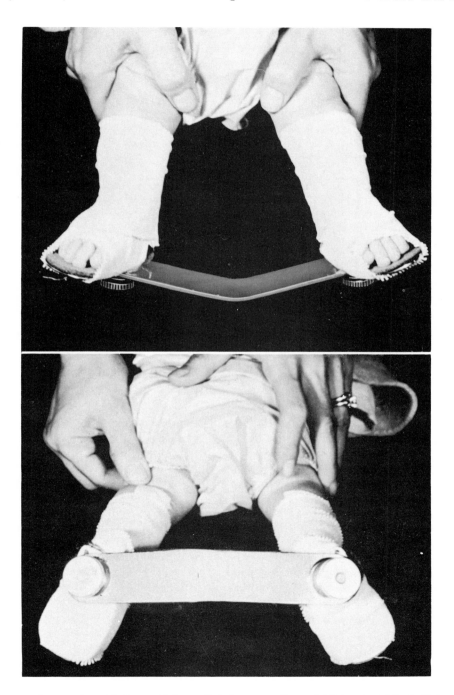

Figure 10-5. Strapped-on kicking splint applied for correction of bilateral clubfeet. Note valgus bend in middle of bar to evert feet. Recommended bend in bar for correction of unilateral clubfoot is shown in Figure 10-6C.

served for ten or fifteen minutes to make sure that the external rotation is not excessive and impeding circulation. Once assured of this, the physician may permit the child to go but sees the youngster again one week later for further external rotation of the foot-plates to the bar. A check on the color of the toes is used as the criterion of the degree of correction permitted on each visit.

Generally, except in excessively warm weather, the skin of the foot and leg of the infant will tolerate the same adhesive dressing for three weeks. At the end of three weeks, the foot-plates and adhesive dressing are removed. The skin will generally show slight maceration. To maintain correction and revitalize the skin, a retention plaster is applied over a soft roller dressing after the skin is sprayed with tincture of benzoin. The plaster is removed in one week. At this time the skin has recovered sufficiently so that another strapping of the foot to the foot-plates can be done if further correction is necessary, and it generally is. Experience has shown that it takes about six weeks of the actual strapped-on, crossbar splint to correct equinus.

At this stage, treatment will have been under way for thirteen weeks: Six weeks of plaster casts changed next week, and six weeks of the strapped-on, crossbar splint interrupted at the end of the first three weeks with an interim plaster for one week, and return to the strapped-on splint.

Correction of the equinus component by the use of a wedging cast can be, and usually is, as effective when applied properly. However, in our considered opinion, there is less likelihood of the development of a rocker-bottom deformity with the use of the crossbar kicking splint.

MAINTENANCE OF CORRECTION

If we may now assume that a full correction of the foot has been accomplished in approximately three to four months of the weekly treatment described, the next step in the logical sequence of management is the maintenance of the correction achieved. It goes without saying that, if no method of maintenance of correction is applied, the deformity will recur without exception. This can be guaranteed.

Correction is maintained by substituting the crossbar shoe-splint for the crossbar strapped-on splint. The shoes should be straight-last in design and the maintenance of correction is accomplished by two mechanical factors: One is external rotation of the shoes to the bar, and the other is a bend in the midpoint of the bar to evert the feet in a bilateral clubfooted infant, or an open lazy Z-bend in the bar which will exert a correcting force on the unilateral clubfoot but avoid ligamentous overstretching of the normal foot. These two types of application of the crossbar shoe-splint are illustrated in Figure 10-6.

The parent is advised to maintain the shoe-splint in place twenty-two hours a day, permitting the child two hours daily of freedom from this apparatus. This discipline is continued until the child is ready for walking, at which stage the splint is worn at night and a clubfoot shoe is worn during the day. The clubfoot shoe is a tarsopronator shoe. It is a high shoe with an out-flare, forefoot last to hold the forefoot in abduction. It also has an eighth-of-an-inch outer sole wedge, and a shank and heel wedge to give the foot slight eversion in walking (Fig. 10-7).

In some instances, the mother will call attention to the fact that the foot will not remain in the shoe or that a blister forms on the child's heel from use of the shoe splint. This is a legitimate complaint which requires thoughtful inspection. There are two main reasons for these occurrences. One is that the shoe is too small or too large. The other is that there remains an element of persistent fixed equinus. The former is easily corrected by an accurate fitting of shoe size for the individual foot. The latter indicates that adequate correction of equinus has not been obtained and further treatment of this element of de-

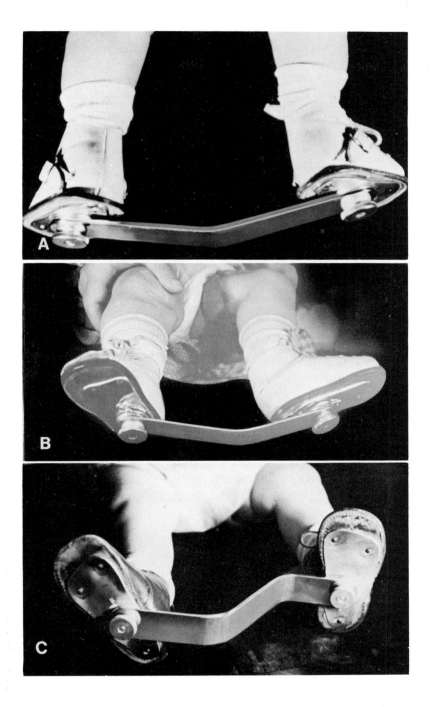

Figure 10-6.   Cross-bar shoe splint.
A.   Maintenance of correction of bilateral clubfeet. Valgus bend middle of bar and optimum external rotation of shoe plates to bar are shown.
   B.   The degree of dorsiflexion of the foot that can be achieved by exaggerated external rotation of the show plate to bar is demonstrated on the left foot.
   C.   Recommended double bend in bar to maintain correction of a unilateral right clubfoot without over-stretching of the normal left foot.
These illustrations are applicable to the strapped-on kicking splint as well.

formity must be undertaken before resorting to the use of the shoe splint. Fixed
equinus and the shoe splint are incompati-
ble. Unless the child's heel engages the
inside bottom part of the heel of the shoe,
the child can thrust with his forefoot in
flexion and work his foot out of the shoe.
It is useless to persist in forcing such a foot

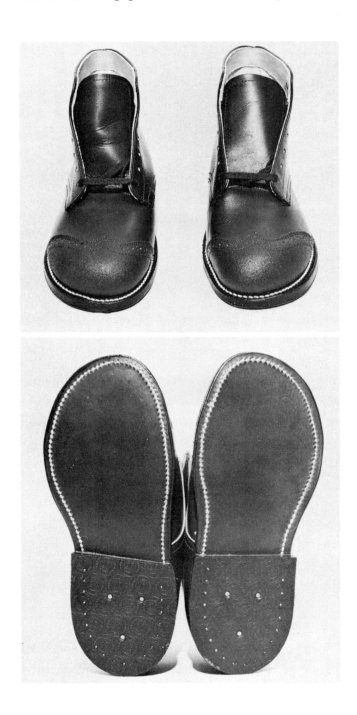

Figure 10-7.   Tarso-pronator shoes with forefoot out-flare last and ⅛ inch outer sole and heel
wedge.

to remain in the shoe by a strap over the tarsus or tight lacing of the shoe. Success in keeping such a foot in the shoe will only result in producing a rocker-bottom deformity of the foot. This is not only undesirable but also productive of an additional deformity which in itself will require special corrective measures to overcome.

If the failure of the foot to stay in the shoe is due to fixed equinus of the foot, correct the equinus by further use of the strapped-on splint, corrective wedging casts or by surgical means and then progress to the shoe splint for maintenance of correction. With equinus eliminated, there will be no difficulty in keeping the foot in the shoe provided the shoe fits properly. These factors also apply to excoriation of the heel with the use of the shoe splint.

The tendency for some children to remove the shoe from the bar can be overcome by setting the circular or wing nut with a wrench or pliers so that the child cannot unscrew it manually. For those children who untie the shoe laces and remove the shoes, there are obtainable barrel-shaped containers which screw together in two halves over the bow knot denying the child access to the knot.

Most infants can be persuaded by patient reassurance to tolerate the shoe splint, although an occasional child will perpetually blow up a storm with its use. This is primarily a matter of parental control of the child. Almost invariably, the child who will not wear the shoe splint will require early surgical intervention to achieve a correction and, even so, it will prove a problem in maintaining correction. Fortu-

nately, such a situation is infrequently encountered.

In a primarily well-corrected clubfoot, correction can be maintained in most instances by the wearing of a shoe splint for twenty-two hours a day until the child starts walking. Then the splint is applied at night and a tarsopronator shoe is worn throughout the day. The child is seen every three months and any indication of recurrence of equinus or varus can be dealt with by a return to serial plaster casts applied weekly to gently correct the recurrent deformity. Occasionally it may be necessary to decide that resistant equinus needs a soft-tissue release behind the heel or resistant heel-varus requires a soft-tissue release at the talonavicular and talocalcaneal joints.

The night splint and the clubfoot shoe should be worn until the child is at least five years of age and possibly longer in those cases treated non-operatively. Discontinuance of this discipline of maintenance of correction in a few patients who have moved out of town and then returned to us a year or two later has consistently shown a recurrence of deformity. This is why we arbitrarily choose the five-year period of this discipline as necessary to avoid recurrence and assure maintenance of correction. It cannot be overemphasized that the chief cause of persistent or recurrent deformity in the clubfoot is failure to achieve an initial full correction or a failure to maintain correction by premature interruption or discontinuance of treatment in the child, two, three and four years of age.

OPERATIVE CORRECTION OF RESISTIVE ELEMENTS OF DEFORMITY

It has been our experience that the previously described methods of conservative treatment of the clubfoot have been successful in well over half of the cases treated. For the remaining cases, it has been necessary to have many operative procedures for the correction of resistive elements of deformity. Each operation has clear-cut indications and contraindications which, if observed, will insure the desired result. There are many operative procedures, advocated for the treatment of the clubfoot.

However, we have stressed standardization of methods of conservative treatment of this deformity. We wish to be consistent and recommend standardized methods of operative correction based on the clinical indications. No attempt shall be made to oversimplify the individual selection of an operative procedure based on experience and conviction or to condemn the trial of many methods to serve a single objective. This would be to alter the nature of investigation and the nature of man. We have sought operative methods which would give consistent and predicable results. In our considered opinion there are three major procedures that we can rely upon to serve these ends. They are suited to correct the three main elements of deformity, namely: Equinus, heel varus and forefoot adduction as fixed deformities unresponsive to conservative correction.

Resistive Equinus

The most commonly encountered element of resistance is equinus. If at six months of age the infant treated by the described methods continues to show resistant equinus, there is little point in pursuing these methods further and operative correction should be undertaken without hesitancy. This is preferable to a continuation of closed methods of obtaining extension with persistent pressure on the dome of the superior articular surface of the talus since this can produce talar articular deformity (table top talus) and restriction of ankle motion. The determining factor regarding early correction of fixed equinus, no matter how desirable such a correction might be by early surgical release, is the age of the child equated to the anesthetic risk for an elective procedure. The decision to delay the operation, when necessary, until the infant is six months of age is based solely on this consideration.

The indication for the operation is resistant equinus which has not responded to a reasonable length of conservative treatment.

The contraindications are:
1. Fixed varus heel
2. Rocker-bottom deformity
3. Structural alteration of the talus.

Fixed heel-varus is characterized by an equinovarus position of the calcaneus beneath talus. This relationship must be corrected by conservative or operative means before proceeding with operative correction of equinus. Lengthening of the Achilles tendon and transverse division of the posterior capsule and ligaments of the ankle joint will correct talotibial equinus at the ankle joint, but will not correct calcaneotalar equinus at the subtalar joint. Therefore, it is necessary to eliminate heel-varus before operative correction of equinus (Fig. 10-8).

A rocker-bottom deformity can occur at the midtarsal or tarsometatarsal joints by attempts to force extension in the presence of fixed heel varus. A varus heel cannot be extended (dorsiflexed) and persistent attempts will force extension to occur elsewhere, usually at the midtarsal joint or, occasionally, as in Figure 10-9, at the tarsometatarsal joints. This iatrogenic deformity must be corrected prior to tendon lengthening and posterior capsulotomy to preserve the mechanical advantage of the foot as a lever in the postoperative plaster. When the forefoot is extended on the hindfoot, which is characteristic of the rocker-bottom deformity, then extension of the foot postoperatively cannot take full advantage of the foot as a lever and the heel will remain in some equinus. Accordingly the major advantage of the operation is dissipated. In the presence of rocker-bottom deformity, it is necessary to immobilize the foot in equinus in a below-the-knee plaster cast until the midtarsal ligaments or tarsometatarsal ligaments "take up," thus correcting the previous overstretching of these ligaments. This generally requires three months of plaster immobilization with the foot in equinus prior to operation.

Another method whereby correction of the rocker-bottom deformity is achieved, is also presented for the reader's consideration. Giannestras manipulates the foot into a position of extension. If the rocker-bottom deformity corrects completely as demonstrated by lateral roentgenograms, the following procedure is applicable. Following tibiotalar capsulotomy and lengthening of the Achilles tendon, insert a Kirschner wire, *centrally positioned* in the tuberosity of the calcaneus. Following closure of the transverse incision, apply downward traction on the wire to correct the equinus position of the os calcis. Simultaneously, apply downward extension pressure on the mid and forefoot to correct the rocker bottom deformity. Then apply a long leg cast with the foot held in the corrected position. The cast should be well-

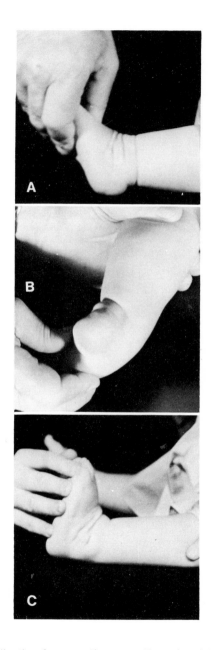

Figure 10-8.   The clinical indication for operative correction of resistant equinus is shown in A and B, but must be confirmed by x-rays taken as illustrated in Figure 10-13.

   A.   Pre-operative fixed equinus unresponsive to conservative management.

   B.   Absence of fixed heel varus. The foot is held with the heel everted to demonstrate that the heel varus has been corrected.

   C.   The same foot following lengthening of the Achilles tendon and transverse division of the posterior capsule and ligaments of the ankle joint.

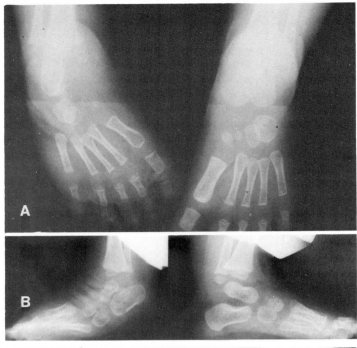

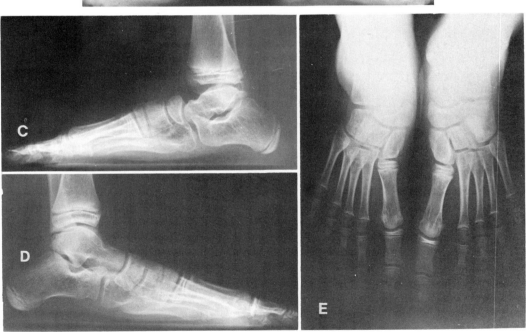

Figure 10-9. Rocker-bottom deformity produced by attempting to correct equinus before correcting varus.

A. Fixed varus of unilateral right clubfoot compared to normal opposite foot. Varus is identified by superimposed longitudinal axes of talus and calcaneus and medial displacement of forefoot at talo-navicular joint.

B. Rocker-bottom deformity at tarso metatarsal joint of the same foot secondary to persistent dorsiflexion of the foot in the presence of fixed heel varus. This iatragenic deformity will occur unless heel varus is corrected before starting correction of equinus. Comparison with normal foot shows equinus of talus in relation to tibia and further equinus of calcaneus in relation to talus.

C. The same foot six years later. The rocker-bottom deformity was corrected by serial changes of plaster for three months with the foot held in correct heel varus and a subsequent lengthening of the Achilles tendon and a posterior capsulorrhaphy at the ankle to correct equinus.

D. Normal opposite foot for comparison.

E. Compare with A. The treated right foot shows correction of the varus deformity and compares favorably with the normal left foot.

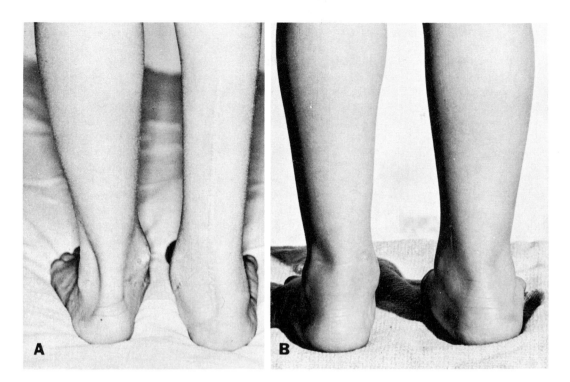

Figure 10-10. Transverse skin incision gives adequate exposure for operative correction of equinus and leaves a vastly superior scar compared with the longitudinal incision.
  A. Longitudinal scar is often longer than necessary and all to frequently becomes keloid.
  B. Barely perceptible scar of transverse incision on left.

molded about the heel, midfoot, and fore-foot with the wire incorporated in the cast. The knee is placed in 45 degrees flexion. Immobilization is maintained for six to eight weeks.

In those instances in which the talar dome is flattened secondary to the deformity or to treatment, it is possible that a tendon lengthening and posterior capsulotomy will not achieve correction of equinus because the architecture of the talus is so deformed that the talus cannot be dorsiflexed in the ankle mortise due to its altered structure.

To recapitulate, in the absence of fixed varus heel, a rocker-bottom deformity or altered structure of the talus, resistant equinus should, according to Gaston, respond most successfully to the following operation.

Lengthening of the Achilles Tendon and Posterior Capsulotomy of the Ankle and Subtalar Joints to Correct Equinus. *Op-*

erative Technique. A transverse skin incision from malleolus to malleolus posteriorly is vastly superior to a longitudinal incision in the axis of the Achilles tendon. The former heals with a barely perceptible scar, whereas the latter all too commonly heals with a keloid scar which, if extended too far distally, can result in annoying ulceration from shoe pressure on the back of the heel. The vertical incision with its keloid scar is particularly unsightly in the female patient. Also, the vertical incision is often made much longer than necessary. As the child grows, the eventual cosmetic result is a long scar up to the lower portion of the midleg, admitting an operatively generous exposure completely unnecessary to the operation and gaining an ugly lifelong cosmetic effect for the patient (Fig. 10-10).

The Achilles tendon is exposed and a lateral crosscut is made halfway through the width of the tendon proximally and a medial crosscut made halfway through the tendon distally. These two crosscuts are joined by a vertical incision through the midline of the tendon. The direction of the crosscuts preserves the lateral portion of the Achilles tendon attached to the os calcis which may be a factor in lessening the varus effect of the pull of this tendon on the os calcis. The distance between the two crosscuts is determined by the amount of correction of equinus desired. A simple rule is that the length achieved will be double the distance between the two transverse half-cuts in the tendon. Generally, 1½ to 2 inches of length between these transverse half-cuts gives a satisfactory lengthening.

Next the peroneal tendons are retracted laterally and the flexor hallucis longus, flexor digitorum communis and posterior tibial tendons with the neurovascular bundle are retracted medially. The posterior capsule of the ankle joint is then divided transversely from one malleolus to the other to include the posterior talofibular and talotibial ligaments. It is this division of the posterior capsule of the ankle which will accomplish the major correction of equinus. It is interesting to see how little is generally gained by the division of the Achilles tendon alone, and how much more is accomplished in terms of a full correction when the posterior capsule of the ankle is divided. If the degree correction is not satisfactory, that is, if the foot does not come up to 80 degrees or better of extension, additional correction can be obtained by dividing the posterior capsule of the talocalcaneal joint as well.

Closure is obtained by connecting the two loose ends of the tendo achillis with a fine chromic or silk suture and closure of the subcutaneous tissues (Fig. 10-11). The author prefers to close the skin with a subcuticular wire suture.

Postoperative Care. Postoperative correction is maintained with a below-the-knee plaster with the foot in as much extension as permitted by the tension on the transverse incision. The suture can be removed in about ten days to two weeks and further correction can be obtained at this time with a new plaster applied with a greater degree of extension of the foot. It is important, of course, to hold the foot in valgus as well as extension. Arbitrarily, about six weeks is chosen for the length of postoperative plaster immobilization to permit the Achilles tendon to heal.

Following removal of the plaster, the crossbar shoe-splint is reapplied, the use of which can be modified by clinical indication. It has been our experience that following this operation the use of the crossbar shoe-splint at night is required for a shorter period of time than in the nonoperated foot. The discontinuance of the night shoe-splint is a matter of clinical judgment depending on the ease of the maintenance of correction. Generally, following early posterior surgical release of equinus, it can be discarded when the child is approximately three years of age. Nevertheless the child must be followed every three months and the shoe-splint again recommended if there is any tendency to recurrence of deformity. While this operation does not permit one to dismiss the child as cured, it does permit modification of the length of treatment.

Resistive Hindfoot Varus

Resistive hindfoot varus is seldom encountered if a standardized, methodical and carefully supervised regimen of conservative treatment is pursued. It is usually seen in those cases in which treatment has been erratic without a design of continuity or methodology and particularly in those resistive cases in which a full correction of heel varus has never been obtained in the early stages of treatment. It is understandable, if a correction has never been achieved, that progression to a maintenance crossbar shoe-splint will fail. It is also understandable, if early correction has never been achieved, that progression to a maintenance crossbar shoe-splint will fail. It is also understandable, if early correction has been accomplished, that premature discontinuance of the crossbar shoe-splint will permit a recurrence of deformity. *We believe that heel varus can be corrected by conservative methods if this*

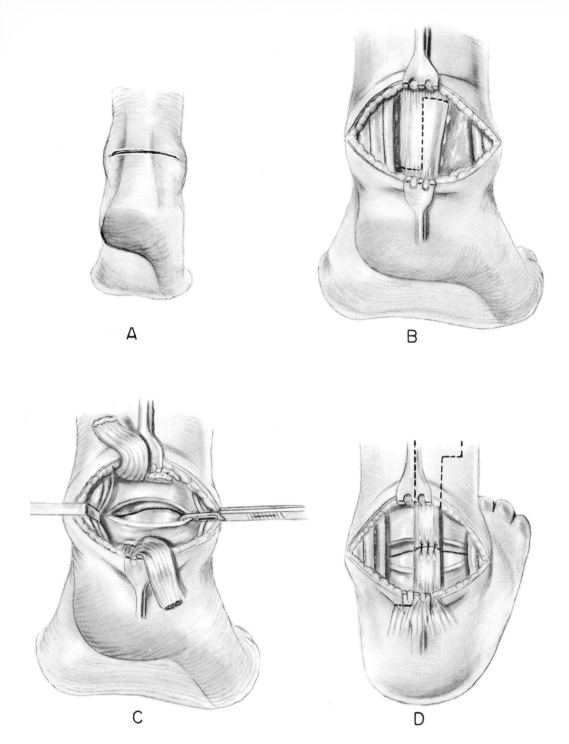

Figure 10-11. Operative technique for correction of resistant equinus.

A. Transverse skin incision at bimalleolar level.

B. Distal medial and proximal lateral half cuts are made in the Achilles tendon. The lateral portion of the tendon remains attached to os calcis.

C. Medial retraction of posterior tibial, flexor digitorum longus and flexor hallucis longus tendons and the neurovascular bundle. Lateral retraction of peroneal tendons. Transverse division of posterior ankle joint capsule and ligaments from medial to lateral malleolus. If necessary, to gain more correction, the posterior talo-calcaneal capsule and ligaments are also transversely divided.

D. Correction of equinus has been obtained. The capsular release is left open. The ends of the lengthened Achilles tendon are sutured and only the subcutaneous tissues and skin are closed.

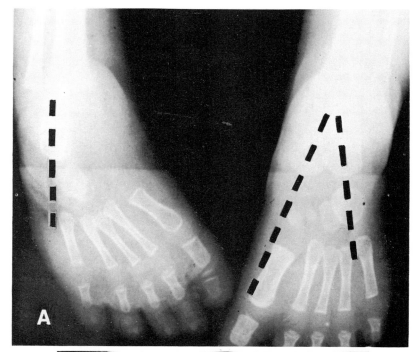

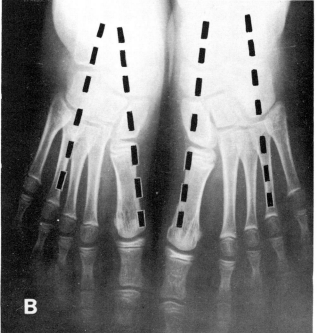

Figure 10-12.   X-ray evaluation of degree of heel varus
    A.   The normal divergence of axes of talus and calcaneus is lost with fixed heel varus and
these axes are superimposed in the anteroposterior x-ray view as seen on the right foot compared
to the normal left foot.
    B.   Same right foot following correction of varus by medial release compared to the normal
left foot.

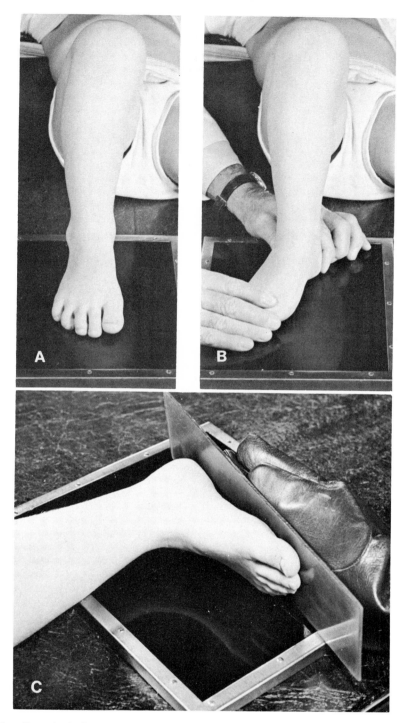

Figure 10-13. X-ray technique.

A. Anteroposterior view with foot in habitual posture, or at rest. The leg is at right angles to the edge of the casette and the sole flat against the surface of the casette.

B. Anteroposterior view with maximum correction of varus. Similar placement of the foot on the casette as in A. with the heel held firmly, the forefoot is forced into abduction. Lead gloves not shown in photograph should be worn.

C. Lateral view. Lateral surface of the foot is flat against the casette and the foot is held at the maximum of forced dorsiflexion by means of a board against the sole of the foot.

element of deformity is kept constantly in mind and its correction or failure of correction monitored by repeated radiologic examinations.

Although one has a clinical appreciation of fixed heel-varus, an anteroposterior roentgenogram of the foot is essential to establish the diagnosis and the degree of varus present. The normal divergence of axes of talus and calcaneus is lost with fixed heel-varus and these axes are superimposed in the anteroposterior roentgenographic view. Furthermore, the long axis of talus corresponds with the long axis of first metatarsal in the normal foot, whereas with heel varus it is directed toward the lateral border of the foot. This talocalcaneal angle with its relationship of axes of the talus and calcaneus to each other, together with the alignment of these axes with the metatarsals, establishes the degree of fixed heel-varus requiring correction. Unless these relationships approach normal, further correction is necessary (Fig. 10-12). The technique for taking these roentgenograms was described by McCauley in 1951 and is illustrated in Figure 10-13.

The indication for operative release of heel varus is a function of the type and duration of previous treatment and the age of the child. We have rarely performed this operation on children under two years of age, believing that conservative methods should be given a full trial in this young group. In those beyond the age of six years, correction of heel-varus by soft-tissue release is difficult to achieve and is not recommended. The ideal time is between two and six years of age, with the best results achieved in the younger child in this age group.

There are no contraindications other than the age of the child. The operation should not be performed to correct functional heel-varus and it will not correct forefoot adduction. Functional heel-varus can be ruled out by manipulating the heel into a position of valgus with anteroposterior roentgenographic confirmation that heel varus is not a fixed deformity. Fixed forefoot-adduction of severe degree requires a different operation and will be described later as the tarsometatarsal ligamentous and capsular release.

Equinus is not a contraindication and can be corrected concomitantly or staged as a later procedure. To follow a rule, however, equinus should never be corrected prior to the correction of heel varus for reasons previously stated.

The operation which has served most satisfactorily to correct this heel varus is the Gaston procedure.

Medial (Soft Tissue) Release for Correction of Hindfoot Varus. *Technique.* An incision is made on the medial side of the ankle and foot starting five cm. above the medial malleolus curving beneath the malleolus at a level with the subtalar joint and extending forward to the first cuneiform. The neurovascular bundle is identified and retracted inferiorly. The posterior tibial tendon is freed from its sheath well up behind the medial malleolus and is lengthened by Z-plasty. Its ends are retracted for subsequent end-to-end suture at the conclusion of the operation. The tendons of the flexor hallucis longus and flexor digitorum longus are released from their sheaths and their thickened and contracted sheaths excised.

The sustentaculum tali serves as a guide to the subtalar joint which lies directly above it. The crux of the operation now presents itself. A capsular and ligamentous release of the talonavicular and subtalar joints is performed to correct medial displacement of navicular on talus at the midtarsal joint and to dissociate the convergence of axial relationship of calcaneus to talus at the subtalar joint. The superior, medial and inferior capsule and ligaments of the talonavicular joint are divided to free the navicular. The calcaneonavicular spring ligament is divided. The medial and posterior capsule and ligaments of the talocalcaneal subtalar joint are divided and the subtalar joint pried open to permit division of the interosseous talocalcaneal ligaments. At this juncture, the forepart of the calcaneus is pushed laterally from its position beneath the head of the talus to occupy a more lateral position in relation to the talus. This maneuver converts the talocalcaneal axial convergence of varus to the axial divergence of valgus and accomplishes the correction by this shift. It is important to emphasize that a *divergence*

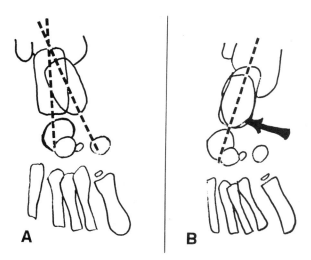

Figure 10-14. The crux of the medial release operation for the correction of fixed heel varus.
A. The purpose of the operation is to achieve divergence of the talo-calcaneal axes to a relationship as nearly normal as possible, together with a correction of the medial displacement of the navicular on the head of talus so that the axis of talus is directed to the first metatarsal and the axis of calcaneus is in line with metatarsals four and five.
B. Following surgical release of the capsular and ligamentous association of talus, calcaneus and navicular, the calcaneus and foot are externally rotated beneath talus on a vertical axis through tibia to accomplish the corrected relationships shown in A.

of the long axes of talus and calcaneus must be surgically accomplished to correct heel-varus (Fig. 10-14).

Prior to closure, a determination of the degree of equinus is made. If there is a significant element of fixed equinus one can, through the same incision, divide the posterior capsule of the ankle joint and lengthen the Achilles tendon. Or, if one prefers, the Achilles tendon lengthening and posterior capsulotomy can be performed six weeks later as a separate procedure. If, in correcting the equinus, it is found that the flexor hallucis longus is tight, thus producing fixed flexion of the great toe when the foot is extended, the flexor hallucis longus should be lengthened behind the medial malleolus.

Closure is accomplished by suturing the ends of the lengthened posterior tibial tendon and closure of the subcutaneous tissues and skin. The amount of valgus in which the heel may be placed is determined by the tension on the skin at the time of wound closure. It may be necessary to achieve less correction than the operation provides at this juncture and get the addi-

tional correction obtainable after the wound is healed in about two weeks.

It should be added that in severe heel-varus, although a correction cannot be obtained with plaster stretching alone, a degree of correction can be accomplished sufficient to permit adaptive skin-stretching on the medial side of the foot. This preliminary stretching of the foot prior to operative medial release will lessen wound healing complications.

Following application of a dressing and webril or sheet wadding, a plaster cast is applied to extend above the flexed knee. This is done with the foot in the degree of abduction and heel valgus permitted by previous testing of wound tension at the time of closure. If a lengthening of the Achilles tendon and division of the posterior capsule of the ankle have been performed concomitantly with the medial release, the foot should also be placed in as much extension as the incision permits. Further correction can be obtained when the wound is healed and the sutures removed by applying a new plaster with the foot in increased valgus and extension.

Postoperative Care. It is recommended

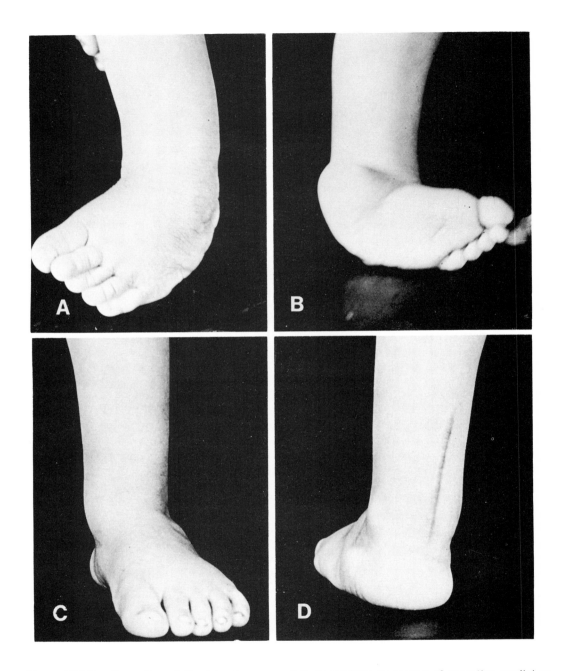

Figure 10-15.   Correction of fixed heel varus and fixed equinus by means of operative medial release and lengthening of the Achilles tendon and posterior capsulorrhapy of the ankle joint.
   A.   Pre-operative front view of the equinovarus deformity in a late case with inadequate treatment.
   B.   Pre-operative back view of the same foot. This is a classic example of the inadequately
treated equinovarus foot, demonstrating the potential for persistence of deformity or recurrence
of deformity if treatment is interrupted or terminated in a young child.
   C. and D.   Correction of varus and equinus by means of an operative medial release and Achilles
tendon lengthening and posterior ankle joint capsulorrhaphy at two years of age. Note keloid vertical scar in D.

that following a medial release postoperative immobilization of the foot in plaster be of at least twelve weeks' duration. If Achilles tendon lengthening and posterior capsulotomy are chosen as staged procedures, the foot can be reoperated for this indication six weeks following the medial release. This is followed by an additional six weeks of plaster immobilization, completing three months for the medial release and six weeks for the tendon lengthening and capsulotomy.

Having described an operation to correct fixed heel-varus, it might appear paradoxical to warn that too much correction of the varus can be achieved by this operation. An overcorrected varus is an unsightly deformity and the child walks with marked heel-valgus and marked prominence of the medial malleolus. Care should be taken during postoperative casting to prevent too much valgus. Moderate heel-valgus is desirable as an end result. but exaggerated heel-valgus is to be avoided.

Following removal of the plaster three months after operation, the crossbar shoe-splint is again used at night but should be monitored carefully so as to prevent overcorrection. The length of time that it is used in terms of the age of the child is a matter of clinical judgment. It is usually sufficient to observe the child until he is seven years of age. During the daytime, the clubfoot shoe is worn in both the non-operated and operated cases until a stable and permanent correction is achieved (Fig. 10-15).

Resistive Metatarsus Adductus

Some slight degree of residual metatarsus adductus is accepted in correction of the clubfoot. Also, some degree of hallux varus is frequently seen and is not important. However, if there is severe metatarsus adductus as a residual deformity, it should be corrected.

Definition of metatarsus varus and metatarsus adductus should be clarified. Generally, one sees pure adduction of the forefoot as a deformity once a major correction of the entire foot has been achieved. The term varus indicates an element of supination as well as adduction and this is infrequently seen in the overall corrected clubfoot.

Persistent metatarsus adductus is generally most apparent when the child first walks and, at this age, correction of the forefoot adduction by serially applied stretching plasters is extremely difficult, if not impossible to accomplish. Furthermore, the use of the crossbar shoe-splint does not accomplish a correction of fixed metatarsus adductus. In fact, inasmuch as the crossbar shoe-splint is used every night and the metatarsus adductus persists, it is proof enough that the device will not correct this deformity. If the metatarsus adductus is of such a degree that it is unsightly and produces a marked in-toeing gait, it should be corrected operatively. In our hands the most successful operation for this purpose has been the ligamentous and capsular tarsometatarsal release of Heyman.

Tarsometatarsal Ligamentous and Capsular Release (Heyman Procedure) Heyman and his co-authors have not established either an upper or a lower age limit at which the operation may be indicated or at what age it will no longer be effective. They reported their conclusions following 20 operations for the correction of metatarsus adductus as a residual deformity in clubfoot cases spanning ages from two-and-one-half years to seven years, with most of their cases between three years and seven years of age. Since they found that the operation did not endanger bone growth, they could think of no reason why it should not be done earlier than three years of age if necessary. In fact, they favored early operation in patients whose deformity was proving most resistant to correction by other means. They have also noticed that in most of the cases, incongruity of joint surfaces is demonstrable after correction has been achieved by capsulotomy, but that remodeling occurs at a fairly rapid rate. They consider the operation decidedly preferable to radical osteotomy, tarsometatarsal arthrodeses or a bone or joint resection in the still young child.

We have demonstrated an excellent

correction in a child ten years of age with noticeable incongruity of the tarsometatarsal articulating surfaces at the time of capsulotomy. This did not preclude an excellent result one year following operation. Roentgenograms showed adaptive modeling of the previously observed joint incongruities.

It is important to point out that this procedure is designed solely for the purpose of correcting resistant forefoot adduction. Other procedures may be necessary, such as a soft-tissue medial release to correct heel varus, or a later triple talar arthrodesis to correct heel deformity in the older child. This should be emphasized. *The soft-tissue medial release is designed for the correction of heel varus and will not correct forefoot adduction. The tarsometatarsal release is designed for the correction of forefoot adduction and will not correct heel varus.* There is a separate indication for each procedure. Heyman and his co-authors have done both a soft-tissue medial release and tarsometatarsal capsulotomy as a single procedure and advise against it because of the extensive dissection and long incision. It was found to be too much surgery for a single procedure on a small foot. This would also apply to performing the Heyman procedure in an older child simultaneously with triple talar arthrodesis. The operations should be staged, each with its individual indication. It would be our choice to correct the heel varus first by medial soft-tissue release or triple talar arthrodesis, depending on the child's age, and then assessing the residual deformity of forefoot adduction and correcting it by the Heyman procedure later.

Operative Technique for Tarsometatarsal Capsular and Ligamentous Release. The operative technique of Heyman and his co-authors has been adhered to by us. Diagrams of the operation are available (see reference in bibliography at the end of this chapter). A transverse curvilinear incision with the curve projected distalward is made from the first metatarsocuneiform joint to the fifth metatarsocuneiform joint on the dorsum of the foot. This incision is in the skin lines of the foot and has been free of wound healing complications. The anterior tibial tendon is identified and protected. A longitudinal incision is made in

the deep fascia over the first metatarsocuneiform joint. The dorsal and interosseous ligaments and joint capsule are cut by a deep incision carried about the base of the first metatarsal, taking care not to injure the anterior tibial tendon. The metatarsal is flexed so that a knife may be inserted across the joint to cut the capsule and ligaments on the plantar aspect. It is also important to cut the intermetatarsal ligaments. Another vertical incision is made between the second and third metatarsals, taking care not to injure the extensor tendons. The second metatarsocuneiform joint is found with care and patience just proximal to the level of the first metatarsocuneiform joint. Once this relationship is established, the other tarsometatarsal joints are not difficult to identify. The same procedure is carried out on the dorsal, interosseous and intermetatarsal ligaments and the plantar capsule and tarsometatarsal ligaments of the second and third metatarsals. Next, a longitudinal incision is made between the fourth and fifth metatarsals. The metatarsocuboid joints are identified and their ligaments and capsules similarly divided. During the dissection one should excercise great care to identify the medial, intermediate, and lateral dorsal cutaneous nerves of the foot.

After the ligaments and joint capsules of the intermetatarsal and tarsometatarsal articulations are cut through thoroughly, the forepart of the foot will swing outward at the tarsometatarsal joints without much resistance. The skin is then closed and a well-padded plaster cast is applied with the forepart of the foot held in as much abduction as possible, with care taken to avoid eversion of the heel.

Two weeks following operation, the plaster and sutures are removed. If additional correction is desirable, it can be obtained at this time. It has been recommended by Heyman *et al.* that the foot be immobilized in a plaster cast for three months following operation. Unpublished communications with other surgeons and our own experience recommend that the plaster cast be worn for a minimum of four months to prevent recurrence of deformity. It has been suggested that, at the time of operation, a transfixion wire can be placed from the first metatarsal into the first cuneiform to prevent recurrence of deformity, but this has not been our practice to date. Following removal of the sutures and reapplication of the plaster cast, the child should be encouraged to bear weight. Such a practice has not had a deleterious effect on the correction or

healing and it seems a desirable measure.

The results of this procedure have been uniformly good and have provided a foot which appears normal or which is satisfactory to both surgeon and parents. Any slight residual forefoot adduction has proved insignificant, both in the appearance and function of the foot.

CORRECTION OF DEFORMITY IN THE OLDER CHILD

The prevention of residual deformity in the older child by utilization of the methods of treatment thus far described is superior to the methods of correction available for the older age group. However, certain cases within our own experience, as well as other cases which come to us late with residual deformity, demand correction and we must provide methods to salvage these cases.

The non-operative and operative methods already described should, by the time the child is six years of age, have accomplished a corrected foot granted continuity of care and prompt surgical intervention when indicated. Once the child is six years of age, the correction of equinus and heel-varus by a soft-tissue procedure can be very difficult and can give less than a desirable result or fail completely. As mentioned, the tarso-metatarsal release can be performed in the child older than six years of age. This is not true for the correction of equinus because of architectural changes in the talus which, beyond the age of six, may prevent extension of the foot at the ankle because of the articular incongruities of the talus and the ankle mortise. The oldest child operated for correction of equinus by soft-tissue technique was nine years of age. He had had a previous lengthening of the Achilles tendon and posterior capsulotomy of the ankle joint. In the standing position his heel failed to touch the floor by approximately 1 inch. Roentgenograms of the talar dome showed that it was not flattened and, as the equinus was of an undesirable degree, correction was undertaken. In addition to lengthening the Achilles tendon and division of the posterior capsule and ligaments of the ankle and talocalcaneal joints, it was also necessary to lengthen the peroneus brevis and peroneus longus and the flexor digitorum longus and tibialis posti-

cus to bring the foot to 90 degrees of extension. The result was satisfactory and the patient walked with his heel engaging the ground.

A medial release is difficult to perform in a child past the age of six because of the established relationship between the talus and calcaneus and the difficulty encountered in doing a ligamentous release sufficient to effect a correction of heel-varus. It has been suggested, although it is not within our experience, that in patients past six, a medial release can be performed if the subtalar joint is approached through bilateral incisions and bilateral dissection of the talocalcaneal ligaments.

We do not recommend surgical correction of persistent equinus or persistent heel-varus between six and ten years of age. We have no alternative surgical approach to the correction of these deformities until the child is ten and reaches sufficient bone maturity to warrant a triple talar arthrodesis. From procedures described in the literature and through personal communications we are aware of astragalectomy, calcaneal osteotomy and excision of the calcaneocuboid joint. We have no experience with these procedures.

Astragalectomy, whatever it may accomplish in correction of deformity in a growing child, can subsequently present a serious problem to the adult. If tibiocalcaneal fusion is necessary in the adult, due to pain and malfunction following astragalectomy during childhood, it is a difficult fusion to accomplish. We have rejected any procedure in the growing child which, although it may be currently of corrective value at the time of operation, may in the adult present a serious problem in the area by loss of working stock for a later and better reconstructive procedure.

We cannot lend support to calcaneal wedge osteotomy as described by Dwyer because it is a contradiction in principle. The operation proposes an osteotomy of the calcaneus and insertion of a wedge to correct heel-varus and equinus independent of the altered relationship of calcaneus to talus at the subtalar joint and navicular to talus at the midtarsal joint. Conceptually, it is difficult to visualize how a procedure can succeed when it basically disregards the morbid anatomy of the deformity. It can only succeed in replacing one deformity with another, leaving the talocancaneal and talonavicular malalignment unresolved. A more logical choice of treatment, which deals directly with the distorted anatomy, is a medial and posterior soft-tissue release in the child two to six years of age and a triple talar arthrodesis in the child ten years of age or older.

Dillwyn Evans reports satisfactory results with excision of the calcaneocuboid joint, combined with a medial and posterior soft-tissue release. He performed this operation in the age group from three to fourteen years with most of the 30 feet operated in the group in children four to seven years of age. This operation adheres to full recognition of the elements of deformity and adds wedge excision and rotation of the calcaneocuboid joint to correct cavus, rockerbottom deformity and midtarsal joint varus as indicated. We have no experience with this operation, but it is another procedure advanced to accomplish the same result which we feel can be accomplished in the younger child by the posteromedial release alone and by triple talar arthrodesis in the older child. Further experience with the Evans procedure may earn it a firm place in the management of the equino-varus residual deformity in the child six to ten years of age.

However impatient one may be to do something for the patient between the ages of six and ten, the reward of patience is to preserve the working stock and make possible a procedure which is anatomically sound in the correction provided and clinically predictable and permanent in the result achieved. Therefore, with children between the ages of six and ten, we do not operate on the residual deformity in the hindfoot, including the midtarsal joint malalignment. We prefer to wait and do a triple talar arthrodesis when they reach the age of ten, or as soon thereafter as bone maturity permits. The one exception is a tarsometatarsal and intermetatarsal capsular and ligamentous release for significant forefoot adduction. This is an excellent procedure for this age group when indicated.

TENDON TRANSPLANTATION

The proponents of tendon transplantation endorse the theory that the recurrence of deformity in a previously corrected clubfoot is due to muscle imbalance. They reason that the peronei are weakened by improper development or improper innervation, either of which could develop in utero, or to over-stretching due to the fact that the peronei occupy the dorsal and lateral aspect of the convexity of the varus foot. On the other hand, the tibialis anticus and tibialis posticus are inserted in a much more straight-line relationship with the medial concave side of the deformed foot and are not so influenced in the attenuation of their length and strength. Such reasoning is subject to critical evaluation: Whether or not the peronei are weak, causing the clubfoot, or are weak as a result of the deformity. Or, stated another way, the anterior tibial and posterior tibial muscles and their tendons constitute a deforming force. Either argument justifies tendon transfer if muscle imbalance is the main causative factor in the recurrence of a previously corrected clubfoot.

Tendon transplantation has been used infrequently in our clinic and we have been pleased with our results without need of tendon transplantation. We, therefore, feel justified in substituting our clinical experience for a theory.

The maintenance of correction of a clubfoot depends primarily on accomplishing a full correction, both clinically and radiologically in the first instance. In those resistant cases in which non-operative methods have failed to accomplish a full correction, we have been able to accomplish a correction, confirmed radiologically, by means of the soft-tissue medial release and lengthening of the tendo achillis and posterior capsulotomy of the ankle joint. We have also insisted that the crossbar shoesplint be used at night following surgical correction to maintain the correction. Under such circumstances, we have found that the strength of the peronei improved and, subsequently, the child could evert the foot against moderate resistance. With these facts known to us, we cannot subscribe to the idea that weakness of the peronei permits a recurrence of deformity nor can we justify tendon transplantation with one notable exception.

A fully-corrected foot is plantigrade in the stance phase of gait. Such a foot may show some inversion and supination of the forefoot in the swing phase of gait. This inversion of the foot in the swing phase of gait does not interfere with the function of the foot, but may offend the observer's eye. If this is to be an indication for tendon transplant, it is, indeed, an extremely sophisticated one. However, there is no question that transplantation of an invertor muscle and tendon to the lateral border of the foot will correct this situation. We repeat that we do not believe that the recurrence of the deformity is as much a function of muscle imbalance as failure to achieve a full correction. We do believe that the posterior tibial tendon is a deforming force and we do believe that the triceps surae is a deforming force. However, we are assuming that by medial release and Achilles tendon lengthening and posterior capsulotomy these deforming forces have been negated or they have been successfully overcome by non-operative correction of the clubfoot. Rather than transplant a tendon to prevent recurrence of the deformity, it would be our choice to do an adequate soft-tissue release behind the heel, or on the medial side of the heel, or both when indicated.

The need for a surgical procedure is the outgrowth of a surgeon's choice of coping with a clinical situation as he finds it. We have found that tendon transplantation is seldom necessary if the methodical adherence to the standardized treatment described is patiently and painstakingly followed.

TIBIAL OSTEOTOMY

The need for derotational osteotomy of the tibia for internal tibial torsion in the clubfoot is infrequently encountered. The indication for such an operation would be a significant degree of internal tibial torsion in the absence of any residual deformity of the foot. Any element of internal tibial torsion accompanying the clubfoot deformity should correct by the use of plaster casts and the crossbar splint. On rare occasions in children already walking with all elements of the foot deformity corrected, one may find an unsightly and bothersome in-toeing gait due entirely to internal tibial torsion. In such instances, a derotational osteotomy of the tibia is indicated and we have employed the technique described by O'Donoghue. Needless to say, this procedure is not indicated for and should not be used for correction of the in-toeing gait due to femoral torsion.

SUMMARY

Successful treatment of the clubfoot requires knowledge of its morbid anatomy. To know what one is trying to correct simplifies the application of methods aimed at achieving a correction. Continuity of care by one doctor from start to finish is desirable. Methodology is essential. Recognition of resistive elements of deformity should be prompt and corrective measures instituted according to specific indication. A clubfoot is not fully corrected beyond any possibility of recurrence of deformity until the child is at least seven years of age and, in some instances, even older. Periodic follow-up examinations are as important as the continuity of active treatment. A good result can be expected if these tenets are observed.

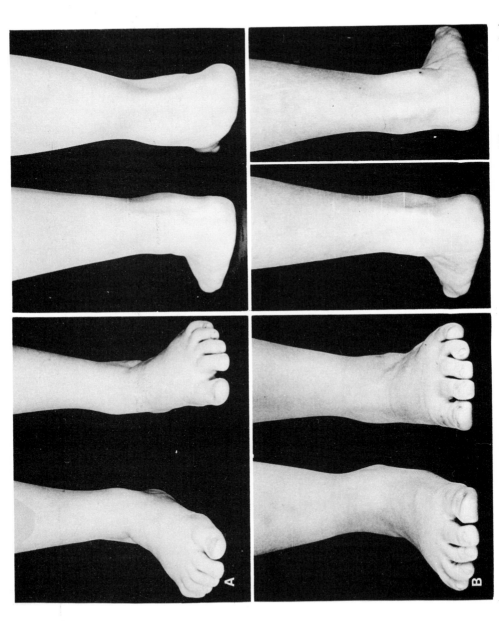

Figure 10-16.   These two cases are illustrative of the result which can be anticipated in more than 50 per cent of cases treated non-operatively, and are submitted as examples to substantiate the methodology recommended for the conservative treatment of this deformity.
A.   Correction of deformity in a unilateral left clubfoot. Note permanent lessening in girth of calf.
B.   Correction of deformity in bilateral clubfoot.

Treatment is begun when the infant is two weeks old. Forefoot and heel varus are corrected with below-the-knee stretching plasters changed every week. Usually at six weeks sufficient correction is obtained to permit progression to the strapped-on crossbar splint. Equinus is corrected by this splint with this phase of treatment generally requiring six to nine weeks. If the equinus persists, the splint is used for a longer time—until the child is six months of age. If at this age equinus still persists, an operative posterior release is performed. In either event, maintenance of correction is provided by the crossbar shoe-splint worn twenty-two hours a day until the child is walking, and then worn only at night with a clubfoot shoe worn during the day. This discipline is continued for five years or until the program is altered in the light of clinical judgment monitored by periodic follow-up examinations. Once correction is achieved, the child is seen every three months to detect any evidence of recurrence so that prompt corrective methods can be employed. Beyond age seven, yearly visits suffice for check-up (Fig. 10-16).

There are three basic operative procedures for correction of resistive elements of deformity in a child under six years of age. They are listed with their indications as follows:

1. Lengthening of the tendo achillis and posterior capsulotomy of the ankle and talocalcaneal joints for equinus.

2. Soft-tissue medial release for the correction of resistant heel-varus.

3. Tarsometatarsal and intermetatarsal capsular and ligamentous release for resistant forefoot adduction.

Between ages six and ten the only recommended operative procedure is capsular and ligamentous tarsometatarsal release for severe metatarsus adductus. Beyond age ten a triple talar arthrodesis is recommended for correction of significant residual varus and equinus deformity.

There are a number of other surgical procedures as well as other conservative regimens for the congenital clubfoot. It is not our intent to imply that these other forms of treatment are valueless merely because we have not included them in this chapter. We wish only to say that the conservative and surgical management recommended in this chapter has proved to be the most effective and satisfactory in our experience.

BIBLIOGRAPHY

Dwyer, F. C.: The Treatment of Relapsed Club Foot by the Insertion of a Wedge into the Calcaneus. J. Bone Jt. Surg. 45B, 67-75 (Feb.) 1963.

Evans, D.: Relapsed Club Foot. J. Bone Jt. Surg., 43B, 722-733 (Nov.) 1961.

Heyman, Clarence H., Herndon, Charles H. and Strong, Joseph M.: Mobilization of the Tarsometatarsal and Intermetatarsal Joints for the Correction of Resistant Adduction of the Fore Part of the Foot in Congenital Clubfoot or Congenital Metatarsus Varus. J. Bone Jt. Surg., 40A,

Kite, J. Hiram: The Club Foot, N.Y., Grune & Stratton, 1964, pp 67-79.

299-310 (April) 1958.

McCauley, Jr., John C.: Surgical Treatment of Clubfoot. Surg. Clin. North America. 563, (April) 1951.

O'Donoghue, D. H.: Controlled Rotation Osteotomy of the Tibia. South. Med. J., 33:1145-1149 (Nov.) 1940.

Stewart, Steele F.: Club Foot: Its Incidence, Cause and Treatment. J. Bone Jt. Surg., 33A, 577-588 (July) 1951.

Wynne-Davis, Ruth: Family Studies and the Cause of Congenital Club Foot. J. Bone Jt. Surg. 46A, 445-463 (Aug.) 1964.

= 11 =

Management of the Poliomyelitic Foot

Jack K. Wickstrom, M.D.

Although the incidence of poliomyelitis has decreased greatly during the past decade, residua from viral infections of this type often create abnormalities of the foot and, consequently, of locomotion. Since the principles and techniques of reconstructive surgery of the foot were developed primarily from experience with paralytic feet, careful consideration of these problems can be of value in understanding such basic principles.

CORRELATIVE PATHOLOGY

The symptoms and the severity of poliomyelitic infections of the central nervous system vary so much that differential diagnosis is often difficult and the prognosis at the onset of this disease is uncertain. Several factors explain this variability. Bodian observed wide variation in severity of injury to the affected nerve cells. Some were destroyed completely; some survived without infection, and some regained functional activity after initial damage. Hodes, Peacock, and Bodian also noted sensitivity to poliomyelitis by variably sized motoneurons and that the most vulnerable of these were the large anterior horn cells.

Although the distribution of damage to motoneurons supplying specific muscles had been described prior to 1955, Sharrard's correlation of spinal cord changes and clinical patterns of paralysis and paresis further clarified the relation between motoneuron damage and the pattern and severity of paralysis. Sharrard also confirmed the observation by Hodes and associates that the large anterior horn cell neurons were the most vulnerable. All sections of the spinal cord showed evidence of previous inflammation, even when clinical evidence was lacking. In his study, "cell charts" developed from serial sections of the lumbosacral cord were used to plot the position, size, number, and distribution of residual motoneurons in the anterior horn cell columns and were compared with similar "cell charts", from normal spinal cords. By studying the muscle function charts of patients from whom the spinal cords were obtained and correlating these with "cell charts", Sharrard found the number of motoneurons surviving to be directly proportional to the muscle strength. Somewhat surprising, however, was his finding of as much as 60 per cent loss of motoneurons supplying muscle which had been rated clinically normal.

The most important finding was the focal rather than diffuse destruction of motor cells. Sharrard noted that each focus was limited to part of one or two segments with unaffected interposing gray matter. Most severely affected were the second, third, and fourth lumbar segments, whereas the lower sacral segments were usually spared.

The motoneurons supplying individual muscles are arranged in columns extending over various levels of the spinal cord. Sharrard found that muscles supplied by columns of motor cells extending over a number of segments, such as the quadriceps, presented a higher incidence of weakness rather than paralysis, whereas the incidence of paralysis of muscles supplied by columns extending over short segments, such as the anterior tibial, was higher. The arrangement of these columns further explained the associated paralysis of one muscle with another to produce the characteristic clinical patterns of paresis and paralysis. All the common patterns of paralysis in poliomyelitis can be explained by the juxtaposition of the motoneuron columns supplying the associated muscles.

The frequency of permanent paralysis of muscles of the lower leg and foot innervated by short motor cell columns accounts for the high incidence of deformities of the foot associated with poliomyelitis. Since paralysis occurs most frequently in the anterior tibial muscle, the most frequent residual deformity is drop foot.

PROGNOSIS

Treatment is based on the presumption that any paralyzed muscle can be expected to recover until the subsequent course of the disease proves this to be incorrect. This presumption is important in planning both the reconstructive surgery and the socio-economic future of the patient.

The severity and extent of initial paralysis at onset are crude indications of the intensity of the infection. As a general principle, Green has found that "muscles completely paralyzed two to four weeks after onset have little likelihood of making a sizable recovery, whereas muscles which show some ability to contract at this time have an increasingly good prognosis". Improvement can be expected over a period lasting sixteen to twenty-four months.

Sharrard found that from an inital rate of recovery of 54.5 per cent during the first month, improvement of muscle function gradually became less noticeable. Less than 5 per cent of the muscles improved after the first year and none after the end of the second year, except when a deformity of a joint was corrected to allow better performance by a muscle working at a disadvantage. The uniformity of recovery in 142 patients allowed him to predict further recovery in any given muscle from knowledge of the functional grade one month after the onset of paralysis: he could estimate an average of the final grade of a muscle in the lower extremity by adding two grade units to its functional grade one month after the onset of the acute illness; one and one-half units to the grade at two months; one unit to the grade at four months, and three-quarters unit to the grade at six months. Children between four and ten years of age, and to a lesser extent those between the ages of two and four, recovered most rapidly, whereas the recovery rates of those ten to twenty years of age were near the mean for all groups. Recovery was lowest in those over twenty-one years of age.

These observations have important clinical applicability. A patient with rather scattered paralysis at six months, with most muscles still capable of moving a joint with or without gravity, will probably recover completely. On the other hand, patients with complete paralysis of certain muscle groups at the end of six months will probably have no return of strength in those muscles, although function may improve by the adaptation of new methods of using existing power.

Hertz, Madsen, and Buchtal, in a study of electromyographic characteristics of paralyzed muscles as an index of return of function, concluded that an increase in the duration of mean action-potential was the poorest prognostic sign. In muscles in which duration of mean action-potential was 30 per cent above normal at onset of paralysis, no signs of recovery were evident a year later. Fibrillation potential was first noted thirteen to twenty-one days after on-set of the disease and was highest in the acutely affected muscles which showed poorest return of function. Moreover, during the initial stage of the disease intramuscular temperature fell significantly in severely affected muscles, which later showed no improvement, by comparison with normal muscle or muscles that did recover. The temperature differential persisted for a year. These are both important prognostic signs, although variations in interpretation of electromyograms somewhat restrict their practical application.

TREATMENT

Nonoperative Treatment. During the subacute or sensitive stage of paralytic poliomyelitis, three manifestations which produce deformity and dysfunctions are pertinent: (1) muscle paralysis, (2) muscle hyperirritability and tenderness to palpation and attempted motion, and (3) hypertonic contracture of spasm of the antagonist of the paralyzed muscles. During this sensitive stage, muscles in spasm pull the joints into abnormal positions, which, in the presence of paralysis, opposing muscles cannot prevent, and the deformity thus increases. If such hypertonic contracture persists, the muscle becomes shortened and fixed.

During this subacute phase, treatment is directed toward relieving pain and preventing deformity by protective positioning, with use of bivalved casts or braces which protect weakened muscles and maintain functional attitudes. Application of hot packs encourages relaxation and affords considerable relief of pain. As pain subsides, the joints of the affected part are gently moved through an ever-increasing range to overcome hypertonic contractures and to prevent myostatic contractures.

During this stage, muscle reeducation by concentration on the part of the patient and stimulation of the involved tissues by the physical therapist is considered important by most authorities. Before ambulation is permitted, standing balance should be well developed. As further strength returns and as the patient's condition permits, ambulation with assistance of appropriate apparatus (parallel bars, walkers, crutches, braces, or pool therapy) will increase the range of mobility. Careful supervision of ambulation is important to insure development of as near a normal gait as possible and to avoid deformed joint positions.

The therapy must be extremely gentle when stretching hypertonic or myostatic contractures. Undue force can result in tearing of muscles, with the subsequent development of myositis ossificans which often follows such unwarranted stretching. This phase of therapy may be short if muscle function returns rapidly, or it may be extremely prolonged. In the latter instance treatment will require considerable patience, reinforcement and encouragement by the physician and the therapist.

Prevention of Deformity. In addition to muscle spasm, paralysis and weakness, other factors, such as growth, persistent muscle imbalance and habitual faulty position, contribute to the development of deformities. Prevention of deformity requires complete cooperation among the orthopaedist, therapist and patient — or if the patient is a child, his parents — with careful observation of the condition at regular intervals. Correction of deformities is important. This is achieved by wedging in plaster casts to overcome myostatic contracture, followed by appropriate bracing. Repeated inventory of muscle return is essential during this phase.

In treating deformities of the foot the entire limb must be considered. That both gait and alignment of the limb contribute to foot deformity can best be illustrated by the effects of a tight iliotibial band. In addition to the hip flexion deformity, valgus of the knee and external rotation of the lower leg with a laterally directed ankle, a varus deformity of the foot often results. This is particularly true when a long leg-brace with attached pelvic band has been used to control rotation. Conversely, the effect of the position of the foot and the ankle on the rest of the limb is important. A common example is the effect of a fixed equinus of the ankle and foot which contributes to the stability of the knee in the presence of a weakened quadriceps. Discrepancies in leg length must also be considered and appropriate epiphysiodeses planned at the proper time to insure equality in leg length.

Surgical Reconstruction. Although paralytic deformities have been recognized since antiquity, it was not until the scope of surgery had been broadened by introduction of anesthesia and asepsis during the late nineteenth century that surgical reconstruction of paralytic feet was attempted. Efforts were first directed toward substitution of tendons with muscles that had residual power for those without function — properly termed tendon transfer. Nicoladoni's description of this procedure in 1880 was followed by reports by Codivilla and others. These attempts stimulated others to use braided silk as artificial ligaments to correct drop foot and other paralytic deformities. These materials successfully acted as check-reins which supported the foot at the proper angle but proved inadequate because of incompatibility with bone and inability to adjust to growth. Gallie later advocated tenodesis in preference to these artificial ligaments and described techniques for correcting both drop foot and calcaneal deformities by attaching tendons of paralytic muscles to the tibia. Albert is credited with having performed the first stabilization procedure of the foot — fusion of the ankle. Many others soon reported their experience in ankylosis of joints to correct the deformities and stabilize the foot. Nierny first advocated arthrodesis of the subastragalar joint as a means of controlling inversion and eversion as well as of correcting deformity. These efforts have been reviewed extensively by Hart.

Today most surgeons use a combination of procedures. The fundamental differences in techniques of arthrodesis are in the amount of bone removed. Some orthopaedists prefer excising a great deal of bone with the articular cartilage to create broad, flat surfaces. This technique can be accomplished rapidly, but often results in considerable decrease in the size of the foot. Others prefer removing only articular cartilage and minimal subchrondral bone. In the latter technique sufficient bone may not, however, be removed to allow easy correction of the foot deformity. In 1952, Grice introduced a technique of arthrodesis in which a bone block is ·inserted across the articular surface of the subastragalar joints. This procedure can be used in young patients without causing cessation of growth of the talus or the calcaneus.

Preoperative Consideration. In spite of expert care, deformities may develop which can be corrected only by surgery, particularly when the acute stage of the disease occurs with severe muscle involvement early in life. Subsequent growth of the child may produce deformity in spite of bracing, dynamic splinting and expert physical therapy. Surgery is still indicated primarily when the anticipated results can be expected to improve function, correct deformity, reduce the amount of bracing or remove the necessity of braces. Occasionally, an operation is necessary to correct a deformity that prevents bracing or makes it difficult.

Since improvement in function during the convalescent stage can be anticipated for about sixteen to twenty-four months, all corrective surgery should be delayed until after this time. Generally, surgery should be postponed until the end of the growth period, except in patients in whom gross deformity, uncontrolled by bracing, greatly impairs function. *Tendon transfers in the foot are usually more successful if delayed until the age of eight years.* Operation on bone designed to stabilize parts should generally be delayed until loss of articular cartilage from which the tarsal bones grow will not greatly reduce the size of the foot. *Ideally, such joint stabilization is delayed until the age of twelve years,* but can be done after the osseous age of nine or ten years.

Although currently not as popular as in the past, the basic principle of correcting as much deformity as possible by preliminary bracing or wedging in plaster casts can often reduce the extent of the necessary operation and increase the ease with which correction can be accomplished. Before surgery, special attention must be given to the condition of the skin of the extremities that have been in casts or braces since there may be areas of irritation of the skin at the point of contact with the brace or even small abrasions in this area. If the extremity has been immobilized in a cast, then the skin will require repeated cleansing to remove the accumulated layers of dead epitheleal cells.

Operative Procedures. Although tendon transfer was the first operation described for control of paralytic deformities of the foot, the procedure without operative stabilization of the foot has not been universally successful or popular, probably because *transfer of the deforming tendon is incapable of correcting the deformity after bony changes have occurred.* Moreover, the technique for tendon transfer is more exacting. Although some orthopaedists use transfer of tendons to prevent progression of deformity, it has been found that *combined stabilization with later appropriate tendon transfers (about six weeks after the initial osseous surgery) results in a better functioning foot.* However, each patient should be evaluated individually. The decision as to early initial tendon transfer, or later combined bone and tendon surgery, also depends upon the individual orthopaedist's experiences.

Bone surgery to correct deformity or to stabilize paralytic feet requires careful planning and selection of patients, procedure and timing. Accurate determination of residual muscle power based on repeated examination, analysis of gait and evaluation of alignment are the foundation upon which reconstructive surgery must be planned. Of particular value are roentgenograms of the foot deformity and development of tracings by which one can accurately determine the amount of bone to be removed and soft tissues to be released, especially if the surgeon's experience is limited or the deformity is unusual. Once a decision to operate has been made, a detailed note should be inserted in the patient's record. This should summarize residual muscle function, persistent deformity, surgical procedures planned, together with their sequence and anticipated postoperative treatment. Such a note is important to the surgeon, his aides and the patient's family, and prevents confusion about the precise extent of each stage once initial operation has altered the foot's appearance and mobility.

All operations are carried out with the extremity exsanguinated and a pneumatic tourniquet applied, preferably before final skin preparation rather than after draping. Since the length of time that tissues in the lower extremity can remain anoxic has not been accurately determined, ischemic contractures of the muscles and damage to the nerves may occur. The wound should be temporarily occluded and the tourniquet released after seventy-five to ninety minutes to avoid development of an ischemic contracture.

This text does not attempt to include every recommended operative procedure for the treatment of foot deformities due to poliomyelitis. Rather, certain basic principles and certain basic operations will be described which can be applied in all instances and which can be modified when necessary. It is suggested that the reader refer to other texts (such as *Campbell's Operative Orthopedics*) for specific modifications of these basic procedures.

The technique which we recommend for stabilizing paralytic feet has evolved from the individual techniques of Ryerson, Dunn, and Hoke through several modifications of Caldwell, Brewster and Lambrinudi. No matter what type of a triple arthrodesis or other corrective osseous surgery of the foot is performed, it should be carried out only after careful planning. Particularly when performing a triple arthrodesis, the operator should try to visualize in his mind's eye that the foot is a three dimensional anatomical entity. He should have an exact preconceived idea of the size and shape of the wedges of bone that he will excise. He should remove each wedge as one single piece rather than in several small fragments. A triple arthrodesis, and for that matter, any other bone surgery of the foot, is not difficult to perform providing the operator has learned to think of the foot as a three dimensional unit and has learned to remove the deforming pieces of bone as single units.

We have routinely used a straight or slightly curved lateral incision over the sinus tarsi, extending from a point immediately lateral to the long toe extensor tendons posteriorly and inferiorly to below the lateral malleolus. Occasionally it is curved under the lateral malleolus when more exposure of the posterior portion of the talocalcaneal joint is desired. Trauma to the peroneal tendon sheaths and peritenon of the extensor tendons must be avoided to reduce restriction of tendon mobility by adhesions, particularly when subsequent tendon transplants are anticipated. Great care must be exerted to prevent skin damage by too vigorous retraction. The periosteum, lateral joint capsule and areolar tissue from the sinus tarsi

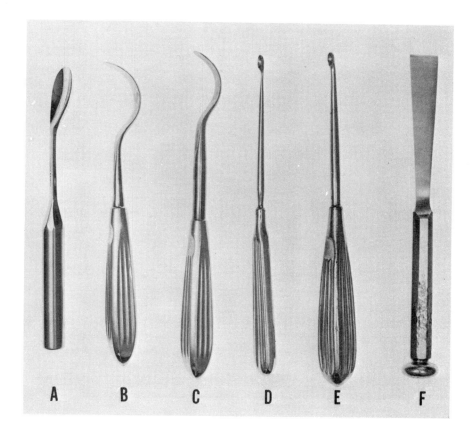

Fig. 11-1. Instruments particularly valuable in performing triple arthrodesis: A. Hatt spoon, adapted from similar instruments of Hoke's, facilitates stripping capsule from superior and medial surfaces of the talonavicular joint.

B and C. Crego retractors of different widths and curves are used to stabilize joint, strip capsule, and protect sutures on opposite side of joint during removal of cartilage and subchondral bone.

D and E. Shallow currettes are of particular value in removing remnants of cartilage from depth of wound of the sustentaculum tali without damaging adjacent soft tissues.

F. Thin sharp osteotome is well adapted to requirements of precise removal of cartilage and bone necessary to shape contiguous surfaces accurately.

should be dissected from the astragalus and os calcis as a distally based flap and reflected together with the short toe extensor muscles. If handled gently, this flap furnishes viable tissue to fill subcuticular dead space and improve the blood supply to the skin after closure of the wound. Next the extensor tendons are carefully elevated and the capsule of the talonavicular joint is incised. A curved Crego retractor or Hatt spoon is then inserted to free the capsule from the superior and medial sides of the talar neck (Fig. 11-1). Sufficient cartilage and subchondral bone are then removed from the talar head and the tarsonavicular to correct or to compensate for the joint deformity. Care must be taken in the removal of the cartilage from the navicular, particularly in the foot with a varus deformity in which the navicular is displaced to the medial side of the talus and is difficult to reach. Incomplete or inadequate removal of the cartilage will result in insufficient correction and in nonunion of the talonavicular arthrodesis. Hoke's technique of removing the talar head facilitates this step. Removal consists of osteotomizing the talus at the junction of the head and neck and carefully and gently removing the head. After the apposing articular surfaces of the navicular and the talar head have been denuded of all cartilage, the head is temporarily replaced in order to obtain an idea of the amount of correction gained. It is then removed, wrapped in a moist sponge until the remaining joints have been corrected, and then reinserted. The subtalar joint is next explored, the cartilage being removed from the distal and medial articular facets first, and a Crego retractor is then inserted into the capsule posteriorly to determine the obliquity of the proximal or posterior facet and to protect the structures on the posterior and medial side of the talus. Use of a modified lamina spreader to distract or open the joint facilitates removal of the cartilage and the subchondral bone. A currette should be used to remove the cartilage from the sustenaculum tali and the medial facet of the os calcis in order to minimize damage to the structures on the medial side of the subtalar joint. The articular surfaces of the calcaneocuboid joint are re-

moved in a similar manner with a thin osteotome and the apposing flat bony surfaces of the navicular, cuboid, talus, and calcaneus are approximated, and foot alignment is tested. Additional bone may have to be removed to correct residual deformity or to insure congruity of adjacent bony surfaces. The foot should fall into the corrected position without any difficulty and the apposing bony surfaces should be congruous. It should not require any particular force to hold the foot in the corrected position, but the foot should easily fall into place. In some deformities, such as a calcaneovalgus type foot, an additional incision on the medial side of the foot facilitates removal of a wedge on the medial side of the subtalar joint and the proximal medial portion of the navicular needed to correct the valgus of the heel and to relieve the prominence on the medial border of the foot.

At the time of stabilization, the foot is aligned with the ankle and is usually displaced slightly posteriorly, depending upon the pattern of residual muscle power. Weakness of the calf group can be compensated by moving the foot slightly posteriorly on the talus to increase the length of the posterior lever arm. The calcaneus must be positioned in the midline and the forefoot in very slight pronation to allow weight to be transferred off the medial side of the foot and great toe. Residual varus of either the heel or forefoot is *not acceptable,* because either deformity forces weight transfer over the lateral border of the forefoot, which exerts an increased varus thrust on the forefoot with each step. Other deformities of the extremity, such as genu valgus or external rotation of the tibia, must be corrected at a later stage to align the foot with the entire extremity (Fig. 11-2). The importance of alignment of the foot with the ankle cannot be overemphasized.

Variations in technique are indicated, depending on the deformity present and the residual muscle power. Calcaneocavus deformities are corrected by removal of a generous wedge from the proximal posterior facet of the calcaneus, together with a dorsal wedge from the head of the talus and navicular, and release of the plantar

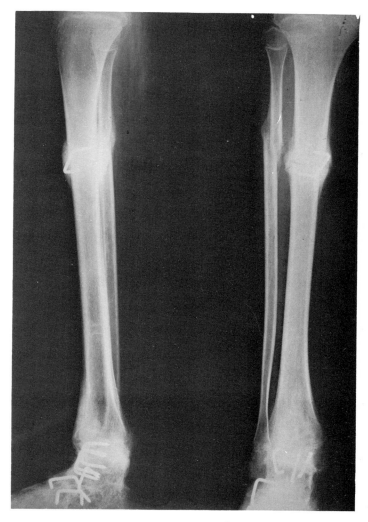

Fig. 11-2. Osteotomy through proximal tibia and fibula to allow proper alignment of foot and ankle by derotation. Similar surgical procedures are frequently necessary to correct malalignment after aligning of the foot with the ankle at the time of stablization. We now utilize a single Kirschner wire protruding through the skin to transfix osteotomy temporarily during application of cast to insure maintenance of position.

fascia from the calcaneus (Fig. 11-3). The cavus is thus corrected, and the forefoot is aligned with the calcaneus (Fig. 11-4). A fixed deformity can be corrected most adequately by the Lambrinudi procedure which consists primarily of resection of the anterior dorsal surface of the head of the talus, resection of the anterior portion of the body of the talus and the calcaneus and upward displacement of the navicular on to the top of the beak of the talus (Fig. 11-5). In performing a Lambrinudi procedure it is most wise to procure a lateral x-ray film of the foot in an equinus position, cut out the outline of each of the bones consisting of the talus, os calcis, navicular, and cuboid, and then place the cutouts on each other in the corrected position so that the operator can estimate approximately how much bone is required to be removed from the head of the talus, as well as from the calcaneal joints in order to achieve the desired result.

We have successfully used the Grice-Green extra-articular fusion, as modified by Young, with two fibular grafts across

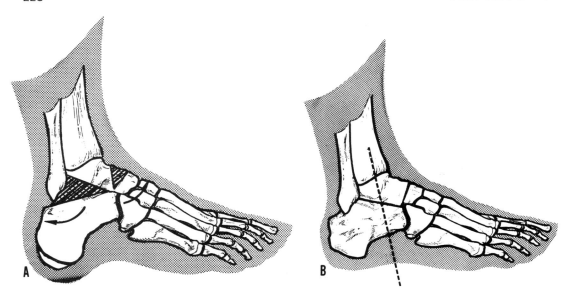

Fig. 11-3. A. Correction of a calcaneal deformity requires removal of a generous wedge of bone from the posterior portion of the calcaneous along with a dorsal wedge from the navicular and head of astragalus to allow the calcaneus to assume a horizontal position and the forefoot to be aligned with it. Release of the plantar fascia from the calcaneus facilitates correction of the cavus deformity.

  B.   The dotted line indicates position of the Kirschner wire used for temporary transfixation.

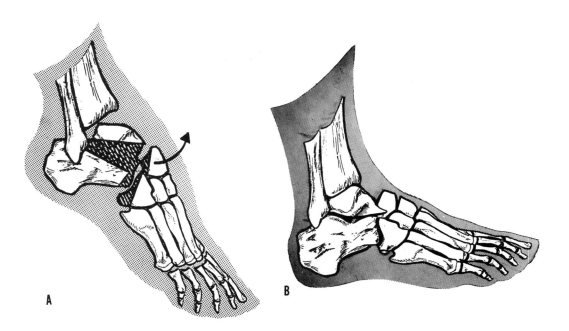

Fig. 11-4.   A. Lambrinudi stabilization requires resection of distally based wedge, principally from the inferior surface of the talus and partly from calcaneus. The notch created in the proximal inferior surface of the navicular is impaled on the beak of the talus.

  B.   Appearance of corrected foot. To maintain correction of equinus obtained at operation some active muscle tendon must be transferred forward or the anterior capsule of the ankle joint will stretch out, lose its check rein effect and the equinus recur.

the subastragalar joint, in the paralytic flat (calcaneovalgus type) foot (Fig. 11-6). Because it produces stability without stopping growth of the tarsal bones, this excellent procedure can be used in very young children.

In feet that are rigid, cavus deformities have been treated by release of the plantar fascia from the calcaneus, combined with the removal of a dorsal wedge of bone from the tarsals. In this procedure, following sectioning of the plantar fascia through a medial plantar incision (Steindler opera-

tion), the talonavicular and calcaneocuboid joints are exposed through the usual incision. Little, if any, bone is removed from the talus or the os calcis. The bony wedges to correct the cavus are removed principally from the cuboid and navicular bones. We have not had personal experience with the osteotomy of the os calcis described by Dwyer to correct nonrigid cavus deformities by correcting the varus of the heel, but the results reported by Dwyer indicate that this procedure has merit.

In performing a pantalar arthrodesis for

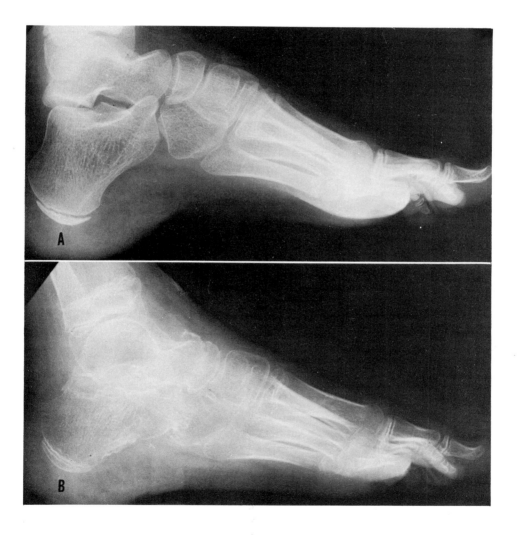

Fig. 11-5. A. Lateral views of right foot with calcaneus deformities. Note vertical position of calcaneus and cavus deformity correctable by resection of appropriate wedge from proximal facet of calcaneus and adjacent surfaces of talar head and navicular.

B.   Appearance of foot at first change of cast about six weeks after stabilization.

flail feet, either the two-stage Steindler procedure can be used or the one-stage Lorthoir method. In the latter, the talus is excised, the articular cartilage is removed from all of the apposing articular surfaces, the talus is denuded of cartilage and replaced. Both methods have proved successful.

The use of some form of fixation to maintain bony alignment and contact during closure of wounds and application of casts was discussed with the various contributors to this book. Some of them used staples or other forms of internal fixation routinely, and others did not. There was no general consensus. Staples are not used as frequently as they were up until 1958 or 1960 since in many instances it became necessary to remove them subsequent to surgery. More recently, some of the contributors have relied on a single Kirschner wire inserted through the middle cuneiform and navicular and into the talus to maintain the foot during routine triple arthrodesis, particularly when performing a Lambrinudi procedure. A Kirschner wire, similarly inserted through the calcaneus into the talus and occasionally into the tibia, has been used when correcting the calcaneal deformity in a triple arthrodesis. The wire is allowed to protrude through the skin and is covered with plaster over sterile dressings. It has caused no complications and has the advantage over other forms of fixation of removability to allow manipulation of the foot should realignment be required immediately after operation. The wires are routinely removed when the first cast is changed at four weeks. Some of the contributors recommend the use of a long leg-cast for the first four weeks following surgery. Others feel that a short leg-cast extending from the tips of the toes to the tibial tubercle is sufficient to hold the posterior tarsal joints and the foot in a corrected position. At the end of four to six weeks, the long leg-cast can be removed and a short leg-cast applied. At the end of eight weeks after surgery, the short leg-cast is removed and a walking cast is then applied for a period of another four to six weeks, depending upon the progress of union that has been demonstrable by roentgenograms at the end of eight weeks.

Prior to wound closure a Snyder hemovac unit is inserted in order to aspirate the excessive blood which accumulates in the soft tissues following release of the tourniquet in the triple arthrodesis. The wound is closed by careful reattachment of the areolar muscle flap proximally with fine sutures of chromic collagen or Number 000 chromic catgut. The subcuticular layer of the skin is then approximated with fine chromic collagen or Number 000 plain sutures and skin closure depends upon the orthopaedist's training and desires. The use of subcuticular stainless steel wire has proved quite satisfactory. Cast application should be carefully carried out. The foot should not be wrapped with an excessive amount of sheet wadding. In fact, it is preferable to use Webril, since it tends to conform more snugly and more satisfactorily to the foot and one can better visualize the position in which the foot is held. The cast is applied snugly, but not tightly, from the tips of the toes to the knee with the foot held in the corrected position. The tourniquet is released after suction has been applied to the hemovac unit. The hemovac unit is allowed to remain in the foot for a period of forty-eight hours. It is removed at the end of this period of time. It is recommended that a sedative be administered prior to removal of the hemovac plastic tubes from the foot since this procedure is painful. We have found that the administration of 50 mg. of Demerol (meperidine) intravenously, administered within a period of one to two minutes is quite efficacious.

Tendon Transfers. The efficacy of tendon transfers is difficult to determine because of variations in techniques, selection of patients, and criteria for evaluation. According to Green, the need for stabilization of the foot can be significantly reduced if proper tendon transfers are done earlier. Mortens and associates reported greatest success in correcting equinovarus and medial cavus foot deformities with tendon transplants alone, but improvement in only 50 per cent of the calcaneovalgus feet and less than 25 per cent of the planovalgus deformities by tendon transfers. Hagelstam had difficulty obtaining correction of varus deformities without arthrodesis, whereas

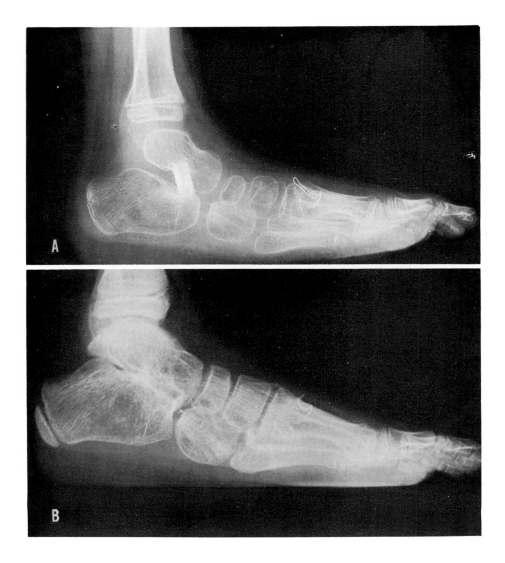

Fig. 11-6. A. Grice-Green subtalar fusion to correct planovalgus deformity after operation.

B. Three years later, note progression of fusion as growth of talus and calcaneus continues. Similar bone block technique for arthrodesis of other tarsal joints has been used by Green to minimize loss of growth by conservation of articular cartilage.

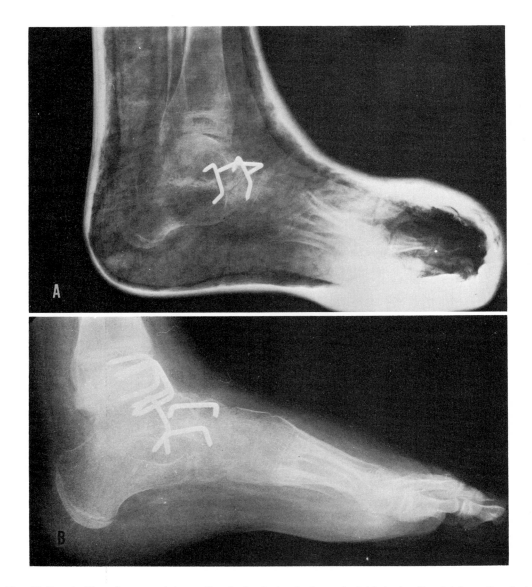

Fig. 11-7.   A. Two-stage pantalar arthrodesis. Lateral view of right foot after triple arthrodesis secured by three staples to maintain bone contact.

B.   Lateral view after tibiatalar arthrodesis with staples in place to maintain bone apposition. Note epiphyseal plate has not been disturbed and can continue to add to leg length.

he was able to correct valgus deformities by transfer of tendons. He was able to restore active motion as well. Westin obtained 92 per cent satisfactory transfers when they were combined with stabilizations, but less than 82 per cent satisfactory tendon transfers alone.

We recommend that tendon transfers be performed six weeks after stabilization. From 1944 to 1958, 67 patients had tendon transfers without stabilization to correct or prevent deformities in 89 feet. Results indicate that tendon transfers were successful in 6.6 per cent of calcaneovalgus feet

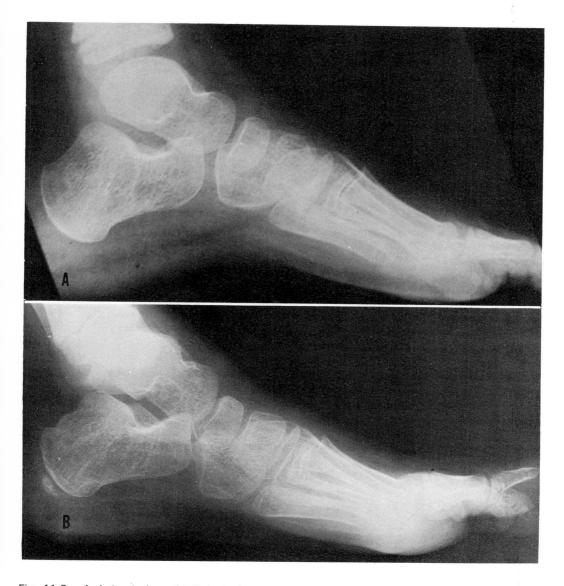

Fig. 11-8.   A. Lateral view of left foot shows early calcaneal deformity at time of transfer of anterior tibial and both peroneals into the calcaneus.

B.   View of same foot three years after transfer. Note deformity forces are now correcting forces and have maintained almost normal alignment of foot. Although no stabilization was necessary in this patient, satisfactory alignment has not been maintained in most other patients without osseous stabilization.

(Fig. 11-8) and about 20 per cent of planovalgus and equinovarus feet (Table 11-1). In contrast, reexamination of 276 feet in 174 patients in whom bony stabilization was accompanied, preceded, or followed by various tendon transfers, indicated that function was far superior (Fig. 11-9) (Table 11-2). Reidy, Broderick, and Barr reported similar success in their review of tendon transfers. As Barr and Record found, most failures were due to instability of the ankle (Fig. 11-10) or, less often, to

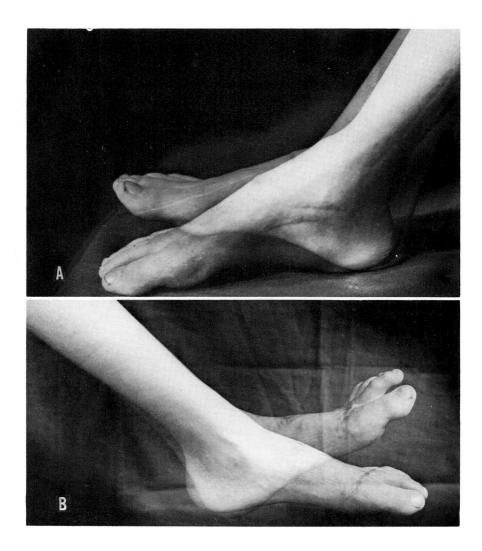

Fig. 11-9.   Range of motion two years after bilateral Lambrinudi procedures to correct fixed equinus with weak triceps surae.

A.   Range of motion of right foot after transfer of posterior tibial tendon forward through interosseous membrane with peroneus longus to middle cuneiform.

B.   Range of motion of left foot after transfer of peroneus longus forward to middle cuneiform and extensor hallucis longus and long toe extensors to metatarsal necks.

stretching or tenodesis of the tendon transfer. Although tendon transfers are obviously useful in reducing deforming forces and in restoring balance and function in selected patients with partial paralysis of muscles controlling the foot, the results are more predictable and superior when the transfers are accompanied or preceded by stabilization procedures.

Barr stipulated several prerequisites for successful tendon transfers. Among these requirements are a free range of joint motion without deformity and sufficient power in the muscle attached to the tendon to act as a substitute for, or at least reinforce, the weakened action of the muscle for which it is being substituted. Moreover, the line of pull of the transferred tendon should be as direct as possible and should follow the course of the muscle and tendon for which it is being substituted whenever possible. Agonist transfers were more satisfactory than antagonist, and results were better if the tendon had a similar or identical range of excursion as the one being supplanted. Mayer stressed the importance of preserving the gliding mechanism of the tendon by inserting the transfer through the tendon sheath of the substituted tendon or

through fat or other tissue to allow it to glide. Tendons should be handled carefully to prevent damage and subsequent adhesions. Obviously, the blood and nerve supply of the muscle whose tendon is being transferred must be preserved during dissection if it is to function.

The Bunnell technique of tendon suture, in which a double-armed stainless steel wire attaches the tendon to the bone or recipient tendon with a pull-out suture, has been used routinely. The wire should pass out through the skin of the sole of the foot and be anchored over a pressure dispersal button (Fig. 11-11).

In addition to the principles already outlined, each tendon transfer has some slight variation which must be carried out in order for the operative procedure to succeed. Therefore, as each transfer is discussed, any technical variations associated with the procedure will be presented. Tendon transfers are particularly effective in reinforcing mild to moderate weakness or paralysis of a muscle. Whenever a muscle is transferred, it loses some of its power. The exact amount of this loss has not been

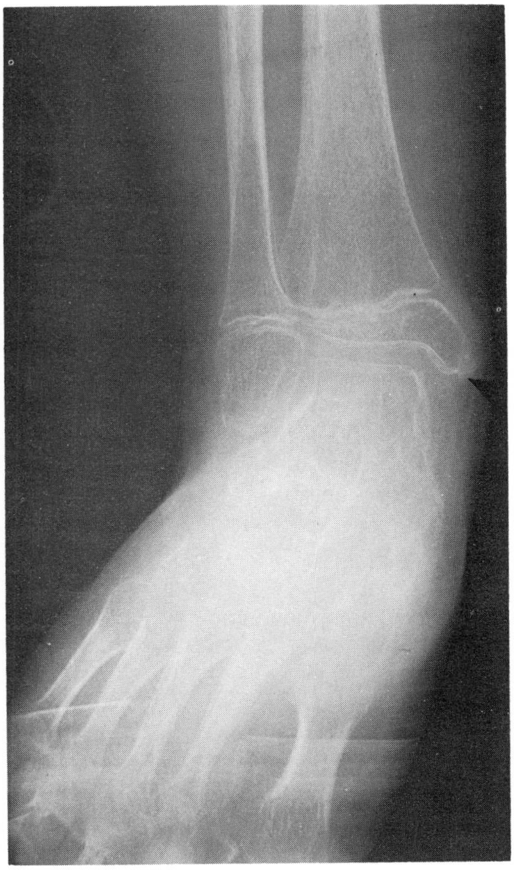

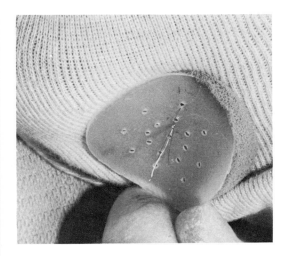

Fig. 11-10. Medial instability of ankle after triple arthrodesis, which was sufficiently disabling to require use of a short leg brace with a T strap to control pronation. Ankle instability was the most common cause of unsatisfactory results in patients after foot stabilizations.

Fig. 11-11. Pressure dispersal button consisting of plastic disc with underlying foam rubber disc. Although this is a prototype there has been no incidence of pressure necrosis when this type button has been used on the plantar aspect of the foot. It can be incorporated inside the cast with no maceration of the skin.

accurately charted up to the present time, but unquestionably some loss does occur. With active isometric exercises following transfer, a good portion of this power can be regained. If a muscle is totally paralyzed or presents only a trace of power, tendon transplantation of even a normal muscle will be relatively ineffective. Transplantation of a muscle with fair power as a substitute for, or as reinforcement for a muscle also with fair power, will almost invariably lead to failure.

The tendon transfers which are most frequently effective, as well as the deformities which they are intended to correct, are discussed below:

Cock-up Deformity of the Great Toe. This deformity is produced in a poliomyelitic foot by either of two muscle imbalance problems. In one, the extensor hallucis longus is used to substitute for a weakened tibialis anterior. Examination of the patient walking barefoot with this type of a drop foot gait reveals that during the swing phase, the extensor hallucis contracts, producing the cock-up deformity. When the patient is standing at rest, this deformity is usually absent. In the second situation, this type of deformity of the great toe occurs in the propulsive or push-off phase of walking when the flexor hallucis longus, along with the other long toe flexors, is used to substitute for a markedly weakened gastrosoleus group.

Several procedures for correction have been recommended, but the one most frequently used and almost universally accepted is the *modified Jones procedure*:

1) Expose the interphalangeal joint through a reversed L-shaped incision extending transversely just distal to the interphalangeal joint and proximally along the dorsomedial side of the great toe for half the length of the proximal phalanx. Reflect the skin proximally, exposing the extensor hallucis longus tendon and cut the tendon 2 cm. proximal to the joint. One can either arthrodese the joint or perform a tenodesis. In the former method, the apposing cartilagenous surfaces are denuded and the underlying cortices are roughened. A Kirschner wire is first passed retrograde through the center of the cortical surface of the distal phalanx, emerging at the tip

of the great toe until at least a length of Kirschner wire 10 cm. long is protruding. After the drill is detached, the wire is cut obliquely at the proximal end just proximal to the cortex, thus producing a relatively sharp point. By reapplying the drill to the end protruding beyond the tip of the great toe, the wire is then spun into the proximal phalanx (but not into the metatarsophalangeal joint) after the two surfaces of the interphalangeal joint are fitted snugly together. At the point where the wire protrudes beyond the skin at the tip of the toe, bend the wire to a right angle, leaving approximately 0.5 cm. beyond the right angle bend and clip off the remainder. By performing this small step, intrusion of the wire into the soft tissues is prevented. When fusion of the interphalangeal joint has taken place (usually four to six weeks), remove the wire.

If one prefers to perform a tenodesis, the proximal end of the severed distal portion is buried into the proximal phalanx by developing a transverse slot in the dorsal cortical surface. A drill hole is also made into the dorsal cortex 0.5 cm. proximal to the slot. Next, pass a mattress suture through the proximal end, pass both ends through the slot, and out the drill hole, thus pulling the tendon into the slot, pass each suture end separately through the tendon, and tie the suture. One must make certain that the distal tendon is pulled snugly so that the interphalangeal joint remains in the exact neutral position.

2) Expose the neck of the first metatarsal through a 2.5 to 3 cm. dorsomedial incision beginning from the level of the proximal transverse skin crease and extending proximally. The extensor hallucis longus tendon is then exposed and delivered into the new incision, care being taken not to injure the short toe extensor tendon. The sheath of the long tendon is completely excised. A drill hole, large enough to permit the tendon to pass through, is made beginning at the inferomedial surface of the first metatarsal neck, transversely and emerging on the dorsolateral surface. The tendon is passed through, pulled snugly (with the foot in maximum extension) and sutured on itself. Chromicized collagen interrupted sutures are preferred. In the

standard Jones procedure, one long dorsal incision is used. It is not as desirable as the two shorter incisions since there is a tendency to thick scar formation with the single incision. Pseudoarthrosis of the interphalangeal joint occasionally does occur, and for this reason, tenodesis is preferable.

Postoperative care consists of immobilization of the foot in the neutral position with the cast extending from the tips of the toes to the tibial tubercle. The cast is removed at the end of six weeks as is the wire, should the latter have been used for the immobilization of the interphalangeal joint. Active physical therapy is then begun to reconstitute the power of the transplanted muscle.

The *Dickson and Diveley* transfer of the extensor hallucis longus to the flexor hallucis longus, accompanied by arthrodesis or by tenodesis of the extensor hallucis longus tendon to correct flexion at the interphalangeal joint, is another method of correcting clawing of the great toe due to weakness of either the extensors or the short flexors of the great toe. In this procedure, the flexor hallucis longus tendon is exposed through a 4 to 5 cm. incision along the medial border of the head of the first metatarsal. The incision should begin just distal to the metatarsophalangeal joint. The second dorsal incision is then made along the extensor hallucis longus tendon which extends from the base of the first metatarsal to the neck of this bony structure. Isolate the tendon of the extensor hallucis longus and divide it just proximal to the interphalangeal joint. A tunnel is then made in the soft tissues on the medial side of the first metatarsal, proximal to the head, and the proximal end of the extensor tendon is rerouted through this tunnel to the plantar aspect of the foot. A slit is then made in the flexor hallucis longus tendon just proximal to the head of the first metatarsal and the extensor hallucis longus tendon is passed through it and sutured on itself with interrupted chromicized collagen sutures. Arthrodesis or tenodesis of the interphalangeal joint is carried out in the usual manner. Immobilization is also carried out in the usual manner.

Dropfoot Deformity Due to Loss of the Tibialis Anterior Muscle Power. In this type deformity the triceps surae muscle group becomes contracted as well as the plantar fascia. If the posterior tibial tendon is intact, restoration of active dorsiflexion can be expected by its transfer anteriorly to the central cuneiform through the interosseous membrane, combined with transfer of the extensor hallucis longus tendon to the first metatarsal, as well as release of the tight plantar fascia and lengthening of the sortened heel cord that usually accompanies this deformity.

Transplantation of the tibialis posterior to the dorsum of the foot through the interosseous membrane is not a difficult procedure, but it does require meticulous dissection of the muscle, adequate splitting of the interosseous membrane, and subcutaneous transfer of the tendon to the middle cuneiform. It is necessary to make four skin incisions. The method of transfer is a slight modification of Barr's technique:

Make a small incision on the medial aspect of the foot beginning at the level of and just plantar to the navicular tubercle, extending distally to the first metatarsophalangeal joint. Identify the posterior tibial tendon and dissect it free from the medial plantar surface of the navicular. Follow the tendon down to its plantar insertion and detach it, thus gaining as much length as possible. Next, make the second incision beginning 2 to 3 cm. proximal to the tip of the medial malleolus and posterior to it, extending proximally for a distance of 8 cm. just posterior to and parallel to the tibia over the region of the musculotendinous junction of the tibialis posterior. Deliver the tendon into the second incision.

The third incision is next made on the anterior aspect of the leg. This incision should be 8 to 10 cm. long, beginning just above the level of the distal tibiofibular syndesmosis and extending proximally just lateral to the edge of the tibia. Split the fascia exposing the underlying tibialis anterior and the extensor hallucis longus muscles. Retract the former medially and the latter laterally exposing the interosseous membrane along the entire incision. The dorsalis pedis artery should be identified and preserved. The interosseous membrane should then be carefully cut along the entire length of the incision from the level of the syndesmosis, extending proximally as high as possible. It should not be stripped from the tibia. The more generous the size of the window, the less likelihood there will be of failure of the procedure. The primary cause for failure for this operation is an inadequate window in the interosseous membrane.

When the tibialis posterior tendon is passed through from the posterior incision to the anterior one (which is the next step), the belly of this muscle should automatically herniate through the opening without any restriction. Next, make an incision on the dorsum of the foot over the base of the third metatarsal or the lateral cuneiform, depending upon the length of the tendon available and follow by the development of a tunnel between the fascia and the subcutaneous fat. Barr advises passing the tendon beneath the cruciate ligament. We do not recommend this step since, in a number of instances, there occurred constriction of the tendon under the cruciate ligament. An adequate sized drill hole is then made in the cuneiform or the third metatarsal base. The tendon is passed through with the use of a Bunnell pull-out wire suture as already described, with the foot in maximum extension and the tendon at physiologic tension. In transferring the muscle and tendon, and prior to inserting the tendon end into the tarsal or metatarsal bone, inspect the former carefully to make certain that it is not constricted or twisted. If necessary, lengthening of the tendo achillis by the Hibbs method (or any of the others already described), plus sectioning of the plantar fascia by Steindler's technique, should be carried out prior to the transplantation of the tibialis posterior. Following closure of all incisions in the usual manner, a long leg-cast is applied extending from the toes to the tibial tubercle with the ankle and foot in maximum extension. Cast immobilization should be continued for six weeks.

In the talipes equinovarus type foot due to poliomyelitis the deformity is that of inversion of the heel, adduction and supination of the forefoot throughout the midtarsal joints, and equinus through the ankle joint. If the muscle imbalance should be severe or long standing, there is cavus of the forefoot and, at times, clawing of the toes. This former deformity is the result of weakness or paralysis of the peroneal muscles with minimal to moderate weakness of the tibialis anterior. Since the triceps surae group is strong, equinus results. This, in turn, enhances the power of the tibialis posterior since it places this muscle at a mechanical advantage. The result is the development of hindfoot inversion and forefoot adduction and supination. Furthermore, with a weak tibialis anterior the toe extensors take over a portion of the function of extension of the foot and ankle, resulting in clawing of the toes. At times, external tibial torsion will further complicate the situation.

Of course, treatment in the young child will consist of adequate bracing with an inside iron, outside T-strap and an ankle stop at 90 degrees. However, one must keep in mind the external tibial torsion and see to it that the bracemaker applies the brace to the shoe in an externally rotated position. Failure to do so may increase the torsion. If the deformity should increase appreciably in spite of the brace, as may occasionally happen, early tendon surgery, as just described, may be necessary if the foot is not physiologically mature enough to allow a triple arthrodesis at first. Should this step be necessary, re-apply the brace after such soft tissue surgery until one can re-educate and rebuild the muscle power. We prefer waiting until the foot is, if necessary, barely mature enough to permit the performance of a triple arthrodesis and Steindler stripping, and then carry out the soft tissue procedures six weeks later, rather than reversing the operative sequence even if the former plan should lead to a slight increase in the deformity.

Paralysis of the Tibialis Anterior and Posterior Muscles. In patients with more severe paralysis affecting the posterior and anterior tibial muscles and the long toe extensors, the best results are obtained by transfer of both peroneal muscles anteriorly into the cuneiforms after tarsal stabilization. Muscle reeducation through intensive physiotherapy should be instituted following removal of the cast.

Hemigastrosoleus Transplant (Caldwell Procedure). Caldwell described transferring half of the gastrosoleus muscle and tendon forward into the cuneiforms to act as an extensor in patients without other active muscles available for transfer anteriorly. His best results were obtained when he transferred the medial half of the muscle and the tendon after closing the cut surfaces of the muscle and tendon edges and bringing them together to form a tube which presented no raw soft tissues surfaces. In this procedure an incision is made beginning at the level of the os calcis and the tendon is split proximally to the musculotendinous junction. The muscle group itself is split to the medial half of the gastrosoleus belly as far proximally as possible without interference with the neurovascular bundle. The aponeurotic portion of the gastrosoleus to be transplanted is tubed by a simple continuous suture of Number 000 plain catgut, as is the tendon.

Through a dorsal longitudinal incision, (Fig. 11-12A) expose the middle cuneiform bone and fashion an opening large enough to accommodate the end of the tendo achillis. A channel for the transplant is then developed between the subcutaneous fat and the deep fascia extending around the medial aspect of the tibia to the dorsum of the foot. This channel should be well delineated anteriorly and wide enough to accommodate the muscle belly in order that the medial half of the gastrosoleus can be transposed anteriorly as far as possible to effect a direct pull on the dorsum of the foot. The tendo achillis and the muscle are then drawn through this previously prepared channel to the dorsum of the foot and implanted into the cuneiform with the usual pull-out wire suture. The foot should be extended to a maximum amount prior to implantation of the end of the tendon into the opening in the middle cuneiform. Following closure of the soft tissues, the incisions are closed with subcuticular wire sutures and a long leg-cast is applied extending from the toes to the midthigh with the foot in maximum extension and with the knee at 90 degrees flexion.

Immobilization is maintained for a period of six weeks after which the cast is removed and physiotherapy is instituted. Ambulation is begun two weeks following removal of the cast. Active physical therapy for re-education of this muscle is necessary. One will observe at the beginning that the transplant will contract when the patient is requested to flex the foot. Gradually, over a period of several months, reversal of muscle action will take place and one will find that, although the lateral half of the gastrosoleus group will flex the foot, the medial half will extend it (Fig. 11-12B).

Combined active extension and flexion of 10 to 20 degrees has been the result of this procedure. Young reported continued success with this operation in correcting drop foot in 20 patients. We have had success in 7 patients using this same technique. In 2 patients, however, although active dorsiflexion did not return, the transplanted tendon acted as a tenodesis and controlled the drop foot deformity.

Calcaneovalgus Deformities of the Foot. In calcaneovalgus deformities, our best results have been achieved by transplanting the anterior tibial tendon through the interosseous membrane according to the technique of Peabody, and transferring the peroneal tendons and posterior tibial tendon, if they present good muscle power, into the os calcis or the tendo achillis. Unless some muscle power for extension of the stabilized foot remains anteriorly, a fixed equinus deformity can result. Such extension can usually be accomplished by transfer of the long toe extensors.

Jacob's modification of Gallie's tenodesis to control calcaneovalgus deformities has been most successful. After the Achilles tendon is severed proximally and split longitudinally, the two ends are passed through a large transverse hole drilled in the tibia. They are then sutured to each other with the foot in equinus. This technique is particularly valuable when tendons with sufficient muscle power are not available for transfer.

Bickle and Moe described transfer of the intact peroneus longus through a longitudinal groove in the os calcis to correct calcaneovalgus deformities. Although we have not had personal experience with this procedure, we have observed excellent function in several patients so treated.

A similar result can be obtained by performing a triple arthrodesis of the foot followed by transplantation of the anterior

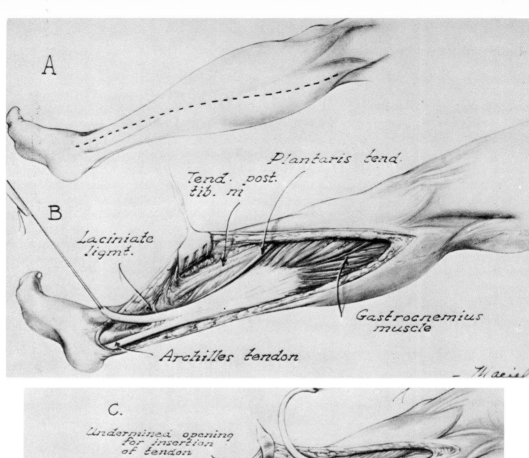

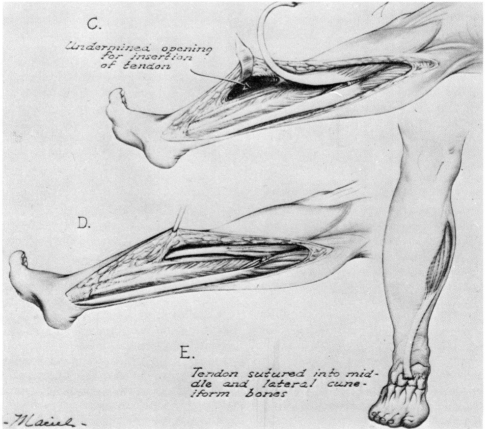

Fig. 11-12. Hemigastrosoleus transplant (Caldwell Procedure): Procedure is used to correct paralytic foot drop.

A. Various steps in the performance of this procedure. (Caldwell, Clin. Orth., Courtesy of J. B. Lippincott Co.)

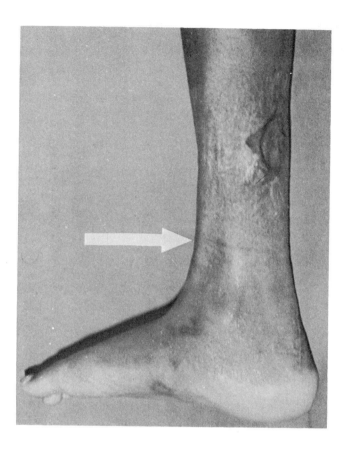

B.   Postoperative result of this procedure. Note the range of extension of the foot and ankle in a previous drop foot deformity.

and posterior tibial and the peroneus longus tendons to the os calcis (Fig. 11-13A & B).

Clawing of the Toes. Clawing of the toes with hypertension of the metatarsophalangeal joints and flexion of the interphalangeal joints is characteristic of two patterns of muscle imbalance. Clawing occurs most often when the long toe extensors are used to aid extension of the forefoot, as already mentioned, particularly when the heel cord is short. It is most pronounced at the beginning of the swing phase. Less often clawing results when the long toe flexors are being substituted for a weak triceps surae. In this case, clawing is present during the stance phase and increases at the point of push-off, when the toes exert maximum pressure on the ground. Non-fixed clawing deformity can be corrected either by transferral of the toe flexors into the extensor hood as described by Taylor, or by transferral of the long toe extensors around the neck of each metatarsal as described by Forbes. The Girdlestone-Taylor transfer corrects the deformity and improves the function in the presence of both extension weakness and triceps surae weakness, whereas the transfer of toe extensors around the metatarsal neck is applicable only in patients with weakness of the extensor muscle group.

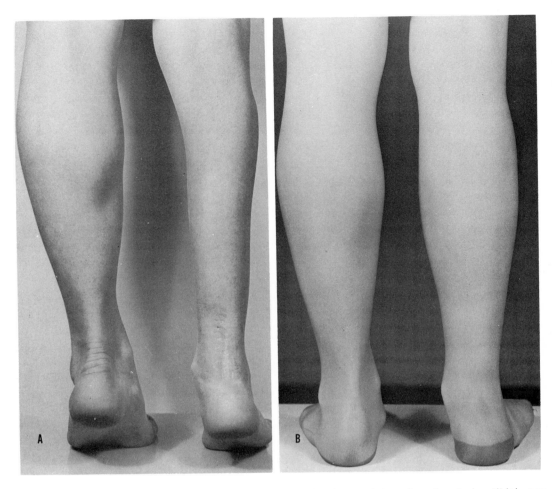

Fig. 11-13.   A. View of calves eight years after stabilization and transfer of anterior tibial, posterior tibial and peroneus longus into calcaneus. Note ability to bear weight on forefoot and the asymmetry of the calves.

B.   Cosmetic prosthesis applied to right calf restoring symmetry, a factor of considerable importance to a nineteen-year-old co-ed.

In the Girdlestone-Taylor procedure, a 3 cm. dorsolateral incision is made (beginning at the level of the neck of the metatarsal to the lateral side of the distal interphalangeal joint of each involved toe) exposing the extensor tendon. The dissection is then carried down between the metatarsal heads, and the transverse capitellar ligaments are severed to expose the short and long toe flexors of each corresponding toe. These two tendons are then delivered into the wound by hooking a small blunt hook around them and are cut at their insertions. This portion of the procedure should be carried out on the lateral side of the proximal phalanx so that the tendons are delivered into each incision. Next, suturing is carried out of both the long and short toe flexors into the distal end of the extensor expansion by the buttonhole technique. This will correct the clawing of each toe. After closure of the soft tissues and with the ankle and foot in maximum extension, the cast should first be applied from the tibial tubercle to the midmetatarsal region. After this portion of the cast has set, the remaining portion of the cast should be applied and molded in such a manner that each corrected digit will be maintained in a position of 10 degrees flexion at the metatarsophalangeal joint level. By placing the toes in this position, the interphalangeal joints will automatically correct themselves into the neutral position. Before either type of transfer for extensor weakness is performed, contracture of the heel cord must be corrected or the transferred tendons will be unable to function.

Hibbs described transfer of the long toe extensors en masse into the dorsal surface of the cuneiform for claw toe deformity associated with the modified Jones procedure to correct clawing of the great toe.

Dorsal Bunion of the First Metatarsal. Dorsal bunion of the first metatarsal results from muscle imbalance, usually weakness of the peroneus longus with a strong anterior tibial tendon and strong toe flexors. It can be corrected by arthrodesis of the midtarsal and tarsometatarsal joints of the first ray, accompanied by transfer of the anterior tibial to the plantar surface of the navicular. Transfer is also performed of the flexor hallucis longus into the dorsum of the first metatarsal and metatarsophalangeal joint through an oblique tunnel from the plantar to the dorsal surface of the first metatarsal as described by Lapidus. According to Riordan, in feet with persistent normal intrinsic muscle power, transfer of the abductor hallucis muscle and tendon into the long toe flexor after release of the flexed metatarsophalangeal joint will also correct the deformity. Hammond transfers all deforming tendons (except the flexor hallucis longus) to the dorsum of the foot in the midline and then uses a plantar wedge osteotomy at the base of the first metatarsal to force it into plantar flexion. We have had no personal experience with this method, but have observed excellent results in patients so treated elsewhere.

Postoperative Care. The principle of postoperative management is maintenance of the corrected position obtained at operation without disturbing circulation until after stabilization or attachment of the tendon has occurred. The extremity is usually immobilized in a long leg-cast applied over sterile sheet cotton. If fixation has

been used to maintain apposition of bony surfaces and is satisfactory, it may suffice to use a pressure dressing with molded plaster splints to maintain the position of the knee and foot. One advantage of this method is quick relief of pressure by cutting the dressing with bandage scissors should edema or circulatory insufficiency ensue. Because of the frequency of swelling after operation, many advocate splitting of the cast before the patient leaves the operating room so that the cast can be spread and the sheet cotton cut if circumstances indicate. The particular regimen followed after the operation will vary according to the effectiveness of the nursing and house staffs. Such personnel should be repeatedly reminded that complaint of severe pain after a reconstructive operation on the foot is indication for *immediate decompression* rather than increased sedation.

Elevation of the part to promote venous drainage and to reduce arterial pulse pressure can best be accomplished by elevation of the knee, rest, and raising of the end of the mattress at least 12 to 18 inches above the level of the thorax. Reducing the temperature of the part by applying ice bags will also add to the patient's comfort if nursing service is adequate to keep the bags free of air and filled with crushed ice instead of luke warm water.

Although a tendon transfer can be expected to become attached within three weeks, it should be protected in a cast, as should the stabilization for at least an additional six weeks after transplant. This is followed by bracing for three to six months to prevent overstretching and to assist in reeducation of the muscles of the transferred tendon. Certain transfers require careful supervision, whereas others regain function in their new position without difficulty. If the muscle of the transferred tendon must work out of phase, as in transfer of the anterior tibial tendon posteriorly to correct a calcaneovalgus deformity, reeducation alone will effect successful function. Transfer of the long toe extensors into the metatarsals to assist in extension seldom requires any training whatsoever, since these muscles are working in phase in their new position.

Once stability has been attained and all residual muscle power transferred to the midline either anteriorly or posteriorly by appropriate tendon transfers, other reconstructive operations can be done to correct deformity and alignment of the extremity. Most patients with paralysis of the lower extremity can be rendered brace-free if the hip and foot can be made stable.

TABLE 11-1.   TENDON TRANSPLANT FOR FOOT IMBALANCE

| | Stabilized Later | | Not Stabilized | | | | Total |
| | | | Poor Result | | Good Foot and Function | | |
	no.	(%)	no.	(%)	no.	(%)	no.
Calcaneovarus							
Anterior tibial, posterior tibial, peroneals	11	(73.4)	3	(20)	1	(6.6)	15
Planovalgus or paralytic pronation							
Peroneals forward and extensor hallucis	5	(50.0)	3	(30)	2	(20)	10
Equinovarus							
Anterior tibial, posterior tibial to midline	12	(31.0)	17	(42)	10	(27)	39
Anterior tibial to midline or cuboid	7	(47.0)	5	(33)	3	(20)	15
							79

TABLE 11-2.   RESULTS OF 276 STABILIZATION PROCEDURES IN 174 PATIENTS

| | Good | | Fair | | Poor | | Total |
	no.	(%)	no.	(%)	no.	(%)	no.
Equinovarus—triple arthrodesis							
Without tendon transfer	8	(43)	2	(14)	8	(43)	18
With tendon transfer	98	(80)	5	(4)	20	(16)	123
							141
Equinus—Lambrinudi							
Without tendon transfer	1	(12.4)	0	(0)	8	(87.6)	9
With posterior tibial forward	9	(50.0)	5	(27.8)	4	(22.2)	18
With posterior tibial and peroneals	28	(71.7)	6	(15.3)	5	(13.0)	39
							66
Calcaneal foot—triple arthrodesis							
Anterior tibial transer posteriorly	10	(47.6)	5	(23.8)	6	(28.6)	21
Anterior tibial, posterior tibial and/or peroneals	20	(71.4)	6	(21.4)	2	(7.2)	28
							49
Pantalar arthrodesis	16	(72.7)	4*	(18.2)	2†	(9.1)	22
							276

*Metatarsalgia
†Tarsal metatarsalgia

BIBLIOGRAPHY

ALBERT, E.: Einige Fälle künstliche Ankylosenbildung en paralytischen Gliedmassen, Wien. Med. Press. 23:1882.

ALDREDGE, R. H. AND RIORDAN, D. C.: The Use of Staples and Bone-chip Grafts for Internal Fixation in Foot Stabilization Operations, J. Bone Jt. Surg. 35A:951-957 (Oct.) 1953.

BARR, J. S.: The Management of Poliomyelitis: The Late Stage, Poliomyelitis, First International Poliomyelitis Conference, Philadelphia, J. B. Lippincott Co., 1949, pp. 201-232.

BARR, J. S. AND RECORD, E. E.: Arthrodesis of the Ankle for Correction of Foot Deformity. Surg. Clin. North America. 1281-1288 (Oct.) 1947.

BARTOW, B. AND PLUMMER, W. W.: The Use of Intra-articular Silk Ligaments for Fixation of Loose Joints in the Residual Paralysis of Anterior Poliomyelitis. Amer. J. Orthop. Surg. 9:65-71, 1911-12.

BICKEL, W. H. AND MOE, J. W.: Translocation of Peroneus Longus Tendon for Paralytic Calcaneus Deformity of Foot, Surg. Gyn. Obst. 78:627-630 (June) 1944.

BODIAN, D.: Poliomyelitis: Pathologic Anatomy, Poliomyelitis. First International Poliomyelitis Conference. Philadelphia, J. B. Lippincott Co., 1949, 62-84.

BREWSTER, A. H.: Countersinking Astragalus in Paralytic Feet. New Eng. J. Med. 209:71-74 (July) 1933

CALDWELL, G. A.: Arthrodesis of the Feet. Am. Ac. Orth. Surg. Instructional Course Lectures. 6:174-177, Ann Arbor, J. W. Edwards Co., 1949.

CALDWELL, G. D.: Correction of Paralytic Footdrop by Hemigastrosoleus Transplant. Clin. Orth. 11:81-84, 1958.

CAMPBELL, W. C.: An Operation for the Correction of "Drop-foot", J. Bone Jt. Surg. 5:815-825, 1923.

CLOSE, J. R. AND TODD, F. N.: The Phasic Activity of the Muscles of the Lower Extremity and the Effect of Tendon Transfer. J. Bone Jt. Surg. 41A:189-208 (March) 1959.

CODIVILLA, A.: Il trattamento chirurgico moderno della paralys i infantile spinale, Policlinco. 7: 110-144 (Feb.) 1900.

COLE, W. H.: Treatment of Claw-foot, J. Bone Jt. Surg. 22:895-908 (Oct.) 1940.

DAVIS, G. G.: Treatment of Hollow Foot (Pes Cavus), Amer. J. Orth. Surg. 11:231-242 (Oct.) 1913.

DICKSON, F. D. AND DIVELEY, R. L.: Operation for Correction of Mild Claw Foot, Result of Infantile Paralysis. J.A.M.A., 87:1275-1277 (Oct.) 1926.

DUNN, N.: Stabilizing Operations in Paralytic Feet. Proc. Roy. Soc. Med. 15 (3) 15-22 (Dec.) 1921.

DWYER, F. C.: Osteotomy of the Calcaneum for Pes Cavus, J. Bone Jt. Surg. 41B:80-86 (Feb.) 1959.

ELLIOTT, H. C.: Studies on Motor Cells of Spinal Cord, Position and Extent of Lesions in Nuclear Pattern of Convalescent and Chronic Poliomyelitis Patients. Amer. J. Path. 21:87-97 (Jan.) 1945.

Studies on Motor Cells of Spinal Cord, Poliomyelitic Lesion in Spinal Motor Nuclei in Acute Cases. Amer. J. Path. 23:313-325 (March) 1947.

FORBES, A. M.: Clawfoot, and How to Relieve It. Surg. Gyn. Obstet. 16:81-83 (Jan.) 1913.

GALLIE, W. E.: Tendon Fixation; A Preliminary Report of a Simple Operation for the Prevention of Deformity in Paralytic Talipes. Ann. Surg. 57:427-429 (March) 1913.

Tendon Fixation in Infantile Paralysis: A Review of 150 Operations. Amer. J. Orth. Surg. 14: 18-29 (Jan.) 1916.

GILL, A. B.: An Operation to Make a Posterior Bone Block at the Ankle to Limit Foot Drop. J. Bone Jt. Surg. 15A:166-170 (Jan.) 1933.

GOLDTHWAIT, J. E.: Operation for the Stiffening of the Ankle Joint in Infantile Paralysis, Amer. J. Orth. Surg. 5:271-275 (Jan.) 1908.

GREEN, W. T.: The Management of Poliomyelitis: The Convalescent Stage. Poliomyelitis First International Poliomyelitis Conference. Philadelphia, J. B. Lippincott Co., 1949, 165-185.

GRICE, D. S.: An Extra-articular Arthrodesis of the Subastragalar Joint for Correction of Paralytic Flat Feet in Children. J. Bone Jt. Surg. 34A: 927-940 (Oct.) 1952.

HAGELSTAM, L.: Muscle and Tendon Transplantations in the Lower Limb in Poliomyelitis, Acta. Orth. Scand. 27 (sup) 49:63, 1957.

HAMMOND, G.: Elevation of First Metatarsal Bone with Hallux Equinus. Surg. 13:240-256 (Feb.) 1943.

HART, V. L.: Arthrodesis of the Foot in Infantile Paralysis. Surg. Gyn. Obst., 64:794-805 (April) 1937.

HASLAM, E. T. AND WICKSTROM, J. K.: Single Kirschner Wire Fixation in Triple Arthrodesis, South. Med. J. 48:767-774 (July) 1955.

HERTZ, H., MADSEN, A., AND BUCHTHAL, F.: Prognostic Implications of Electromyography in Acute Anterior Poliomyelitis. J. Bone Jt. Surg. 36A: 902-911 (Oct.) 1954.

HIBBS, R. A.: An Operation for Claw Foot. J.A.M.A., 73:1583-1585 (Nov.) 1919.

HODES, R., PEACOCK, S. M., JR., AND BODIAN, D.: Selective Destruction of Large Motoneurons by Poliomyelitis Virus, Size of Motoneurons in Spinal Cord of Rhesus Monkeys. J. Neuropath. & Exper. Neurol. 8:400-410 (Oct.) 1949.

HOFFMAN, P.: An Operation for Severe Grades of Contracted or Clawed Toes. Amer. J. Orth. Surg. 9:441-449 (Feb.) 1912.

HOKE, M.: An Operation for Stabilizing Paralytic Feet. J. Ortho. Surg. 3:494-507, October, 1921.

HUNT, W. S. AND THOMPSON, H. A.: Pantalar Arthrodesis, J. Bone Jt. Surg. 36-A:349-362 (April) 1954.

JACOBS, JOHN T.: Personal Communication.

JONES, R.: The Soldier's Foot and the Treatment of Common Deformities of the Foot, Part II: Claw-Foot. Brit. Med. J., 1:749-753 (May) 1916.

LAMBRINUDI, C.: New Operation for Drop-foot. Brit. J. Surg. 15:193-200 (Oct.) 1927.

LAPIDUS, P. W.: "Dorsal Bunion": Its Mechanics and Operative Correction. J. Bone Jt. Surg. 22:627-637 (July) 1940.

LEGG, A. T.: The Early Treatment of Poliomyelitis and the Importance of Physical Therapy, J.A.M.A., 107:633-635 (Aug.) 1936.

LORTHOIR: Huit cas d'arthrodèse du pied avec extirpation temporaire d'astragale. Ann. Soc. Belge de Chir. pp. 6-7, 1911.

LOVETT, R. W.: A Plan of Treatment of Infantile Paralysis, J.A.M.A., 67:421-424 (Aug.) 1916.

MAYER, L.: The Physiological Method of Tendon Transplantation. Surg. Gyn. Obstet. 22:182-197 (Feb.) 1916.

MORRIS, H. D.: Personal Communication.

MORTENS, J., GREGERSEN, P., AND ZACHARIAE, L.: Tendon Transplantation in the Foot After Poliomyelitis in Children. Acta. Orth. Scand. 27:153-163, 1957.

McCARROLL, H. R.: Role of Physical Therapy in Early Treatment of Poliomyelitis. J.A.M.A., 120:517-519 (Oct.) 1942.

McCARROLL, H. R.: Foot Deformities Resulting from Irrepairable Nerve Lesions. Am. Acad. Ortho. Surg., Instructional Course Lectures. Ann Arbor, J. W. Edwards Co., 1944, 149-168.

NICOLADONI, K.: Uber sehnentransplantationen, Versammi. Deutsch Naturforsch. u. Artzte im Salsburg, 54. 1880.

NIERNY, K.: Zur Behandlung der Fussdeformitäten bei ausgedehnten Lahnungen, Arch. f. Orthop. u. Unfall Chir. 3:60, 1905.

PEABODY, C. W.: Tendon Transposition in the Paralytic Foot. Am. Acad. Orthop. Surg. Instructional Course Lectures. 6:178-188, Ann Arbor, J. W. Edwards Co., 1949.

PEERS, J. H.: Pathology of Convalescent Poliomyelitis in Man. Amer. J. Path. 19:673-695 (July) 1943.

RANSON, S. W. AND SAMS, C. F.: A Study of Muscle in Contracture: The Permanent Shortening of Muscles Caused by Tenotomy and Tetanus Toxin. J. Neur. & Psychopath. 8:304-320 (April) 1928.

REIDY, J. A., BODERICK, T. A., AND BARR, J. S.: Tendon Transplantations in the Lower Extremity, J. Bone Jt. Surg. 34-A:900-914 (Oct.) 1952.

RIORDAN, D. C.: Personal Communication.

RYERSON, E. W.: Arthrodesing Operations on Feet. J. Bone Jt. Surg. 5:453-471 (July) 1923.

SHARRARD, W. J. W.: Muscle Recovery in Poliomyelitis, J. Bone Jt. Surg. 37-B:63-79 (Feb.) 1955.

The Distribution of Permanent Paralysis in the Lower Limb in Poliomyelitis. J. Bone Jt. Surg. 37-B:540-558 (Nov.) 1955.

STEINDLER, A.: Stripping of Os Calcis. J. Orth. Surg. 2:8-12 (Jan.) 1920.

Treatment of Flail Ankle: Parastragaloid Arthrodesis. J. Bone Jt. Surg. 5:284-294 (April) 1923.

STEPHENS, R.: Dorsal Wedge Operation for Metatarsal Equinus. J. Bone Jt. Surg. 5:485-489, 1923.

TAYLOR, R. G.: The Treatment of Claw Toes by Multiple Transfer of Flexor into Extensor Tendons, J. Bone Jt. Surg. 33-B:539-542 (Nov) 1951.

WESTIN, G. W.: Tendon Transfers About the Foot, Ankle, and Hip in the Paralyzed Lower Extremity. Am. Acad. Orth. Surg. Instructional Course Lectures. J. Bone Jt. Surg. 47-A:1430-1443 (Oct.) 1965.

WHITMAN, R.: The Operative Treatment of Paralytic Talipes of the Calcaneus Type. Amer. J. Med. Sci. 122:593-601 (Nov.) 1901.

YOUNG, B. H.: Personal Communication.

= 12 =

The Foot in Cerebral Palsy

Frank H. Bassett, III, M.D.

DEFORMITIES of the foot in patients with cerebral palsy and related central nervous system conditions are similar to those resulting from other neuromuscular diseases, but because of complicating central nervous system factors, such as muscle spasticity, they differ in their response to treatment. Therefore, one cannot predict the results of therapy programs for patients with cerebral palsy as is possible with patients who have poliomyelitis, meningomyelocele, Charcot-Marie-Tooth disease, or other neuromuscular disorders.

In cerebral palsy, the sense of balance, sight, and hearing are often impaired. In addition to spasticity and athetosis, mental retardation of varying degrees is frequently present. Any therapeutic program for the cerebral-palsied child must be directed toward meeting his overall needs and potentials. The treatment of deformities is only one part of the problem. The complete spectrum of social, educational, mental, emotional, and physical capabilities must be evaluated in each instance and management instituted according to need.

The decision to treat a foot deformed by cerebral palsy must take into account the patient's potential for ambulation. When ambulation is not the primary goal, the need for correction of the deformity is lessened, but correction may still be important for the benefit of sitting, bracing, and particularly, cosmetic effect. When there is a possibility of ambulation, a well-planned rehabilitation program may promote a bedridden or wheelchair patient to partial or independent ambulation. Indicated surgery can be effective in the correction of refractory deformities and, when performed early, can prevent fixed deformities, eliminate long and expensive periods of bracing, and avoid the development of bad habits of locomotion. Early age is not a contraindication to corrective surgery.

PATHOGENESIS OF DEFORMITIES

Hypoxia, cerebral hemorrhage, Rh factor and other blood incompatibilities, various prenatal and postpartum infectious processes, and prematurity all have been im-plicated as causative factors of cerebral palsy. No consistent cause-and-effect pattern has been established. Frequently associated findings are: prematurity with spastic diplegia, kernicterus with athetosis, anoxia neonatorum with athetosis, and trauma with spasticity. Regardless of the cause, when there is sufficient damage to any of the suppressor areas in the central nervous system, the result is uninhibited function of the gamma motor system.

The arrangement of the nerve pathways in the gamma motor system, with afferent nerve endings located in muscles and tendons, is thought to be responsible for maintaining proper muscle tone. When central control over this motor system is lost, the muscles exhibit an increased response to stimulation. There is increased muscle tone and spasticity and smooth, coordinated neuromuscular control is lost. In cerebral palsy, voluntary effort by the patient can be thwarted by clonus, exaggerated stretch reflex, tension, or overflow. The basic underlying pathology responsible for the various neuromuscular dysfunctions is not clear, nor is the etiology of the several forms of cerebral palsy adequately understood. Despite extensive investigations, autopsy findings have not revealed any consistent pathologic patterns.

The spastic type of cerebral palsy is characterized by an exaggerated stretch reflex, clonus, and increased deep tendon reflexes. A patient with athetosis, on the other hand, presents uncontrollable, purposeless movements of which there may be many patterns. Muscle tension is often associated with athetosis. The anti-gravity muscles are usually the more severely involved. Extensor thrust, consisting of equinus, knee extension, and scissoring, are usually present in both types of palsy. The antagonist muscles are seldom involved to the same degree of spasticity or tension. The resultant muscle imbalance tends to increase. The antagonist muscles, although involved, become additionally stretched out and weakened. The resulting deformity can become fixed with permanent bone and joint changes.

Equinus, the result of involvement of the triceps surae, is the most common deformity of the foot in patients with cerebral palsy. When the peroneals, posterior tibial, or toe flexors are also involved, they contribute to the deformity and create a valgus or varus foot in association with the equinus. Spasticity or tension in the toe flexors causes flexion or curling of the toes, particularly when the foot is extended.

EVALUATION OF DEFORMITIES

In evaluating foot deformities in a patient with cerebral palsy, one must recognize that such deformities can be either primary, secondary to deformities elsewhere, or the result of overflow. An evaluation of the entire trunk and all extremities must be included in any critical effort to determine the etiology and type of muscle imbalance, contracture, or deformity, and to ascertain whether the involvement is fixed or is due to spasticity without true shortening. The patient should be examined both while at rest and while ambulating or attempting to do so, and one should remember that osseous, as well as fibrous soft tissues, may be involved.

Foot deformity may be secondary to proximal deformities of the hip and knee.

When the more proximal deformities are present, tests should be carried out to determine, when possible, which is the primary offender. For example, the gastrocnemius muscle can produce both equinus and knee flexion. When a knee flexion contracture is present, the part played by the gastrocnemius must be evaluated by relaxing the hamstrings, which can be done by hyperextending the hip and flexing the knee. With the extremity so positioned, and the foot in extension (dorsiflexion), if full knee extension is not possible, the degree of gastrocnemius involvement can be estimated fairly accurately by the amount of plantar flexion required to gain knee extension.

When equinus and knee flexion occur in

combination with a hip flexion contracture, a careful appraisal of the hip deformity is obligatory. Until correction is obtained of the often complex hip deformity, erect posture cannot be achieved. In fact, as a result of attempts to maintain an upright posture, the patient may experience a recurrence of the foot and knee deformities.

When ankle extension is limited by a tight Achilles tendon, and the patient attempts to place the heel on the floor during ambulation, the tibia acts as a lever and can thrust the knee into genu recurvatum.

Foot deformities frequently result from overflow. This is a phenomenon in which involuntary contraction of one muscle group results from stimuli brought on by attempts of voluntary contractions of another group. Muscles which do not appear excessively spastic or strong on the examining table may produce disabling de-

formities on attempts at ambulation when affected by overflow. For example, as the result of overflow from spastic quadriceps or adductor muscles, the triceps surae, while not found tight on the examining table, may produce marked equinus when the child is on his feet. The patient with clonus and hyperactive reflexes in the antigravity calf muscles, who has only mild limitation of abduction of the hips on the examining table, may demonstrate scissoring with attempts at ambulation. Only by observing the entire dynamic muscle picture with the patient ambulating or attempting to do so, can overflow and its influence in the production of foot deformities be properly evaluated. Observation of attempted activity allows simultaneous evaluation of the functional relationship of all the muscles of the lower extremities and the trunk.

MUSCLE TESTING

Neither spasticity nor tension can be measured accurately. The standard muscle tests employed to determine muscle weakness do not provide reliable estimates of muscle power in cerebral palsy. Some of the reasons for this relative unreliance are:

1) When a spastic muscle is stimulated by active contraction or passive stretching, the excitable stretch reflex system produces a contraction of unpredictable degree. Clonus or repetitive rhythmic contractions may occur.

2) The degree of spasticity in a given muscle varies from time to time. Emotional excitement, strange environment, or the presence of crowds often aggravate muscle hypertonicity or tension.

3) In patients with a brief attention span, the cooperation necessary for accurate muscle testing is often lacking.

When variations in muscle imbalance exist, a full study of the overactive muscle and its antagonist is a prerequisite for rational therapy. Such evaluation may be difficult, particularly of the multiple-joint-action muscles, such as the triceps surae, hamstrings, and quadriceps. The muscle analysis must include tests for strength,

muscle length, clonus, tension, rigidity, resistance to rapid passive stretch, and resistance to slow steady pressure. Before instituting therapy, the physician must decide whether the malfunction is due to muscle imbalance, structural shortening, tension, or spasticity without true shortening.

The muscles, which play a direct role in the production of foot deformities, are the triceps surae (composed of the gastrocnemius, the popliteus and the soleus), the posterior tibial, the flexor and extensor hallucis longus, flexor digitorum longus, peroneus longus, and peroneus brevis. The common toe extensors and the intrinsic muscles of the foot rarely play a significant role in the production of deformities.

To separate the triceps surae into its component parts, one must analyze the involved muscles with the knee extended initially and then in the flexed position. Since the gastrocnemius portion of the triceps surae takes its origin from the femoral condyles, it is partially relaxed when the knee is flexed, and therefore can be eliminated from the analysis. With the patient's knee flexed, one can test the soleus muscle alone by applying an extending (dorsiflexing) force to the os calcis. To test the part played by the gastrocnemius, the examination is repeated with the knee extended. Employing an extending force at the forefoot brings the peroneals, posterior tibial, and toe flexors into play, and thus a true evaluation of the calf muscle group cannot be achieved. Therefore, one must grasp the heel and exert the necessary extension force in order to test the triceps surae group.

In association with an equinus deformity, one often finds a varus or valgus positioning of the heel. The latter is the more common. It usually results from the bowstring effect of the heel cord on the ankle and subtalar joints, preventing normal extension of the foot. In the face of this re-

striction of extension by the tight heel cord, the calcaneus is rotated posterolaterally from beneath the talus; the sustentaculum tali loses its normal supporting position, and a rocker-bottom deformity results (Fig. 12-1). Although the heel may appear to be in contact with the ground, in actuality, the calcaneus is plantar-flexed and everted, and the talus is standing on its head (plantar flexed or vertical talus). The apparent extension occurs at the midfoot. When spastic or tension-involved peroneal muscles contribute to this deformity, their hyperactivity produces taut tendons which can be palpated posterior to the lateral malleolus. The tendons often migrate from their normal position and subluxate later-

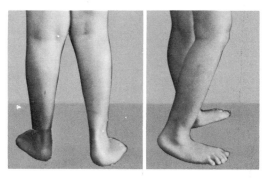

Fig. 12-1.   Rocker-bottom deformity of right foot resulting from tight soleus with bow-string effect on the ankle and subtalar joint resulting in rotation of the os calcis posterolaterally.

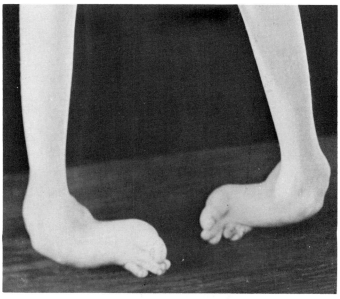

Fig. 12-2.   Untreated thirteen-year-old with spastic diplegia and severe equino-varus deformity bilaterally. What would you do to correct these feet? See Figure 12-8.

ally. Light, passive attempts to correct the valgus deformity often produce a clonus or exaggerated stretch reflex of the peroneals.

Equinovarus deformities, on the other hand, may result from overactive posterior tibial and toe flexor muscles (Fig. 12-2). Weight bearing or extension of the ankle in such feet leads to tightening of the posterior tibial tendon in its groove behind the medial malleolus, causing it to stand out as a tight band. A forefoot varus deformity may be seen in such cases associated with a tendency for internal rotation of the entire extremity.

Spasticity or tension of the toe flexor muscles must be differentiated from primary involvement of the posterior tibial muscle. If, when extension is applied to the foot, the toes curl, involvement of the toe flexors is present. The tendons can be felt

to tighten in the interval between the posterior tibial tendon and the pulse of the posterior tibial artery.

The active function of the extensor muscles of the foot should be evaluated. Often these structures have been stretched out and weakened by the more powerful antigravity muscles of the calf. In most cases, voluntary function of the anterior tibial muscle cannot be elicited. In many instances, with active flexion of the hip, extension of the foot will result along with flexion of the knee. This maneuver brings out a reflex action associated with ambulation sometimes referred to as "confusion". If, during the training period, the anterior tibial muscle can be developed, equinus can often be controlled. By taking advantage of "confusion" in early training programs or postoperative periods, occurrence or recurrence of equinus may be prevented.

SURGICAL TREATMENT

In the properly selected patients with cerebral palsy, surgical correction of foot deformities can offer beneficial results. Achieving such benefits depends upon restoration of muscle balance, joint alignment in the proper weight-bearing position, and correct posture. The ideal goal is a foot with a well-developed longitudinal arch, balanced muscle function, and a brace-free extremity with a heel-toe gait and adequate push-off. *In most instances surgery to correct a foot deformity should be considered only in the patients who are ambulatory or have a potential for ambulation.* Usually, muscle rerouting procedures are more successful than tendon transfers, but in children with the spastic type of cerebral palsy, who are carefully evaluated and who have fair to normal intelligence, tendon transfers can be carried out with excellent results. Tendon transfers should not be performed in the patient whose mental evaluations at most demonstrate appreciable impairment. Furthermore, one should not depend solely on the mental test in determining the patient's intelligence. He should evaluate the youngster's motivation. An attitude of over-protection on the parents' part should be corrected to one of encouragement.

Equinus. Numerous surgical procedures

and techniques have been employed to correct pes equinus. In 1913, Stoffel advocated selective motor branch neurectomy of the overactive muscle. Theoretically, any desired level of flaccid paralysis can be produced by this technique, but the results are unpredictable and a weakened push-off can be the consequence.

In 1924 Silfverskiold reported that muscles, which cross two joints, could, when spastic, produce not only movement at one joint, but also associated movement at the other joint. To permit function only at the primary joint, he reduced the action of the muscle by recession. Equinus, present with the knee extended and correctable by flexing the knee, was improved by recessing the heads of the origin of the involved gastrocnemius. More recently, other and perhaps more effective operations have been described. These are based on the principle of decreasing the function of the offensive gastrocnemius. Strayer advocates the release of the gastrocnemius muscle belly from its aponeurotic insertion. Baker prefers to lengthen the middle third of the gastrocnemius aponeurosis by a tongue-in-groove method (Fig. 12-3). Both these procedures relieve much of the stretch reflex and afford neurologic as well as mechanical advantages.

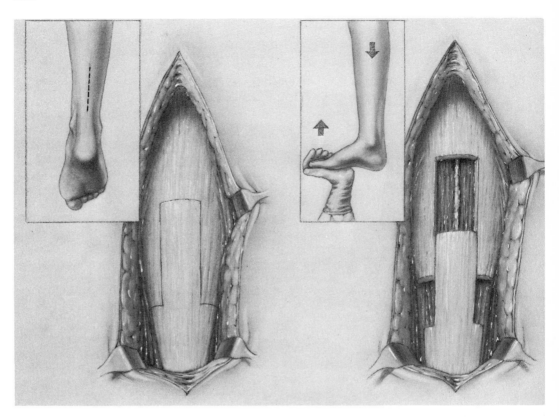

Fig. 12-3. Baker tongue in groove lengthening of the gastrocnemius tendon when this portion of the triceps surae is responsible for the equinus deformity of the foot.

Achilles tendon lengthening can correct an equinus deformity when the triceps surae is contracted, rather than when the gastrocnemius, alone, is involved. Success has been achieved with a coronal or sagittal plane "Z" lengthening. Banks and Green use multiple properly-spaced hemisections of the tendon, similar to the procedure described by White, to assure severance of each fiber at one level or another. Midcalf aponeurosis lengthening is preferable to the non-specific lengthening of the Achilles tendon since it avoids adherent scars over the Achilles tendon, allows selectivity, avoids the soleus, and affords less chance of weakening push-off.

Equinovalgus. In a high percentage of children with cerebral palsy, valgus of the heel and pronation of the foot accompany equinus. Only in the mild cases, those without fixed bone and joint changes, can one hope to accomplish permanent realignment of the foot with correction of the equinus

element alone. Not until the calcaneus has been restored to its normal position with the sustentaculum tali supporting the posterior portion of the talus can equinus be accurately corrected. All elements of equinovalgus should be treated. To leave a valgus, pronated foot untreated is to invite progression of the deformity with the future problems of joint pain, shoe fitting, and ineffective gait.

To accomplish permanent correction, muscle balance must be restored, a dictum long-recognized in the treatment of flaccid as well as spastic paralyses. When peroneal muscle overactivity contributes to the valgus, as is usually the case in spastic equinovalgus deformities, the antagonist muscle which is responsible for maintaining eversion and inversion balance, is usually weakened and stretched out. Tenotomy of the offending peroneal tendons may allow the antagonist to take over, but a varus deformity may develop as a result of this procedure.

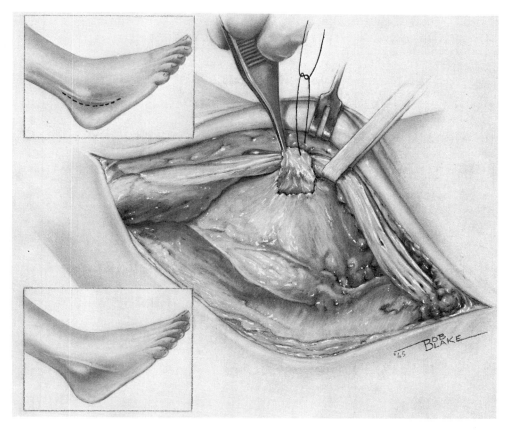

Fig. 12-4. Subcutaneous rerouting of the peroneus longus and brevis muscles to correct mild to moderate spastic valgus of the foot when there is no roentgenographic evidence of a plantar flexed or a vertical talus.

Lengthening of the peroneal tendons may aid in better muscle balance but, here again, the results are unpredictable. Subcutaneous rerouting of the peroneals (well to the front of the lateral malleolus) has appeared to overcome this complication. In this procedure (Fig. 12-4) an 8- to 10-cm. curvilinear incision is made posterior to the lateral malleolus with the halfway point of the incision at the level of the tip of the lateral malleolus. The annular ligament and the tendon sheath are opened proximally and distally for a sufficient distance to allow the rerouted peroneal tendons to be positioned subcutaneously in a straight line parallel to the pull of the peroneus tertius tendon and well in front of the malleolus. A raised flap of fascia sutured to the subcutaneous tissue will aid in stabilizing the tendons in the new, desired position. After closure of the skin with subcuticular wire

sutures, a cast is applied for four weeks with the foot held in mild inversion. Active exercises under the supervision of a physiotherapist are instituted following removal of the cast. Supervised ambulation is also permitted after cast removal. This procedure is indicated in the mild equinovalgus foot which on roentgenographic examination does not demonstrate a rocker-bottom deformity with a vertical talus.

In the severe equinovalgus deformities, extra-articular arthrodesis of the talocalcaneal joint is indicated with or without lengthening of the gastrocnemius, depending upon whether the shortness of the tendo achillis is due to tightness of the gastrocnemius when the muscles of the triceps surae group are the offenders. When necessary, the type of lengthening preferred is the Baker tongue-in-groove method (Fig. 12-3). An 8-cm. incision is made at the level of the musculo-tendinus junction of the calf. The overlying sheath is split; the gastrocnemius is identified and gently separated from the soleus. The tendon to the gastrocnemius is incised (Fig. 12-3) and extension is applied to the foot slowly but firmly until the desired length is achieved. The soleus is not disturbed. If, on the other hand, the contracture is due to the entire calf muscle group, then lengthening of the tendo achillis is per-

formed by one of the several methods already described. The type of arthrodesis employed is preferably the Grice type. This is described in detail in Chapter 7. The incision is made over the sinus tarsi, beginning from the level of the head of the talus and extending plantarly and slightly posteriorly to the palpable edge of the os calcis. The sinus tarsi is exposed, the fat removed, and the origin of the short toe extensors attached to the beak of the os

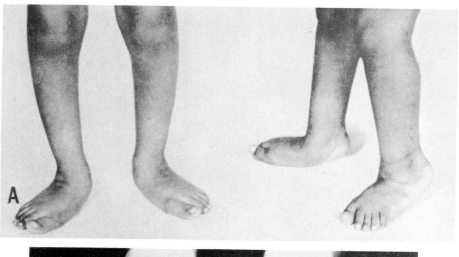

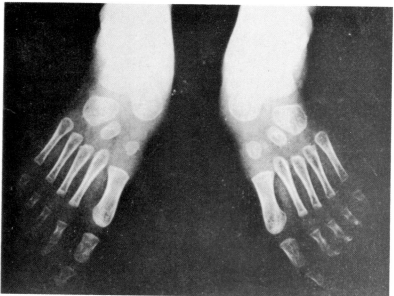

Fig. 12-5.   A.   Photographs of the feet of a child, three years old, with spastic quadriplegia, showing typical equinovalgus deformities.

B.   Roentgenograms of the feet shown in Fig. 12-5A. Note severe bilateral eversion of the calcaneus, vertical talus with resultant rocker soles, and valgus deformity of the fore part of both feet. This is the type of foot amenable to correction by lengthening of the gastrocnemius aponeurosis combined with Grice subtalar arthrodesis or a horizontal osteotomy of the posterior articular process of the calcaneus with lateral wedge grafts (see Fig. 12-5D). (See page 255 for C and D.)

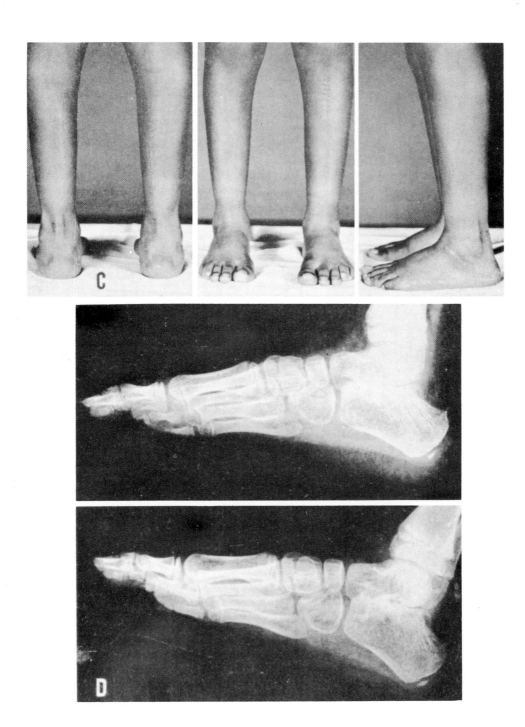

Fig. 12-5. Continued
    C. Photographs of the feet of the patient shown in Fig. 12-5A three years after lengthening of the gastrocnemius aponeurosis and Grice extra-articular subtalar arthrodesis. At the time of writing, eight years after operation, the feet were rated excellent.
    D. Postoperative lateral roentgenograms of the feet shown in Fig. 12-5C. (Baker and Hill, courtesy of J. Bone & Joint Surg.)

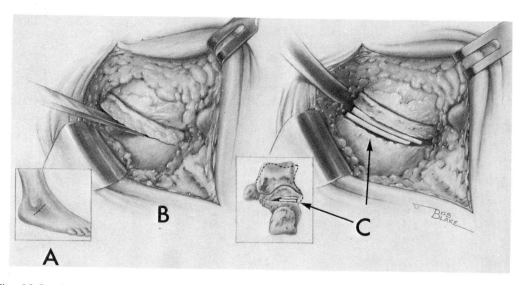

Fig. 12-6. Lateral Open Wedge Osteotomy of the Os Calcis.

Through a vertical incision, taking care not to excise the soft tissues of the sinus tarsi, a horizontal osteotomy is placed just below the posterior articular facet of the os calcis. The medial cortex should not be disrupted. Sufficient fibular cortical grafts are placed in the osteotomy site to hold the heel in the corrected position thus maintaining a well developed longitudinal arch. The deformity must be corrected by surgery and not with a postoperative cast.

calcis (just posterior to the calcaneocuboid joint) is detached and retracted distally.

The sinus tarsi should be thoroughly cleaned of all soft tissue. The os calcis is inverted to attempt to position it in relationship to the talus. If necessary, the lateral capsular structures of the talocalcaneal joint can be sectioned to bring the os calcis in a neutral position at least. In order to raise the head and neck of the talus to its anticipated corrected position, an osteotome should then be inserted between the neck of the talus, just posterior to the cartilaginous border of the head, and the calcaneal groove, just posterior to the beak of the os calcis. If the talus is in a practically vertical position, it is frequently necessary to section the dorsal and the lateral portion of the talonavicular capsule in order to wedge the talus into its properly corrected talocalcaneal relationship. The Grice type of the talocalcaneal arthrodesis is then carried out. This procedure is a rewarding one (Fig. 12-5 A,B,C and D) both from a functional and a cosmetic viewpoint. If the tibialis anterior presents active function, it should be transposed to the plantar aspect of the navicular.

Instead of the Grice operation to correct valgus deformity one may use the lateral open wedge osteotomy of the os calcis. This procedure is ideally suitable in patients with calcaneovalgus feet, whose standing lateral foot roentgenograms demonstrate only a mild plantar flexion of the talus and whose non-weight-bearing lateral x-ray views present an almost normal talocalcaneal relationship. In the severely plantar-flexed, almost horizontal talus the Grice procedure with talonavicular capsulotomy, with or without transplantation of the tibialis anterior to the plantar aspect of the navicular, is the procedure of choice.

In order to perform the lateral wedge osteotomy the incision (a routine vertical one) is made over the sinus tarsi (Fig. 12-6A). Baker states the "soft tissues are divided and not cleaned out of the sinus tarsi as is done in an arthrodesis. A blunt dissector is passed posteriorly beneath the fibular collateral ligaments and behind the posterior calcaneal articular process. This instrument gives adequate exposure and supports the calcaneus during the osteotomy which is made in the horizontal plane with care not to enter the subtalar joint (Fig.

12-6B). The osteotomy extends to, *but not through,* the medial cortex which should be preserved as a hinge. . . . Homogenous split-rib grafts are used as multiple wedges to build a buttress sufficiently thick to hold the foot in the desired position (Fig. 12-6C). Full correction must be achieved at operation; further postoperative correction by manipulation and corrective casts is not feasible. . . . Overcorrection must also be avoided since there is little tendency for the grafts to settle and the pes planus deformity to recur." The end result is a well-balanced foot with no loss of subtalar motion. (Fig. 12-7). Some orthopaedists prefer to take the graft from the fibula since it is a simple matter to expose the mid third-lower third junction of the fibula subperiosteally; resect the amount of fibula desired, split it into multiple grafts and insert the grafts into the defect in the os calcis which is created by the osteotomy. No difficulty will be experienced at the donor site since in a child, the defect will have filled in within a matter of six months.

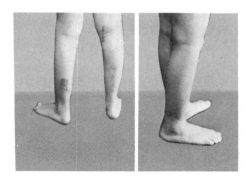

Fig. 12-7. Photographs of patient in Fig. 12-1 following bilateral mid one-third gastrocnemius aponeurosis lengthening and lateral open wedge osteotomies of the calcaneus.

Postoperatively the foot and leg are immobilized in a short leg-cast extending from the tips of the toes to the knee for a period of eight weeks. The foot is held in the neutral position. Following removal of the cast, weight bearing is permitted but under the supervision of the physical therapist. One must keep in mind that a new gait-pattern has been established and the youngster, particularly if he is mentally retarded, will require aid to develop this new stance.

As experience with extra-articular subtalar arthrodesis and lateral calcaneus osteotomy is gained, the short-term results indicate that both procedures are equally effective as far as reestablishment of balance, correction of alignment, and restoration of function are concerned. Osteotomy of the calcaneus, performed in a horizontal plane below the posterior subtalar articular facet, maintains normal contact between the talar and calcaneal joint surfaces, and does not interfere with subtalar motion. For this reason, osteotomy of the calcaneus may be the procedure of choice.

Both of these procedures, when properly performed, have the advantage of eliminating the necessity of a triple arthrodesis at a future date. They can be done on children as young as two years of age and may eliminate the lifetime need for expensive braces. It must be especially emphasized that these procedures do not eliminate the necessity for adequate correction of equinus or inversion-eversion imbalance (Figs. 12-8, 9A and B, 10 A and B, and 11 A and B).

When alignment and stabilization are necessary in the older child or adult, the same principles apply. Triple arthrodesis is accepted as the best stabilizing procedure, particularly in the adult group.

Equinovarus. This deformity, although not as common as equinovalgus, may equally handicap attempts at ambulation. Whether or not the condition is due to excessive lengthening of the formerly overactive peroneals or resulting from primary overactivity in the posterior tibial, the principle of restoring muscle balance should be adhered to. The posterior tibial muscle usually is the major deforming force in the production of the varus component of this deformity and may also participate in producing equinus.

A rerouting procedure of this tendon to the front of the medial malleolus reduces its influence on inversion of the hindfoot and varus of the forefoot. A slightly curved incision, approximately 10 cm. in length is carried out just posterior to the medial malleolus. It should begin along the medial edge of the tibia 5 cm. proximal to the

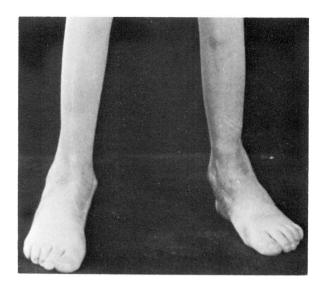

Fig. 12-8. End result of corrective surgery performed on feet illustrated in Figure 12-2 consisting of carefully supervised plaster correction followed by bilateral sectioning of the tibialis posterior tendon, heel cord lengthening and release of the talo-navicular capsule and deltoid ligament. Postoperative immobilization in casts then followed. The patient is now ambulatory and brace free.

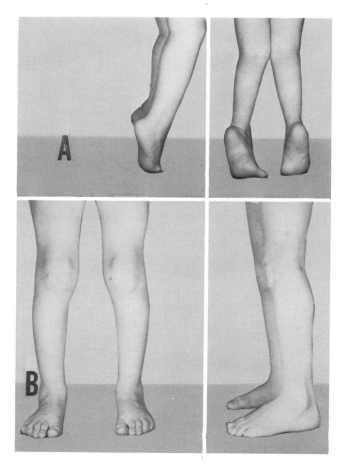

Fig. 12-9. A. Photographs of lower extremities of a two and one-half year old child with spastic diplegia demonstrating severe equinus.

B. Same patient following bilateral mid one-third gastrocnemius aponeurosis lengthening and lateral open wedge osteotomy of the calcaneus.

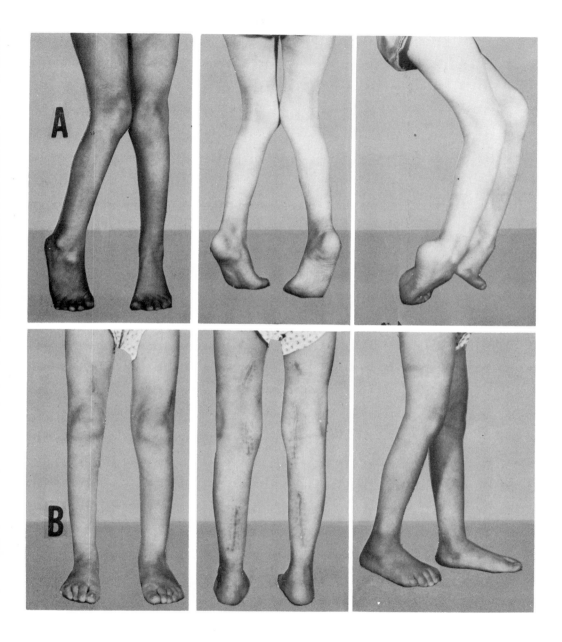

Fig. 12-10.   A. Lower extremities of a six year old child with spastic quadreplegia. Note the equino-varus deformities associated with adduction of the thighs and internal rotation of the extremities.

B.   Same patient following bilateral rerouting of the posterior tibial, peroneus longus and brevis tendons and mid one-third gastrocnemius aponeurosis lengthening. Proximal surgery included bilateral adductor longus myotomy, gracilis tenotomy, and transfer of the semi-tendinosus tendon to the anterolateral aspect of the femur to act as an external rotator.

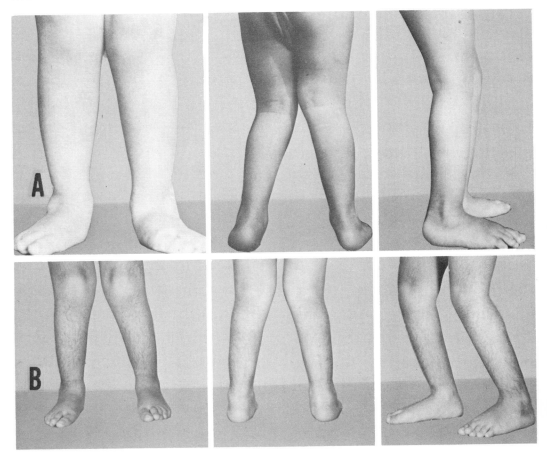

Fig. 12-11.   A. Feet of a three year, three month old patient with spastic diplegia demonstrating pes equino-valgus deformities with pronation.

   B.   Same patient following bilateral lateral open wedge osteotomies of the os calcis, rerouting of the peroneal tendons and gastrocnemius aponeurosis lengthening.

malleolus and extend distally along the medial surface of the foot over the navicular tubercle and beyond it to the medial cuneiform-metatarsal joint (Fig. 12-12). The annular ligament and the tendon sheath are divided. The tendon is then carefully separated from its insertion into the medioplantar aspect of the navicular tubercle; one must make certain to maintain continuity of the tendon with its remaining plantar insertions. The subcutaneous tissues and the skin on the dorsomedial aspect of the ankle and tarsal region are undermined sufficiently to permit the tendon to move to its new position parallel and close the anterior tibial tendon. The rerouted tendon should follow a straight course to the point where it passes to the

plantar aspect of the foot. A flap of fibrous tissue sutured to the subcutaneous tissues may be necessary to maintain the desired direction of pull.

The postoperative regimen is similar to that described for rerouting the peroneal tendons. Greater success is achieved when the tendon follows the new course along or adjacent to the tendon of the anterior tibial muscle. Not only does the rerouted tendon act as a dorsiflexor, thereby helping prevent recurrence of the equinus, but it may correct the internal rotation of the entire extremity so frequently seen in association with inversion of the foot.

Another procedure which can be performed to correct this deformity is the transplantation of the tibialis anterior

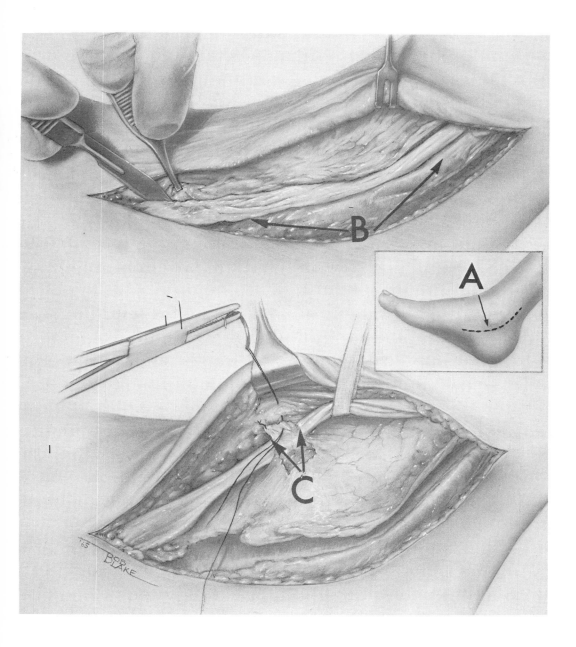

Fig. 12-12.   Posterior tibial tendon rerouting to overcome varus deformity of the foot.
   A.   Shows line of incision.

   B.   Demonstrates splitting of the annular ligament and the tendon sheath and separating the tendon from its proximal area of insertion in the navicular tubercle. Care should be exercised in order not to sever the tendon.

   C.   Demonstrates rerouted tendon on dorso-medial aspect of foot close to and parallel with the tibialis anterior.

through the interosseous membrane to the dorsum of the foot. Although this is a more complicated surgical procedure, the end results warrant the added effort necessary to transplant this tendon. The first incision is made over the medial aspect of the foot at the level of the navicular tubercle. It is 4 to 6 cm. in length and through it the posterior tibial tendon is detached from the navicular tubercle and from its insertion in the underlying structures of the foot.

To expose the tibialis posterior tendon and muscle, a second incision, approximately 10 cm. in length, is then made on the posterior medial aspect of the leg (beginning 3 cm. above and behind the medial malleolus). The musculotendenous junction is identified, the tendon is delivered into the second incision, and very careful dissection of the muscle belly is carried out up to the level of the neurovascular bundle which is usually at the junction of the upper and lower halves of the muscle belly.

The third incision, usually 6 to 8 cm. in length, is then made on the anterior aspect of the leg just lateral to the tibia begining at the level of the distal tibiofibular syndesmosis. The fascia is split and the tibialis anterior muscle is retracted medially and the extensor hallucis longus laterally, exposing the interosseous membrane. The interosseous membrane is incised and a large window is made extending the entire length of this third incision.

The success of the transfer depends quite a great deal on constructing a window large enough to permit the entire belly of the tibialis posterior to "herniate" anterior to the interosseous membrane. In other words, this requires detaching the interosseous membrane from the level of the tibiofibular joint distally and extending as far up as possible. The window can never be made too large. After the tibialis posterior tendon and muscle belly are delivered through the window, the tendon is passed subcutaneously down to the foot where it can be inserted either into the middle or the lateral cuneiform, depending upon whether the surgeon desires to have a neutral pull or a pull in slight valgus. The decision will depend upon how active the tibialis anterior is. If the tibialis anterior demonstrates little, if any, activity, then the tendon should be inserted into the midportion of the foot. If the tibialis anterior demonstrates some muscle power, then the tibialis posterior tendon should be transferred to the midlateral portion of the foot. Following closure of the soft tissues with absorbable type sutures and the skin with subcuticular wire suture, the foot is immobilized at maximum extension in a plaster cast extending from the toes to the knee.

When overactivity of the toe flexors contributes to the equinovarus deformity, a tendon-lengthening procedure of this muscle group is indicated. It should be performed through an incision just above the medial malleolus and posterior to this bony structure.

MISCELLANEOUS DEFORMITIES

Deformities of the forepart of the foot are not as detrimental to ambulation as the deformities previously mentioned in this chapter, but they can be a nuisance in shoe fitting. Hallux valgus is such a deformity (Fig. 12-13). It may result from weight-bearing pressure on the medial side of the great toe in an equinovalgus foot, from adductor hallucis muscle overactivity, or it may be a coincidental deformity not related to the cerebral palsy. When surgery is indicated, the same principle of surgical correction should be followed as in the correction of the same deformity in individuals without cerebral palsy. If the deformity is felt to be secondary to abnormal weight-bearing pressure, the primary deformity should be corrected first.

POSTOPERATIVE CARE

A long and continuing postoperative follow-up is required with particular attention to recurrence of old or the development of new deformities. Every effort to

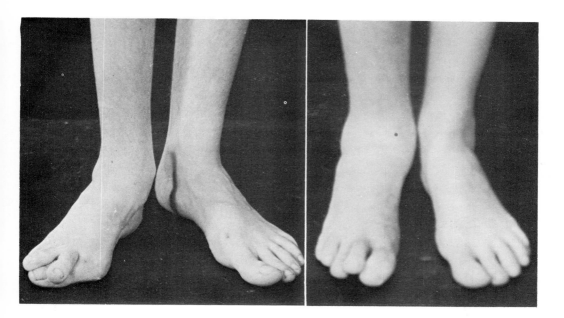

Fig. 12-13.   Hallux valgus deformity in a thirteen-year-old spastic hemiplegic corrected by transfer of adductor hallucis to neck of first metatarsal, exostectomy, and capsuloplasty. Any of the standard hallux valgus procedures can be employed but the adductor hallucis **must** be transferred.

prevent or discourage these undesirable developments should be made.

Precise application of the postoperative cast is one of the most important facets of a thorough, continuing care program. The surgeon should be especially alert while applying the postoperative cast to avoid excessive correction of equinus deformities; a weakened calf prolongs therapy and in itself is a greater handicap than equinus. The position in which the foot is immobilized will depend on the preoperative strength and degree of spasticity of the corrected muscles. When the muscles are judged to be of normal or good strength, slight overcorrection in plaster may be desired. In patients with weak muscles, one should immobilize the foot in neutral position.

When an extra-articular subtalar fusion or lateral calcaneal osteotomy is done, full correction must be fulfilled by the surgery and not with the postoperative cast. If additional correction by plaster is subsequently required to achieve the desired position, the surgery was inadequately done.

Following tendon surgery, plaster immobilization is necessary for four to six weeks. The period required for adequate skeletal consolidation following fusion or calcaneal osteotomy is eight to twelve weeks. A below-the-knee cast is sufficient immobilization. To maintain adequate lengthening of the gastrocnemuis following procedures to correct equinus, the plaster should extend to the groin with the knee in extension. To avoid neurovascular complications, hyperextension of the knee should be prevented. Excessive padding of the cast should be avoided. Little or no plaster should be applied over the posterior aspect of the heel. Even in well-molded casts, uncontrollable movement of the foot occurs, and friction of the heel against the cast in this area may be a source of troublesome blisters or pressure sores. The presence of a painful sore behind the heel delays therapy, postpones the comfortable use of braces and splints, and needlessly prolongs hospitalization.

NONOPERATIVE TREATMENT

Following plaster removal, therapy is aimed at restoration of joint function, gait improvement, and prevention of recurrence of deformity, keeping in mind the need for bracing. In patients with lesser degree of involvement, improvement in gait and function may be achieved without surgery. However, it should be particularly emphasized that a long, expensive rehabilitation program of physical therapy, bracing, and medication is not indicated when surgery can be used advantageously to shorten such programs.

Nonoperative treatment is also indicated in the child who has not begun to show reciprocal movements. It is often difficult to predict which child will be a candidate for ambulation, and until he reveals his potential for ambulation, a home program for muscle stretching and splinting should be provided to encourage muscle balance and prevent fixed deformities. Braces, night splints, Dennis-Browne splints with outriggers, or plaster posterior splints, can be used effectively in the prevention of deformities. If correction cannot be achieved with these methods, one should not hesitate to correct the deformities with a single or a series of plaster casts, and then maintain correction with the appliance of choice.

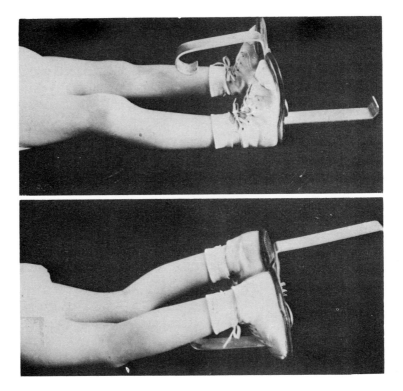

Fig. 12-14. Pre-walker brace using principles of Dennis-Browne bar. Anterior and posterior outriggers are attached to maintain ankle in neutral extension both in supine and prone position. Outrigger should be detachable to allow for standing when possible.

The Dennis-Browne splint (Fig. 12-14) with outriggers has advantages over the conventional right-angle splint or brace. It is inexpensive, easy to apply, and controls adduction of the thighs as well as foot equinus. When varus or valgus complicates the picture, proper alignment of the heel can be obtained by bending the aluminum cross bar the desired degree. A similar effect can be achieved by bradding the patient's shoes 8 inches apart on a piece of plywood. The plywood outriggers should lie flat on the bed at 90 degrees to the spreader piece, extending toward the foot of the bed, and they should be of sufficient length to prevent equinus.

Bracing is an important aspect of any therapeutic program. A well-fitting posterior stop of Klenzac brace, with T-straps as needed to control inversion and eversion, is often effective in preventing or controlling deformities. This is especially true in the postoperative period of gait training. The Klenzac brace allows push-off, maintains the foot at the desired angle of dorsiflexion, and is to be preferred to the conventional posterior stop brace.

Probably the most common reason for a recurring deformity is an inadequate or insufficiently prolonged postoperative period of splinting and bracing. Although the goal for each child is a brace-free extremity, the presence of active, strong extensors of the ankle is the primary standard by which the decision is made whether or not to discard the brace. With active extensors, equinus seldom recurs.

So often there is a tendency to discard braces when the deformity has maintained its correction for a year or two. One should not be lulled into a false sense of security, particularly when the child is quite young, for the tendency to recurrence due to growth is greater than in the older child. If braces are eliminated, close and periodic examination is mandatory.

The treatment of foot deformities in children with cerebral palsy and adults with spasticity following a cerebral vascular accident must be kept in proper perspective, based on the patient's need and potentials. In any therapy program for brain-damaged individuals, the treatment of deformities, although important, attends to only one facet of the patient's needs. There is no question, that deformities consequent to brain injury, particularly in children, are now among the most common orthopaedic problems.

Many orthopaedic procedures have been devised for these unfortunate youngsters, but only those operations have been described which have been in our experience the most successful in combating the more common problems.

BIBLIOGRAPHY

BAKER, L. D.: A Rational Approach to the Surgical Needs of the Cerebral Palsied Patient. J. Bone Jt. Surg. 40A:1359-1370, 1958.

BAKER, L. D. AND DODELIN, R. A.: Extra-Articular Arthrodesis of the Subtalar Joint (Grice Procedure). J.A.M.A., 168:1006, 1958.

BAKER, L. D. AND HILL, L. M.: Foot Alignment in Cerebral Palsy Patients. Bone Jt. Surg. 46A:1, 1964.

BANKS, H. H. AND GREEN, W. T.: The Correction of Equinus Deformity in Cerebral Palsy. J. Bone Jt. Surg. 40A:1359, 1958.

GRICE, D. S.: Extra-Articular Arthrodesis of the Subastragalar Joint for Correction of Paralytic Flatfeet in Children. J. Bone Jt. Surg. 34A:927, 1952.

SILFVERSKIOLD, NILS: Reduction of the Un-Crossed Two-Joint Muscles of the Leg to One-Joint Muscles in Spastic Condition. Acta Chir Scand. 56:315, 1924.

STOFFEL, A.: The Treatment of Spastic Contractures. Amer. J. Orthop. Surg. 10:611, 1913.

STRAYER, L. M., JR.: Recession of the Gastrocnemius. An Operation to Relieve Spastic Contractures of the Calf Muscles. J. Bone Jt. Surg. 32A: 671, 1950.

Gastrocnemius Recession. J. Bone Jt. Surg. 40A: 1019, 1958.

WHITE, J. W.: Torsion of the Achilles Tendon. Its Surgical Significance. Arch. Surg. 46:784, 1943.

13

Hallux Valgus and Hallux Rigidus

HALLUX VALGUS

THE term "bunion" or, the more sophisticated one, "hallux valgus" still leaves a great deal to be desired in describing a deformity which at various stages involves not only the first metatarsophalangeal joint, but also the soft tissues surrounding it, the first tarsometatarsal joint, and the sesamoids on the plantar aspect of the first metatarsal head. Furthermore, to attempt to introduce a new, more descriptive term would only confuse a situation which is already sufficiently confused. If one were to list all of the procedures that have been written for the correction of this deformity of the great toe, one would not contribute anything to the sum total of human endeavor, but would confuse the issue even further. Suffice it to say that a review of the literature reveals that up to the present writing there are at least 78 different procedures for the correction of hallux valgus. Furthermore, when one analyzes them, 75 per cent of them are modifications of certain basic operations. Such a descriptive "arbeit" will be left to others. This chapter will cover certain basic principles and will present certain basic therapeutic procedures, both

non-surgical and surgical, as well as minor modifications of operations which can be used to fit specific problems pertaining to bunion surgery.

Causes. Ill-fitting shoes have been considered as the principle cause of bunions by many authors, but this oversimplified statement is not exactly correct. People who have never worn shoes have been known to develop a hallux valgus deformity and, conversely, many people have worn what I would term "poorly-fitted shoes" yet have not developed bunions. Haines and Mc-Dougall reported that the incidence of hallux valgus in Egypt is related to social classes. It does not exist among poor people who usually walk barefoot. Schlegel reported that in Japan hallux valgus is becoming more frequent since the wearing of modern footwear (*i.e.* European) has become widespread. Our considered opinion is that there is a basic structural defect of the foot which predisposes to the development of this deformity and that ill-fitting shoes accentuate the situation and speed up the development of the bunion.

One may see a congenital hallux valgus,

but such a deformity is indeed rare. Heredity, on the other hand, plays a definite part and in the majority of instances a detailed history will reveal a strong familial diathesis, not only as to the type of valgus deformity, but also as to its unilateral or bilateral occurrence.

There are certain basic intrinsic factors which predispose to hallux valgus. The pes planus or flat foot is certainly one of these. If one should observe carefully the patients who present themselves with a symptomatic hallux valgus, he will find that a considerable number of them demonstrate a pronated foot. Jordan and Brodsky consider the majority of hallux valgus and hallux rigidus as acquired deformities resulting from foot pronations. The role of footwear is secondary serving to aggravate an existing mild deformity.

The next most common suggested cause of hallux valgus is a comparatively longer first toe. This, of course, is understandable. In a patient whose great toe is much longer than the rest, the excessive length cannot be compensated for in the modern shoe. The toe will be squeezed into the shoe, deviation will occur, and the vicious cycle leading to hallux valgus will be initiated.

Lapidus in 1934 coined the term "metatarsus varus primus" to indicate a primarily developmental type of entity as a cause for the hallux valgus deformity. In this clinical entity, there is abduction of the first metatarsal shaft and head and subsequent valgus deformity of the great toe along with plantar rotation. He feels that this deviation of the first metatarsal is a developmental one due to posteromedial slanting of the distal articular surface of the medial cuneiform. However, Lapidus states that even in this deformity improper shoes precipitate the development of the valgus deformity.

One also sees a hallux valgus deformity associated with muscle imbalance or over-activity of muscles as in postpoliomyelitic paresis of the foot or in cerebral palsy. Inflammatory disturbances of the first metatarsophalangeal joint as in rheumatoid arthritis or metabolic diseases such as gout, are also predisposing factors.

In the final analysis, one can definitely state that in a large majority of instances in both the male and the female there is present an instigating, developmental factor of either congenital or hereditary nature. However, in the female there is a greater incidence of hallux valgus because of the shape of the shoes into which women force their feet. In fact, the ratio of female to male incidence of this condition is approximately 40 to 1.

Symptoms. The symptomatology consists primarily of pain on the dorsomedial aspect of the first metatarsal head or directly over the medial exostosis. The patient will frequently complain about recurrent "swelling of the big toe". However, upon careful evaluation of the history, the examiner will find that this complaint does not apply to the joint itself, but simply to the bursa overlying it. Occasionally, the individual may complain of pain on the plantar aspect of the first metatarsophalangeal joint. Quite frequently, because of the concomitant subluxation or dislocation of the second metatarsophalangeal joint (which occurs due to displacement of the second toe dorsally as the first drifts laterally), the chief subjective symptom will be pain in the soft tissues underlying the second and/or third metatarsal heads with the formation either of a painful callus or an even more distressing plantar keratosis. In addition, the average patient will also state that the entire foot becomes uncomfortable as the forefoot, in general, becomes more fatigued and symptomatic, and this discomfort or pain may radiate to the leg and to the knee.

One specific query which the examiner *must* make is to ask the patient if there is any pain *in* the first metatarsophalangeal joint itself. One will be greatly surprised to find, even in patients with a severe hallux valgus, that the greater majority will have no pain in the articulation per se in spite of marked disalignment of the articulating surfaces. A few patients who present themselves in the office with even a moderately severe bunion will have no symptoms referable to the hallux valgus but will complain of discomfort on the lateral aspect of the fifth metatarsal head, or of generalized foot discomfort associated with pronated feet. Others will complain that only certain shoes produce pain in the feet. Obviously these will be the high style, high-heeled shoes into which the female patient will have been cramping her feet.

Examination. In the examination, one should not only consider the obvious deformity of the foot, but also the patient as a whole. There are some patients who are not properly motivated and no matter how excellent the operative result may be, the patient will still continue to complain. Therefore, evaluate the patient, the symptoms, and lastly, the deformity. If the patient complains only of metatarsal pain, obviously correction of the hallux valgus does not automatically indicate that the patient will be relieved of her metatarsalgia. In other words, to quote an old cliché, "Don't lose sight of the forest for the trees."

It is incumbent upon the surgeon to inform a patient that the postoperative period of convalescence is a minimum of six weeks on the average and in some instances, depending upon the extent of the surgery, even longer. Should the patient express surprise at the length of this period, simply remind him that bony and capsular tissues have a slower healing rate, particularly when a joint is involved. Furthermore, during a certain phase of ambulation, the joint in question will bear a large portion of the entire body weight and, therefore, will tend to require a longer period of partial weight-bearing.

Next, circulation in the foot should be evaluated. Primarily this requires palpation of the dorsalis pedis and the posterior tibial pulsations, as well as the evaluation of temperature of the foot in general. In the absence of pulsations and the presence of a cool foot, one does not necessarily infer that surgical correction for a symptomatic bunion is contraindicated. On the contrary, if surgery is indicated, it should be performed but without the use of the tourniquet. By the same token, diabetes is not a contraindication to surgical intervention as long as the medical problem is well-controlled. In this instance also, a tourniquet is not employed.

With regard to the *deformity* of the great toe, one should measure the deformity and record the amount in degrees. It is also necessary to note whether or not the great toe is over-riding or under-riding the sec-

ond toe. The range of motion should be carefully recorded since marked limitation of motion will determine the type of procedure to be performed. A marked restriction of active extension or flexion of the first metatarsophalangeal joint precludes the performance of certain types of procedures. There must be at least 25 degrees of extension since limited mobility and/or crepitation suggests involvement of the articulating surfaces that may not be demonstrated even by roentgenography. The state of the skin overlying the deformity should be evaluated. It is important to determine whether or not there has been any recent inflammatory reaction of the overlying bursa, since such inflammation would preclude the consideration of any surgical procedure for at least three months.

The rotation of the nail and the toe itself should be observed and recorded. If they are rotated medially, one should determine if this is due to abduction of the first metatarsal. This is done by compressing the forefoot and observing whether this axial rotation corrects spontaneously and the toe resumes its normal axial position. Some investigators feel that this rotation is due to the shift of the abductor hallucis plantarward with associated shifting of the sesamoids laterally. However, we are not in total agreement with this concept since in the great majority of hallux valgus deformities, which present no such axial rotation of the great toe, the sesamoids are still displaced laterally. The examiner should also palpate the plantar aspect of the first metatarsophalangeal joint to determine whether or not there is tenderness underlying the sesamoids which might indicate arthritic involvement of the articular surfaces of these bones. The tendon of the extensor hallucis longus should be inspected to determine the extent of the bow-stringing effect of this structure.

Next, the adjoining toes should be evaluated. Is there a subluxation or dislocation of the second or third metatarsophalangeal joints? Can the subluxation be reduced passively without too much discomfort to the patient? How short are the extensor tendons to these digits, and how contracted is the dorsal capsule of the metatarsophalangeal joints? Are the metatarsal heads prominent plantarly and is there an underlying tender callus or a plantar keratosis?

The patient should next be asked to stand since in the standing position additional information can be gained as to the amount of deformity of the great toe, the amount of splaying of the forefoot, the degree of pronation of the foot, and the manner of weight distribution of the entire foot. Frequently one finds that in a standing position the patient's weight is shifted toward the lateral side of the foot with the presence of a painful callus or keratosis under the fifth metatarsal head. Also one should observe whether or not there is a symptomatic exostosis on the lateral aspect of the fifth metatarsal head. Compression of the forefoot should be carried out to determine the amount of splaying present.

Roentgenograms. Roentgenographic examination should include at rest and standing dorsoplantar views, a lateral standing view and an oblique at rest view. Occasionally, in patients complaining of tenderness under the sesamoids, a sagittal view of the sesamoidmetatarsal joints is also necessary. The dorsoplantar views should be superimposed to determine the amount of splaying of the forefoot. Each film should also be examined for any degenerative changes that may be present. Any sclerosis of the arterial tree of any consequence will also be visible and if it is extensive, the possibility of conservative therapy only should be seriously considered.

Treatment. Conservative therapy is not to be decried in the care of the mildly symptomatic, mildly deformed, great toe. Furthermore, one must remember that, in a certain percentage of people, complaints are referable to the metatarsal region only even with a severe bunion deformity. In such instances every attempt should be made to relieve the symptomatology by conservative means. There are all manner of "bunion pads", plasters, toe separators, etc., which are commercially manufactured but, by and large, these are useless. At times, relief can be procured by the use of a combination shoe-last wherein the shoe is wider in the forepart than in the heel as, for example, a "C" width in the forepart and an "A" width in the heel, along with the insertion of a specially constructed pad.

The pad consists of a combination comma-shaped metatarsal pad (on the average 3/8 inch thick) with bunion flanges built into the metatarsal pad. These pads should be custom built. An outline of the foot should be drawn with the patient in a standing position. The point just behind the head of the first and fifth metatarsals should be marked on the outline in order to determine the leading edge of the bunion flange (Fig. 13-1). An outline of each foot should be procured and each foot individually marked since no two feet are alike. This type of pad is available and is custom made by the various manufacturers of foot supports. It can be fitted in a properly selected shoe and will provide fairly

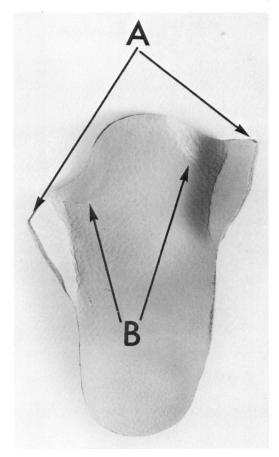

Fig. 13-1. Arch support with medial and lateral bunion flanges (A) which fit just proximal to the medial exostosis of the first metatarsal and lateral exostosis of the fifth metatarsal. Comma shaped metatarsal pad (B) which fits just proximal to plantar aspect of the metatarsal heads to relieve metatarsalgia.

moderate relief in a minority of patients.

There are a large number of patients who are reluctant or unwilling to undergo surgery and although one may feel that such padding will not afford adequate relief, they should be given "the benefit of the doubt" and be permitted to try them. If the pads should fail to give the required relief, the patient will then be more amenable to surgical intervention. Nor is surgery without its pitfalls. Not all surgical results end happily and, therefore, surgical procedures should be considered only after conservative therapy has been given at least a fair trial. In addition to prescribing the use of the pad, the physician should also have a blood uric acid determination carried out. This is advisable since in more than an occasional patient, the uric acid level will be elevated and with the use of uricosuric drugs the foot can be rendered asymptomatic without resorting to surgery. (See Chapter 16).

Preoperative Care. If the decision to operate has been made, the status of the patient should be thoroughly evaluated. Upon admission to the hospital, a fasting blood sugar should be ordered routinely along with the usual laboratory studies. The preparation of the foot the evening prior to surgery should consist of a complete pedicure, shaving of the extremity from the dorsum of the toes to the knee, and gentle scrubbing of the leg and foot for five minutes with water and one of the surgical detergent soaps. The foot is dried with a sterile towel, but not wrapped. Under general anesthesia at the time of surgery, the extremity is elevated and "milked" with an elastic bandage. Following the application of a pneumatic thigh tourniquet (except if contraindicated) the skin is again gently scrubbed with sterile sponges for five minutes with the same type of soap. The soap suds are blotted with a sterile towel and the skin is painted with an aqueous antiseptic solution beginning from the toes and progressing proximalward. The foot and the distal two-thirds of the leg are encased in a sterile stockinette through which the surgery is performed.

Operative Procedure. Up to the present portion of this chapter, it is doubtful if

there has been much, if any, disagreement with the statements that have been made, but we now arrive on the battleground. Of the seventy-odd procedures described in the literature, which to choose? Of course, many of them have been discarded, but there are still ardent proponents as well as opponents for the 15 to 20 operative procedures still in vogue. No attempt will be made to describe all of them. A poll of the various contributors to this book was carried out and the general consensus is that no one specific procedure is a cure-all for all patients who present themselves with a symptomatic hallux valgus. In addition, no matter what procedure the surgeon may perform, the results will be good-to-excellent in only about 85 per cent. Each case should be evaluated individually and each procedure to be performed should be fitted to the clinical as well as the roentgenographic findings. It is our considered opinion that the following criteria and surgical procedures have given the best overall results.

In patients under the age of thirty who present this deformity, it is obvious that in addition to the valgus of the great toe, there will be abduction of the first metatarsal. Therefore, the Lapidus procedure or an osteotomy of the shaft of the first metatarsal (the Mitchell operation) is the procedure of choice when the angle between the first and second metatarsals is 12 degrees or more. In order that there may be no confusion or misinterpretation each of these procedures will be quoted verbatim.

The Lapidus Procedure (Fig. 13-2). This procedure, as described by the originator, is as follows: "The operation over the big toe is performed first. A straight longitudinal incision about 3-1/2 to 4 inches (9 to 10 cm.) long is made along the medial aspect of the big toe and the first metatarsal. The subcutaneous veins are ligated. The medial cutaneous nerve frequently seen in the wound is identified and retracted. The bursa over the bunion is opened, and further dissection is carried proximally in the same plane, as the tissues here have few blood vessels. The fascia covering the abductor hallucis muscle is incised longitudinally just below the insertion of this fascia along the first metatarsal shaft. The muscular belly of the abductor hallucis pops into the wound. Its loose connection with the first metatarsal shaft may be separated by blunt dissection. As a rule, in nearly all bunions, the abductor hallucis is found displaced plantarly, blending with the medial belly of the flexor hallucis brevis and acting as a plantar flexor of the big toe rather than its abductor (Fig. 13-2). These muscles are separated from each other also mostly by blunt dissection.

"The slender tendon of the abductor hallucis is then followed distally and separated from the capsule of the metatarsophalangeal joint down to its insertion on to the base of the proximal phalanx, care being taken not to sever this tendon or to open the joint capsule. The tendon is retracted plantarly, and a U-shaped flap is made in the medial capsule, with its base attached to the proximal phalanx. This flap usually is about 3/4 of an inch (2 cm.) long and 3/8 of an inch (1 cm.) wide at its distal base, tapering proximally to the neck of the first metatarsal. The capsular flap is reflected distally, care being taken to dissect it from the medial aspect of the first metatarsal head, preserving its full thick-

ness. Usually a small artery is cut over the metatarsal neck. The joint now is opened by reflecting the flap distally. The neck of the metatarsal is exposed. The 'sagittal groove', so well described by Haines and McDougall (1954) is noted. It runs in dorsoplantar direction, separating the normal lateral cartilagenous articular surface that remains in contact with the laterally subluxated proximal phalanx from the fibrously degenerated cartilage of the medial part of the head. This groove often is quite deep in marked cases of bunions and is reddish, containing denuded rough bone. The 'bunion' itself is represented usually by the dorsomedial prominence of the first metatarsal head. This prominence is shaved off so that the medial, the dorsal, and to a certain extent, the medial plantar flare-up of the first metatarsal head is removed. Now the medial part of the head is in the same plane and is a continuation of the cortex of the neck and the shaft of the metatarsal. Occasionally, there is a dorsal prominence over the first metatarsal head, which likewise has to be shaved off. Small wood carving chisels, obtainable in any hardware store in a set together with a sharpening stone, have been used by the

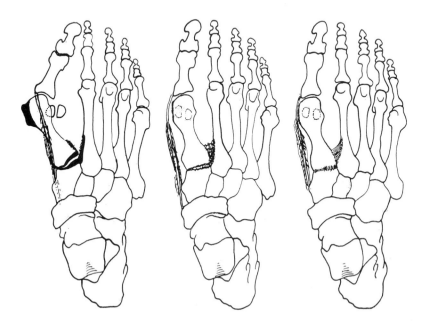

Fig. 13-2. The principal operative steps of the Lapidus Procedure. (Lapidus, courtesy of Surg. Obst. & Gynec.)

author (Lapidus) for many years and are indispensable, particularly for resection of the first metatarsocuneiform joints. They are sterilized together with the stone and sharpened just before the operation. When resecting the medial part of the first metatarsal head, care should be taken to preserve its round shape, and especially its part covered with the normal cartilage, without excising too much bone.

"We usually replace the capsular flap and the skin and palpate through them to be sure that no bony prominences are left.

"The subcutaneous tenotomy and capsulotomy then are performed over the fibular aspect of the first metatarsophalangeal joint from a dorsal approach, while the big toe is forced gently into varus (10 to 15 degrees) position. A sharp, stout tenotome should be used for this, and it should be inserted to hug the bone and the joint closely, as the blood vessels and nerves pass more superficially to bone in surrounding soft tissues. The medial tongue-shaped flap of the capsule is sutured to the tendon of the abductor hallucis longus with considerable tension, several number 00 chromic stitches being used. The plantar and dorsal capsular wounds are also closed. At the same time the abductor hallucis belly, together with its tendon, is shifted dorsally, running now along the medial aspect of the first metatarsal head instead of plantarly to it, and its action as an 'abductor' now is re-established (Fig. 13-2). The closing of the capsule should be performed carefully and judiciously.

"All capsular slack produced by resection of the medial part of the head should be removed, but at the same time the capsule should not be sutured so tightly as later to cause limitation of motion of the big toe; a good balance between adduction and abduction and dorsal and plantar flexion should be created. As a rule, the big toe in hallux valgus is in internal rotation, so that both big toe nails face each other. This also has to be corrected. In ordinary cases no removal of the bursa is ever attempted unless suppurative bursitis is present. In a few of our patients, there was a communication of the infected bursa with the joint. In these cases after thorough debridement of the infected tissue, we were able, also,

to perform the bunion operation with primary union of the wound and used antibiotics postoperatively. Occasionally, there is a communication of the bursa with the joint also in cases without infection. . . . The skin is closed without suturing the subcutaneous structures. If the procedure is carried out adequately, the big toe remains well corrected without any external support. . . . If, however, the correction of the metatarsus varus primus is indicated, it is carried out as a second step following completion of the operation on the big toe. A longitudinal incision about 3-1/2 inches (9 cm.) long is made along the dorsum of the first metatarsal and the first cuneiform. The first metatarsocuneiform joint is exposed by retracting the tendon of the extensor hallucis longus medially and that of the extensor hallucis brevis laterally. The cutaneous nerve branches are identified and protected. A V-shaped space between the first and second metatarsal bases is exposed by dissection, hugging the first metatarsal closely. The perforating plantar branches of the dorsalis pedis vessels are retracted distally and fibularward with the soft tissues when exposing the second metatarsal base. Occasionally, the veins are ruptured, but we have never had any complications from that.

"The cortex from the adjacent surfaces of the base of the first and second metatarsals is removed, leaving the bone ships *in situ*. The first cuneiform-metatarsal joint is opened on its dorsal aspect. The adjacent cartilagenous articular surfaces of the first metatarsal and the first metatarsal and the first cuneiform are shaved off. Here a small wood carving chisel about 5 inches (13 cm.) long and about 3/8 of an inch (about 1 cm.) wide is indispensable! We learned that no real wedge dissection was necessary, that mere shaving off of the articular cartilage down to subchondral bone was not only enough, but also essential, in order to produce close linear coaptation of the resected joint surfaces and insure prompt 'primary union' of the bones.

"One has to become familiar with this bean-shaped joint which measures almost 1-1/8 inches (2.9 cm.) in dorsal plantar direction, and approximately 1/2 of an inch (1.3 cm.) from side to side in its widest dimension. It also faces plantarward and medially. The articular facet of the first metatarsal is slightly concave, while that of the first cuneiform is correspondingly convexed in a sagittal plane. There is also a similar concavity of the first metatarsal and convexity of the first cuneiform in the horizontal plane. A snug fitting and close approximation of the resected surfaces should be obtained. A hole is then made with a shoemaker's awl over the dorsolateral part of the first metatarsal base and a number 0 chromic catgut is passed through it, using a curved needle. Proximally the needle is introduced through the strong dorsal ligamentous structures between the first and second cuneiforms. When this stitch is tied, a close approximation is obtained. The pieces of bone obtained from the first metatarsal head are denuded from soft tissue and cartilage and cut in small bone chips which are inserted abundantly between the denuded bases of the first and second metatarsals. They later form a bony bridge that maintains permanently the correction of the first metatarsus varus.

"Skin is closed with silk without suturing the subcutaneous tissue. A 5 inch (about 12 cm.) long and 5/16 of an inch (7 mm.) wide steel corset stay is used as a splint and is inserted along the medial aspect of the first metatarsal over well padded dressings. The big toe is strapped to it at about 10 degrees of varus and in slight external rotation. The first dressing should be done snugly, but not too tightly. After adequate correction, one will find on postoperative roentgenograms complete correction of the metatarsus varus primus without tight bandaging across the forefoot. Likewise, the splinting of the big toe should be done most carefully in order to avoid pressure over the suture line. This is very important. One should depend primarily upon an adequate surgical correction, the splinting being aimed only at maintaining it, rather than on increasing the correction. . . . Usually, we change the dressing on the second or third post-operative day and replace carefully the steel corset stay maintaining the big toe at 10 degrees of varus. . . . The stitches usually are removed at the end of two weeks and snug bandaging and adhesive

strapping across the metatarsal heads over an adequate padding are continued for about four to six weeks. The splinting of the big toe may be discontinued three or four weeks after the operation, depending upon the amount of correction. During the first two weeks there may be slight overcorrection with a few degrees of varus of the big toe. This should not be allowed to remain permanently. Controlled postoperative dorsoplantar roentgenograms are taken to ascertain the amount of the approximation of the first and second metatarsal heads and the relation of the big toe to its metatarsal. Also, they show the amount of bone bridge-formation between the first and second metatarsal bases and the degree of fusion of the first cuneiform metatarsal joint. Both are usually quite solid at the end of three months, with subsequent roentgenograms showing further consolidation of the intermetatarsal bridge.

"At first, special canvas shoes or wool socks with leather soles are worn. During the second postoperative month the patient may wear wide soft shoes or sandals. After that time he is able to use regular well-fitted, but perhaps slightly larger shoes. Housewives, as a rule, can resume their work about two months after the operation; patients having to do a great deal of walking or standing require another week or two before going back to their eight-hour-workday.

"Hammer toes and overlapping hammer toes frequently associated with bunions usually are corrected at the same sitting."

The Mitchell Procedure. The rationale is based on the premise that to correct only the deformity of the toe without simultaneous correction of the metatarsus varus primus when it is present to an abnormal extent, *i.e.*, over 10 degrees, will lead to a recurrent deformity in many patients. The operative procedure is as follows: "This procedure may be described as an osteotomy of the distal portion of the first metatarsal, lateral displacement and angulation of the head of the metatarsals, with exostectomy and medial capsulorrhaphy.

"A dorsal medial incision is made on the foot curving above the bursa and callous (Fig. 13-3A).

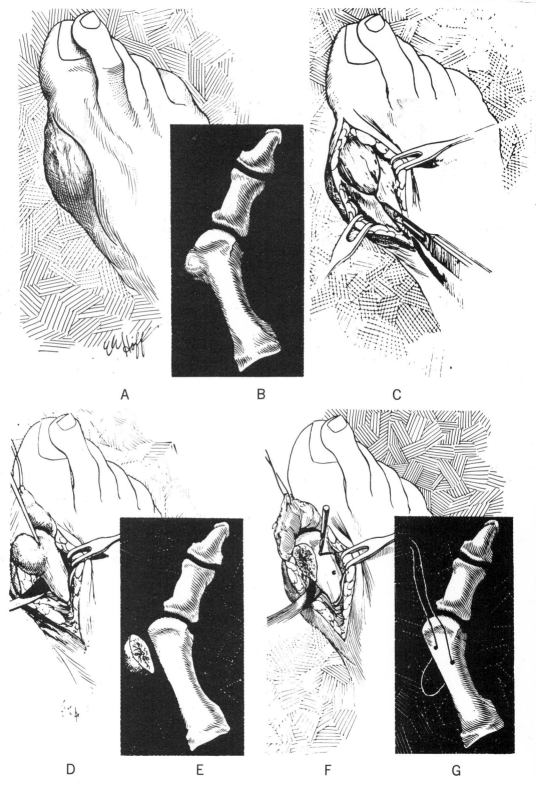

A   B   C

D   E   F   G

Fig. 13-3.   Operative technique for the Mitchell Procedure. (Mitchell, courtesy of J. Bone & Jt.
Surg.)

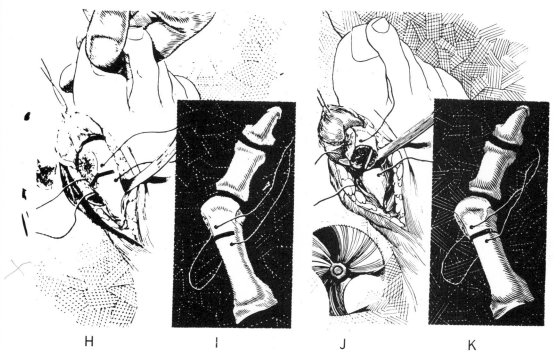

H   I   J   K

Fig. 13-3. Continued.

"A Y-shaped incision (Fig. 13-3B) is made through the medial capsule and the periosteum of the first metatarsal. The arms of the Y should meet 1/4 of an inch proximal to the metatarsophalangeal joint. If the arms of the Y extend too far proximally, insufficient tissue is left to obtain secure medial capsulorrhaphy.

"The neck and the shaft of the metatarsal are then stripped subperiosteally (Fig. 13-3C). The lateral capsular attachments are not disturbed, for these structures are the only remaining source of blood supply to the metatarsal head. The exostosis is removed flush with the shaft of the metatarsal.

"Two holes are drilled, one being 1/2 inch and the other 1 inch from the articular surface (Fig. 13-3D). The distal drill hole is slightly medial so that the holes will be in line when the lateral shift of the head is accomplished. Care is taken to place these holes perpendicular to the metatarsal shaft. A number 1 chromic catgut suture is placed through the holes by means of a ligature carrier or straight needle.

"A double incomplete osteotomy is then done 3/4 of an inch from the articular surface between the drill holes and perpendicular to the shaft (Fig. 13-3E). The thickness of the bone between the two cuts depends upon the amount of shortening of the metatarsal which will be necessary to relax the contracted lateral structures. Usually about 2 to 3 mm. (1/8 of an inch) of bone is removed. The size of the lateral spur depends upon the amount of metatarsus primus varus to be neutralized by the lateral shift of the metatarsal head. In a moderate deformity one-sixth of the width of the shaft is left to form the lateral spur, while in a severe deformity, one-third of the shaft remains. The osteotomy is completed proximally with a thin saw blade (Fig. 13-3F).

"Then the metatarsal head is shifted laterally until the lateral spur locks over the proximal shaft (Fig. 13-3G). The head is angulated slightly laterally so that its articular surface parallels the axis of the second metatarsal. Slight plantar displacement or angulation is desirable at this stage for reasons that will be discussed. The suture is tied giving surprising stability to the osteotomy site.

"Medial capsulorrhaphy is carried out

with the hallux held in slight over-correction (Fig. 13-3H). Chromic number 00 is commonly used for the capsular repair. The toe is then released and examined. It should stay in complete correction as a result of the capsulorrhaphy. If it does not, the distal capsular flap should be shifted further proximally and resutured. Postoperative splinting will not provide correction that is not obtained at the operating table.

"Splints made of padded tongue depressors are applied to the toe in slight over-correction and in 5 degrees plantar flexion to avoid dorsal displacement or angulation of the osteotomy site (Fig. 13-3I). The splint is worn for ten days. Following suture removal, a short walking-cast is applied to the leg, incorporating the great toe. Again, care is taken not to displace or angulate the osteotomy site dorsally."

Technical failures are due primarily to the fact that occasionally the osteotomy is performed too far proximally. This, of course, leads to a prolongation of disability because of the prolonged period required to achieve union. Instability of the osteotomy can be due either to an asymmetrical lateral spur on the distal fragment or the drill holes are improperly placed in relation to the osteotomy site. Another technical failure is sometimes due to the incomplete correction of the metatarsus varus primus because of neglect to angulate the head of the metatarsal laterally. Dorsal angulation or displacement of the metatarsal head should be avoided. When dorsal angulation occurs, occasionally postoperative second or third metatarsalgia develops. In some instances, aseptic necrosis of the metatarsal head occurs as a result of excessive stripping of the lateral capsule. In dissecting the lateral capsule, a great deal of care must be exercised to avoid circulatory embarrassment to the head. The walking cast is usually worn for a period of from four to five weeks. At the end of this time, the cast is removed and roentgenograms are taken and if the osteotomy site is clinically united, weight bearing is instituted immediately. On the other hand, if union is not present, then another walking cast should be applied. The period of convalescence is usually anywhere from four to twelve weeks following surgery.

Although in the original article Mitchell recommended avoidance of dorsal angulation because of the possible development of metatarsalgia, in a personal communication he stated it is advisable that the distal fragments be slightly angulated dorsally if the foot presents a cavus deformity or an exceptionally high arch. However, if the foot is pronated, the distal fragment and head should be slightly angulated plantarly.

Joplin has reported good to excellent results with his procedure in the same type of foot.

In patients between the ages of thirty and fifty-five the situation is somewhat different. If examination reveals that the extension and flexion of the metatarsophalangeal joint is only slightly limited (that is; 10 to 15 degrees limitation of extension and 5 to 10 degrees limitation of flexion), and who have no complaint of pain in the metatarsophalangeal joint, itself, and whose roentgenographic findings demonstrate a relatively normal articulation, the surgeon again has a choice of two procedures which have withstood the test of time. One is the author's modification of the Akin procedure and the other is the McBride.

Giannestras' Modification of Akin Procedure. This operation is based on the simple principle that it is not necessary to attempt to realign the metatarsophalangeal joint and to correct this misalignment which has existed for quite a long period of time. To put it plainly, the joint has been functioning asymptomatically with only minimal limitation of motion in spite of its malposition for quite a number of years. Therefore in my opinion, it is asking too much of such a joint to attempt to replace the proximal phalanx on a metatarsal head whose medial one-third of the articular cartilage has become quite thin and eroded because of lack of contact with opposing cartilage. Hence, why not leave the joint in its present position and simply correct the deformity of the great toe as well as remove the exostosis of the first metatarsal head?

Preoperative standing photographs and radiographs of both feet should be pro-

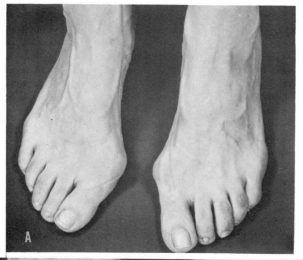

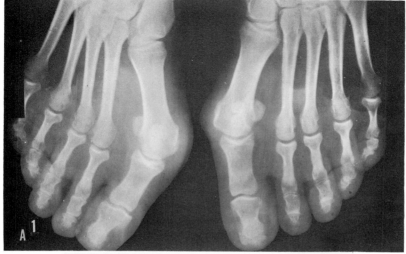

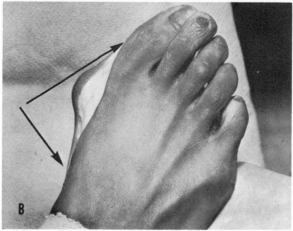

Fig. 13-4. Giannestras' modification of Akin bunion procedure for patients between thirty-five and fifty-five years of age.

A. Standing photograph of bilateral Hallux Valgus in forty-eight-year-old patient whose chief complaint is pain on the dorso-medial aspect of each first metatarsal head when ambulatory for more than thirty to forty-five minutes; standing roentgenogram of some feet.

B. The incision extends from mid-shaft of the first metatarsal on medial aspect, then curves up over the dorsal aspect of the first metatarso-phalangeal joint, and then dips to the medial surface of the great toe to the level of the interphalangeal joint.

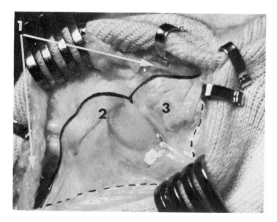

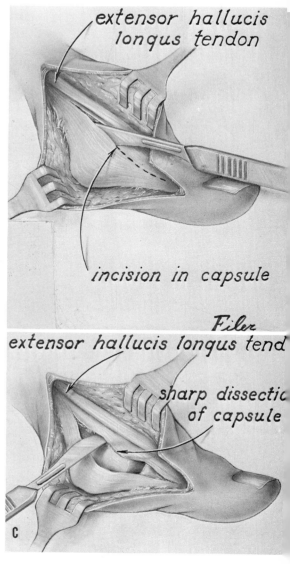

Fig. 13-4. Continued. C. Capsule reflected along with periosteal layer (1) to expose dorsal and medial aspect of first metatarsal head and exostosis (2) and proximal two-thirds of dorsomedial surface of the proximal phalanx (3). Diagrammatic sketch of same.

cured (Fig. 13-4A). The procedure is carried out under tourniquet control. The incision begins on the medial side of the first metatarsal 4 cm. proximal to the metatarsophalangeal joint. It curves dorsomedially (Fig. 13-4B) and extends distally to the level of the interphalangeal joint. No attempt is made to remove the bursa. The subcutaneous tissues are gently retracted medially and laterally to expose the capsular structures. The capsule is incised (Fig. 13-4C) to expose the exostosis and the incision is continued distally to expose the proximal two-thirds of the phalanx. The capsule is carefully dissected from the medial and dorsal surfaces of the metatar-

sal head and the phalanx. The removal of the exostosis and the adjoining bone must be carried out carefully in any of these procedures.

The foot should be properly lined up in the dorsoplantar position. The osteotome should be at least 1-1/2 cm. wide, *thin* and sharp. The amount of bone removed should include the entire exostosis and the medial portion of the head to the sagittal groove which runs in a dorsoplantar direction. The cut should be in a line parallel to the shaft (Fig. 13-4D). If there is a slight dorsal exostosis, this is shaved off. Following removal of the exostosis the head is rounded off with particular attention be-

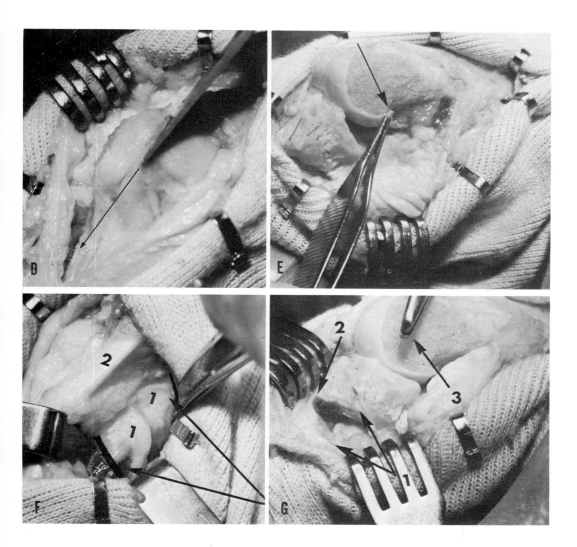

Fig. 13-4. Continued. D. Exostosis being excised along with small portion of first metatarsal head at level of "sagittal groove" which runs dorso-plantarly along course indicated by arrow.

E. Plantar exostosis which must be searched for and removed thus smoothing the plantar articular edge of the head.

F. Tendon (1) of both heads of adductor hallucis isolated prior to tenotomy through the same incision. Note extensor hallucis longus tendon (2) retracted medially.

G. Medial wedge osteotomy of the proximal phalanx (1) which extends up to but not through the lateral cortex (2). It is performed with a needle nosed rongeur (3) just 1cm distal to the articular surface.

ing paid to the small spur or exostosis on the plantar aspect of the head (Fig. 13-4E). The subcutaneous tissues are reflected on the dorsal surface to expose the lateral side of the metatarsophalangeal capsule, the transverse metatarsal ligament is sectioned, and the adductor hallucis tendon is brought into view.

The tendon is carefully delineated and tenotomy of the entire tendon is performed

(Fig. 13-4F). The base of the proximal phalanx is exposed and a wedge of bone is removed with the base located medially (Fig. 13-4G). This can best be carried out with a narrow, practically needle-nosed, rongeur and should be performed approximately 1 to 1.5 cm. distal to the metatarsophalangeal joint. The osteotomy is carried up to, but not through, the lateral cortex of the phalanx. The lateral cortex

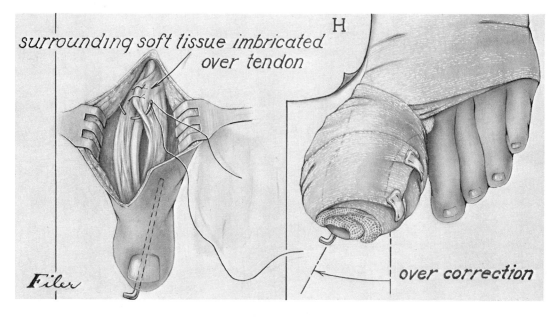

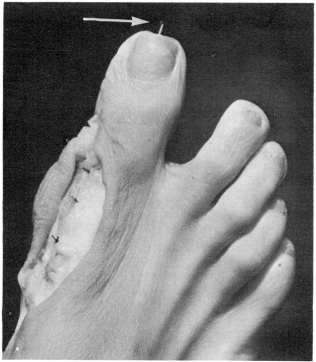

Fig. 13-4. Continued. H. Immediately following osteotomy of phalanx, insertion of Kirschner wire (note arrow) and closure of capsule. The toe is well corrected.

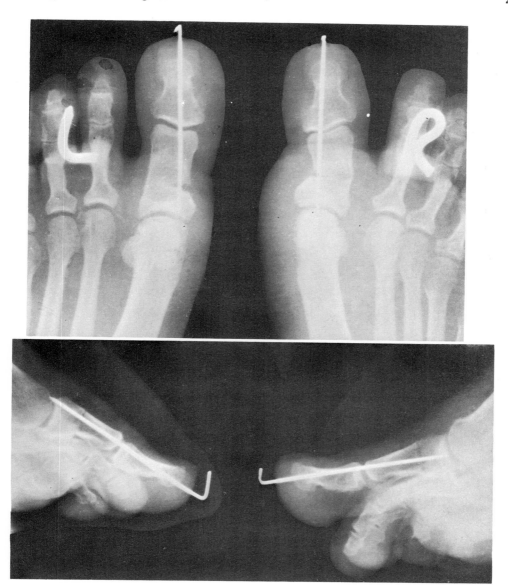

Fig. 13-4. Continued. I. Postoperative roentgenograms. Note osteotomy closed, wire well placed, and exposed portion of wire bent at right angle to prevent inward migration.

is broken in a greenstick-like fashion to realign the great toe in relation to the first metatarsal and the foot in general. Any axial rotation of the great toe can also be corrected. Under direct vision a threaded Kirschner wire is then inserted through the distal phalanx and the distal portion of the proximal phalanx, the osteotomy closed, and the wire then driven into the proximal fragment, care being taken not to drive it into the metatarsal head (Fig. 13-4H).

I prefer to have the tourniquet released at this time and all major bleeding controlled. This step, although somewhat tedious, will materially aid in the primary healing of the skin incision since, as we have all experienced, there is occasionally delayed healing of the skin incision. The capsule is closed with interrupted number 00 chromic sutures, care being taken that the medial half of the capsule be brought up toward the dorsal surface and the redundant portion resected. If the extensor hallucis longus tendon is still producing a

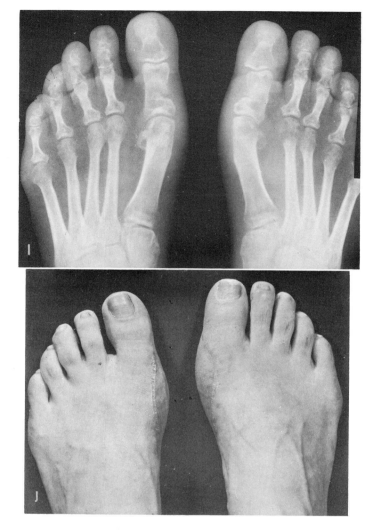

J. Postoperative photographs and roentgenograms of same feet. Note that metatarso-phalangeal joint relation is unchanged. Joints are asymptomatic and demonstrate full range of motion. (One year after surgery.)

bow-stringing effect, it can be lengthened by the usual multiple step-cut method and, if necessary, the surrounding areolar tissues imbricated about the tendon. The skin incision is closed with a subcuticular wire suture. A telfa dressing is applied over the incision and after the application of a roll of 4-inch sheet wadding, a 3-inch ace bandage is applied firmly, but not snugly. The foot is redressed in forty-eight hours, with the sheet wadding discarded upon this subsequent dressing. The patient is encouraged to ambulate on the fourth or fifth postoperative day in a thong-type sandal

which helps to maintain the great toe in slight varus.

If the second toe presents either a hammertoe deformity or a subluxation, or a dislocation of the second metatarsophalangeal joint, this is corrected through a separate L-shaped incision over the second metatarsophalangeal joint by resecting the proximal one-half of the proximal phalanx. A threaded Kirschner wire is passed retrograde and distalward through the medullary canal of the remaining portion of the phalanx with the toe held in the corrected straight position. The wire is then spun back into the second metatarsal head with the defect between the head and the remaining portion of the phalanx moderately separated. If the Kirschner wire is used, the circulation of the toe should be observed carefully for the next twenty-four hours. If there is the slightest suggestion of circulatory embarrassment of the second toe, the Kirschner wire should be removed immediately. In order to prevent migration of the wire into the toe, the wire is bent back as illustrated (Fig. 13-4 I). The sutures are removed only when the incision appears healed. The wire or wires are re-

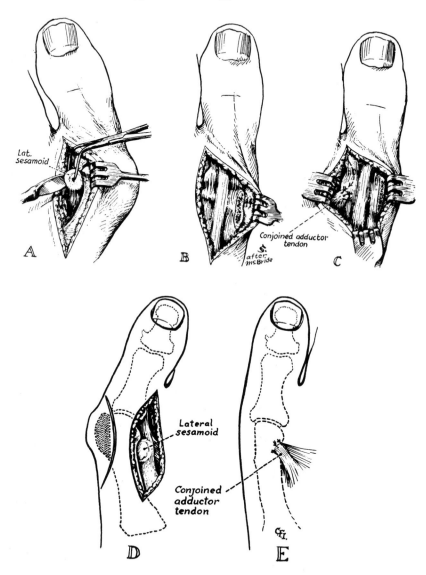

Fig. 13-5. McBride operation. **Top,** original technique with one incision. A, Lateral sesamoid is being excised. B, Exostosis has been resected from the medial aspect of the metatarsal head, and the medial part of the capsule plicated. C, Conjoined adductor tendon has been detached from the proximal phalanx and fixed to the metatarsal neck. **Bottom,** The technique we use with two incisions. D, Lateral sesamoid and the conjoined adductor tendon have been exposed through the lateral incision. **Stippled area** denotes the exostosis, which is to be resected through the medial incision. E, Sesamoid and the exostosis have been excised, and the conjoined adductor tendon has been fixed to the metatarsal neck. (B, Redrawn from McBride, E. D.; J.A.M.A.; A, C, D and E, from Campbell's Operative Orthopedics, A. H. Crenshaid, Editor, courtesy of the C. V. Mosby Co.)

moved in three weeks. The foot is then fitted with a loose broad-toed shoe for another three to four weeks until the swelling has subsided. The patient should be advised that at least two or three months will elapse before a dress shoe can be worn. In our experience, there have been no non-unions of the proximal phalanx of the great toe (Fig. 13-4J).

The McBride Procedure. "The incision starts slightly laterally to the great toe immediately above the web and extends directly upward and slightly inward on the dorsum of the foot for 1-1/2 inches, then curves more medially and downward about 3/4 of an inch (Fig. 13-5). This curve permits retraction of the incision medially in order to reach the bursa. (It is not necessary to make two incisions, but there is no objection to two, if the surgeon prefers this method over the single incision.) As the incision curves medially and downward, it crosses the extensor hallucis longus tendon so that the surgeon must use caution to prevent lacerating the tendon. It should *not* be necessary to tenotomize it if this operation is correctly done.

"The *adductor hallucis* is exposed at its insertion to the lateral aspect of the base of the proximal phalangeal joint of the great toe. The fatty fascial covering is removed by a scraping-like movement with a scalpel blade in order to bring the outline of the adductor distinctly into view. The tendon is then excised from its insertion, separated from its fascial attachment, and the end pulled well back between the first and second metatarsal bones where it is clamped until the surgeon is ready to transplant it. As the plantar aspect of the adductor is separated from the bone, the medial side of the sesamoid may be observed.

"Removal of the *sesamoid* has become much easier with less surgical trauma since the discovery (by McBride) of a little trick in enucleating it. With a number 15 Parker blade, enucleation of the sesamoid starts *laterally,* removing it from the fascial attachment of the flexor brevis tendon. When it has been loosened as much as can be accomplished through lateral dissection, it is firmly grasped *in its center* with the modified prongs of the towel clamp. The

surgeon who has been standing lateral to the table now changes places with his assistant and steps around to the end of the table. With a towel clamp held firmly in the left hand, the surgeon continues to enucleate the sesamoid bone until he reaches the *intersesamoid ligament.* He then turns the sharp edge of his blade toward the dorsal surface of the foot and cuts upwards between the two sesamoids. The intersesamoid ligament is very tenacious, but if one will cut *straight upward* between the two sesamoid bones and, at the same time, rotate the sesamoid outward with the left hand, its removal becomes easy. The lessening of the surgical trauma in this respect is greatly to be desired. The *lateral sesamoid,* only, is removed unless there is a painful bursitis with deformity of both sesamoids; then both may be removed.

"The skin incision is now retracted medially to freely expose the *bursal prominence.* It is found preferable to open the bursa by making first, a plantar-to-dorsal cut through the central thickened portion in line with the joint. A *proximal flap* is then made by a dorsal and a plantar cut extending upward slightly between the bone prominence. This flap is easily torn by manipulation of the osteotome because it is very thin at its upper end. If it is not kept intact, it will become difficult to suture firmly to the distal flap after excision of the bone prominence. As a result the lapse of the toe into valgus may occur.

"The *excision of the bone prominence* should be in a line parallel to the shaft. A one-inch, very thin osteotome is used. Before starting the excision, one should retract and expose the joint sufficiently to observe the slight groove on the end of the first metatarsal and make sure that the portion of the bone prominence removed *includes the lateral margin of the groove.* Otherwise, it may be difficult to reduce the toe medially and to maintain correction.

"*To shorten the capsule,* the toe is now manipulated into free overcorrection. If necessary, the capsule may be tenotomized on the lateral aspect. The toe should be held in about *10 degrees overcorrection.* While it is in this position the edges of the bursal flaps are brought together and *overlapped* to measure the portion to be excised

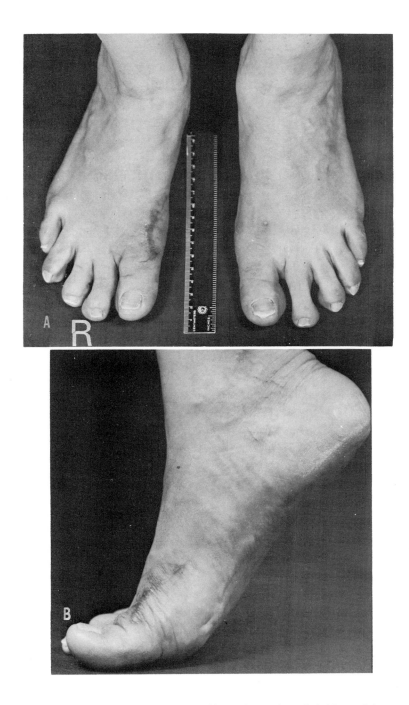

Fig. 13-6. A. Postoperative Keller procedure. Note shortening of right great toe.

B. Amount of extension of great toe following Keller procedure.

in order to hold the toe in correction. Usually, it requires a one-eighth to 1/4-inch excision and this is taken preferably from the *distal flap.* The two flaps of the bursa are then firmly sutured with number 000 chromic catgut. If the capsule has been torn, the shreds should be picked up and sutured to firmly close the capsule. *If too much shortening of the capsule occurs, it will cause overcorrection and this is a very undesirable complication.*

"*To transplant the adductor tendon,* a 1/2-inch incision is made in the periosteum and fascia on the lateral side of the distal shaft of the first metatarsal. The periosteum is elevated, the bone scarified so that the adductor tendon can be brought into direct contact with the cortex. The tendon is pulled into contact with the bone by passing a suture from the periosteum through the tendon and back through the tendon into the periosteum and tied quite firmly. The author (McBride) has not found it necessary to transplant the tendon in any other manner. To do so is undesirable, added, surgical trauma.

"To approximate the first to the second metatarsal, there are two methods:

"A) The usual technique is to pass a number 1 chromic catgut suture through the deep fascia about the head and neck of the second metatarsal from downward and upward through the fascia of the neck and head of the first metatarsal. The foot is squeezed firmly by the assistant while the knot is tied.

"B) The circumferential suture is used occasionally when there is necessity for greater force in holding the metatarsals to-gether. When this occurs, one should investigate the bases of the second and third metatarsals to determine if there is an anomaly that should be corrected. When the circumferential suture is used, and before the capsule or any other sutures are taken, a number 2 chromic catgut suture on a Reverdin needle is passed around the neck of the first metatarsal beneath the extensor hallucis and up around the second metatarsal under the extensor tendon. Before closure of the fascia and skin, the suture is tied while the foot is firmly squeezed to bring the metatarsals together.

"*At closure* all small bleeding points are electrocoagulated during the operation. Still there will be some bleeding on removal of the tourniquet. It is well to let the wounds 'bleed out' before applying the final dressing. The deep and superficial fascia are closed with a few number 000 plain catgut sutures, fine silk or number 32 wire may be used to close the skin. *It is very important* to make smooth, well-approximated skin edges which are of cosmetic perfection.

"The foot is dressed by fitting fine mesh-gauze between the toes, then wrapping the foot in four or five thicknesses of sheet wadding. A two-inch elastoplast bandage is applied rather loosely up to the ankle, with two or three spica laps around the great toe to hold it in about 5 to 10 degrees of overcorrection.

"Postoperatively, in bed the feet are elevated. The patient may stand on his feet within three or four days. The sutures are removed within seven to eight days and a light, protective, cotton bandage is applied

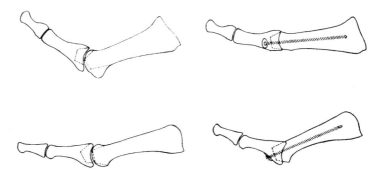

Fig. 13-7. Schematic drawing showing the amount of bone removed and the angle of fixation in both places. (McKeever, courtesy of J. Bone & Joint Surg.)

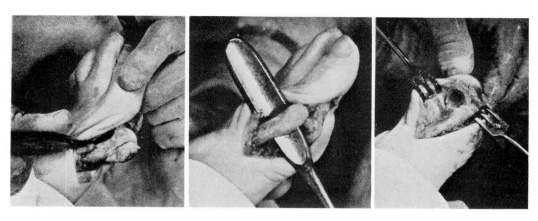

Fig. 13-8. A. The head of the metatarsal bone is disarticulated. B, Metatarsal after removal of bone. C, A hole is drilled and reamed out at the base of the proximal phalanx. (McKeever, courtesy of J. Bone & Joint Surg.)

with adhesive strapping in spica manner to support the position of the great toe. Sandals provide the best footwear for two or three weeks. If sandals are not available, the great toe portion of a pair of oxfords may be cut out to give room for the straightened toe."

In patients over the age of fifty-five, and in those with hallux rigidus, it is the unanimous opinion of the contributors to this volume that the Keller procedure has more to offer than any other, and if one does not care to employ the Keller technique, then McKeever's arthrodesis of the metatarsophalangeal joint could be considered. Usually in those past the age of fifty-five to sixty, the great toe is in marked valgus position, rotated on its axis and either overriding or underriding the second toe. The metatarsophalangeal joint presents moderate to extensive degenerative changes.

The Keller Procedure. Through the standard dorsomedial incision, the metatarsophalangeal joint is exposed. The exostosis of the first metatarsal head is removed as described in the previous two procedures. Then by sharp dissection, the capsule is dissected free from its attachment to the proximal phalanx. The capsule should be detached with a pointed scalpel as far dorsolaterally and plantarlaterally as possible. The toe should then be forcibly plantar-flexed and the phalanx dislocated, thus permitting detachment of the lateral plantar capsule. Care should be ex-

ercised that the dissection is carried close to the bone to avoid sectioning of the flexor pollicis longus tendon which has been known to happen. The proximal half of the proximal phalanx is delivered into the wound. The base is grasped with a towel clamp and stabilized while a Gigli saw or a narrow rongeur is used to resect the proximal one-half of the proximal phalanx. A Kirschner wire is passed retrograde through the distal portion of the proximal phalanx and through the distal phalanx. Traction is applied to the great toe in line with the metatarsal to maintain the gap created by the removal of the phalanx as recommended by Fitzgerald. Removal of the sesamoids is an optional matter. Some orthopaedists do and others don't. I feel that the sesamoids should rarely be excised and usually only in those instances where the patient presents definite symptoms indicative of painful sesamoids. Again, it is wise to remember not to treat the roentgenograms, but the patient. If the patient has no pain or tenderness under the sesamoids, even though they may be markedly displaced roentgenographically, leave them alone. The tourniquet should be released and hemostasis secured. Following closure of the capsule and the skin, a firm but not snug pressure-dressing should be applied. The toe should not be overcorrected (Fig. 13-6A and B Refer also to Fig. 13-13).

The McKeever Arthrodesis. Although arthrodesis of the first metatarsophalangeal

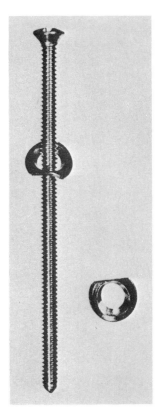

Fig. 13-9. Screw and special washer. The narrow side of the washer goes toward the bone and away from the plantar surface. (McKeever, courtesy of J. Bone & Joint Surg.)

joint was described in the last decade of the 19th century, McKeever devised and popularized the present method of fusion of this articulation. To quote McKeever, "this technique is presented here for general consideration; however, it must be stressed that it is the arthrodesis and its position that is important, and not the method by which it is produced (Fig. 13-7). The author (McKeever) prefers a medial linear incision slightly toward the plantar surface. The incision may also be made directly medial or toward the superior surface. This incision may be extended from the interphalangeal joint proximally to about the central portion of the first metatarsal, or a somewhat shorter incision may be made over the joint, with a small separate incision on the plantar surface for the insertion of the internal fixation screw. The proximal one-fourth of the proximal phalanx on the medial side and the distal one inch of the metatarsal are denuded of periosteum and ligaments and the joint is disarticulated (Fig. 13-8A). The distal end of the metatarsal is then cut down to a wide point with an osteotome (Fig. 13-8B). The first metatarsal is osteotomized in a distal direction in order to avoid splintering.

"The procedure requires the removal of a large quantity of bone around the head

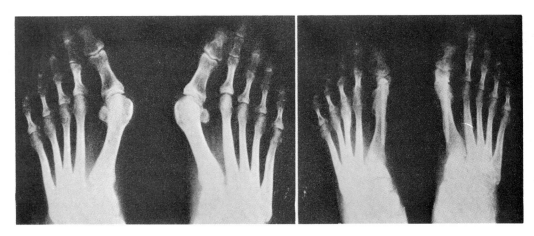

Fig. 13-10. Preoperative and postoperative roentgenograms made while the patient was bearing weight. Note correction of varus of the first metatarsal. (McKeever, courtesy of J. Bone & Joint Surg.)

of the first metatarsal. The tip, when finished, slopes at about 3/8 of an inch in diameter and slopes at a rather sharp angle back to the neck of the metatarsal. A hole 1/4 of an inch in diameter is then drilled in the base of the proximal phalanx. This hole should not be over 3/8 of an inch in depth. With a small motor driven reamer it is then reamed out to a conical shape corresponding to the end of the first metatarsal (Fig. 13-8C). This bone is extremely hard and must be cut slowly to avoid overheating. A Kerrison punch may be found useful here. Exposure of the plantar surface of the proximal phalanx is obtained either by means of extending the single incision or by making a small separate incision.

"It is now necessary to determine the angle of arthrodesis between the first metatarsal and the proximal phalanx. This is determined in the sagittal plane, by pressing the first metatarsal as close as possible to the second metatarsal and then putting the first and second toes side by side. In the coronal plane the angle varies according to the anticipated function (Fig. 13-9). In men it will be approximately 15 to 20 degrees of extension. In women who habitually wear shoes with medium heels, it will be from 15 to 25 degrees of extension, and in women who wish to wear high heels at all times, it may be as high as 35 degrees.

"While the toe is held in the position required, a hole is drilled which starts at the middle of the plantar surface of the proximal phalanx and crosses into the medullary canal of the shaft of the first metatarsal. A stainless steel screw with small curved oval washer is then inserted into the drill hole (Fig. 13-10). The screw should be long enough to extend almost the full length of the shaft of the first metatarsal, as rigid fixation is difficult to obtain with a short screw because of lack of purchase on the first metatarsal. The washer is necessary in order to prevent the head of the screw from pulling through the thin cortical bone on the plantar surface of the proximal phalanx. Lack of foresight in these matters resulted in five failures in the writer's (McKeever's) series. The incision is then closed and any superfluous skin and subcutaneous tissue are resected

to insure a smooth closure. There is usually a considerable amount of resection as the entire joint and the medial side of the foot have been made smaller. If the medial sesamoid seems to interfere with the closure, it then may be removed; it is the author's (McKeever's) custom to do so, although it is not necessary.

"A pressure bandage is applied to the foot. This bandage is loosened after four to six hours. It is replaced with a small dressing on the third or fourth day when weight bearing in a cutout shoe is permitted. The only precaution used is that the patient is not allowed to place his full weight on the toe at the end of the step for six weeks. The patient is cautioned strongly about this and is given specific instruction in walking. As soon as the stitches have been removed and the swelling is sufficiently reduced, the foot is put into a shoe which is not cutout. After six weeks a normal gait is resumed and any type of shoe may be worn. About 50 per cent of patients require no alteration in their shoes after the operation. The other 50 per cent may require some metatarsal padding temporarily and a few will require some metatarsal padding permanently.

"It is necessary to call attention to the fact that in many cases the hallux valgus operation alone is not sufficient to produce a good result. Such deformities and conditions as hammer toe, digital neuroma, soft corn, complete subluxation of lesser metatarsophalangeal joints and marked discrepancies between the lengths of the metatarsals must be taken into consideration and corrected at the time when the operation for hallux valgus is performed."

In the final analysis these thoughts should be kept in mind: No operative procedure will yield excellent results every time that it is attempted. Conservative therapy should be given a fair trial when ever possible. *No single procedure should be adopted for all types of hallux valgus deformities.* Each patient represents an individual problem and careful evaluation of the clinical and roentgenographic picture should be carried out before surgery is decided upon. A short postoperative convalescent period should not be used as the criterion for the selection of the procedure to be performed.

Last but not least, the blood uric acid should always be checked.

HALLUX RIGIDUS

Hallux rigidus, a term designating a stiff great toe, was first used by Cotterill in 1888. Although the expression is descriptive, it fails to indicate the underlying pathological condition, which is a degenerative osteoarthrosis of the first metatarsophalangeal joint. Throughout the years, other names have been suggested as substitutes for this term since hallux rigidus is not too scientific an appelation. In fact, Lapidus suggested the substantive "dorsal bunion", but even this substitute does not fully describe the condition.

Primary hallux rigidus can best be described, therefore, as being primarily a localized arthritic process of the first metatarsophalangeal joint. It is usually, but not necessarily, unilateral. The cause of this degeneration is almost invariably post-traumatic, although the average patient may be very hard put to recall the various episodes of minimal or mild trauma which might have initiated the process. Occasionally, an individual may recall one specific incident of acute trauma of moderate severity which, in his mind, precipitated the gradual, but progressively increasing disability of the great-toe joint. Pronation of the foot, overweight, as well as mechanical disalignment are also given as contributory factors in the production of this condition.

Secondary hallux rigidus is the type usually found in association with degenerative changes due to rheumatoid arthritis, gout or various other metabolic diseases. Clinically, the patient with primary or secondary hallux rigidus gives a history of a slowly progressive, almost imperceptible, loss of extension and/or flexion of the first metatarsophalangeal joint. The individual concerned will also state that in addition to the pain, he has noticed a gradual increase in the size of the joint. The articulation is most painful when the patient is required to walk for any distance or to stand for any period of time. The subjective symptomatology is never so acute as to completely disable an individual but is one of chronic discomfort, progressively increasing ever so gradually until the patient becomes intolerant of it and, therefore, seeks relief. The patient is most often a young adult, more commonly a male than a female.

On physical examination several or all of the following changes may be found:

1. There may or may not be an exostosis on the head of the first metatarsal. If an exostosis is found, it is usually located dorsally or dorsomedially.

2. The metatarsophalangeal joint is enlarged circumferentially.

3. Valgus deviation of the toe beyond normal is found only occasionally.

4. On palpation there is generally found osteophytic ridging of the base of the proximal phalanx and of the articular edge of the first metatarsal head.

5. Passive as well as active motion is limited and painful both in flexion and in extension, but the maximum limitation is in extension. The normal range of passive flexion of the metatarsophalangeal joint in a young adult has already been described. The loss of motion may be moderate, but in the majority of instances passive extension is totally absent.

On roentgenographic examination one finds either narrowing or almost total obliteration of the joint space (Fig. 13-11). Spur formation may be slight or, on the other hand, quite extensive with an occasional intra-articular loose body. Quite frequently on surgical exposure of such a joint, the changes will be even greater than those found on the roentgenograms. In instances where roentgenographically the articular space does not appear to be appreciably narrowed, one usually finds extensive erosion of the hyaline cartilage.

Treatment. In most circumstances, hallux rigidus of moderate to severe degree requires surgical intervention. Various conservative measures are frequently quite helpful and in many instances obviate the necessity of surgery in the less symptomatic cases and in those in which there is a slight to moderate loss of motion. The injection

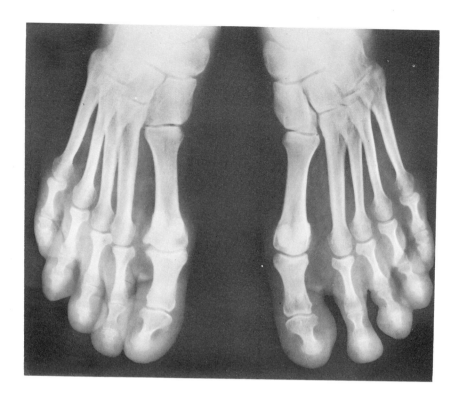

Fig. 13-11. Narrowing of the right first metatarsophalangeal joint with spur formation. Compare the difference between the right and left first metatarsalphalangeal joints.

of 0.5 cc. of one of the various intra-articular steroids given initially once every seven days; following relief of the symptomatology, only as the pain necessitates reinjection, aids in the elimination of the subjective symptomatology. Dr. Frederick R. Thompson in a personal communication several years ago drew my attention to an effective means of relieving the patient of his symptoms through application of a Chinese finger-trap to the great toe and the suspension of the foot through the finger-trap, thus applying traction to the hallux for five minutes daily. Although this maneuver may sound unphysiological and implausible, it has proved to be efficacious. The use of a transverse metatarsal bar is only mentioned to discontinue its applica-

tion. An arch support to control pronation has proved to be of help to some patients.

Surgical Intervention. Surgical intervention is successful when conservative means have failed and when the findings, both subjective and objective, are extensive enough to warrant this type of definitive therapy. Here again, as in hallux valgus, various operative procedures have been recommended from time to time over the years. In our opinion only two procedures are worthy of consideration: a) The Keller Operation, and b) arthrodesis of the metatarsophalangeal joint. Of the two the Keller technique is preferable (Fig. 13-12, A, B, and C). Both operations have been described earlier in this chapter for the correction of hallux valgus in the older patient.

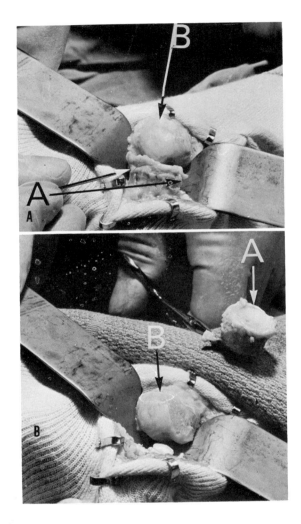

Fig. 13-12. A. (A) Demonstrates exposure of the proximal end of the proximal phalanx with extensive arthritic lipping of the proximal articular edge. (B) Note ridging along articular edge of metatarsal head.

B. (A) Resected proximal one-half of proximal phalanx. (B) Osteophytic ridging of the metatarsal head, as well as dorso-medial exostosis removed.

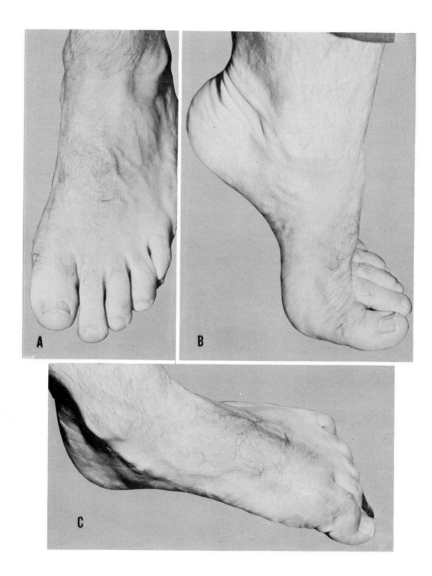

Fig. 13-12. Continued. C. Photographic appearance of foot one year following surgery. Note shortening of great toe but it is now asymptomatic with an almost normal range of motion.

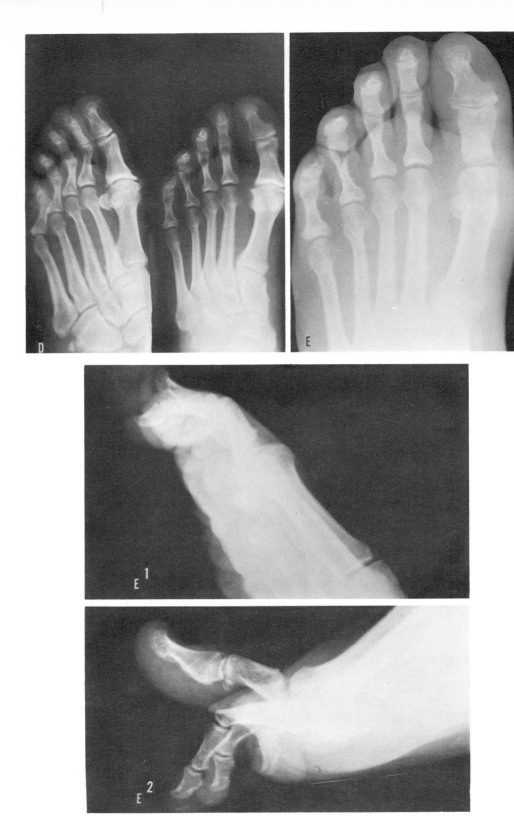

Fig. 13-12. Continued

    D.   Preoperative appearance of the first metatarsophalangeal joint. Note osteophytic production.

    E.   Postoperative appearance of same joint one year later. Note range of active flexion and extension.

BIBLIOGRAPHY

AKIN, O. F.: The Treatment of Hallux Valgus—A New Operative Procedure and Its Results. Med. Sentinel, 33:678-679, 1925.

ALLAN, F. G.: Hallux Valgus and Rigidus. Brit. Med. J., 1:579-581, 1940.

BUTTERWORTH, R. D. AND CLARY, BEVERLEY, R.: A Bunion Operation, Virginia Med. Monthly, 90, 10-14 (Jan.) 1963.

COTTERILL, J. M.: Stiffness of the Great Toe in Adolescents. Brit. Med. J., 1:1158, 1888.

FITZGERALD, W.: Hallux Valgus, Jour. Bone Jt. Surg., 32:139, 1950.

HAINES, R. W. AND McDOUGALL, A.: The Anatomy of Hallux Valgus. J. Bone Jt. Surg., 36:272, 1954.

JOPLIN, R. J.: Sling Procedure for the Correction of Splay Foot Metatarsus Varus Primus, and Hallux Valgus. J. Bone Jt. Surg., 32:779, 1950.

JORDAN, H. H. AND BRODSKY, A. E.: Keller Operation for Hallux Valgus and Hallux Rigidus A.M.A. Arch. Surg., 62:586-596, 1951.

KELLER, W. L.: Further Observations on the Surgical Treatment of Hallux Valgus and Bunions. N.Y. Med. J., 95:696, 1912.

LAPIDUS, PAUL W.: The Author's Bunion Operation from 1931 to 1959. Clin. Orth. 16:119-135, 1960.

The Operative Correction of Metatarsus Primus Varus in Hallux Valgus. Surg. Gyn. Obstet., 58: 183-191, 1934.

McBRIDE, EARL D.: The Surgical Treatment of Hallux Valgus Bunions. Amer. J. Orth. 44-46 (Feb.) 1963.

McKEEVER, DUNCAN D.: Arthrodesis of the First Metatarsophalangeal Joint for Hallux Valgus, Hallux Rigidus, and Metatarsus Primus Varus. J. Bone Jt. Surg., 34A:129-34, 1952.

MITCHELL, C. LESLIE: Personal Communication.

MITCHELL, C. LESLIE, et al.: Osteotomy, Bunionectomy for Hallux Valgus. J. Bone Jt. Surg., 40A, 41-60 (Jan.) 1958.

PIGGOTT, HARRY H.: The Natural History of Hallux Valgus in Adolescents and Early Adult Life. J. Bone Jt. Surg. 42:749-760, 1960.

THOMPSON, FREDRICK R.: Personal Communication.

14

Other Problems of the Forefoot

In addition to the problems of the great toe there are other deformities of the forefoot, either in association with those of the hallux, or separate from the first metatarsophalangeal complex. At times there is a definite interrelationship between the deviations of the first toe and the malalignment of the remainder of the forefoot. On other occasions these malformations will be individual, unrelated problems.

The correction of the major ones when associated with hallux valgus was presented in the previous chapter; but what of their therapy when they are unrelated to hallux valgus or hallux rigidus? Such conditions include the isolated hammer toe, syndactylism, varus deformity of the third digit (congenital curling), supernumerary digits of either the first or fifth toes, plantar keratosis, and other disorders. The nature and management of these problems will be discussed in this chapter.

However, at the start it is essential to recognize one basic dictum: In such cases, *never amputate a toe and leave a defect because the adjoining toes located medial to it will drift and valgus deformity of the toes will develop.*

HAMMER TOE

This deformity (Fig. 14-1), when severe enough, can be disabling because of the pain resulting from shoe pressure. Such pressure leads to the formation of a painful clavus on the dorsal surface of the involved interphalangeal joint. In addition, when the deformity is severe enough to produce subluxation or dislocation of the metatarsophalangeal joint, resulting pressure develops on the skin underlying the corresponding metatarsal head. This leads to the development of a painful callus or a disabling keratosis on the plantar surface. Although the use of various types of pads and sling appliances affords relief, these devices do not correct the deformity. Therefore, surgical correction is eventually necessary.

Operative Procedures. There are three recommended operative procedures, any one of which will produce good results

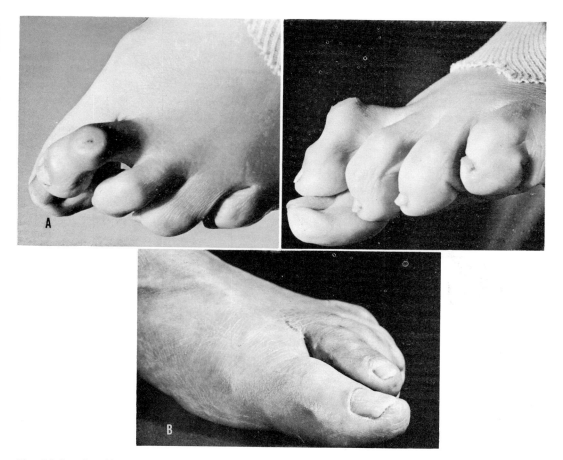

Fig. 14-1.   A.   Hammer toe deformity. Dorsal and lateral views. Note flexion at the proximal interphalangeal joint and extension at the metatarsophalangeal joint.

B.   Postoperative result one year later.

in the properly selected cases. In all cases a thigh tourniquet is used when not contraindicated by circulatory impairment.

Arthrodesis of the Interphalangeal Joint. This procedure is primarily recommended for patients under thirty-five to forty years of age who present a typical hammer toe deformity with no displacement of the metatarsophalangeal joint. It is carried out through a hockey-stick incision, beginning 0.5 cm. distal to the involved joint, extends 1.5 cm. proximally, and then transversely proximal to the metatarsophalangeal joint (Fig. 14-2). The total length of the incision, therefore, should be between 2 to 2.5 cm. This affords excellent exposure, does not place a longitudinal scar on the dorsum of the digit and the scar does not cross the transverse crease. The digital nerves are protected. The capsule and the extensor tendon are incised transversely and the articular surfaces are exposed. The use of an osteotome and mallet to excise the cartilage and the underlying bone is frequently troublesome because of the difficulty in maintaining stability and counter pressure on the toe. The technique for performing the arthrodesis consists of drilling a hole into each articular surface of the interphalangeal joint large enough to accommodate a small currette. The articular cartilage and the underlying cortex are thus excised. If, upon extending the interphalangeal joint, the toe is too long, it is shortened by resection of a portion of one of the phalanges. A Kirschner wire is passed

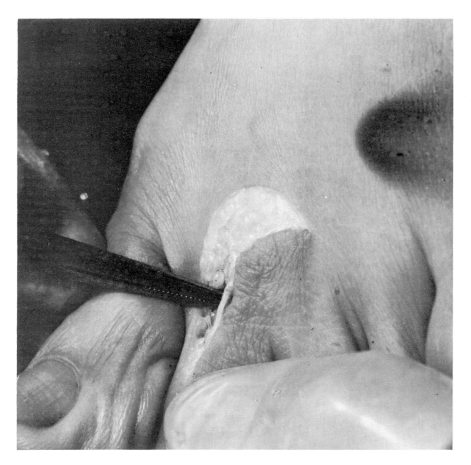

Fig. 14-2.   Utility incision for correction of hammer toe. With this type of incision the proximal interphalangeal joint as well as the metatarsophalangeal joint can be exposed. Note branch of dorsal digital nerve.

retrograde through the middle and distal phalanges and then with the digit in complete extension into the proximal phalanx down to its base, but not through it. The capsule and the tendon are closed with one or two catgut sutures.

The clavus (corn) overlying the interphalangeal joint is usually excised. Even if it is not, it will gradually disappear spontaneously. The skin is closed and a small Kling pressure dressing is applied. The wire is left *in situ* until the fusion is demonstrable roentgenographically, but it is removed by the end of six weeks. The toe should be well covered at all times in order to avoid pin-track infection. If fusion is not present in six weeks, remove the wire since the fibrous union is, almost invariably, sufficiently strong to maintain the correction.

If, in addition to the hammer toe deformity, the soft tissue structures of the corresponding metatarsophalangeal joint are contracted to the extent that the toe does not spontaneously correct completely, tenotomy of the extensor tendon, with or without dorsal capsulotomy, can be performed. Ambulation is permitted as soon as the patient shows a desire to walk and certainly by the fifth postoperative day.

Resection of the Proximal Half of the Proximal Phalanx. Resection of the proximal half of the proximal phalanx is indicated in patients over thirty-five to forty years of age who not only demonstrate a hammer toe deformity, but in addition, present marked subluxation or dislocation of the metatarsophalangeal joint of the same toe. The metatarsophalangeal joint is approached through a hockey-stick incision beginning transversely at the base of the toe 1 cm. proximal to the web, either medially or laterally, and extending distally for a distance of 3 cm. The skin and subcutaneous tissues are reflected exposing the extensor tendon to the toe. Two catgut sutures are applied 0.5 cm. apart and the tendon is severed between them to facilitate excision of the phalanx. The capsule is incised with a pointed type scalpel blade and is then dissected free from the base of the phalanx dorsally, medially, and laterally. The toe is flexed bringing into view the plantar surface of the proximal phalanx, the capsule detached, and at least the proximal one-half of the proximal phalanx resected. The two catgut sutures are tied loosely approximating the tendon but not under tension. If the tendon ends do not meet, have no concern. They will establish continuity later. The skin is closed and a firm pressure dressing applied.

Some orthopaedists are critical of this method, claiming that the toe is unstable and flail, and that "even if it touches the proffered surface, it cannot press down on it with sufficient force to obtain purchase." This has not been my experience. A large number of patients who have undergone this procedure were questioned about this loss of purchase, but none of them appeared to notice a disturbance of the gait because of it. It is true that the joint is unstable, but this, too, does not seem to be of concern to the patients.

Kelikian's Surgical Syndactilia. Kelikian's surgical syndactilia is indicated in patients who have adjoining hammer toes along with marked subluxation or dislocation of the metatarsophalangeal joints. This operation requires meticulous attention to detail and, therefore, will be presented verbatim. The only criticism of this procedure is that the originator recommends it for single hammer toe deformity and from that standpoint to quote an old cliché, "It's like running a mile to jump a foot ditch." The procedure follows. (Fig. 14-3). Kelikian, Clayton, and Loseff have treated numerous toe deformities, congenital as well as acquired, with surgical syndactilia. . . . The foot is prepared in the usual manner; hemostasis is secured with the aid of a pneumatic tourniquet. A silk thread is passed through each pulp of the two neighboring toes; the strands of the thread are brought together and clamped with a hemostat. The assistant puts traction on these forceps to straighten the toes and pulls them apart to bring the web space into full view. The area is now delineated by three sets of incisions: a web-bisecting incision, a pair of paradigital incisions, and a pair of connecting, or what we like to call "sartorial", skin cuts.

The web-bisecting incision starts on the dorsum of the forefoot in the selected intermetatarsal groove; it passes distally, dips plantarward and bisects the web. The incision ends at about the same point posteriorly on the plantar aspect of the forefoot as it does on the dorsal. The two paradigital incisions, one for each toe, fork out from the point where the web-bisecting cut begins to dip in a plantar direction. These incisions are extended lengthwise along the adjacent side of each toe; they terminate on the side of the distal phalanx at a point below and just proximal to the base of the nail. When one toe is short, as in the case of the fifth, the incision on the side of its neighbor is of commensurate length. By placing the paradigital incision slightly closer — but not too close — to the plantar border of the toe, one can insure a semblance of interdigital groove after surgical syndactilia. The sartorial cut connects the terminal point of the paradigital incision on either side with the plantar end of the web-bisecting incision. The intervening triangular patch of skin is dissected and discarded. In undermining the skin in this area care is taken not to puncture the plexus of veins ordinarily present.

The partial or total resection of the proximal phalanx is effected through the paradigital incision. The shaft of the phalanx is sought, and a small retractor is passed dorsally to protect the extensor tendon. The long flexor on the plantar aspect is enclosed in a fibrous sheath which blends with the periosteum on either side. The toe is rotated until the junction of the fibrous sheath and the bone is seen. The pointed scalpel penetrates the sheath, and hugging the inferior surface of the phalanx, it sweeps toward the metatarsophalangeal

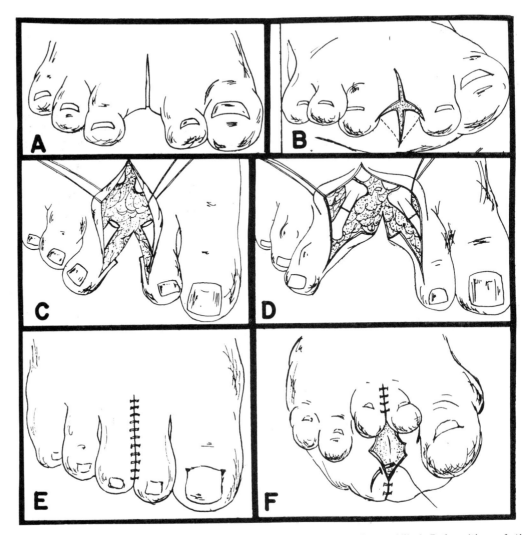

Fig. 14-3.   Kelikian's Syndactilic Procedure. (Kelikian—Hallux Valgus, Allied Deformities of the Forefoot and Metatarsalgia, courtesy of W. B. Saunders Co.)

   A: Dorso-plantar incision. Begins at metatarsophalangeal dorsally and extends plantarly to same level.

   B.   Paradigital incisions. Each begins at level of nail bed and extends to the initial incision. Dotted line indicates portion of skin to excised after it is undermined. It extends from distal end of paradigital incision to the end of the plantar portion of the dorsoplantar incision.

   C.   Resection of proximal half of each proximal phalanx.

   D.   Appearance of operative site after resection of the proximal half of each phalanx.

   E.   Dorsal closure of skin.

   F.   Plantar closure of skin.

joint. After the fibrous sheath is severed, another small retractor is introduced to protect the plantar soft tissues. The phalanx is divided at the desired level. A small paddle screw is inserted into the medullary cavity of the proximal fragment. The transfixion screw is used as a lever to lift the bone out of the wound. The proximal segment is dissected free and discarded. Rarely, the entire phalanx is enucleated. As a rule, the proximal half or two-thirds is removed.

After bone resection the surgical wound is packed with a moist sponge and the pneumatic tourniquet is deflated. It is advisable to wait a few minutes until post-tourniquet hyperemia subsides; the bleeders are clamped and ligated. The terminal points of the paradigital incisions are approximated by a number 34 stainless steel wire suture. The strands of the wire are temporarily twisted, the two toes are brought together, and the level of the nails is scrutinized. Eversion and inversion of the toes are avoided; if necessary, the wire suture is removed and reapplied. We usually approximate the dorsal skin edges with fine silk or nylon and use number 0000 plain catgut to bring the plantar margin together.

VARUS DEFORMITY OF THE FIFTH TOE

Whenever one is faced with this little problem (Fig. 14-4), the Lantzounis procedure is ideal. The operative procedure consists of exposure of the fifth metatarsophalangeal joint, tenotomy of the extensor digitorum longus tendon at the distal end of the incision, and release of the capsule of the joint dorsally, medially and laterally. The capsule is plicated plantarly by passing a #0 chromic catgut mattress suture proximal to the joint from the lateral to the medial edge, thence from medial to lateral distal to the joint and the suture tied with the toe flexed plantarly. The extensor tendon is transplanted into the neck of the fifth metatarsal. The subcutaneous and skin layers are then closed and the toe is maintained in the corrected position for three weeks. The author does not agree with Kelikian's statement that "replacement and realignment of the toe as a free functioning unit is next to impossible and at best highly unsatisfactory."

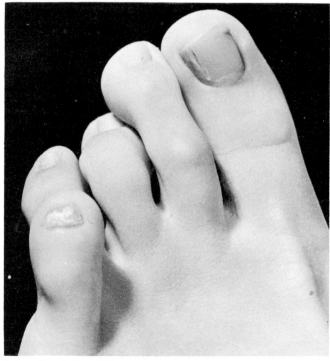

Fig. 14-4.   Varus deformity of the fifth toe.

CLAWTOE DEFORMITY

Rarely does one see a clawtoe deformity of a forefoot unassociated with a cavus or a cavovarus deformity of the rear foot. Occasionally it will be found unilaterally. It is not seen as frequently on a unilateral basis as it was prior to the poliomyelitis vaccine era. If this deformity is associated with a cavus foot and is bilateral, one should evaluate the patient's neurological background since it is usually due to one of the neuromuscular dystrophies, *e.g.*, Charcot-Marie-Tooth disease or Friedreich's ataxia. The reader is advised to refer to the chapter on neurological diseases for further information pertaining to such problems since a deformity of this type affects the foot primarily and the toes secondarily.

In a patient suffering a clawtoe deformity, whose primary difficulty is the fitting of shoes and who has only a minimal amount of discomfort in the toes, Hibbs' extensor tendon transplant is quite adequate a procedure. The toes should be carefully evaluated. One should determine the flexibility and correctibility of the digits. With the knee in 90 degree flexion, finger pressure should be applied on the plantar surface of the toes just proximal to the second and third metatarsal heads. If complete or almost complete extension of the toes occurs, Hibbs' procedure will give adequate correction.

The operation consists of transplanting the extensor tendons of the lateral four toes into the middle cuneiform through a dorsal curvilinear incision. The extensor hallucis longus is transferred into the neck of the first metatarsal and tenodesis of the interphalangeal joint of the great toe is also carried out (Jones Suspension Procedure). The only modification that I would suggest is the method of transplantation of the tendons into the middle cuneiform. Hibbs recommended the drilling of two holes into the middle cuneiform with the two medial tendons passed through the medial to the lateral opening, and the two lateral tendons passed in the opposite direction, followed by suturing the tendons to each other.

An easier method is to drill an opening large enough to accommodate all four tendons, pass a number 2 chromic suture through all four tendons to form a "figure 8"; using two straight needles, pass the needles through the opening to the plantar aspect of the foot, pull the tendons into the middle cuneiform with sufficient tension to hold the foot in neutral position by the transferred tendons after the suture is tied. The two ends of the suture are tied on the plantar aspect of the foot over a plastic pressure dispersal disk with foam rubber interposed between the skin and the disk. This is done to distribute the pressure even-

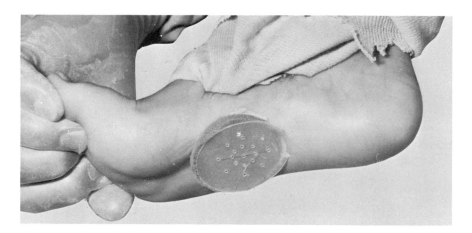

Fig. 14-5.   Plastic pressure dispersal disc over which tendon suture is tied. Pressure is distributed over large area preventing development of pressure area on plantar aspect of foot which developed almost invariably when ordinary button was used in order to tie suture.

ly and prevent some of the complications which formerly ensued when the suture was tied over an ordinary button. A Bunnell pull-out wire suture complex can also be used if one so desires, but here again, the wire should be tied over a pressure dispersal disk (Fig. 14-5). The extensor hallucis longus is sutured on itself after it has passed through the neck of the first metatarsal through a separate incision on the dorsum of the first metatarsophalangeal joint. Tenodesis of the interphalangeal joint of the great toe is carried out by suturing the proximal end of the distal 2-1/2 to 3 cm. of the tendon into the base of the proximal phalanx with the interphalangeal joint held in complete extension. A plaster cast is applied extending from the tips of the toes to the knee, with the ankle in neutral right angle position and the toes in moderate flexion at the metatarsophalangeal joints and complete extension in the interphalangeal joints. This can best be carried out by applying the cast in sections: First, from the knee to the midfoot and after this portion of the cast has set, the remaining forefoot part of the cast can be applied with the toes in the desired position and parallel to one another. The cast *must* extend to the tips of the toes in order that they be held in the corrected position.

When the same clawtoe deformity is encountered in an adult whose toes are not flexible and present fixed contractures at both the metatarsophalangeal joints and the interphalangeal joints, the procedure of choice is proximal phalangectomy of all five toes through a transverse incision and insertion of Kirschner wires through all five digits in retrograde fashion. Subsequently, the wires are spun into each metatarsal head with each toe in complete extension through the interphalangeal joints and 5 degrees flexion at the metatarsophalangeal level with the defect created by the phalangectomy partially maintained by the wires. If a medial exostosis presents itself on the first metatarsal head, this is excised as well. If the great toe is not involved in the clawing, it is left alone and only the lateral four toes are corrected. The tourniquet is released and after the application of pressure over the incision for a five-minute period to control a good deal of the bleeding, the major bleeders are ligated. A firm pressure dressing is applied and a plaster of paris splint, or a piece of cardboard extending beyond the toes for protection, is incorporated into the dressing. Weight bearing with crutches or a walker is permitted within five days. The dressing is not changed for a period of one week. The Kirschner wires are left *in situ* for three weeks.

During this period, walking should be concentrated on the rear foot with the use of crutches, but preferably with a walker. Occasionally, one encounters circulatory embarrassment when the clawtoes are corrected and a Kirschner wire is inserted to maintain correction. The postoperative orders should always include instructions to pull out the Kirschner wire immediately should such circulatory difficulties occur. This will relieve the tension on the surrounding soft tissues and permit circulation to be reestablished in the involved digit or digits.

BUNIONETTE OF THE FIFTH TOE (TAILOR'S BUNION)

The term "tailor's bunion" to describe an exostosis on the lateral aspect of the fifth toe (Fig. 14-6) was coined many years ago since it was found predominantly in people who sat in a cross-legged fashion, as tailors were apt to do. If the lesions are symptomatic or particularly unsightly, resection is easily performed through a dorsolateral curvilinear incision similar to the procedure described for exostectomy of the first metatarsal head.

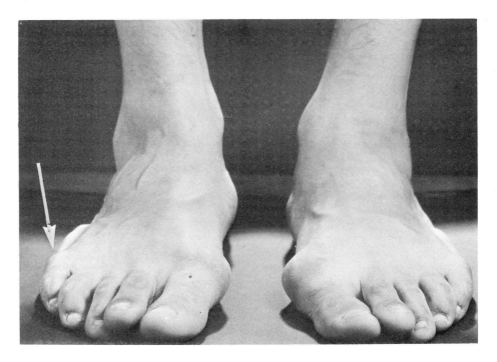

Fig. 14-6. Tailor's Bunion. Exostosis is located on the dorso-lateral aspect of the fifth metatarsal head (arrow). It can be either unilateral or bilateral and is frequently found in conjunction with hallux valgus.

CONGENITAL SYNDACTYLISM OF THE TOES

Congenital syndactylism of the toes, when partial, should not be corrected under any circumstances and should a patient request correction, the individual should be discouraged from such a procedure unless he may be required to pass some physical examination in which separation of all toes is absolutely required. Even in this latter instance a letter should be written advising whomever it may concern that such a syndactylism will in no way contribute to any disability of the foot and that surgical correction would improve the cosmetic appearance but not the function of the foot.

If the syndactylism is complete, it is usually associated with congenital shortening of the metatarsals. In the male surgical correction should most definitely be discouraged since, again, it will not improve the function of the foot. In the female, the occasion may arise in which the patient or the parents wish to have the syndactylia corrected for cosmetic reasons. Such corrective surgery is not recommended.

CONGENITAL GIGANTISM WITH OR WITHOUT MACRODACTYLIA

Congenital gigantism of one or more toes is a rare deformity in which a digit or digits are longer and larger than normal. When such a problem presents itself, the procedure to be selected will depend upon the evaluation of the digit by the examiner. Correction of the condition should be attempted in two stages. The operation should be planned carefully and meticulously. If the second digit is involved, which is most frequently the problem, it is approached first from the lateral side with the incision made according to Kelikian's technique for syndactilism. The lateral side

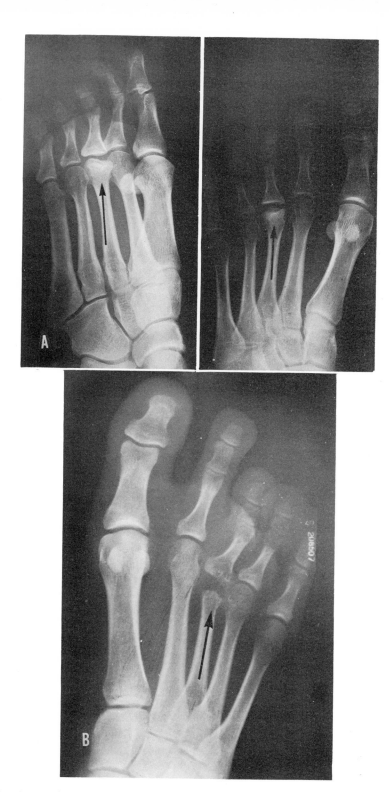

Fig. 14-7. A. Infraction of the metatarsal head (Frieberg's disease) roentgenographic appearance. The head is flattened. A loose body may or may not be found in the metatarsophalangeal
joint along with the capital changes.

B. Postoperative roentgenograph appearance of the same foot fourteen months following resection of the metatarsal head.

of the toe is completely defatted; the entire proximal phalanx, and as much as is necessary of the middle phalanx, is excised to shorten the toe adequately to place it in normal relationship with the first and third toes. The skin flaps are closed and permitted to heal. Six weeks later the medial side of the same digit is approached, defatted, and syndactylized to the great toe.

At times one or two toes are found to be longer than normal. These are usually the second and/or the third. The procedure consists of excision of as much as is necessary of the proximal phalanx, sometimes total excision, to achieve the necessary amount of shortening.

METATARSALGIA

As the term denotes, metatarsalgia is pain in the metatarsal region of the foot. It is very rarely seen in children. When a child or a teenager complains of pain in the plantar metatarsal area, it is most frequently due to trauma or to an osteochondritis of the second metatarsal head, commonly known as Freiberg's disease, or infraction of the second metatarsal head. If it is traumatic in origin, after appropriate roentgenograms have been procured, the usual rest and supportive circular wrapping with an ace bandage are sufficient.

In Freiberg's disease (Fig. 14-7) the situation is an entirely different one. When Dr. Albert H. Freiberg first described this entity in 1914, he suggested that trauma was the causative factor since the patients who had presented themselves all gave a history of having "stubbed the second toe". Later on, Freiberg reported that he was not certain trauma was the principal cause of this condition. Over the years many theories have been propounded, but as yet the cause of this deformity of the head is still theoretical. It can occur at almost any age, and has been reported from the age of thirteen to the age of sixty. In the patients seen by me the youngest has been twelve and the oldest nineteen.

In my cases conservative therapy with the use of a comma-shaped metatarsal pad (Fig. 14-8) has given only temporary relief in that as soon as the pad was discarded, the symptoms reappeared. However, conservative therapy should first be attempted. Should it fail, and the patient should be advised of this likely possibility, then excision of the metatarsal head should be conducted through the usual dorsal hockey-stick incision used to approach the metatarsophalangeal joint. One will fre-

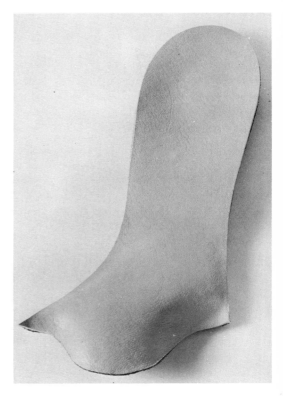

Fig. 14-8. Comma-shaped metatarsal pad. Maximum elevation is placed just proximal to the involved metatarsophalangeal joint.

quently find not only flattening and an increase in the size of the head but a loose osteocartilaginous ossicle. Weight bearing is permitted as soon as the acute postoperative pain subsides.

Metatarsalgia in the adult, however, is a painful entity which can be due to any number of causes. Any disturbance which can affect feet — circulatory, metabolic, neurogenic, static, traumatic, or infectious — can first manifest itself in the plantar

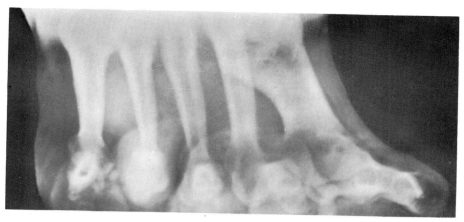

Fig. 14-9.   Roentgenogram of forefoot in standing position. Note that all five metatarsal heads participate in weight-bearing. There is no metatarsal arch. The same conformation is also present when the weight is borne on the forefoot as in high heel shoes or in the forward thrust phase of a step.

metatarsal or dorsal metatarsal region of either one or both feet. The more common causes are disturbances of the sesamoids, stress or "march" fracture of either the second or third metatarsal shaft (rarely the fourth), plantar keratosis, Freiberg's disease, pes cavus, pronated feet, hallux valgus, plantar fibromatosis, interdigital neuroma, and other plantar nerve entrapment syndromes. The last two will be discussed in the chapter dealing with neurological diseases of the foot. As regards the various systemic diseases, metatarsalgia, as it relates to them, will be discussed in their appropriate chapters. In this section the causes of metatarsalgia due to the more common static reasons will be presented.

One fact must first be reiterated before going on and that is that *there is no metatarsal arch* as has been contended in the past. In a standing position with or without a raised heel, the plantar aspect of each of the five metatarsal heads is in contact with the underlying surface (Fig. 14-9). The weight is borne equally on all five heads. The foot is not a tripod with the weight being borne on the plantar aspect of the heel and the first and fifth metatarsal plantar surfaces.

Most often, the patient complaining of static metatarsalgia will complain of pain on the weight-bearing surface only. It may be unilateral or bilateral. It will be located usually under the second, third, and/or the fourth metatarsal heads. The patient

may or may not give a history of prolonged standing on this region of the foot, as for example on a step ladder, or in high-heeled shoes. The condition is most frequently caused by poorly-fitted shoes as when the forepart of the foot has been squeezed into too narrow a shoe. Often times, the appearance of these symptoms is spontaneous.

On examination there is tenderness located directly under the plantar surface of the metatarsal head. There is no swelling or inflammation. Usually there will be some pain on passive manipulation of the metatarsophalangeal joints. Upon standing, the foot may or may not be pronated or splayed. Frequently there is a mild or moderate pes cavus associated with this symptomatology rather than a pronated foot. The arterial pulsations will be normal. The corresponding toes may or may not display a hammer toe deformity or mild clawing. The roentgenograms will be negative on examination.

Treatment.   Treatment consists of the procurement of an outline of the foot or feet in a standing position and the manufacture of a comma-shaped metatarsal pad (Fig. 14-8). This pad should be 3/8 of an inch in thickness. The comma-shaped pad is preferred to the oval one. The pad should be fitted in a low-heeled shoe. This will present no problem for the male, but the average female will balk at the idea of having to wear low-heeled oxford tie shoes, but if her pain is intense enough, she will do so. The patient should be advised to wear the support or supports constantly until the symptomatology subsides. Following relief, the pad is worn only when he or she will stand for long periods of time. Again, the male patient will make no protest, but the female will wish to know how soon she can discard the pads. This, of course, will depend upon how long the symptomatology persists.

If the patient should present a static deformity of the foot, such as a pes cavus, a mild clawtoe, or a hammer toe deformity, or pronation of the foot, the patient may have to wear such pads permanently because, upon discontinuing their use, the symptoms will recur. By and large it is surprising how many patients will be content to continue wearing such an apparatus in their shoes. The use of an anterior metatarsal bar rather than a pad is recommended by some orthopaedists and/or some clinical groups. This is mentioned, only so that one may be cognizant of the use of an anterior metatarsal bar. I have not found it necessary to use it since prescribing the comma-shaped metatarsal pad in its stead. The pads will require replacement annually and, therefore, the patient should be placed on an annual follow-up basis after he has been fitted initially and is comfortable. Occasionally after careful examination and fitting, the patient will still be dissatisfied. One must take the time and the patience to work with the individual and to do the utmost to find what is wrong and to try alleviate the problem. It is true that one cannot relieve the discomfort for every patient, but success in at least 90 per cent of the cases is an acceptable average.

Much has been written about the use of exercises to relieve the pain of metatarsalgia. Such a regimen is nothing more than a mental cathartic for the patient and in actuality does no good. The patient, however, feels that he is accomplishing something by performing these exercises.

Occasionally, the symptoms will occur under the first metatarsal head only. Here, again, the metatarsal pad will be of help, but the maximum elevation should be under the region of the first metatarsal head, tapering off to nothing in the region of the fifth metatarsal area. Frequently, when a patient complains of pain under the first metatarsal head, the roentgenograms of the foot will reveal that one of the sesamoids presents a line or lines through it. This finding does not indicate that it is fractured, but that it is bipartite, or sometimes tripartite. The medial sesamoid is affected more frequently than the lateral one. In order to sustain a fracture of one of these ossicles, sudden violence is required, such as jumping or falling from a height and landing on the forepart of the foot. Occasionally such a fracture will be found as a fatigue-type fracture in dancers who land rather forcibly on their toes. The fragments remain separated and do not heal with callus formation, if at all. Since bipartite sesamoids are usually bilateral, a roentgenogram of the opposite foot may be helpful. In a fresh fracture the lines will be sharp and possibly serrated, whereas in a bipartite sesamoid the lines will be smooth. Axial views of the first metatarsophalangeal joint should be procured as well to determine whether the pain under the metatarsal head is due to arthritic changes or chondromalacia of the sesamoids, rather than to involvement of the plantar aspect of the metatarsal head itself. Metatarsalgia under the great toe, associated with degenerative findings of the sesamoid articular surfaces, is relieved by surgical intervention. This can be carried out through an incision beginning on the medial aspect of the first metatarsal at the level of the neck, extending distally to the plantar crease of the great toe, and transversely to the lateral edge of this digit. The abductor hallucis tendon should be retracted dorsally and the capsule incised longitudinally. The metatarsophalangeal joint should be flexed permitting plantar retraction of the capsule and bringing the sesamoids into view. They should then be removed by sharp dissection.

On rare occasions one may find on roentgenographic examination a calcific deposit within the flexor hallucis brevis tendon either proximal or distal to the sesamoids. It should be treated as one would treat a calcareous tendonitis of the supraspinatus tendon in the shoulder, either by multiple needling and the injection of 1 cc. of one of the steroid preparations or with radiation therapy. As yet I have not found it necessary to extirpate the deposit surgically.

CALLUSES, CLAVI, AND KERATOSES

Calluses. Calluses are found in any portion of the forefoot where there is abnormal pressure or excessive friction. They are formed as a defense mechanism of the skin to protect it from excessive irritation and/or blistering. They can be found under any of the metatarsal heads, on the medial aspect of the first metatarsal head area, the lateral aspect of the fifth metatarsal head area, on the dorsal surface of a toe or toes, or on the tips of the toes. By and large, they are due to improperly-fitted shoes or to abnormal pressure in a well-fitted shoe if there is a deformity of the foot present. Relief can be procured by the elimination of the cause whether it be a poorly-fitted shoe or a deformity of the toe or toes. In the plantar metatarsal area the use of the same type of comma-shaped metatarsal pad will afford comfort. With the elimination of the abnormal pressure and with careful shaving of these calluses or rubbing with a pumice stone, the hyperkeratotic lesions can be gradually eliminated.

Clavus. The clavus, a synonym for the corn, is found on the toes wherever there is an underlying bony prominence upon which pressure is exerted by the shoe. The clavus is nothing more than a localized response of the skin to abnormal pressure from without against a bony prominence from within. Microscopically there is central hyperkeratosis with a thickening of the underlying rete pegs.

The clavus is usually located over an interphalangeal joint, most frequently on the fifth toe, or on the dorsal prominence of the hammer toe. In some instances, in addition to the one on the dorsolateral aspect of the fifth digit, there may be opposing clavi on the interdigital surfaces between the fourth and fifth toes. At times they can be extremely painful as well as disabling.

Conservative treatment consists of nothing more than the relief of the pressure by wearing properly-fitted shoes or corn pads. The use of various unguents containing primarily either salicylic acid or one of the tissue destroying chemicals may give temporary relief since these medications cause an excoriation of the hyperkeratotic area, but as mentioned, such alleviation is transitory. In order to remedy the situation permanently it is necessary to excise the underlying exostosis by surgery.

The surgical procedure consists of excision of the center of the clavus through an elliptical incision and exposure of the underlying small exostosis which is usually located on the dorsolateral surface of the head of one phalanx and the base of the adjoining distal phalanx. The exostoses should be removed with a small osteotome similar to the type used in hand surgery. Closure of the exposed articulation is unnecessary. The skin is closed in the usual manner and a dressing is applied. When there are apposing clavi, as between the fourth and fifth toes, both must be excised and the exostoses underlying each of them must also be removed.

Plantar Keratosis. This lesion was first described microscopically by the author in 1954. The plantar keratosis is the lesion which for years has been misdesignated as a "plantar wart". A microscopic differential diagnosis between it and the verruca plantaris was presented (Fig. 14-10 A and B). Microscopically the verruca plantaris (Fig. 14-10 A) presents central hyperplasia of the squamous epithelium surrounded by severe hyperparakeratosis. The rete pegs are elongated and appear to spread upward and outward from the center in a wart-like fashion. There is increased vascularity through the central portion of the lesion. The corium is normal in appearance.

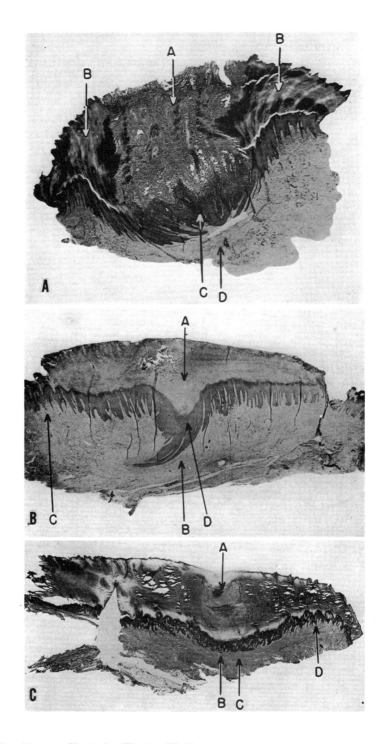

Fig. 14-10. A. Verruca Plantaris (Plantar Wart).

B. Plantar Keratosis.

C. Plantar Keratosis previously treated with fulguration and roentgenotherapy. (Giannestras, courtesy of J. Bone & Joint Surg.)

The plantar keratosis on microscopic examination (Fig. 14-10 B) presents the following findings: The epithelium on the central portion of the lesion is indented and there is striking hyperkeratosis of the center in comparison to the marginal portions. There is localized elongation of the rete pegs which extend into the corium in contrast with the pegs underlying the marginal normal portion of skin. Throughout the thickened stratum corium many small shrunken nuclei can be seen. The corium does not show any abnormality.

Thus it is obvious that the two lesions are unrelated. The verruca plantaris is considered to represent a viral response, whereas I consider the plantar keratosis to be a response to pressure.

The two types of lesions also differ on clinical examination. The plantar keratosis is found primarily in adults and not necessarily only "in older individuals with established forefoot deformities" as sometimes claimed. The pain is present after the individual has been walking for a short period of time, particularly if the individual has been wearing high-heeled shoes. The lesion is found predominantly in the female on the plantar surface of one or, at most, two metatarsal heads or metatarsophalangeal joints. It is heavily cornified and when trimmed it presents a small pearl-gray avascular center. If the keratosis is of long duration, small hemoserotic areas may be found within this center, but no true blood vessels are seen. If there is bleeding when the keratosis is trimmed, it occurs at the periphery of the pearl-gray center. It is tender to direct pressure by the palpating finger.

The verruca plantaris, on the other hand, is found on any portion of the foot and occurs in children as well as in adults. It may occur as an isolated solitary lesion or in clusters. Its center is soft and is covered by a thin layer of epidermis. The true verruca is extremely vascular and upon even the slightest trimming will bleed profusely from its center. The plantar wart resembles the plantar keratosis only in that it is tender to direct pressure. It differs in that it is also painful upon lateral compression. It responds well to any type of tissue-destroying therapy whether it be electrical, chemical, or irradiative.

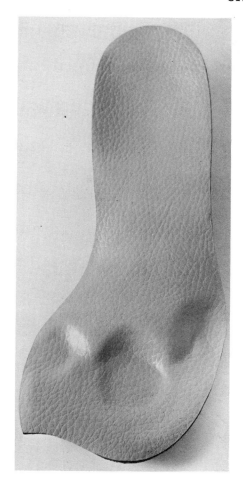

Fig. 14-11. Metatarsal pad with depression constructed into the pad to relieve pressure on the plantar keratosis and alleviate pain.

The treatment of the plantar keratosis should be conservative to begin with, but should conservative measures fail, surgical removal of the overlying pressure should be considered. Conservative therapy is aimed at reducing or eliminating the pressure on the plantar aspect of the keratosis. In many instances this can be carried out by the manufacture of a comma-shaped metatarsal pad with a depression constructed in the center where the keratosis is located (Fig. 14-11). This can best be accomplished by taking a standing outline of the foot with methylene blue or a similar dye applied to the keratosis so that an imprint is left on the pedograph. The individually designed pad is then fitted into the shoe.

Along with the insertion of the pad, the patient is instructed in the use of a pumice stone or an emery board with which to scrape the keratosis and thus thin it down. For men this plan of therapy has been successful in most instances since it is not difficult for them to wear a sensible broad-toed shoe. With female patients such is not the picture. They may wear a low-heeled shoe for a portion of the time with the supportive pad, but as soon as the acute pain subsides and the discomfort is tolerable, they will return to the use of the high-styled, high-heeled shoes. Cryotherapy (by the use of carbon dioxide snow and other tissue destroying chemicals such as salicylic acid) can be used if one wishes, but in a large number of patients this type of therapy fails. Roentgenotherapy may be used for one series only, since occasionally the lesion may respond, but the patient should be warned against repeated series. Occasionally, elliptical excision of the lesion, followed by careful primary closure and no weight bearing for a period of three weeks may produce a satisfactory result. There are a few more successful local therapeutic measures that have been prescribed over the years. By and large, however, if the orthopaedist concerned should follow the patients who are suffering from a plantar keratosis carefully, he will find that conservative therapy in the large majority of patients fails.

In my considered opinion, conservative therapy should be given a trial with the patient clearly understanding *from the outset,* that there is a good probability of failure with this nonoperative regimen and that shortening of the metatarsal head to eliminate the pressure may eventually be necessary. It is absolutely essential that a good rapport be established with the patient. If any or all of the conservative measures have failed, then surgical intervention should be recommended. Criticism has been leveled by some that this is a major procedure for a minor lesion, but for the patient who has had to live and to suffer with this condition it is a major disabling factor.

DuVries recommended condylectomy or resection of the plantar half of the metatarsal head, but no adequate follow-up on his end-results had been presented up to the early part of 1965. McElvenny in a personal communication in 1956 had performed the DuVries procedure in a series of cases with a careful follow-up study and although he was quite enthusiastic in the beginning, when he reviewed his end-results, he discarded the procedure altogether because of the large percentage of recurrences. Metatarsal shortening for the treatment of plantar keratosois was recommended by McKeever. The shortening, however, was performed at the junction of the head with the neck of the metatarsal. Although in my experience the end-results were satisfactory, there developed in many patients limitation of function of the metatarsophalangeal joint, as well as a flexion contracture deformity at the metatarsophalangeal joint.

In 1964 I mailed a questionnaire to each member of the Academy of Orthopaedic Surgeons in order to determine whether or not the method of treatment recommended in 1954, which consisted of shortening of the metatarsal by the step-cut method of osteotomy, was of any value in the recalcitrant cases of plantar keratosis. Approximately one-third of the members replied. Of these, 201 stated that they had used the procedure in cases of plantar keratosis which had failed to respond to other conservative therapy. Twelve of the 201 reports had to be discarded from the study because of insufficient information. In two or three instances the discarding was regrettable as the respondees had treated a number of patients by this method and were enthusiastic about the results. Thirty-four preferred resection of the offending metatarsal heads, but several of them stated that the end-result was not always satisfactory because of the development of a hammertoe deformity in some instances and a flailtoe deformity in others with or without a recurrence of the plantar keratosis.

A large number felt that with conservative means and patience, surgery could be avoided. Therapeutic measures recommended by this group were properly-fitted shoes, metatarsal pads, frequent trimming of the lesion, use of warm applications to soften the lesion, twice daily soaking of the feet in water as hot as could be tolerated, daily use of an abrasive soapstone, and padding with mole skin. Many of these

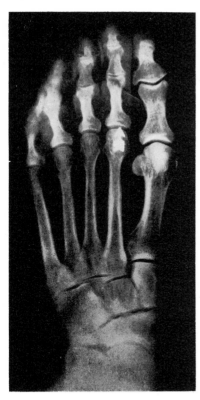

Fig. 14-12. Lead marker to indicate location of plantar keratosis. (Giannestras, courtesy of J. Bone & Joint Surg.)

respondees stated that in their experience the plantar keratosis has never become a major disabling factor. However, this group of respondees stated that 767 patients had undergone metatarsal shortening because of failure of all conservative measures. In this entire series known nonunion developed in 18 metatarsals or a nonunion rate of 2.03 per cent. Of these 18, 4 were symptomatic, and in only one were the symptoms severe enough to warrant bone grafting. Nonunion occurred only in the second, third, and fourth metatarsal shafts. Apparently, therefore, nonunion per se is not a major disabling factor when it occurs at the base of the metatarsal. No nonunions were reported in patients who underwent shortening of the first or fifth metatarsal shafts.

The contraindications to this procedure are clear-cut. This technique should not be performed in patients who have cavus feet. It is also contraindicated in patients suffering from such neurological diseases as Friedreich's ataxia, Charcot-Marie-Tooth disease, and similar disorders. In an elderly patient in whom the circulatory function of the lower extremity may be highly impaired, one should give careful consideration to the patient's activity, as well as the

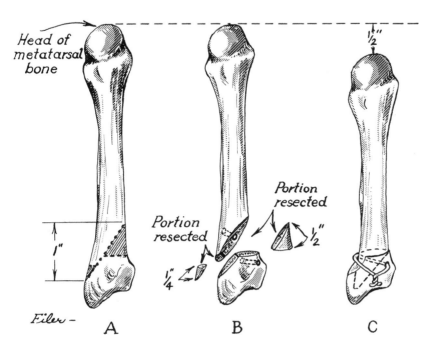

Fig. 14-13. Oblique Osteotomy of the Metatarsal Shaft. (Giannestras, courtesy of J. Bone & Joint Surg.)

severity of the impairment of the circulation before considering such an operative procedure. In a diabetic with recurrent trophic ulcer under the metatarsal head, which heals with rest and reappears with weight bearing, one should not consider a metatarsal shortening under any circumstances. In this instance the ideal therapy is excision of the entire ray.

Operative Procedure. In a patient who has had various types of local therapy and is still seeking relief from this disability, the plan of therapy is as follows: The foot is carefully examined and a standing x-ray film is procured with a lead marker placed under the plantar keratosis (Fig. 14-12) in order to determine whether or not the lesion is located under the metatarsal head or the metatarsophalangeal joint. If the lesion is not in the above mentioned area, then surgery should not be considered since it will be of no value.

Through a dorsal 5 cm. incision beginning at the tarsometatarsal joint and extending distally, the proximal two-thirds of the metatarsal shaft is exposed subperiostially. An oblique osteotomy is carried out beginning 1/2 to 3/4 of an inch from the tarsometatarsal joint of the offending metatarsal. The technique of the operative procedure is as follows: With the use of a 3/32 of an inch drill point, multiple small drill holes are made preparatory to the oblique osteotomy which is 1 inch in length (Fig. 14-13). A thin, narrow osteotome similar to that which is employed in hand surgery is then used to complete the osteotomy. One-quarter inch of the shaft is resected from the distal fragment and 1/2 inch from the proximal fragment. A drill hole is made obliquely from cortex to cortex in the proximal fragment 1/4 inch from the cut edge. A similar drill hole is made through the distal fragment 1/4 inch proximal to the cut end of the shaft. Through the same incision the deep transverse metatarsal capitellar ligaments are severed both medially and laterally to facilitate telescoping of the distal fragment into the proximal one. If the proximal end of the distal fragment cannot be easily fitted into the base because of the width of the shaft, the shaft can then be tapered by using a rongeur and carefully biting off small fragments of the shaft until it will telescope into the proximal fragment. A number 30 stainless steel wire is passed through one cortex of the base and then through the shaft and then distally through the other cortex. The distal shaft is grasped

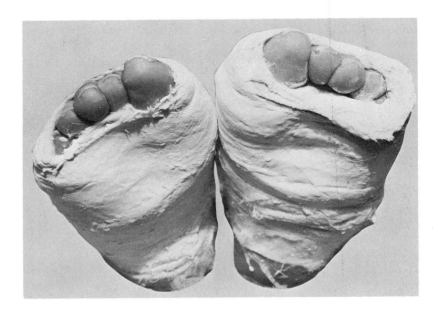

Fig. 14-14. Casts applied following metatarsal shortening. Note flexion of the toes plantarly and molding of casts on the plantar surface.

with a large Kelly clamp and pushed into the proximal one and the wire is tightened and tied. The ends of the wire are then folded flat against the medial or the lateral surface of the metatarsal base.

In the past if the keratosis had been exposed to a great deal of tissue destroying therapy, it was excised at the same time. However, it has been found that this no longer was necessary and, therefore, the plantar keratosis is no longer excised. Following closure of the softo tissues a plaster cast is applied from the tips of the toes to the midleg. The cast should be molded over the toes so as to place the metatarsophalangeal joint in plantar flexion. This maneuver is carried out in order to prevent the development of any contracture of the dorsal capsular structures of the metatarsophalangeal joint (Fig. 14-14). Furthermore, in order to displace the osteotomized metatarsal head slightly dorsally, the plantar surface of the cast is molded proximal to the plantar keratosis.

Postoperative Care. On the fifth postoperative day a walking heel is applied and the patient is permitted to ambulate with or without crutches. Four weeks postoperatively the cast is removed and irrespective of the absence of firm union radiographically of the osteotomized metatarsal, weight bearing is permitted.

Following removal of the cast and as soon as the swelling of the foot has subsided, the patient is fitted with a metatarsal comma-shaped pad which he or she is encouraged to wear for a period of at least three months. This routine is standard in our treatment of plantar keratosis located under the second, third, and fourth metatarsal heads. I have not found it necessary to shorten the fifth metatarsal head for symptomatic plantar keratosis. With a properly-fitted comma-shaped metatarsal pad, which can be fitted even into high-heeled shoes, the pressure on the plantar keratosis almost invariably can be relieved and the foot become asymptomatic. Furthermore, most lesions under the fifth metatarsal head develop from improper weight bearing and an attempt by the patient to prevent weight bearing on the second or third heads where another plantar keratosis usually exists. Therefore, by correcting the initial lesion

on the mid-portion of the foot, the patient then resumes normal weight bearing and this, in addition, helps to relieve pressure under the fifth metatarsal head, leading to irradication of the plantar keratosis.

When the lesion is under the first metatarsal head, sesamoidectomy has been valueless in my hands. If the keratosis is located under the first metatarsal head, a careful examination of the foot should be carried out from the standpoint of whether or not the patient's foot in a standing position demonstrates either a pronation, a mild cavus deformity, or a normal conformation. If the patient has a pronated foot, in addition to shortening of the first metatarsal, the distal fragment should be flexed. On the other hand, if the patient's foot presents a mild cavus deformity, the distal fragment should be extended. If the foot presents a normal appearance of the longitudinal arch, then only shortening of the metatarsal shaft should be carried out.

Results of Operative Treatment. In the series of patients I reviewed and reported in the Journal of Bone and Joint Surgery in January, 1966, the longest follow-up was twelve years and the shortest six months. In 51 of these patients the shortest follow-up was six years. In 86.1 per cent of this series of patients the results were excellent. In the other 13 per cent only 3.9 per cent can be considered absolute failures in that the lesion recurred under the same metatarsal head. Among the remaining 10 per cent, many of the patients were pleased with the end-result in spite of the development of a plantar keratosis or a callus under an adjacent metatarsal head, since this recurrence was not the major disabling factor which the original lesion had been. In some instances when a symptomatic disabling keratosis did develop under an adjacent metatarsal head, the patients of their own volition requested that the same procedure be performed to irradicate the subsequent lesion rather than first undergo the various forms of conservative therapy. There is no question that conservative therapy is definitely indicated and will relieve a large number of patients who are disabled by this lesion. On the other hand, for those few individuals in whom all conservative therapy has failed, shortening of the metatarsal shaft should be considered.

SUPERNUMERARY FIRST AND FIFTH TOES

Supernumerary digits are rare. They almost invariably involve either the hallux or the fifth toe. Involvement of the fifth toe is much more frequent than the first. The deformity results primarily in the duplication of the phalanges. The head of the involved metatarsal may, on occasion, be slightly larger than normal. In one case only I found reproduction of a separate fifth metatarsal head and a portion of the fifth metatarsal shaft. Furthermore, the accessory digit, when found on the great toe, is almost invariably located on the medial aspect, whereas on the fifth toe it is located on the lateral aspect. Usually the supernumerary toe is syndactylized to the normal one, but on occasion the digits may be entirely separate and again the tendency for such an occurrence is more frequent on the fifth toe.

The treatment consists of total amputation of all of the supernumerary parts after roentgenograms have been procured to determine the amount of osseous reproduction present.

INGROWN TOENAIL — ONYCHOCRYPTOSIS

This affliction of the toenails almost invariably involves the great toe. Numerous reasons have been given as to the cause of ingrown toenails. Of these, two seem to be the more acceptable ones: improper pedicure with abnormal convexity of the toenail, and improperly-fitted shoes. The nail should be trimmed or cut in a straight line across the edge with the corners squared. Cutting down into the edges of the nail predisposes to local improper growth of the nail as well as local irritation which finally leads to the development of a localized infection. Usually the patient does not appear at the office until such time as there is a well-developed infectious process along either one or both nail edges with purulent discharge and chronic edematous granulation tisssue.

When the patient is initially seen presenting such an infection, the treatment is conservative, consisting of hot packs every three hours, application of a topical antiseptic and the use of clean sterile dressings between soaks. If the granulation tissue is exuberant, silver nitrate should be applied by the physician every other day until the infection has subsided. In addition, if the patient is cooperative, an attempt should be made to cut the corner of the nail which has grown deeply into the side and temporarily remove the local irritative factor. After the infection has subsided and has remained quiescent for two or three weeks, the patient should undergo partial ony-chectomy unilaterally or bilaterally as may be indicated. Total onychectomy for an infected toenail is seldom indicated. To achieve a successful end-result following surgery, it is necessary to remove not only a fair portion of the nail, but also the entire underlying matrix which is exposed following sectioning of the nail.

The operative procedure consists of beginning a skin incision 0.5 cm. proximal to the lunular edge of the nail and extending distally through the nail through the anterior pulp of the toe to the plantar surface. The operative procedure is carried out under local infiltration of 1 per cent Xylocaine anesthesia injected at the base of the great toe providing the patient has no allergic predisposition to any of the local anesthetics. Ten cc. of this agent is a sufficient amount to encircle the base of the toe. A rubber band, applied to the digital base, is used as a tourniquet.

The skin and subcutaneous fat should be reflected to expose the ingrown portion of the nail and the matrix (Fig. 14-15A). The nail and matrix, as well as the soft parts, are excised (Fig. 14-15B) completely in a block to expose the underlying edge of the phalanx, particularly at the base. It is important to make certain that all of the matrix under the proximal end of the nail and proximal to the nail edge is removed. I prefer to use a small curette to remove all of the soft tissues down to the phalanx, particularly in the proximal corner (Fig. 14-15C). A small amount of 5 per cent penicillin ointment is inserted in the defect and the skin flap is closed both proximally and distally with one or two dermalon sutures (Fig. 14-15D).

The dressing should be snugly applied to help produce some modicum of hemostasis since bleeding tends to be rather profuse. The tourniquet is released following the application of the telfa pressure dressing. The dressing is changed on the fourth day to a less voluminous one and the sutures are usually removed on the seventh post-operative day. Ambulation is permitted within twenty-four hours.

If a total onychectomy should be necessary for any reason for which the surgeon believes such a procedure is warranted, resection of the distal one-fourth of the distal phalanx will also be necessary to permit closure of the defect. A Syme type amputation repair is carried out.

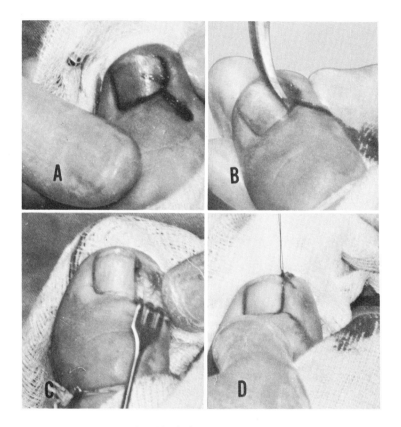

Fig. 14-15. Ingrown Toenail Operative Technique.

   A. Oblique incision at lunula of nail.

   B. Medial one-fourth of nail being excised to include the matrix.

   C. Nail and matrix removed and underlying phalanx exposed.

   D. Closure of wound.

BIBLIOGRAPHY

Du Vries, H. L.: A New Approach to the Treatment of the Verruca Plantaris (Plantar Wart). J.A.M.A., *152*:1202-1203, 1953.

Freiberg, A. H.: Infraction of the Second Metatarsal Bone—A Typical Injury. Surg. Gyn. Obstet. *19*:191-193, 1914.

Giannestras, Nicholas J.: Shortening of the Metatarsal Shaft and the Treatment of Plantar Keratosis and End Result Studies. Bone Jt. Surg. *40A*:61-71 (Jan.) 1958.
Shortening of the Metatarsal Head for Correction of Plantar Keratosis. Clin. Ortho. *4*:225-231, 1954.
Plantar Keratosis, Treatment by Metatarsal Shortening, Operative Technique and End-Result Study. Bone Jt. Surg. *48A*:72-76 (Jan.) 1966.

Hibbs, R. A.: An Operation for "Claw-foot". J.A.M.A., *75*:1583-1585, 1919.

Hadgert, G. E.: The Conservative and Surgical Treatment of Plantar Warts. Surg. Clin. North America, *14*:1211-1218, 1934.

Jones, A. R.: Discussion on the Treatment of Pes Cavus. Proc. Roy. Soc. Med. (Sec. of Orthopaedics) *20*:1118-1132, 1927.

Kelikian, H., Clayton, L., and Loseff, H.: Surgical Syndactilia of the Toes. Clin. Ortho. *19*:208-231, 1961.

Lantsounis, L. A.: Congenital Subluxation of the Fifth Toe and Its Correction by a Periosteo-Capsulo-Plasty and Tendon Transplantation. Bone Jt. Surg. *22*:147-150, 1940.

McElvenny, Robert T.: Personal Communication.

McKeever, D. C.: Arthrodesis of the First Metatarsophalangeal Joint for Hallux Valgus, Hallux Rigidus, and Metatarsus Primus Varus. J. Bone Jt. Surg. *34A*:129, 1952.

Morton, D. J.: *The Human Foot,* New York, Columbia University Press, 1935.

Pipkin, J. L., Layman, C. F., and Resmann, A.: The Treatment of Plantar Warts by Single Dose Method of Roentgen Ray. South. Med. J. *42*: 193-202, 1949.

=15=

Surgical Treatment of the Rheumatoid Foot

MACK L. CLAYTON, M.D.

RHEUMATOID arthritis is a chronic inflammatory disease of unknown etiology and pathogenesis. It is systemic in nature and characterized by the typical manner in which it involves the joints. There is not complete agreement as to which conditions should be included or excluded from the present concept of rheumatoid arthritis. Therefore, any definition must be regarded as provisional until more complete knowledge is obtained of the etiology and pathogenesis of the disease.

The term collagen disease (connective tissue disease) has come to be applied chiefly to rheumatoid arthritis, rheumatic fever, disseminated lupus erythematosus, periarteritis nodosa, dermatomyositis, and scleroderma. Pathologically the group reveals widespread involvement of connective tissue throughout the body. A relationship among these diseases had been postulated but as yet remains unproven. There is considerable overlap of these conditions, particularly between rheumatoid arthritis and disseminated lupus erythematosus. However, from the standpoint of orthopaedic treatment, this is of no clinical significance.

All the patients discussed in this chapter have met the criteria for diagnosis of "classical rheumatoid arthritis" required by the "1958 Revision of Diagnostic Criteria for Rheumatoid Arthritis", compiled and published by the The American Rheumatism Association.

To establish the diagnosis of rheumatoid arthritis requires that seven of the following criteria be met. In criteria 1 through 5, the joint signs or symptoms must be present continuously for at least six weeks.

1. Morning stiffness.
2. Pain on motion or tenderness in at least one joint (observed by a physician).
3. Swelling (soft tissue thickening or fluid—not bony over-growth) in at least one joint (observed by a physician).
4. Swelling (observed by a physician) of at least one other joint (any interval free of joint symptoms between the two joint involvements may not be more than three months).
5. Symmetric joint swelling (observed by a physician) with simultaneous involvement of the same joint on both sides of the body (bilateral involvement of mid-

phalangeal, metacarpophalangeal or meta-tarsophalangeal joints is acceptable without absolute symmetry). Terminal phalangeal joint involvement will not satisfy this criterion.

6. Subcutaneous nodules (observed by a physician) over bony prominences, on extensor surfaces or in juxta-articular regions.

7. X-ray changes typical of rheumatoid arthritis (which must include at least bony decalcification localized to or greatest around the involved joints and not just degenerative changes). Degenerative changes do not exclude patients from any group classified as rheumatoid arthritis.

8. Demonstration of a positive agglutination test of the "rheumatoid factor" by any method that, in two laboratories, has been positive in not over 5 per cent of normal controls; or positive streptococcal agglutination test.

9. Poor mucin precipitate from synovial fluid (with shreds and cloudy solution).

10. Characteristic histologic changes in synovial membrane with three or more of the following: marked villous hypertrophy; proliferation of superficial synovial cells, often with palisading; marked infiltration of chronic inflammatory cells (lymphocytes or plasma cells predominating) with tendency to form "lymphoid nodules"; deposition of compact fibrin, either on surface or interstitially; foci of cell necrosis.

11. Characteristic histologic changes in nodules showing granulomatous foci with central zones of cell necrosis; surrounded by proliferated fixed cells, and peripheral fibrosis and chronic inflammatory cell infiltration, predominantly perivascular.

Rheumatoid arthritis is seen in patients of all ages up to eighty. Females are involved at a ratio of about 3 to 1. (Rheumatoid spondylitis is not included with "classical rheumatoid arthritis"). Males generally have a less severe form of rheumatoid arthritis with less involvement of the joints than females and the average involvement is not as severe. There appears to be a familial tendency to the disease, but there is not enough evidence to establish any hereditary factor as responsible for it. Onset is usually gradual although it may be abrupt. Joint involvement at onset is evenly divided between large and small joints in about 40 per cent of the cases. In 16 per cent of the cases, the process begins in the feet and in 4 per cent in the ankle. About the same percentage experience the condition initially in the hands as in the feet. This observation tends to disprove the statement that in a majority of patients, rheumatoid arthritis is first apparent in the hands, or in the feet and hands. Although 30 per cent of the cases begin with unilateral involvement, eventually 95 per cent become bilateral. One large series showed that the metatarsophalangeal joints were involved in 46 per cent of the cases; tarsals in 46 per cent; toes in 23 per cent; ankles in 68 per cent; knees in 78 per cent; and metacarpophalangeal joints in 71 per cent.

Drs. Charles J. Smyth and Mack L. Clayton, working in conjunction at the Arthritis Clinic at the University of Colorado during the last twelve years, feel that there are two definite clinical subtypes of chronic rheumatoid arthritis. The first is the group in which the joints tend to stiffen with gradual loss of motion, even progressing to ankylosis. The predominant aspect is joint involvement (stiff type). The second type is the group in which soft tissue and bursal involvement predominate and cause secondary joint deformity. In this group joint destruction is slow and does not always lead to ankylosis. In fact, there may be gradual destruction of the joint with developing instability (loose type). This loose type predominates in patients with hand and foot involvement. Whether or not steroid treatment may play a causative role in the development of this feature is still open to question.

However, Smyth and Clayton are not certain if a definitive subclassification can be established along these lines since the microscopic pathologic changes are the same in both groups and, of course, many cases overlap. Nevertheless, quite definite cases are seen representing each extreme. These two "subtypes" may account for the marked difference in the results obtained with reconstructive surgical procedures in rheumatoid arthritis. In the first type, ankylosis is prone to occur and arthrodeses are easy to obtain, but mobility may be hard to regain after arthroplasty. In the latter type, arthrodesis may be more difficult to obtain than in an ordinary case.

Many articles in the literature, even in the last few years, make the statement, "Surgery should not be performed until the arthritis is 'burned-out' or 'quiescent'". The various authors have found it difficult to define the term "burned-out" or to determine if a patient's disease is "quiescent".

There are three main clinical forms of rheumatoid arthritis, based on a cyclic progression of the disease. The first group is the one with a single cycle lasting over a period of a number of months and then subsiding with no further attacks of arthritis. Such cases would not fall into a group considered for surgery. The second group is a polycyclic one with periods of activity followed by remission, and then more activity and remission, and a gradual heightening of the activity. The third group has slow, but steadily progressive, active involvement.

The large majority of chronic cases that are seen for surgical treatment will continue to smoulder on indefinitely, producing progressive deformity and disability. Experience has borne out the conclusion that it is not advisable to wait for the disease to "burn-out" before surgery is performed. Surgery is performed at any time indicated, provided the patient is not in an extremely acute exacerbation and there is no general medical contraindication. The decision to operate is not based on the outcome of a sedimentation rate test. There is no evidence that surgery in any way alters the course of the underlying disease. In a patient with a polycyclic type disease, surgery may occasionally appear to have temporarily caused a general change in either direction. However, no permanent alteration in the course of the disease has been noted in long-term evaluations.

This is not entirely a new concept, since Smith-Petersen, Aufranc, and Larson have recommended surgery even when the disease is still active.

HISTORICAL REVIEW

Hoffman in 1911 reported on "An Operation for Severe Grades of Contracted or Clawed Toes". Several of his cases were "infectious arthritis" (now called rheumatoid arthritis). His description of a suitable case was, "The toes are strongly dorsiflexed at the metatarsophalangeal joints and plantar flexed at their interphalangeal ones and are retained in this position by shortening through adaptation of tendons, ligaments, and other soft structures and by bone changes due to long-continued new relationship of articular surfaces." This is still an excellent description of the rheumatoid foot. His operation consisted of excision of the heads and if necessary, parts of the necks of the metatarsal bones of all of the affected toes through a transverse curved plantar incision just behind the web of the toes. In the closing discussion, Hoffman stated, "The operation is simply to get rid of the metatarsal heads, because they make the patient's life miserable. Every step he takes hurts him so, he is afraid to get up from his chair. Mild grades of contracted toes should not be operated upon in this way." This is an excellent paper with many valid principles. It represents the basic paper in the literature on surgery of the rheumatoid forefoot.

T. C. Thompson in 1937 outlined surgical procedures useful in correcting deformities of the arthritic foot, such as the Keller procedure (exostectomy and proximal hemiphalangectomy of the great toe to correct hallux valgus and/or hallux rigidus); dorsal dislocation of the toe at metatarsophalangeal joint corrected by excision of the metatarsal head; hammer toe with painful corn corrected by excision of the corn and fusion of the interphalangeal joint; painful hammer toe with pressure on toenail corrected by terminal Syme amputation removing the toenail and the distal phalanx; clawtoe projecting dorsally corrected by excision of the proximal phalanx.

Aufranc and Larson presented a series of chronic rheumatoid arthritic feet at the Boston Orthopedic Club in 1949. In such instances, surgery has been performed with varying degrees of metatarsophalangeal joint resections through multiple dorsal incisions.

J. Albert Key in 1950 reported on "Surgical Revision of the Arthritic Feet" and mentioned a number of surgical procedures with a certain amount of excellent philosophy regarding the care of the arthritic foot. "I find it possible to benefit a greater number of patients to a greater degree by a few relatively simple operations on the feet than by any of the elaborate procedures on the larger joints which occupy so much of the time and thought of the modern orthopaedic surgeon."

He recommended a Keller operation for bunions and hallux valgus and occasionally used a proximal osteotomy of the first metatarsal to narrow the metatarsus primus varus. Hammer toe was corrected by dorsal capsulotomy of the metatarsophalangeal joint, excision of the corn transversely and excision of the distal half of the proximal phalanx. For marked depression of the metatarsal heads, either the base of the phalanx, the metatarsal head, or both, were excised. "The surgery tends to be destructive or at least ablative and should be moderately radical. Deformities are corrected by extensive removal of bone and movement is restored to joints by wide excision rather than by meticulous arthroplasties. . . . Many patients with deformed and painful arthritic feet can be greatly benefitted by multiple relatively minor surgical procedures."

Larmon in 1951 discussed "Surgical Treatment of Deformities of Rheumatoid Arthritis of the Forefoot and Toes". He felt that the deformity was accounted for by contracture of the long and short extensor tendons with a loss of function of the lumbricals and interossei. For the severe, typical deformity he recommended a Keller procedure on the great toe, excision of the entire proximal phalanges of the small toes, and exostectomy of the individual metatarsal heads rather than complete excision of the heads. The procedure was performed through three dorsal incisions. He recommended amputating the small toe if necessary.

Campbell's *Operative Orthopedics* has a small section on rheumatoid arthritis of the feet. "The relief of foot discomfort affords a degree of overall improvement of function all out of proportion to the extent of the surgical procedures." Multiple procedures are recommended to be used as indicated, often involving ten separate, but relatively minor procedures on the feet.

In 1956 Leavitt presented two cases. In one case he removed the phalanges from the four lateral clawtoes and performed a bevel ostectomy of the plantar aspect of the metatarsal heads and a Keller procedure. He recommended never shortening the first metatarsal heads. Other procedures recommended were arthrodesis of painful tarsal joints or occasionally of other joints; excision of bunionettes, adventitious bursae, and hyperplastic synovial tissue.

Kuhns and Potter in 1960 presented a well-organized description on both the prevention and conservative treatment and the operative treatment of deformity of the forefoot with operative procedures outlined to correct hallux valgus, hammer toe and dislocation of metatarsal heads.

In 1959 Fowler reported "A Method of Forefoot Reconstruction" in which metatarsal heads and bases of phalanges were removed through a dorsal incision which divided skin, veins, and extensor tendons. Twelve of the patients had rheumatoid arthritis and he reported satisfactory results in these instances.

In 1960 Flint and Sweetnam reported a procedure for amputation of all toes through the metatarsophalangeal joints. In 12 patients with rheumatoid arthritis, they reported 6 excellent, 4 good, and 2 fair results. (Other authors have reported that this is often unsatisfactory since the metatarsal heads still remain prominent in the sole of the foot.)

Aufranc in 1961, in an instructional course, detailed an operation he had used for a number of years. This consists of excision of the four smaller metatarsophalangeal joints through a S-shaped dorsal incision, excising the metatarsal heads and bases of the phalanges of toes, two, three, and four, and metatarsal head only of five. Through a separate longitudinal dorsal incision, a Keller procedure was performed and excision of the first metatarsal head if necessary. The fifth phalanx was not resected in an attempt to prevent lateral deviation of the toes postoperatively.

Potter in an exhibit on "Rheumatoid Arthritis of the Foot" in 1961, presented the following findings. A forefoot spread due to involvement of the intermetatarsal ligaments was noted in 40 per cent of the cases. Hallux valgus was noted in 28 per cent of the cases. In some simple cases a simple exostectomy was recommended; in cases with a marked metatarsus primus varus, bunionectomy and a distal osteotomy of the first metatarsal was recommended. In some severe cases fusion of the metatarsophalangeal joint was preferred. Flexion deformities of the toes were present in 50 per cent of the cases. Severe cases of depressed metatarsal heads with cock-up toes were treated by the Hoffman procedure of excising the metatarsal heads through a plantar approach. Also illustrated were examples of bursitis, tenosynovitis, rheumatoid nodules, and a Morton's neuroma due to rheumatoid involvement.

The author has written several well-documented papers in the conservative and surgical therapy of the rheumatoid foot. Schwartzmann as well as Marmor have recently reported on correction of rheumatoid forefoot deformity by utilizing excisional surgery in the forefoot and other procedures as indicated.

PROGRESSION OF FOOT DEFORMITY

In the early active stages of rheumatoid arthritis manifestation the forefoot is usually "puffy" and tender. There may be mild heat and redness. Increased sweatiness is common. Manual lateral compression of the metatarsal heads is a useful test. Pain between the metatarsal heads indicates involvement of periarticular non weight-bearing structures which are involved in rheumatoid arthritis, but are not usually involved in a mechanical type of metatarsophalangeal abnormality. The exception to this rule, of course, would be a plantar neuroma with its characteristic findings. Due to synovitis, the toes tend to assume a cocked-up position with active and pas-

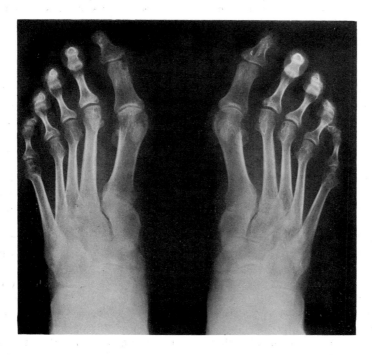

Fig. 15-1. Early rheumatoid arthritic changes with soft tissue swelling. Note erosion of bone at the metatarsophalangeal joints, particularly of the metatarsal heads. Also note the interphalangeal joint of the great toes. Joint spaces are quite well preserved at this stage.

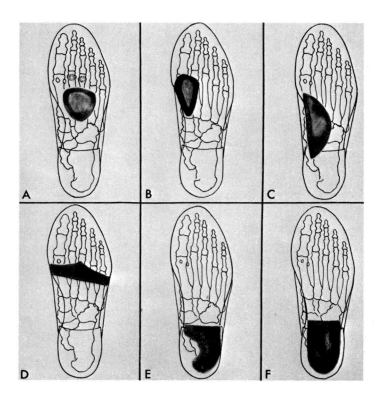

Fig. 15-2. Types of arch supports which have been helpful. The object of their use is relief of pain through mechanical realignment and pressure relief. These pads do not differ too much from those used for other basic orthopaedic problems. The rheumatoid arthritic will require more adjustment and "custom fitting" of the supports.

sive limitation of plantar flexion at the metatarsophalangeal joints. In the early stages roentgenograms (Fig. 15-1) reveal only osteoporosis with soft tissue swelling, but later, soon show surface erosions of the metartasal heads in most cases.

In the early stages, proper shoeing and supports with a graduated exercise regimen is helpful; many of the deformities (Fig. 15-2) can be prevented. Considerable rest and often resting plaster shells are indicated in early acute exacerbations.

Despite conservative measures, many cases progress to severe painful disabling deformities in the forefoot. Deformity of the knees often accentuates foot deformity. Hallux valgus and bunions with forefoot spread and depressed metatarsal heads and varying degrees of cock-up of the toes is the most common combination of deformities. Some toes remain slightly flexible, while others are rigid with dorsal subluxation or complete dislocation of the proximal

phalanges on the metatarsal heads. This increases the height of the forefoot and makes shoeing difficult (Fig. 15-3C). Painful corns develop over the dorsum of the middle joints (Fig. 15-3A, C and D) and calluses (Fig. 15-3B, C) develop beneath the depressed prominent metatarsal heads on the sole of the foot.

With walking, pain arises from abnormal pressure beneath the metatarsal heads on the sole or against the shoe on the dorsum of the toes. Attempts to support the metatarsal area often produce increased pressure on the dorsum of the toes due to the inflexibility. There is contracture of the soft tissues, including muscles, tendons, fascia and skin; this often leads to fibrous ankylosis. However, spontaneous bony ankylosis of the metatarsophalangeal joints is rare (two joints of over 500 metatarsophalangeal articulations). When active synovitis continues, the intrinsic muscles are overpulled by the long extensors and flexors and the

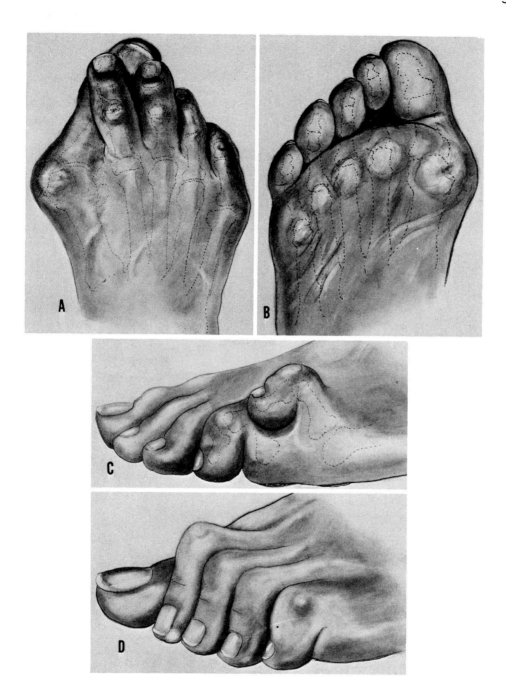

Fig. 15-3.   A.   Note hallux valgus with overlying second toe and dislocation of the second metatarsophalangeal joint.

   B.   Because of hammer toe deformity and subluxation or dislocation of the metatarsophalangeal joints, note abnormal amount of pressure exerted by the metatarsal heads on the plantar
surface of the skin resulting in painful calluses and/or plantar keratoses.

   C.   Occasionally only the fifth digit may be involved.

   D.   Involvement of the lateral four digits at the interphalangeal joints with resultant plantar
keratoses at the tips of the toes.

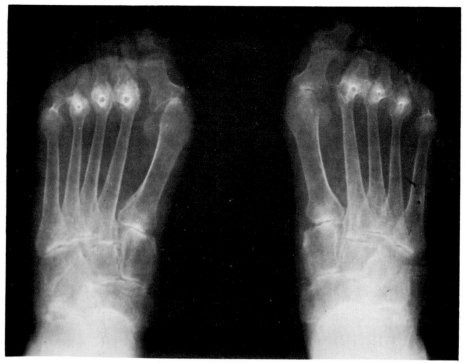

Fig. 15-4.   Note extensive erosion of first metatarsal head. Observe "gun barrel" sign due to marked dorsal dislocation of proximal phalanx on metatarsal head.

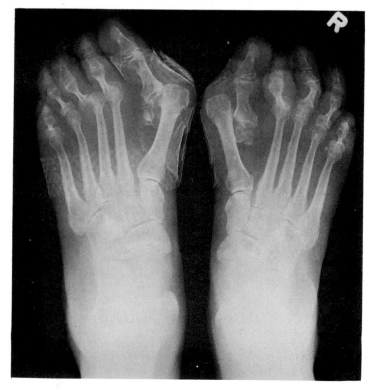

Fig. 15-5.   Preoperative deformity of forefoot with dislocation of metatarsophalangeal joint of great toe and several smaller toes.

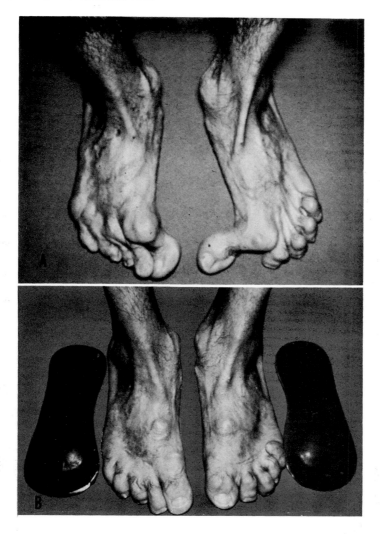

Fig. 15-6. Hallux varus plus other unusual deformities seen in rheumatoid arthritis. Following bilateral forefoot resection, note the simple metatarsal pads which are the type most commonly used.

cock-up deformity of the toes is similar to that often seen with paralysis of the intrinsics of the foot. This defect does not resemble the so-called intrinsic plus deformity commonly seen in rheumatoid arthritis of the hand.

Of course there are many variations of pathology in the involved tissues which would give rise to other deformities, but the majority have the basic pattern of hallux valgus, bunion, and cock-up toes with depressed metatarsal heads. X-rays help reveal the deformities as noted clinically more erosion of the metatarsal heads or bases of the phalanges than that suspected on clinical evaluation. Joint spaces are narrowed; subluxation to actual dislocation of the metatarsophalangeal joints is noted and this can be seen on anteroposterior films by overlap of the proximal phalanx over the metatarsal head. In the marked dorsal dislocation, when the phalanx is actually located at almost 90 degrees to the metatarsal (Fig. 15-4), a "gun barrel" sign can be noted. This is simply an axial view of the proximal phalanx in which the bony cortex is outlined as if it were a gun barrel. Varying degrees of osteoporosis are present in cases of this type.

Two cases in this group had complete

spontaneous dislocation at the first metatarsophalangeal joints (Fig. 15-5) and the
writers have seen this only with rheumatoid arthritis. The deformity represents
spontaneous rupture of the dorsal portion
of the capsule and the adductor hallucis
tendon, caused by rheumatoid synovial involvement and aided by friction against the
underlying irregular first metatarsal head.
The pull of the unopposed muscles dislo-
cates the proximal phalanx in a fibular
direction. This is illustrated by the sesamoids following the base of the phalanx on
the x-ray. This dislocation greatly increases
the metatarsus varus primus with pressure
on the bunion of the first metatarsal head
and gives rise to large painful bursae which
tend to drain intermittently.

Two unusual feet with a spontaneous hallux varus (Fig. 15-6 A and B), which is an
unusual deformity in untreated feet, are
also presented. The varus deformity was
due to a rupture of the adductor hallucis by
rheumatoid synovitis which was identified
at surgery. Similar tendon ruptures as a
cause of certain hand deformities are well
known.

Hindfoot deformity is usually a progressive valgus (loose type) with changes first
in the subtalar joint and later through the
midtarsals. In other cases the deformity is
minimal but there is limited motion with
pain in the hindfoot due to arthritic joint
changes (stiff type).

Bursitis (or tenosynovitis) may develop
around the Achilles tendon insertion area
or the plantar fascia insertion. Tenosynovitis of the various tendon sheaths may occur. The most commonly involved are those
of peroneal or of extensor tendon groups
beneath the dorsal retinaculum at the ankle
with the same pathologic condition as that
so commonly encountered in the hand and
wrist.

INDICATIONS FOR SURGERY

We feel that the conservative measures
of proper shoeing with simple ordinary
orthopaedic supports should be used in
early cases with a proper exercise regimen

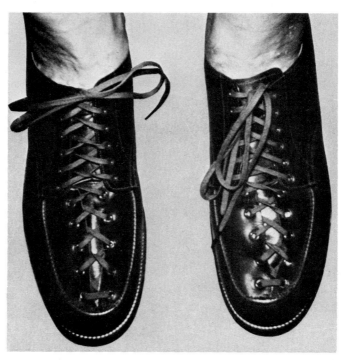

Fig. 15-7. Basic type of shoe used for everyday wear. By adding eyelets to the toes, it can
be used for postoperative care also.

to keep the toes flexible. Simple, low to medium heel, basic oxford shoes with closed toes and heels are recommended (Fig. 15-7); to these are added metatarsal pads, long arch pads, or heel wedges when indicated. (Specially constructed shoes are occasionally indicated.) Arch supports are usually of firm rubber and leather covered. Steel, alone, is usually too rigid for the rheumatoid foot. The supports must be custom made for each patient, and frequently require secondary alterations for pressure relief.

The same care must be used in postoperative supports, which are necessary in practically all cases. These are simply the same basic orthopaedic supports used for mechanical foot deformity of any other cause.

A brace may only occasionally be necessary for the valgus deformity of the hindfoot. However, this will give only temporary relief at best, and if the arch supports do not suffice, surgical stabilization may be

necessary. A simple, outside iron, short leg-brace with an inner "T" strap has been used where the ankle joint is not particularly painful. If the ankle is painful, a double upright brace with limited ankle motion may be used.

Surgical procedure is indicated when there is increasing deformity of the foot with painful weight bearing in spite of conservative measures. In such advanced cases, relief of the abnormal weight-bearing pressure can be obtained by surgery. Such joints are extensively damaged and the feet are already "weak". The toes have lost their usual function. Not only do these patients lack the "takeoff" to their gait, they even avoid pressure on the forefoot. Surgery on the forefoot does not further weaken the damaged arthritic foot or further impair the patient's gait; in fact, the gait is improved. With the improved gait there is often a decrease in pain from involved knees and hips.

ANESTHESIA

Surgery to correct arthritic defects in the feet is usually performed under general anesthesia, although regional anesthesia has been used occasionally with good success. The majority of the patients have been on steroid medication at the time of surgery or had received steroids in the past. Supplementary steroid medication should be given at the time of general anesthesia to prevent "adrenal insufficiency" from stress. All patients receiving supplementary steroid medication at the time of surgery receive varying amounts of preoperative and postoperative steroids. The dosage prescribed

depends upon the judgment of the internist supervising the patient's medical regimen. No definite difference has been found in the various regimens used in the different cases. No difficulty in healing of the soft tissues was attributed to the steroids either in the immediate operative phase or postoperatively as long as supplementary steroids were given. Wound healing was not affected. The patient should be carefully watched and additional medication should be administered when indicated to prevent "adrenal insufficiency". Antibiotics have not been used routinely.

FOREFOOT SURGERY

The marked contracture of soft tissues accompanying these deformities demands adequate bony resection for correction and pain relief. The basic procedure has been metatarsophalangeal joint resections of varying degrees, excising an adequate amount of bone for correction of the deformity. In the more markedly involved cases, the tendency has been to resect all the metatarsal heads and a portion of the necks. The proximal half of each of the proximal phalanges

is also removed as indicated. The distal joints of the toes have been manipulated straight to correct cock-up deformities, but fusion of the distal joints of the small toes has not been performed.

As many as ten toes have been corrected at one operative procedure in a number of the patients. Sometimes a metatarsal head that does not have a callus must be resected because it would otherwise remain too prominent after removal of the offending

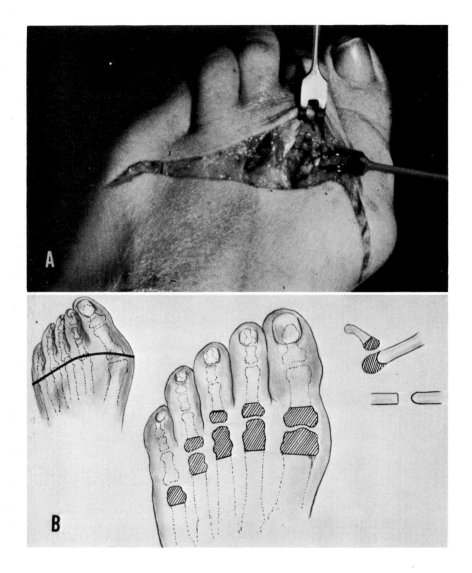

Fig 15-8.   A.   Transverse incision beginning at dorsal aspect of fifth metatarsophalangeal joint and extending to medial aspect of first metatarsal head.

B.   Note average amount of bone which is removed and the contouring of the ends of the metatarsals.

adjacent head. The surgical procedure is tailored to fit the individual case. The recent tendency, however, has been to operate on more toes at one time. The first cases were done through multiple longitudinal dorsal incisions (Fig. 15-8 A and B), but now it is considered preferrable to operate on all toes through one transverse dorsal incision at the base of the toes because the major blood and nerve supply to the toes enters through the plantar aspect. Exposure is also easier than through multiple dorsal incisions.

Two surgical teams working simultaneously can help to shorten the anesthesia and operative time and diminish the stress placed on the patients. An Esmarch bandage may be used as a tourniquet around the ankle or a mid-thigh tourniquet can be applied. A transverse dorsal incision is made at the base of the toes curving slightly proximally over the first and fifth metatarsal heads. The small toes are manipulated straight. In the usual case, without the marked rigid deformity, the extensor tendons are retracted and the base of each proximal phalanx is exposed. The bases of the proximal phalanges are excised except for the fifth toe and subsequently the metatarsal heads are easily delivered and adequately resected. *The plantar aspect of each of the lateral four metatarsals is beveled to give a smooth weight-bearing surface.* The second toe is operated first and then one moves laterally to the third, fourth, and fifth, thus leaving the great toe last. The fifth toe is rarely dislocated and in most cases only the fifth metatarsal head is excised. This also helps in preventing later fibular drift of the toes. After the smaller toes are corrected, the entire incision can be drawn slightly medially and exposure of the first metatarsal head and proximal phalanx is simplified. The proximal one-third to one-half of the proximal phalanx

of the great toe is resected and usually the first metatarsal head is resected to a varying degree. The dorsal surface should also be beveled to prevent later pressure. Through the single incision the exact contour of the distal metatarsals can be determined and adjusted as desired. Small double-action bone cutting forceps and rongeurs simplify the procedure. We recommend that the best alignment is for the first and second metatarsal stumps to be approximately the same length, with gradual tapering evenly across the third, fourth, and to the fifth. A small piece of oxycel gauze may be placed over the raw end of the first metatarsal or the excess capsule of the great toe, interposed and closed with a few chromic catgut sutures. At this stage all of the toes can be placed in the desired position; it is desirable to shift them slightly medially (Fig. 15-9) and only the subcutaneous tissues and the skin are closed. Intramedullary Kirschner wires may help give stability, particularly where deformity of the first and fifth is marked. These can be removed when sutures are removed.

In the markedly severe cases with quite

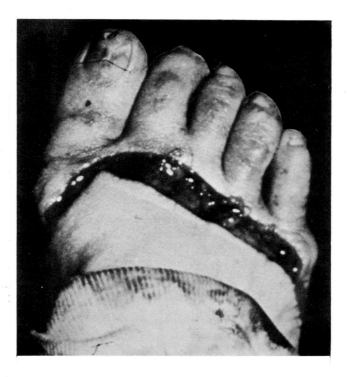

Fig. 15-9. Toes shifted into desired position before closure.

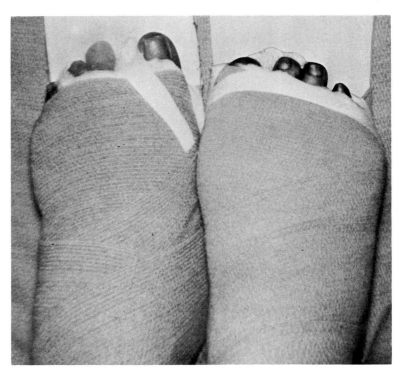

Fig. 15-10. Postoperative dressing. The toes are carefully bandaged with gauze between each toe and a large compression dressing applied to hold toes in desired position.

a rigid forefoot, the same dorsal transverse incision is preferable but all of the extensor tendons are also divided exactly in line with the incision. Excellent exposure is obtained by flexing the toes downward. In closing the incision it is not necessary to suture the tendons except for one small suture in the great toe extensor followed by closure of the skin and support of the toes. Loss of extension does not occur.

The postoperative dressing (Fig. 15-10) is most important and is applied to give a large compression dressing holding the toes *exactly* in the desired position. Care should be taken not to separate the first and second toes too much. Cardboard is incorporated into the dressing to protect the toes from the bedclothes. This dressing is left undisturbed until the sutures are removed at two weeks postoperatively.

Patients are permitted to take a few steps on approximately the fifth or sixth day. There has been no evidence of circulatory difficulty in the toes. The patients have usually been discharged from the hospital after one and two weeks. Rarely has there been a persistent swelling of the forefoot

six to eight weeks following surgery. After removal of the sutures, the forefoot is strapped and the patients fitted into a split oxford shoe (Fig. 15-7), then gradually moved into a simple, medium heel, oxford shoe. Patients who do not require crutches for any other disability do not require crutches after the foot surgery. A metatarsal pad, approximately 3/16 of an inch, and often a 3/16-inch metatarsal bar are recommended for all patients postoperatively because of the altered configuration of the distal metatarsals. As a rule no attempt is made to resect corns, calluses or thickened bursae beneath the metatarsal heads at the time of surgery (Fig. 15-11A, B). With relief of abnormal pressure these corns, calluses and bursae disappear gradually (Fig. 15-11D, E, F, G).

"These feet do not stand surgery well" is a common statement, but it is contrary to our experience and to the experience of other investigators who have performed similar operations.

Isolated procedures are used in the forefoot with less severe deformity, utilizing the same basic principles of adequate bony re-

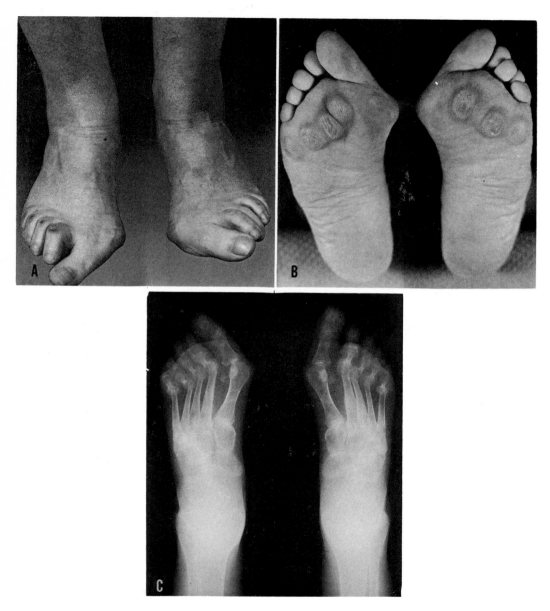

Fig. 15-11. A. and B. Note typical deformity of forefoot with marked callus formation.
  C. Preoperative x-ray.

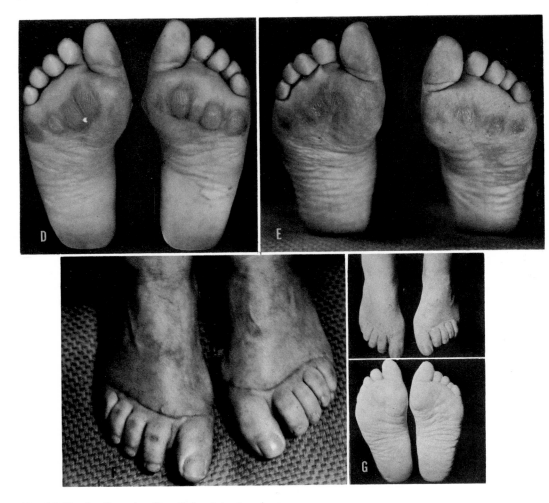

Fig. 15-11. Continued.   D.   Sole at twelve days.

    F.   Three months postoperative.

    E.   Three months postoperative.

    G.   Eighteen months postoperative.

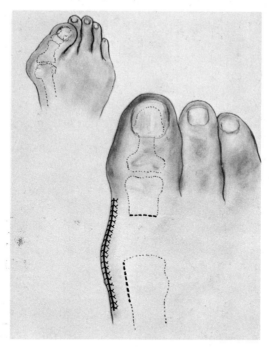

Fig. 15-12. Keller procedure for isolated hallux valgus and bunion. A Kirschner wire is not to be used to maintain the distance between the remaining proximal phalanx and the metatarsal since early active motion is desirable in this type of foot.

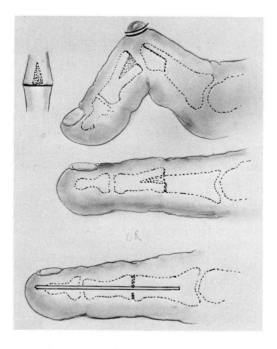

Fig. 15-13. Middle joint resection for hammer toe (whether or not bony ankylosis is obtained is unimportant). Bony resection is the important factor.

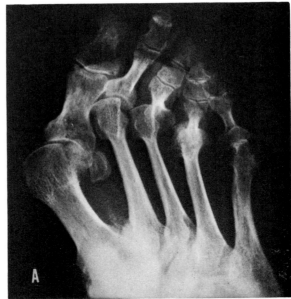

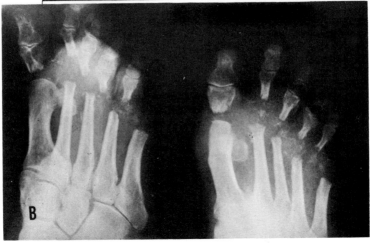

Fig. 15-14.   A.   Severe preoperative deformity. Note comparative shortness of first metatarsal.

B.   Immediate postoperative x-ray. Note contour of distal metatarsals.

section, *e.g.*: Keller procedure (Fig. 15-12) for hallux valgus and bunion; partial proximal phalangectomy or middle-joint resection, with or without arthrodesis, for individual hammer toe (Fig. 15-13); oblique resection of the fifth metatarsal head for a bunionette or intractable callus beneath the fifth metatarsal head. Again, the basic principle remains that of adequate bony resection.

If more than three metatarsal heads require surgery, it is preferable to perform the entire forefoot resection to give a new weight-bearing alignment across the entire metatarsophalangeal portion of the foot. This is determined by the relative alignment of the metatarsal ends. Further decompression is obtained by resecting the bases of the phalanges as necessary for proper realignment without unnecessarily shortening the metatarsals. If the patient has a short first metatarsal, resection of the first metatarsal may not be necessary (Fig. 15-14A and B). It is the final relative length that is important. There is a little more leeway in the exact length of the first metatarsal as the sesamoids are not removed unless they are adherent and immobile. Usually they retract slightly and give a fairly wide area to transmit weight to the first metatarsal head.

Other forefoot procedures in unusual cases have been arthrodesis of the great toe interphalangeal joint (for hyperextension deformity with painful callus beneath the distal condyles of the proximal phalanx but with a well aligned serviceable metatarsophalangeal joint).

Terminal Syme procedure is excellent for marked nail deformity and/or terminal joint deformity (Fig. 15-15).

In an early case of flexion deformity of an interphalangeal joint or of extension deformity of a metatarsophalangeal joint, simple subcutaneous tenotomy of the extensor tendon with manipulation of the toe may give pressure relief in combination with proper support.

While the patient is in the hospital and in bed recovering from the surgical procedure, treatment of other involved joints is carried out by using selected apparatus and regimens. Medical treatment as indicated is also carried out so that "no time is wasted". Often improvement can be obtained in other joints by conservative measures utilizing the necessary period of rest after surgery.

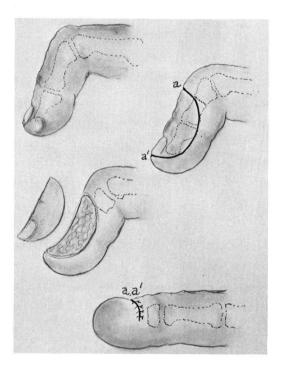

Fig. 15-15. Terminal Syme procedure for nail or terminal joint deformity. Note amount of middle phalanx which is resected in diagramatic sketch (a-a').

HINDFOOT SURGERY

Progressive valgus deformity often resembles a paralytic valgus with its insidious progression. Surgical stabilization is indicated when conservative measures fail to give relief.

If the valgus can be passively corrected and there are reasonably good midtarsal joints, then subtalar arthrodesis alone will suffice. Inlay bone blocks (on the principle of a Grice subtalar arthrodesis) or a Gallie posterior approach are satisfactory since the joint contours are maintained. Subtalar joint

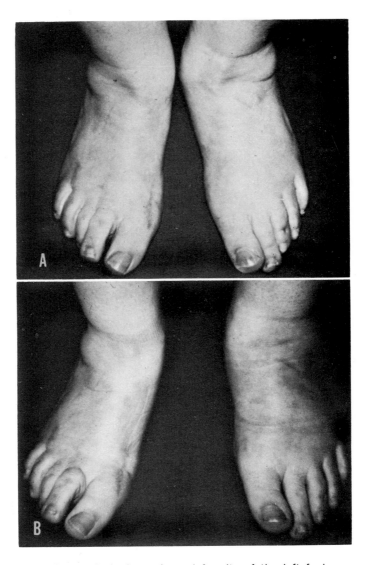

Fig. 15-16. A. Note the marked planovalgus deformity of the left foot.

 B. Following triple arthrodesis.

resection alone would tend to alter the configuration of the talonavicular and calcaneocuboid joints. More feet should have surgery at this relatively early stage as recommended by Larson. However, due to the bilateral nature of the disease there has been some hesitancy in performing hindfoot arthrodeses.

If the valgus deformity is irreducible and or the midtarsal joints are involved, then triple arthrodesis is indicated and it yields the usual satisfactory result (Fig. 15-16A and B). In a rheumatoid arthritic with pronounced deformity it may be difficult to realign the foot in the best position.

Arthrodesis is occasionally indicated in an isolated tarsal joint with slow progressive involvement and pain.

The ankle rarely needs a fusion. Proper shoe supports and the occasional use of a double upright brace usually will relieve ankle pain. Sometimes the patient may later be free of the braces.

In planning a series of reconstructive procedures on a lower extremity, it is preferable to operate on the forefoot first, if the hindfoot is mobile. If the hindfoot requires an arthrodesis, then the hips and knees should be corrected first. Next, the hindfoot is stabilized to bring the foot plantigrade and, finally, forefoot resection is performed. Approximately 10 forefoot procedures will be indicated to one hindfoot procedure. This accounts for the greater attention that has been given to the forefoot.

RESULTS

The object of surgery to correct foot deformities due to rheumatoid arthritis has been to relieve the pain from abnormal weight-bearing pressure and to obtain a weight-tolerant foot. No attempt has been made to retain strong toe function. Active toe motion has not been considered in the postoperative evaluation. In general, the functional and cosmetic results have been gratifying to both the patient and the surgeon. In the experience of orthopaedists who have worked with arthritic patients and have been able to follow them carefully, the consensus is that these patients have been satisfied with the results, while no patient regretted having undergone the operation. Usually such patients have been grateful for the relief of pain. Results of surgery in this chronic progressive generalized disease cannot be compared with that obtained in any other type of static condition, since the goal sought is the attainment of a limited gain in function.

In rating these cases, it seems advisable not to include a category of "excellent" in evaluating the results of this type of excisional surgery. Many times the difference between excellent and good results depends on the patient's overall condition. The criteria for a good result include absence of pain or only minimal pain with no more than mild calluses; ability to wear regular shoes with simple supports; and pain in the forefoot of such a mild degree that it does not interfere with gait. Results are considered fair in those patients who have moderate pain and/or moderate calluses in the forefoot. Such a patient may require special shoes. Only mild improvement has been obtained with the surgery. In any condition other than rheumatoid arthritis, this would be considered a poor result. (A failure is a result regarded as worse than the condition prior to surgery.)

In approximately 10 per cent reoperation is necessary. This is usually for minimal "tailoring" of the length of one of the metatarsals which was either too long initially, or in which a spike of bone has regrown. Rheumatoid arthritics are abnormally sensitive to pressure and there will be some recurrences in time, no matter what the type of surgery employed.

CONCLUSIONS

Surgery of the rheumatoid arthritic foot can give satisfactory results despite the fact that this is a progressive, crippling disease. *Adequate bony excision* at the metatarsophalangeal joint level (forefoot resection) is the basic principle in correction of a severe deformity in the rheumatoid arthritic in order to obtain a *weight-tolerant* foot. The operation is most easily performed through a single dorsal transverse incision. Forefoot resection, as described by the author, has been the most satisfactory procedure in rehabilitation of the lower extremity in patients with chronic rheumatoid arthritis.

The surgical procedures employed to correct foot deformities in rheumatoid arthritics do not differ from the basic orthopaedic procedures performed for similar defects due to other conditions. This is well exemplified in surgery of the hindfoot where the basic procedure is stabilization with a subtalar or triple arthrodesis when necessary.

BIBLIOGRAPHY

AUFRANC, O.: Reconstructive Surgery of the Lower Extremity in Rheumatoid Arthritis. Instructional Course, American Academy of Orthopedic Surgeons, Miami, January, 1961.

AUFRANC, O. AND LARSON, C. B.: Personal Communication

CLAYTON, M. L.: Surgery of the Forefoot in Rheumatoid Arthritis. Arth. and Rheum., 2:84-85, 1959.
Surgery of the Forefoot in Rheumatoid Arthritis. Clin. Orth., 16:136-140, 1960.
Surgery of the Lower Extremity in Rheumatoid Arthritis. J. Bone Jt. Surg., 45-A:1517-1536, 1963.

CLAYTON, M. L., LEIDHOLT, J. D., AND SMYTH, C. J.: Surgery of the Forefoot in Rheumatoid Arthritis. Motion Picture available through the American Academy of Orthopaedic Surgeons, 29 East Madison Street, Chicago, Illinois.

FLINT, M. AND SWEETNAM, R.: Amputation of All Toes. J. Bone Jt. Surg., 42-B:90-96, 1960.

FOWLER, A. W.: A Method of Forefoot Reconstruction. J. Bone Jt. Surg., 41-B:507-513, 1959.

HOFFMAN, P.: An Operation for Severe Grades of Contracted or Clawed Toes. Amer. J. Ortho. Surg., 9:441-449, 1911-12.

KEY, J. A.: Surgical Revision of Arthritic Feet. Amer. J. Surg., 79:667-672, 1950.

LARMON, W. A.: Surgical Treatment of Deformities of Rheumatoid Arthritis of the Forefoot and Toes, Quart. Bull. Northwestern Med. School, 25:39-42, 1951.

LEAVITT, D. G.: Surgical Treatment of Arthritic Feet. Northwest Medicine, 55:1086-1088, 1956.

LEWIS-FANNING, E.: Report on an Enquire into Aetological Factors Associated with Rheumatoid Arthritis. Ann. Rheumat. Dis. 9, Suppl. 94 pp., 1950.

MARMOR, L.: Rheumatoid Deformity of the Foot. Arth. and Rheum., 6:749-755 (Dec.) 1963.

POTTER, T. A.: Rheumatoid Arthritis of the Foot. Exhibit. American Medical Association Meeting, Denver, November, 1961.

POTTER, T. A., AND KUHNS, J. G.: Correction of Arthritic Deformities. In Hollander Arthritis and Allied Conditions, 7th Ed., Philadelphia, Lea & Febiger, 1966, pp. 428-457.

ROPES, M .W., BENNETT, G.A., COBB, S., JACOB, R., AND JESSAR, R. A.: 1958 Revision of Diagnostic Criteria for Rheumatoid Arthritis. Arth. and Rheum., 2:16-20, 1959.

SCHWARTZMANN, J. R.: The Surgical Management of Foot Deformities in Rheumatoid Arthritis. Clin. Ortho., 36:86-95, 1964.

SHORT, C. L., BAUER, W., AND REYNOLDS, W. E.: Rheumatoid Arthritis, 457 pp., Cambridge, Harvard University Press, 1957.

SMITH-PETERSEN, M. N., AUFRANC, O. E., AND LARSON, C. B.: Useful Surgical Procedures for Rheumatoid Arthritis Involving Joints of the Upper Extremity. Arch. Surg. 46:764-770, 1943.

SMYTH, C. J.: Personal Communication.

SPEED, J. S., AND KNIGHT, R. A.: Miscellaneous Affections of Joints. In Campbell's Operative Orthopedics, 2nd Ed., Vol II, St. Louis, C. V. Mosby Co., 1956, pp. 1110-1113.

THOMPSON, T. C.: The Management of the Painful Foot in Arthritis. Med. Clin. North America, 21: 1785-1796, 1937.

=16=

Gout and Allied Disorders

LEONARD MARMOR, M.D.

GOUT

AN historical note of this most ancient disease states in The Scripture, II Chron., XVI, 12: "Asa in the thirty and ninth year of his reign was diseased in his feet . . . Yet in his disease he sought not the Lord, but to the physicians."

The Egyptians knew of this disease and records indicate that to treat it they administered medication derived from crocus and saffron herbs, two plants from which colchicum was extracted. Although gout was familiar to the Ancients, its etiology is no more definitely known today than it was in their day. The earliest recorded history of gout is credited to Hippocrates who in 400 B.C. labeled it as the "unwalkable disease". Among the Ancients it was called *Podagra* from the Greek derivation "πους" meaning foot and "αγρα" meaning attack. However, the term most frequently used at present to describe this disease is *Gout*, a word derived from the Latin word "gutta," meaning a drop. The Ancients proposed that a toxic element drop by drop entered the joint in the foot from the head or some

other part of the body. Galen, in approximately 150 A.D., described a typical tophus. It is generally recognized that Sydenham described the disease in the Seventeenth Century and from this source the modern history of gout has developed.

Quite frequently the orthopaedist is first to see the patient suffering from acute gout with its typical, classical appearance of a swollen, inflamed, excruciatingly painful first metatarsophalangeal joint. He also encounters the more common but more difficult diagnostic problem: the subclinical type of gout wherein the patient gives a history of painful feet with pain radiating into the calves and knees, but not associated with any clinical findings typical of gout, and demonstrating primarily a mildly pronated foot with minimal restriction of motion. When the objective findings of such an examination of the feet are not consistent with the multiple subjective complaints, subclinical gout may be the cause of the disability.

Incidence

Gout, particularly of the subclinical type, is more frequent than is recognized. It is a metabolic disease which is neither uncommon nor unusual. Its reported incidence is directly related to the clinical curiosity of the orthopaedist. Although at one time it was considered a disease solely of males, recent investigators, as well as many orthopaedists with whom we have had personal correspondence, have found that it also occurs among females. Schopf has even reported a case of gout in a five-weeks-old infant with urate deposit in the carpal bones and in the kidneys. There are a number of reported instances in which the disease had been misdiagnosed for several years. An example is that of a seventy-three-year-old Negress, whom one of us recently examined. She complained of almost constant bilateral foot-pain from which she had suffered for over twenty years. She stated that she had worn all types of corrective shoes, arch supports, etc., but with no relief. She had been given numerous types of medications on the basis that her foot pain was due to arthritis, but, again, with no relief of her symptoms. On examination her feet were found to be perfectly normal except for slight stiffness. The longitudinal arch was normal at rest as well as upon standing. Arterial pulsations were within normal limits for her age. There was no evidence of any inflammatory reaction in the various joints of both feet and no pitting edema. The patient stated that at no time had her feet been swollen. There was no family history of gout and her dietary habits were quite normal. Roentgenograms of both feet were completely negative. A blood uric acid was procured as a matter of routine, and the report indicated a blood uric acid level of 9.7 mg./100 ml. When she was placed on a uricosuric drug, her feet became asymptomatic within several days.

Etiology

The etiology of this dyscrasia is not definitely known despite intensive research which has been carried on for many years. The literature on this subject is too voluminous to detail in this text. Therefore, Talbot's book, *Gout,* is recommended to the orthopaedist who may wish to procure more information than will be herein presented.

Gout may be classified as primary and/or secondary. The former type has a definite hereditary tendency. On the other hand, the frequency with which one obtains affirmative information about an hereditary background depends upon the thoroughness of the investigation. In many instances following careful questioning, a definite familial history is established in situations where a positive family history has been previously denied. Asymptomatic hyperuricemia is frequently found in relatives of gouty patients. Bauer and Krane suggest that hyperuricemia is due to a single dominant gene, but that only a small number of those affected by hyperuricemia ever develop gout. The inheritance is not sex linked. A blood uric acid level of 5 to 6 mg. per cent is not uncommon in female relatives of gouty patients, but such an elevation is not usually sufficient to cause the precipitation of urate in tissues and the development of gout. It is the tendency to hyperuricemia, rather than clinical gout, which is hereditary. At present, exact genetic association is not an established fact, nor the previous assumption that it is the metabolic defect that is hereditary and not the disease. Although a high purine diet is a definite precipitating factor of an acute attack in a hyperuricemic patient, there are endogenous factors concerned with the intermediary metabolic function of the purines and the other uric acid precursors which are more responsible for the underlying defect. Of the many theoretical internal and external dysfunctions which are considered to be the cause of an increased concentration of uric acid in the body, three are somewhat reasonably tenable:

1. Diminished enzymatic destruction of uric acid.

2. Diminished renal excretion of uric acid.

3. Increased formation of uric acid through faulty intermediary metabolism.

Secondary gout is a consequence of blood dyscrasias. Hyperuricemia can also occur without arthritis in polycythemia vera, leukemia, pernicious anemia, nephritis, starvation, infections, diabetic acidosis, mongolism, psoriasis, and sarcoidosis.

Pathology

The pathology of gout is characterized by the deposition of uric acid crystals (monosodium urate monohydrate salt) in tissues and joints. The deposition of urate crystals on the articular surface of a joint damages the cartilage. The crystals tend to be precipitated in the avascular area of the cartilage which implies that the urates are deposited from the synovial fluid. It is suspected that minute trauma to the cartilage may initiate the process as urates precipitate easily and once initiated, the deposits will continue to grow. Granulomatous changes occur in the synovium and surrounding joint tissues, producing a fibrous tissue reaction which, at times, can lead to destruction of the articular surface and ankylosis. It can also lead to the roentgenographic appearance of punched-out lesions in the various bones of the foot as tophaceous deposits or urates accumulate. These may be deposited on all surfaces of the foot, producing severe deformities (Fig. 16-1 and 2). They may vary from several millimeters to several centimeters in size.

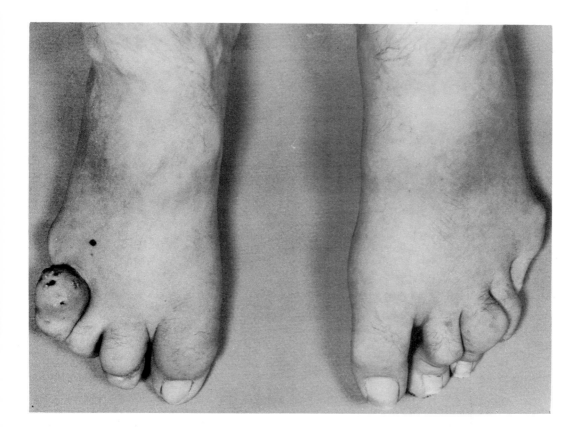

Fig. 16-1. Patient with severe gouty deposits on the dorsum of foot. The deformity of the foot by these deposits actually prevented the wearing of shoes.

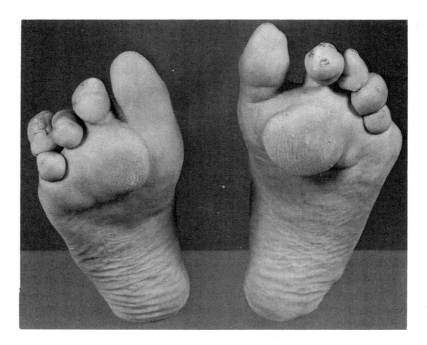

Fig. 16-2.   Large tophaceous deposits were also present on the ball of the foot. The serum uric acid level was 11 mg. per cent.

Clinical Aspects

The disease appears initially in a middle-aged man or woman as an acute monarticular arthritis. In about 70 per cent of the patients the metatarsophalangeal joint of the hallux is primarily involved. Other sites of the foot that may be afflicted are the dorsum of any of the tarsal joints. The onset may come at any time and often the patient experiences the initial attack in the early morning hours. It is frequently an articular pain which is worse upon weight bearing and can be excruciating in character. It increases gradually and as it does, the patient becomes extremely apprehensive and uncomfortable. Within a few hours the skin over the joint becomes edematous, hot, red, and shiny, simulating an infection. The patient may even demonstrate an increase in temperature up to 102° to 103°F. This attack, if left untreated, may last for two or three days or even longer. The swelling will then gradually disappear and the joint will return to normal. However, this is the beginning of a chronic stage. Gout may manifest itself in any joint of the extremities, as well as the spine.

In the chronic stage, gout may affect several joints, or there may be just an aching sensation in the feet. At this stage it may be difficult to make the diagnosis since many of the changes typical of gout are not demonstrable. Many cases of gout remain undiagnosed because of failure to consider the possibility of this diagnosis. The attacks of acute gout may recur and become more frequent. During the early years of the disease, the patient's foot may be asymptomatic between acute attacks, but as the disease progresses and the joints are progressively destroyed by the pathologic progress, the symptoms persist. The patient will often have a premonition of an impending attack of acute gout from two to forty-eight hours prior to its onset. This warning consists of a peculiar sensation of burning and aching in the joint, with or without stiffness.

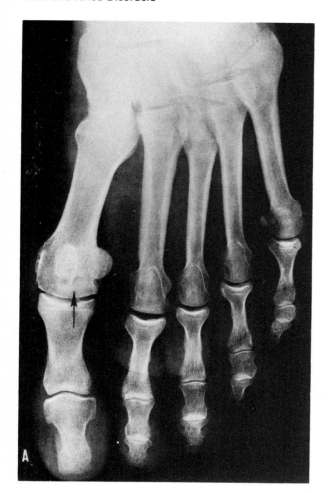

Fig. 16-3. A. The roentgenogram in this early case of gout reveals punched out lesions in the first metatarsal head.

B.   A more advanced case of destruction of the metatarso-phalangeal joint due to uric acid deposits.

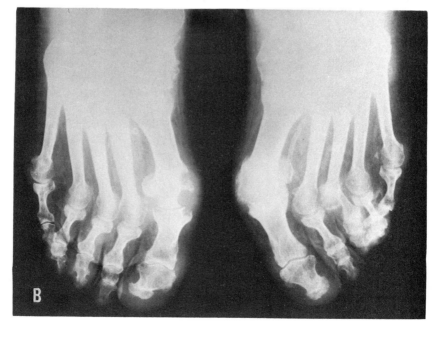

Laboratory Data

The most valuable laboratory test in gout is the blood uric acid determination. The upper limit of the normal will vary with the laboratory performing the test, but in general 6 mg. per cent is the upper limit of normal in the male and 5.5 mg. per cent in the female. It is unwarranted to exclude the diagnosis of gout merely because the serum uric acid level may be normal since it is frequently within normal limits during the initial attack. The physician should make certain that the patient is not ingest-ing a uricosuric drug which may reduce the serum level of uric acid to normal. Furthermore, each laboratory will vary as to what is considered the normal range, and the orthopaedist should be familiar with the particular laboratory normals. Usually, in a patient with gout other laboratory tests are within normal limits except during an acute attack when leukocytosis may be present, as well as an elevated sedimentation rate.

Roentgenograms

During the acute phase of gout and even after many episodes, the roentgenograms may be perfectly normal. It is of interest to note that on roentgenographic examination approximately 35 per cent of patients with chronic gout have lesions that are typical and that the roentgenographic findings in another 30 per cent are merely compatible with gout.

The joints most commonly presenting roentgenographic changes are those of the hands and feet. The lesions are frequently symmetrical. The earliest roentgenographic finding of clinical significance is an area of osteoporosis at the base of the proximal phalanx, usually of the great toe which ap-pears somewhat cystic. Later a "punched-out" lesions is apparent (Fig. 16-3A and B). The lesions are produced by urate crystals and also by fibrosis of the area. As this disease process continues, the corner of the phalanx is lost and marginal articular destruction continues until the articular surface is destroyed (Fig. 16-4).

Tophaceous deposits do not necessarily involve the articular surface but can be deposited beneath the periosteum, thus producing erosion of the shaft of the bone. Occasionally uric acid deposits may expand the end of bone causing an appearance similar to that of a giant-cell tumor.

Diagnosis

The diagnosis of gout should not be difficult, if the orthopaedist remembers that it is a possibility in any case of vague arthralgia or an acute attack of joint pain. A complete history, physical examination, and laboratory tests will facilitate the correct diagnosis. The important facts in the history are as follows:

1) Acute monarticular arthritis of unknown etiology.

2) Awareness of symptoms prior to joint pain.

3) Development of pain in the early morning hours.

4) Family history of gout.

The physical examination of the patient, frequently male, presents the findings of an erythematous, swollen, tender foot or great toe, or, on the other hand, simply an arthralgia of one or both feet, or any other joint or joints.

An elevated uric acid (with a normal blood urea nitrogen to rule out renal disease) suggests a diagnosis of gout. The roentgenograms may or may not be of value, but if they reveal a punched-out or bubble-shaped area in the involved joint, the diagnosis of gout is then even more likely to be correct.

An excellent diagnosic test is the use of colchicine to relieve the acute symptoms. Dramatic response to the drug is invariably pathognomonic of gout.

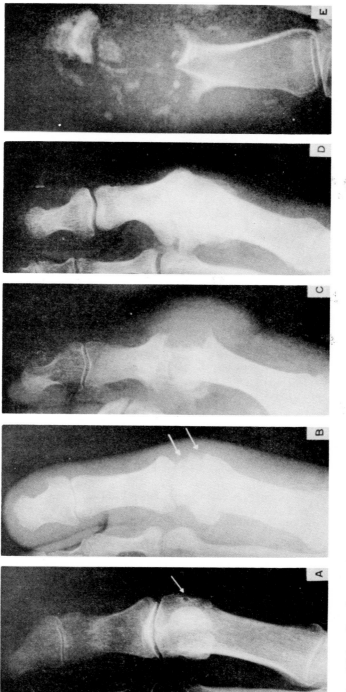

Fig. 16-4. Roentgenograms of the first metatarsophalangeal joint (bunion joint) of 5 gouty patients. Progressive erosion and joint destruction is illustrated from left to right; earliest change is a punched-out area (A), more marked destructive changes (B and C), secondary hypertrophic changes (D), far-advanced destruction (E). (Smyth in Hollander's *ARTHRITIS*, Lea & Febiger.)

Differential Diagnosis

A differential diagnosis must consider the possibility of rheumatoid arthritis, osteoarthritis, sarcoidosis, metastatic tumors, hyperparathyroidism, among other conditions with symptoms similar to those of gout.

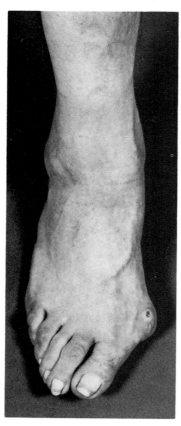

Fig. 16-5. This forty-six-year-old male patient has a history of rheumatoid arthritis with a large bunion with a small ulceration over the bursa. The pathological report was compatible with rheumatoid arthritis.

Rheumatoid Arthritis. At times the differential diagnosis between rheumatoid arthritis and gout may pose a problem, especially when only one joint is involved (Fig. 16-5). Rheumatoid arthritis usually produces gradually progressive bilateral symptoms with systemic manifestations. Early morning stiffness (gel phenomena) may be of importance in diagnosis, as well as evidence of involvement of the temporomandibular joints or the proximal interphalangeal joints, since these findings occur only in rheumatoid arthritis. A positive latex fixation test (indicative of rheumatoid disease) will help in the differential diagnosis if the uric acid test is normal. Occasionally both diseases can occur in the same patient.

Osteoarthritis. Occasionally involvement of the metatarsophalangeal joints by degenerative changes can simulate gout (Fig. 16-6). Osteophyte formation may produce a process which, at times, becomes swollen, tender, and painful. Rarely is the onset acute or the pain excrutiating.

Cellulitis. An infection of one of the toes or the dorsum of the foot may be confusing at first because of the pain, swelling, and erythema. The temperature, sedimentation rate and white count are all elevated. The patient may present a history of trauma or previous abrasion of the skin. If the serum uric acid level is normal and there is no response to colchicine within twenty-four hours, a trial of antibiotics is warranted.

Bunions. A hallux valgus deformity can be confused with gout. The bursa may become acutely inflamed and painful preventing the wearing of shoes. However, the swelling and redness is usually limited to the area of the bursa, and the joint can be moved carefully without pain (Fig. 16-7).

Pseudo-Gout Syndrome. This is a relatively new syndrome described by Gatter and McCarty which tends to resemble gouty attacks involving joints. Recently (1963) 30 cases were reported by these authors with 22 acute attacks, 18 involving the knee. (There have been no cases reported in the great toe.) In this condition calcium pyrophosphate crystals are found within the leukocytes removed from the joint fluid. The menisci and the articular cartilage may be calcified and this phenomenon may be demonstrated by roentgenography. The average attack lasts approximately eight days, and the maximum pain for not more than twenty-four hours. It is more commonly found in diabetics in the age group from thirty to eighty, (with the average age of around fifty). The diagnosis is confirmed both by the roentgenograms and the laboratory tests of the joint fluid which is examined for the presence of calcium pyrophosphate crystals.

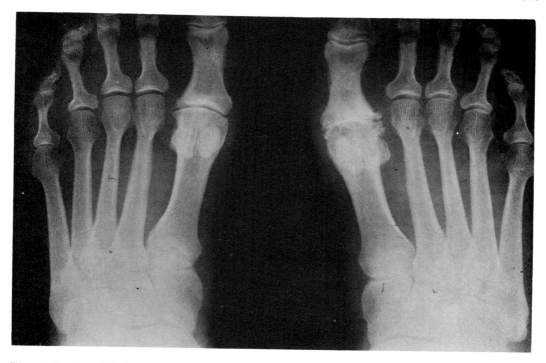

Fig. 16-6. This fifty-two-year-old female patient had a history of increasing pain in her great toe and loss of motion. A diagnosis of osteoarthritis with a hallux rigidus was made.

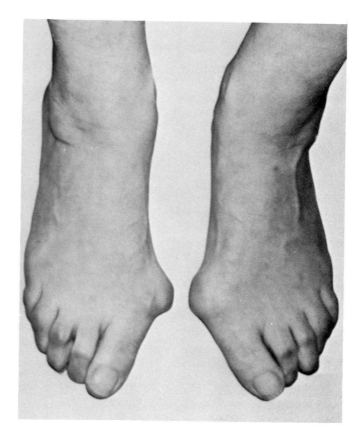

Fig. 16-7. This fifty-six-year-old woman had painful bunions of both feet due to a hallux valgus.

Treatment and Prophylaxis

With adequate prophylaxis and management, acute attacks of gout can, almost invariably, be prevented. Therefore, the management of the prophylactic period will be considered first.

Method of Control. The method of control of prophylaxis is relatively simple and, if followed, permits the affected individual to live a relatively normal life. The regimen may also either slow down appreciably or reverse the progressive effect of this disease. It is the control and handling of the patient during the so-called "intercritical" period which is of much greater importance in controlling the metabolic disturbance than is the actual therapy during an acute attack.

Interception or Between-Attacks Management. The supervision during the interval between attacks demands first the administration of two of the most effective anti-gout medications — Benemid [p-(di-n-prophylsulfamyl)-benzoic acid] and colchicine. The two are synergistic and neither one, individually, is as effective as the combination. Benemid is a uricosuric agent which has proved to be of inestimable value in the treatment of gout during the intercritical period. It is absorbed quite rapidly and effectively by the gastrointestinal tract and carried into the blood stream partially bound by plasma protein. It has a blocking action in the renal tubules, thus permitting an increased excretion of uric acid in the urine, a decreased concentration of the uric acid in the serum, and a decrease in the metabolic pool as long as daily ingestion is maintained. The uricosuric action of Benemid can be neutralized either partially or completely by the concurrent administration of salicylates and, therefore, the latter drug should never be prescribed as part of the therapeutic regimen for gout when Benemid is used. Benemid has another specific action: namely, the decrease in the size of the subcutaneous tophi and the recalcification of the punched-out areas in the affected bones.

Colchicine alone is neither an analgesic nor a uricosuirc. It is suspected, but not proved, that it surpresses phagocytosis and thus has antiphlogistic properties. However, when combining these two drugs, the experience of investigators, who specialize in the therapy of gout, has shown that there is a marked diminution, if not an actual elimination, of acute attacks of gout. Another result of the combined medication is that the patient experiences a sense of well-being not observed when colchicine is the only drug administered. However, one word of warning: during the early stages of this combined therapy (by this, one does not mean the first few days, but rather during the first few weeks) acute attacks can and will recur. Nevertheless, if the patient is informed of this possibility, he will not be discouraged but will take the recurrence or recurrences in stride, since following the one or two episodes there is a gratifying diminution in the number of attacks.

Before placing the patient on this regimen, the blood urea nitrogen, as well as the blood uric acid, should be examined as a matter of routine. Although one may find some evidence of renal dysfunction (this is true in probably 50 per cent of these patients), this does not necessarily contraindicate the institution of the anti-gout regimen, but simply means that the patient must be observed carefully and cautiously given the medication necessary to combat the gout and kept under periodic observation.

In the patients with mild gout the average daily dosage recommended is 1.5 mg. of colchicine and 500 mg. of Benemid. An abundant fluid intake should accompany the medication. The minimum amount should be at least 2,000 to 3,000 cc. daily consisting either of water or mineral waters, but preferably not carbonated beverages.

Patients suffering from moderately severe gout, that is, those with serum uric acid of approximately 9 to 14 mg. per 100 ml., should be given 1 to 1.5 mg. of colchicine and 1.5 gm. of Benemid daily. High fluid intake should be recommended as well. To prevent any gastrointestinal disturbances the patient should be advised to take his Benemid with his meals. The incidence of toxicity from these two medications is clinically insignificant, nor has there been any evidence of bone marrow depression or damage to the liver with these dosages. Occasionally a patient may develop a mild rash, but this is not an indication for discontinuation of the medication. It merely indicates the need to diminish the dosage until the rash subsides. The regular dosage may then be reinstituted. Concurrently with the above regimen it is important to again heed the warning that salicylates should not be prescribed because they will nullify the effect of the Benemid.

A new drug, which holds a great deal of promise in the treatment of gout, is Allopurinol [Allopurinol (4 Hydroxypyragolo (3.4d) Pyrimidine)] which is not a uricosuric, but is a potent inhibitor of uric acid crystal formation, *in vivo*, as well as *in vitro*. In man, it effectively inhibits uric acid formation since it inhibits the formation of xanthine oxidase (the enzyme which catalyzes the conversion of hypoxanthine to xanthine and xanthine to uric acid). In 1963 Rundles and other investigators who first used this drug found it useful and without any serious side reactions. Their findings have since been corroborated by many investigators. Since Allopurinol inhibits uric acid formation, the xanthine and hypoxanthine levels in the plasma are increased and readily excreted through the urine. They are more easily excretable than uric acid and, therefore, can be filtered out more rapidly and with less difficulty.

Of course, the advantage of this drug is twofold. (1) The inhibition of the formation of uric acid. (2) As a result of the first, there is far less likelihood of the development of renal calculi, which is an ever-present possibility when Benemid is prescribed.

Allopurinol is devoid of any antirheumatic properties and is found to be ineffectual in overcoming acute gouty arthritis. Several investigators have found that salicylates can be given concurrently with this drug without interference with its function. The average daily dose is 400 to 600 mg. per day. Other than an occasional diarrhea, there are no significant gastrointestinal, renal, or other toxic effects noted with this drug. With its use, the urinary excretion of xanthine and hypoxanthine is markedly increased in proportion to the diminution of uric acid excretion. It has been found, however, that when Allopurinol is used jointly with a uricosuric, such as Benemid, it further reduces the serum urates and increases the renal excretion of uric acid.

One troublesome complication which has been found with the use of Allopurinol is the frequent precipitation of an acute attack of gouty arthritis, sometimes in spite of the prophylactic administration of colchicine. However, it is anticipated that the problem will be solved as the drug has greater clinical exposure and investigation. From all the evidence derived from the literature and from the producers of the drug, it can be safely concluded that Allopurinol can suppress uric acid production without any toxic hazard. It reduces the plasma urates even in the presence of renal damage of such intensity that the usual uricosuric drugs are contraindicated. It thus secondarily diminishes uric acid excretion and lessens the risk of uric acid urolithiasis.

Dietary Management. What of the dietary regimen during the intercritical period? Diets for the control of gout have been as numerous as the physicians who have treated this condition in the past. Of recent years, particularly since the utilization of isotope techniques, observations by some investigators have caused them to conclude that "proteins may be no worse offenders as precursors of uric acid than are carbohydrates or fats." It is, therefore, no longer considered necessary to place gouty patients on a low protein diet. A well-balanced diet of carbohydrate, fat, and protein is recommended. If, subsequent to the ingestion of some specific food the patient should notice a definite relationship to an acute attack of gout, the constituents of this one particular meal should be investigated and any offending food should be tested by repeatedly administering it to the patient. If it proves to be an inciting factor, it should be eliminated from the diet. *Foods which are high in purine content should be avoided at all times.* However, such a restriction is of no great import since it will impose a hardship only on the epicurean or the Sybarite. Such forbidden items are liver, kidney, spleen, tongue, anchovies, sweetbread, and meat extracts.

There is little corroborating evidence that the consumption of alcoholic beverages in moderation predisposes to aggravation or precipitation of an attack. Occasionally a patient may report that some one type of derivative of a grain or the grape will trigger an acute attack and, of course, this beverage should be avoided if the correlation can be established.

The intercritical management of the patient with gout is quite variable, and is generally dependent upon the severity of the symptoms, the length and frequency of the attack and the attitude of the patient. While the use of drugs is accepted therapy to reduce the attacks of gout, it is extremely difficult to assure a patient's taking the medication, particularly if he has an attack only once every two or three years.

Acute Gout

Acute gout is a disease which requires immediate and practically heroic therapy. There are several drugs available for the treatment of acute primary gout. The choice of the drug may be based on patient's response to the medication or to the side effects of the medication. The "sine qua non" of acute gout therapy is colchicine, which has been the standard therapy for several centuries. It is generally used in over 90 per cent of the cases. Colchicine was originally used as treatment for gout by Alexander Tralles in the sixteenth century. It is believed that a French Army Surgeon, Nicholas Husson, made a potion of colchicine for acute gout. Garrod in 1859 wrote the classic paper on the action of colchicine in gout. The use of this drug in this disease is empirical and the mechanism of the antiarticular action is unknown. It is not uricosuric nor is it a diuretic or a hypouricemic. In an acute attack colchicine is administered orally in 0.6 mg. tablets as soon as possible after the onset, and in one- or two-hour intervals for 16 to 18 doses. It is important to continue the medication until the pain is relieved, or until gastrointestinal symptoms develop, such as diarrhea, nausea, or cramps. The drug should be administered continuously around the clock even if the patient must be awakened throughout the night. The full therapeutic effect of colchicine does not take place in the acute attack until gastrointestinal symptoms develop, nor is there any satisfactory explanation why this cause and effect is necessary to achieve complete therapy.

Once the drug has produced such a response, it should be discontinued for twenty-four hours to allow the gastrointestinal symptoms to subside. Colchicine in 0.6 mg. tablets should then be administered once or twice daily for two weeks; this will help to prevent a recurrence of the acute attack which can occur within twenty-four hours after the drug is stopped.

ACTH has also been utilized in the treatment of acute gout, but it is generally not as effective as colchicine. It should be reserved for patients who do not respond to colchicine and phenylbutazone. Even then, as with other adrenocorticosteroids, ACTH should be administered under careful medical supervision, for it is not without danger.

Phenylbutazone (3.5-dioxo-1, 2 diphenyl-4-n-butyl-pyrazolidin sodium) has also been reported useful in the treatment of acute gout. It should be administered under careful medical supervision, because it, too, is not without danger.

During the chronic phase of the disease, the patient should be under the care of a rheumatologist or an internist. A specific therapeutic regimen, appropriate for the patient, should be established. Furthermore, the patient should be advised that maintenance doses of the drugs will be required for a long period of time, perhaps even for the remainder of his lifetime. The presence of a peptic ulcer is not a contraindication for the use of colchicine or Benemid or a combination of the two, providing the patient is carefully supervised.

Surgery

It is during the chronic phase of the disease, when deformities have developed, that surgical treatment has proved of value. There is much to commend it and it can rehabilitate an incapacitated person. The preoperative care is important because an operation can precipitate an acute attack which may complicate the postoperative management. In addition to the maintenance dose of Benemid, colchicine (0.6 mg.) should be administered twice daily for a week prior to the operation and again as soon as possible after surgery. If necessary, colchicine may be administered intravenously, but under careful supervision. An accidental injection of colchicine subcutaneously can result in sloughing of the tissues or in a severe toxic neuritis.

Large tophi in the foot may be extremely painful if they are on the weight-bearing surface and they can prevent the wearing of a shoe. These tophi may ulcerate and produce draining sinuses which fortunately do not often become infected. Tophi may be removed surgically from the surface but are difficult to extirpate because of the infiltration of the urate crystals within the fibrous septa, but it is necessary to carry out as complete a curretage as possible. It is important to inform the patient that these incisions will heal slowly because of the poor subcutaneous tissue. The lesions are not always as circumscribed as they appear on the surface, and it may be necessary to scrape them out with a curette. It is also important to keep in mind that penicillin is contraindicated because of the possible precipitation of an acute attack. A broad spectrum antibiotic is more desirable.

At times a digit will be so badly destroyed that surgical removal will be necessary to obtain improvement. Ray resection of the foot is not generally recommended since it narrows the weight-bearing surface of the foot.

The first metatarsophalangeal joint may be destroyed with loss of motion and a painful hallux rigidus may develop. In these cases removal of the proximal one-half of the proximal phalanx and of the tophaceous material may bring satisfactory improvement. The sesamoids should be removed.

In severe cases of gout, tendon ruptures can occur since urate crystals deposited in the tendon sheath interfere with proper nutrition of these tissues. Such ruptures can be extremely difficult to repair because of the poor surrounding tissue.

In general, surgery is limited to correction of painful deformities of the foot to allow comfortable weight bearing.

PULMONARY HYPERTROPHIC OSTEOARTHROPATHY

This condition is a syndrome or clinical complex consisting of clubbing of the fingers and/or toes with periosteal new bone formation and arthritic changes. The striking enlargement of the feet may be confused with acromegaly.

Clubbing of the foot was first reported in approximately 400 B.C. by Hippocrates and the deformity of the finger or of the toe is called the "Hippocratic deformity." Bamberger in 1889 described the skeletal changes seen in pulmonary disease. Marie, independently, in 1890 described the same condition. It is, therefore, referred to in the modern textbooks of medicine as Marie-Bamberger disease.

This syndrome is generally associated with pulmonary disease which may actually be the first sign of it. It has been found with primary lung carcinoma, metastases to the lung, pulmonary infections, such as a lung abscess, tuberculosis, bronchiectasis, carcinoma of the stomach, cirrhosis of the liver, and cyanotic heart disease. Gibbs and associates, as well as Aufses, have described hypertrophic pulmonary osteoarthropathy heralding lung metatases. The exact etiology of this syndrome is not clear at this time. The pathologic condition consists of periosteal new bone formation along the shaft of tubular bones which is referred to as osteophytosis. The deposition of bone is most intense along the middle of the shaft. The metatarsals are usually more involved than the phalanges, but the phalanges may show tufting at the ends. Microscopically the osteoperiostitic bone appears to be demarcated from the original cortex of the shaft. As time passes, the two surfaces become less distinct. The joints may also be involved and show thickening and inflammatory changes in the synovia.

There is no specific therapy for this syndrome, but the physician should be cognizant of it to prevent overlooking an occult lesion of the lung or, at least be alerted to the possible diagnosis of periostitis of the tubular bones.

CALCIFIC DEPOSITS

Calcium deposits may occur in and about the tissues of the foot. Calcification may occur either as an isolated lesion or part of a systemic disease.

Amorphous calcification in the soft tissue may be classified according to etiology:

1. Congenital
2. Infectious
3. Neoplastic
4. Traumatic
5. Degenerative

Calcium deposits can be demonstrated in many regions of the body. The most common site of acute deposits are in the rotator cuff of the shoulder and in the tendons and ligaments about the hand and wrist. These same deposits may occur in the soft tissues of the foot and produce a clinical picture of dramatic, acute pain. The dorsum of the foot may reveal some swelling and induration. Commonly the peroneus tertius tendon is involved at its insertion.

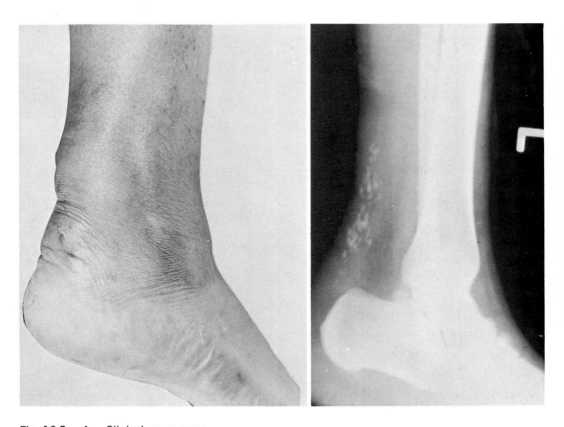

Fig. 16-8.   A.   Clinical appearance.
    B.   Roentgenogram demonstrating calcareous deposits within the tendo achillis.

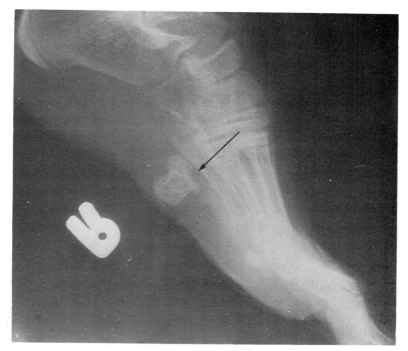

Fig. 16-9.   A large calcified mass was on the plantar surface of the foot. The deposit was circumscribed and nontender, but produced symptoms due to pressure on weight bearing.

Occasionally one may have cause to examine a patient complaining of a mass in the tendo achillis, primarily, but occasionally in other tendons of the foot as well, accompanied by pain and tenderness (Fig. 16-8A). Roentgenographically (Fig. 16-8B) one will find a diffuse calcareous deposit within the tendon. At times the entire tendon will be outlined by this calcareous mass. The exact cause of this condition is unknown. All laboratory studies have failed to disclose any specific, positive results.

The attack may simulate gout and a serum uric acid test may be of value as a diagnostic aid. Roentgenograms may reveal a rounded, calcific deposit in the soft tissue (Fig. 16-9), indicating an acute process.

One might hypothesize that it is nature's attempt to add necessary support to a degenerated tendon since upon exploration the tendo achillis will be found to be infiltrated with this calcific deposit, much the same as in the calcareous tendonitis of the shoulder. Microscopic examination of many of the tendon fibers will disclose various stages of degeneration.

Treatment consists of injection of the deposit with hydrocortisone and a local anesthetic. In the acute attack oxyphenylbutazone may also be of value in those patients who do not want an injection. The treatment of choice is the use of cold packs for the first twenty-four hours followed by heat. The cold tends to reduce the pain and inflammation. The subsequent heat will aid in the reabsorption of the calcium deposit. The use of systemic steroids is contraindicated.

In general, treatment is empirical. In the following illustrated instance the condition was bilateral. One tendon became asymptomatic with conservative therapy of the "shot gun" type consisting of ultrasound treatments and carefully controlled low voltage skin erythema doses of radiation. The corresponding tendon on the opposite side did not respond to conservative treatment. Surgical exploration was attempted but was found unrewarding since it would have been necessary to resect a major portion of the tendo achillis to remove all of the calcific deposit. However, following closure of the wound and immobilization in a cast for six weeks, the symptomatology disappeared. The patient has been lost to follow-up as to the ultimate fate of the calcification within the tendon.

There are several other metabolic diseases which cause deleterious changes in the feet. These include scurvy, hyperparathyroidism, etc., but these conditions present other clinical manifestations which are more striking and more pronounced. Therefore, they are mentioned only in passing in order to make the chapter more inclusive.

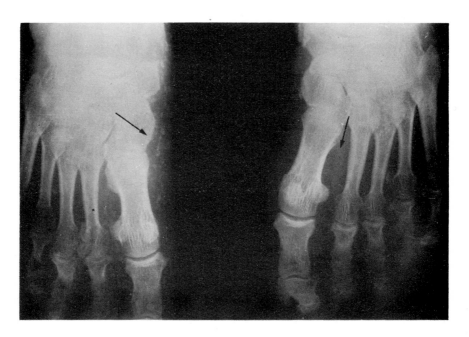

Fig. 16-10.   A young woman with a distribution of soft tissue calcification in both feet due to calcinosis.

CALCINOSIS

Calcinosis, originally described by Weber in 1878, is a rare disease which occurs in two syndromes. The first is the interstitial, or universalis, calcinosis which is diffuse and is said to be found primarily in children. The second is calcinosis circumscripta which occurs in females six times as frequently as in males, and is a localized condition that afflicts adults and/or children.

Calcinosis universalis is a diffuse, systemic disease which may be preceded by an acute infection. The etiology is unknown. Calcium is laid down in the skin, subcutaneous tissues, fascia, muscle, nerve sheaths, tendons, and ligaments. Visceral calcifications are rare. As the calcium salts are deposited in increasing amounts, the depositions gradually enlarge to become evident upon clinical examination, especially about the joints (Fig. 16-10).

Calcinosis circumscripta has an insidious onset in the adult and frequently occurs near joints. Subsequent investigators such as Rothstein and Kilburn feel that the division of calcinosis into the circumscripta and universal forms is undesirable. One cannot state with assurance that one form is truly independent of the other. Such classification does not take into account the many transitional forms of the disease process. One cannot disregard the possibility that the underlying defect which causes the localized calcinosis may in future years result in further calcific deposition elsewhere in the body. Calcinosis has been reported

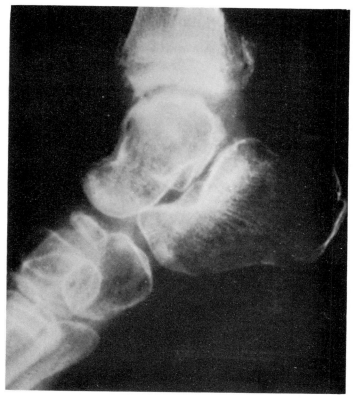

Fig. 16-11.   Seven months after a burn there is evidence of articular destruction involving the talo-calcaneal and talo-tibial joints in the unburned ankle. (Evans, & Smith: courtesy of J. Bone & Jt. Surg.)

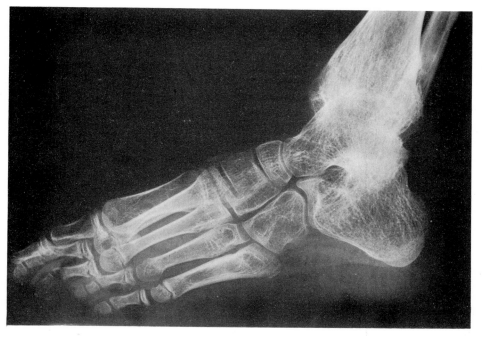

Fig. 16-12.   The talo-tibial and talo-calcaneal bony ankylosis as it appeared 6 years after the burn. (Evans, & Smith: courtesy of J. Bone & Jt. Surg.)

in association with such diseases as scleroderma, Raynaud's disease, lupus erythematosus, and rheumatoid arthritis, as well as
other associated collagen diseases.

Treatment is generally symptomatic relief or excision of a prominence if it is painful on weight bearing.

BURNS

Frequently in severe burns periarticular
soft tissue changes may occur as a late sequela (Fig. 16-11). Three types of changes
have been noted:
1) Osteoporosis and periosteal new bone
   formation
2) Pericapsular calcification

3) Progressive articular destruction and
   ankylosis
These changes occur in approximately 3
per cent of the patients with severe burns
and may involve not the area of the burn,
but distal joints such as the ankle or foot.
This may seriously limit rehabilitation of
such patients (Fig. 16-12).

HEMOPHILIA

Hemophilia is a rare disease that involves
the coagulation mechanism of the blood
and prevents normal clotting. It is an hereditary disorder transmitted by the mother
almost exclusively to the male child. It is a
hemorrhagic disorder characterized by a deficiency of antihemophilic globulin (AHF).
The severity of the disease is related to the
degree of AHF deficiency. There are essentially three main stages in the clotting
of blood, each dependent on many factors.

Stage I — Formation of plasma throm-
          boplastin
Stage II — Conversion of prothrombin
          to thrombin
Stage III — Formation of fibrin

Hemophilia is a defect involving Stage I.
It involves a prolonged clotting time, a
normal one-stage prothrombin, and a normal platelet count, with a clotting time
seldom less than thirty minutes.

Male infants or children usually have
symptoms of hemarthrosis, soft tissue hemorrhage, and excessive bleeding after minor
trauma. Large collections of blood in the
fascial planes may produce severe crippling
deformities even after a solitary episode.
Furthermore, such deep tissue bleeding
should be recognized since it is most often
misdiagnosed as a hemarthrosis.

Treatment of the acute hemorrhage includes rest and immobilization but the only
significant theapy is the use of anti-hemo-
phillic globulin concentrate. In the average
hemophyllic patient, the amount of anti-
hemophyllic globulin concentrate is 1 to 2

per cent of normal. The normal anti-hemophyllic globulin factor in the average individual is over 30 per cent. In order, therefore, to control bleeding which may occur
in an area due to injury and, therefore,
subsequent hemorrhage, one packet of anti-
hemophyllic globulin concentrate (pool)
per 30 pounds of body weight must be administered. Prior to the last two or three
years, the only significant therapy was normal, fresh, pooled lyophilized or fresh
whole blood. In the average individual,
therefore, who suffered hemorrhage due to
hemophylria, it would be necessary to ad-
minister at least five units of plasma in
order to experience the same clotting effect
which five packets of anti-hemophyllic concentrate in 200 cc. of saline solution would
produce.

With the advent of improved management, the survival of the hemophiliac
patient has increased, so that advanced
arthropathy and deformities are less frequently encountered.

The manifestations of disease in the joint
have been pointed out by DePalma and
Cotler and appear to be governed by:
1) The severity of the blood defect.
2) The age of onset.
3) The personality of the patient.
The latter fact is of importance because
some patients will not heed advice and
continue to inflict trauma to their joints
producing further hemorrhage and damage. Once a joint is subjected to hemarthrosis, it often becomes predisposed to

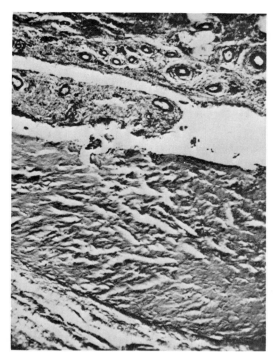

Fig. 16-13. The synovium is markedly thickened and falls into folds and shows evidence of marked hyperplasia and hypertrophy. (DePalma, and Cotler: courtesy of Clin. Orthop.)

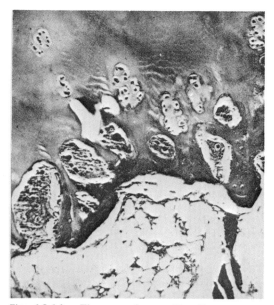

Fig. 16-14. The vascular proliferating connective tissue that seems to cause resorption of the surrounding bone trabeculae. (DePalma and Cotler: courtesy of Clinical Orthop.)

further hemorrhage. The points most frequently involved are the knee, elbow, ankle, and hip. During the acute phase the joint is hot, red, painful, and swollen. The pain results from the acute distension of the capsule and pericapsular tissues by the hemorrhage. With the proper use and administration of anti-hemophyllic globulin concentrate, the various joints of the body can be aspirated without any fear of further hemorrhage.

The basic change within the joint is produced by the presence of the blood which stimulates an inflammatory response with hyperplasia of the synovium (Fig. 16-13), increased vascularity and thickening of the capsule. The synovium can grow across the articular cartilage as pannus, destroying it as well as invading the subchondral bone and destroying it also (Fig. 16-14).

The roentgenographic findings do not usually parallel the clinical changes because the early changes first involve the soft tissues. Some thickening of the synovium and capsule may be evident and

later subchondral cysts occur with punched-out areas in the articular surface. Flattening of the talus, resembling osteochondrosis, has also been described in hemophilia, as well as several cases of ankylosis of the subtalar joint. (Fig. 16-15).

Surgery is possible in this condition particularly with the use of the newly discovered anti-hemophyllic globulin concentrate.

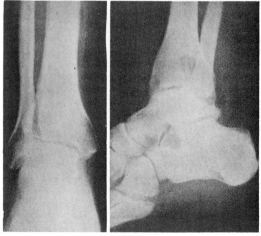

Fig. 16-15. The talus appears flattened and the bone is sclerotic. The talus appears similar to that noted in osteochondritis. (DePalma and Cotler: courtesy of Clinical Orthop.)

BIBLIOGRAPHY

BAILEY, R. W.: Calcinosis Circumscripta—A Local and Metabolic Study. J. Bone Jt. Surg., 39-B, 1957.

V. BAMBERGER, E.: Sitzurgsb. der k.k. Gesellsch, der Arzte in Wien, vom 8, 1889, Wien. klin. Wchnschr, 1889.

BARTELS, E. C.: Unrecognized Cases of Gout. Lahey Clin. Bull., 11:226, 1960.

BAUER, WALTER AND KRANE, STEPHEN M.: Diseases of Metabolism, 5th Ed., Philadelphia, W. B. Saunders Co. 1964, 805-845.

CROCK, H. V., AND BONI, V.: The Management of Orthopaedic Problems in Hemophiliacs, A Review of 21 Cases. Brit. J. Surg., 48:8, 1960.

DE PALMA, A. F., AND COTLER, J.: Hemophilic Arthropathy. Clin. Orth. 8:163, 1956.

EVANS, E. V., AND SMITH, J. R.: Bone and Joint Changes Following Burns. J. Bone Jt. Surg., 41-A:785. 1959.

GALEN, C.: Opera Omnia, ed by Kühn. Leipzig, 1821-1833.

GALL, E. A., BENNET, G. A., AND BAVER, W.: Generalized Hypertrophic Osteoarthropathy. Amer. J. Path. 27:349, 1951.

GARROD, A. B.: Observations on Certain Pathological Conditions of the Blood and Urine in Gout, Rheumatism, and Bright's Disease. Trans. Med. Chir. Soc. Edinburgh, 31:83, 1848.

GARTLAND, J. J.: Fundamentals of Orthopaedics. Philadelphia, W. B. Saunders Co., 1965.

GATTER, R. A. AND McCARTY, D. J.: Pseudogout Syndrome. Clinical Analysis of 30 Cases. Arth. Rheum., 6:271, 1963.

GIBBS, D. D., SCHILLER, K. F. R., AND STOVIN, P. G. I.: Lung Metastases Heralded by Hypertrophic Pulmonary Osteoarthropathy. Lancet, 1: 623, 1960

GRAHAM, W.: Gout and Gouty Arthritis. Postgrad Med., 30:555, 1961.

HOLLANDER, J. L.: Arthritis. 7th Ed. Philadelphia, Lea & Febiger, 1966.

KILBURN, P.: Calcinosis: A Review with Report of Four Cases. Postgrad Med. J. 33:555, 1957.

KOLAR, J. AND VRABEC, R.: Periarticular Soft Tissue Changes as a Late Consequence of Burns. J. Bone Jt. Surg., 41-A:103, 1959.

KRAKOFF, I. H. AND MEYER, R. L.: Hyperuricemia in Leukemia and Lymphoma. J.A.M.A., 193: (July) 1965.

KUHNS, J. G.: The Foot in Chronic Arthritis. Clin. Orth., 16:141, 1960.

LAPIDUS, P. W. AND GUIDOTTI, F. P.: Gout in Orthopaedic Practice. Clin. Orth., 28:97, 1963.

MARIE, P.: De l'Osteo-Arthropathie Hypertrophi-

ante Pneumique. Rev de Med., 10:1, 1890.

McCARROLL, H. R.: Problems of Soft Tissue Calcification as Related to Orthopaedic Surgery. J. Bone Jt. Surg., 38A:1389, 1956.

ROOK, R. W.: Gout in Orthopaedic Practice. South Med. J., 52:1111, 1959.

ROSENQUIST, R. C., SMALL, C. S., AND DEEB, P. H.: Unusual Manifestations of Gout. Arch Path, 68:1, 1959.

ROTHSTEIN, J. L. AND WELT, W.: Calcinosis Universalis and Calcinosis Circumscripta in Infancy and Childhood. Amer. J. Dis. Child., 52:368, 1936.

RUNDLES, R. W., SILVERMAN, H. R., HITCHINGS, G. H., AND ELION, G. D.: Effects of Xanthine Oxidase Inhibitor on Clinical Manifestations and Purine Metabolism in Gout. Amer. Jour of Int. Med. Ann. Int. Med., 60:717, 1964.

V. SCHOPF, E. M.: Gout in a Five-weeks-old Infant: Klin. Wschr., 9:2148, 1930.

SEIDENSTEIN, H.: Acute Pain in the Wrist and Hand Associated with Calcific Deposits. J. Bone Jt. Surg., 32-A:413, 1950.

SELYE, H., GOLDIE, I., AND STREBEL, R.: Calciphylaxis in Relation to Calcification in Periarticular Tissue. Clin. Orth. 28:181, 1963.

STEFANIN, M., BRODERICK, T. F. JR., GOBB, F., AND WHITE, M. T.: Corrective Orthopaedic Procedure in a Severe Hemophiliac. Lancet, 1:1016, 1959.

SYDENHAM, T.: The Whole Works of that Excellent Practical Physician, Dr. Thomas Sydenham, 7th Ed., London: Feales, 1717.

TALBOT, J. H.: Gout. 2nd Ed., New York, Grune & Stratton, 1964.

TENGBERG, J. E., RAMGEN, O., AND PLENGIER, L.: Hemophilic Arthropathy. Acta Phenum. Scand., 6:135, 1960.

THIBODEAU, A. A. AND MALOY, J. K.: Bone Changes in the Blood Dyscrasias. Clin. Orth., 7:136, 1956.

THOMAS, M. D.: Some Orthopaedic Findings in 98 Cases of Hemophilia. J. Bone Jt. Surg., 18: 140, 1936.

TS'AI-FAN YU, AND SUTMAN, ALEXANDER, A. B.: Effect of Allopurinol on Serum and Urinary Uric Acid in Primary and Secondary Gout. Amer. J. Med., 37:833 (Dec.) 1964.

WEBB, J. G., AND DIXON, A. ST. J.: Haemophilia and Hemophilic Arthropathy an Historical Review and a Clinical Study of 42 Cases. Ann. Rheum. Dis., 19:143, 1960.

WEBER, H.: Sklerodermie, Korresp. bl. Schweiz Arz., 20:623, 1878.

=17=

Neurologic Diseases of the Foot

PAUL H. CURTISS, M.D.

Many of the neurologic problems and diseases involving the foot represent primary pathologic involvement of the terminal portions of the peripheral nerves, while others have their origin in the central nervous system. In clinical problems involving neurologic disturbances in the foot, it is necessary to determine whether the origin of the problem is of a mechanical, metabolic, primarily neurologic or post-traumatic nature. A thorough knowledge of the neurologic anatomy of the foot is essential for accuracy of diagnosis.

The dorsum of the lower leg and foot is supplied by the common peroneal nerve (Fig. 17-1A) through its division into the superficial peroneal (musculocutaneous) and deep peroneal (anterior tibial) nerve (Fig. 17-1B). The posterior and plantar aspects of the foot are supplied through the posterior tibial nerve (Fig. 17-2) which below the medial malleolus breaks up into the major terminal medial plantar, lateral plantar, and calcaneal branches. Additional nerves (of entirely sensory function) are the saphenous branch of the femoral nerve to the medial aspect of the calf and longitudinal arch, and the sural (external saphenous) branch of the tibial nerve to the lateral aspect of the foot and the fourth and fifth toes (Fig. 17-2).

Involvement of these peripheral nerves either by acute trauma or by chronic entrapment syndromes has been described. The following are the most commonly observed localized primary neurologic syndromes encountered in the foot.

INTERDIGITAL NEUROMA

In 1876 T. G. Morton introduced the term "metatarsalgia," believing the symptoms of this disorder to be neurologic in origin, due to pressure of the metatarsal heads on the interdigital nerves. In 1940, Betts pointed out the frequency with which the lateral branch of the medial plantar nerve is involved in a so-called neuroma with symptoms in the third and fourth toes. Although a primary arterial change leading

361

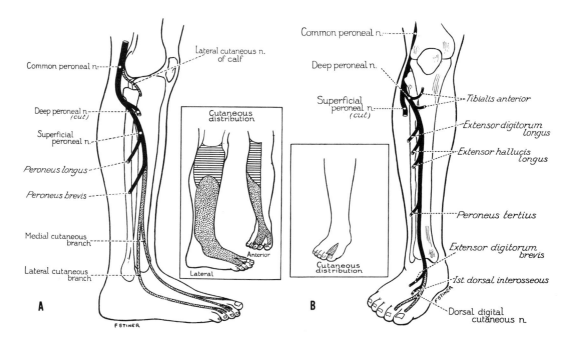

Fig. 17-1. A. Common peroneal nerve with peripheral distribution of the superficial peroneal nerve.

B. Peripheral distribution of the deep peroneal nerve. (Haymaker and Woodhall, Peripheral Nerve Injuries, courtesy of W. B. Saunders Co.)

to ischemic nerve changes has been postulated along with fibrosis and thickening of the nerve at the level of the bifurcation, some investigators have suggested that the primary factor is pinching of the digital neurovascular bundle between the metatarsal heads, causing the damage to the interdigital vessels and fibroneuromatous formation.

An additional factor stems from passage of the interdigital nerve from the sole of the foot dorsalward beneath the deep transverse metatarsal ligament between the metatarsal heads (Fig. 17-3). Forced extension of the toes, such as is encountered in the continued use of high heels, or from a chronically hyperextended metatarsophalangeal joint as is seen in claw toes, will angulate the nerve or the ligament. This is not infrequently found in association with other abnormalities of the foot, such as hallux valgus and in the common partial syndactylism between the second and third toes. A working posture which causes prolonged hyperextension at the metatarsophalangeal joint, such as a carpet layer who

habitually works in a squatting position, is a predisposing cause.

In any event, it is now generally recognized that the lesion is not limited to the nerve to the third and fourth toes but is found between other toes as well.

The development of an interdigital neuroma is accompanied by the appearance of sharp pain between the involved toes, occurring first with activity, but later often present at rest as well. Occasionally there is atypical radiation of the pain, a neuroma between the second and third toes most frequently causing the discomfort that is felt more proximally. A typical feature of such a history is the relief of pain obtained by the patient when he removes the shoe and massages the foot.

On examination there may be found a disturbance of sensation, usually hyperesthesia along the adjacent sides of the involved toes. The most common symptom, however, is localized tenderness between the metatarsal heads, most easily palpated from the pantar surface. Such tenderness

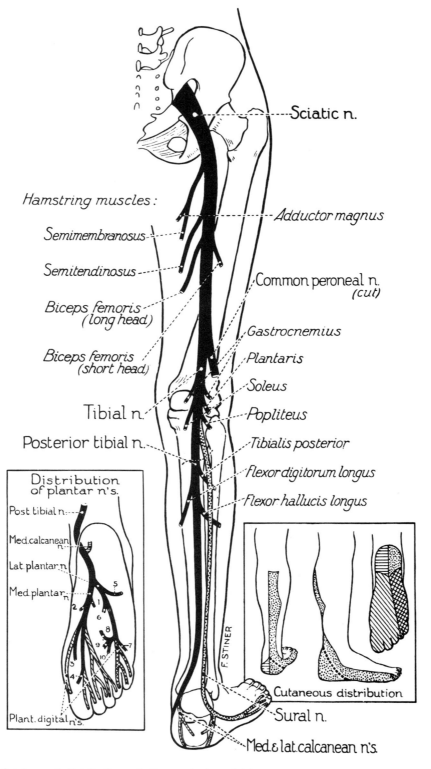

Sciatic n.

Hamstring muscles:
Semimembranosus
Semitendinosus
Biceps femoris (long head)
Biceps femoris (short head)
Tibial n.
Posterior tibial n.

Adductor magnus
Common peroneal n. (cut)
Gastrocnemius
Plantaris
Soleus
Popliteus
Tibialis posterior
Flexor digitorum longus
Flexor hallucis longus

Distribution of plantar n's.
Post tibial n.
Med. calcanean n.
Lat. plantar n.
Med. plantar n.
Plant. digital n's.

F. STINER

Cutaneous distribution
Sural n.
Med. & lat. calcanean n's.

Fig. 17-2. Origin and distribution of the posterior tibial nerve. Inset presents distribution of the plantar nerves. The sural nerve is also illustrated. (Haymaker and Woodhall, Peripheral Nerve Injuries, courtesy of W. B. Saunders Co.)

PLANTAR VIEW

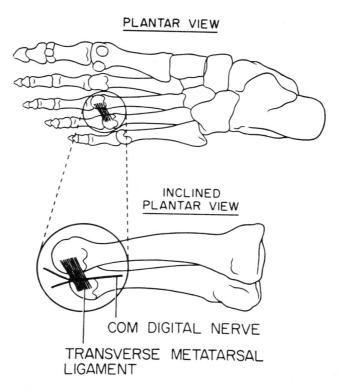

INCLINED
PLANTAR VIEW

COM DIGITAL NERVE

TRANSVERSE METATARSAL
LIGAMENT

Fig. 17-3. Diagrammatic sketch of transverse metatarsal ligament and the position of the inter-digital nerve in relation to the ligament. (Kopel and Thompson, Peripheral Entrapment Syndromes, courtesy of Williams and Wilkins Co.)

should not be confused with that which is commonly known as metatarsalgia and is located directly under the metatarsal heads on the plantar aspect of the foot. Occasionally a large interdigital neuroma may be palpated and found moving between the metatarsal heads on manipulation of the latter. Conservative treatment occasionally suffices. This is directed at increasing plantar flexion at the metatarsophalangeal joints by means of a metatarsal support. However, surgical excision of the neuroma is usually necessary either through a dorsal interdigital incision or a plantar incision. In either approach the neuromatous mass is resected as high as possible. It is recommended that at least 1 cm. of normal appearing nerve be resected both proximally and distally. Failure to do so can result in incarceration of the proximal nerve end in scar tissue or even the development of an

amputation neuroma. It is necessary to section the deep transverse metatarsal ligament in order to expose the mass as well as the proximal end of the nerve if the dorsal interdigital incision is used.

When the dorsal approach is used, a longitudinal incision is carried out, beginning in the web space and extending proximally between the metatarsal heads for 6 to 8 cm. (Fig. 17-4). The soft tissues are gently dissected until the transverse metatarsal ligament is exposed and sectioned. Retraction can be carried out by the insertion of a curved handle end of a small Hibbs retractor around the neck of each metatarsal to separate the heads. By applying pressure to the underlying tissues from the plantar aspect, the neuroma can be easily delivered into the wound. Both distal branches should be dissected free, as well as the main portion of the digital nerve,

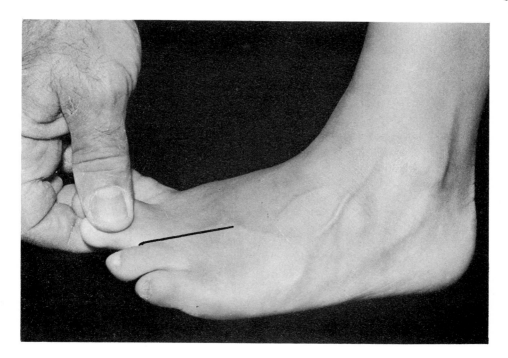

Fig. 17-4.   Location of dorsal incision beginning in web space and extending proximally to expose interdigital nerve and neuroma. The incision should extend at least 3 cm. proximal to the metatarsophalangeal joint.

for at least 1 cm. and all three should be sectioned. Repair of the ligament is not required. Following closure of the soft tissues, a firm pressure dressing (consisting of at least one roll of 6-inch sheet wadding and a snugly, but not tightly, applied ace bandage) will suffice to produce hemostasis. The patient is permitted to ambulate with crutches on the following day and weight bearing is permitted whenever the patient is comfortably able to do so. This is usually within five to seven days. The shoe should fit loosely and comfortably until the swelling has subsided.

When the plantar approach is used, the incision is performed transversely at least 1 cm. distal to the metatarsal heads, thus avoiding a scar on the weight-bearing surface of the foot. The plantar subcutaneous tissues are retracted posteriorly while the toes are simultaneously extended. The neuroma is exposed and excised. Closure and postoperative dressing are the same as in the previous procedure. The dorsal incision is the one used more frequently.

Occasionally, upon exposing the digital nerve, one will find no evidence of a neuroma. In spite of this, the digital nerve should be excised. In addition, there are rare occasions when the patient may have symptoms indicative of a neuroma in two interdigital spaces. Should this occur then both interdigital nerves should be excised.

MEDIAL AND LATERAL PLANTAR NERVES

Burning pain in the plantar aspect of the foot and toes may also indicate an entrapment neuropathy of the plantar nerves (Fig. 17-2-insert) as they each pass through the abductor hallucis muscle directly below the calcaneonavicular (spring) ligament.

Overpronation of the foot, or pressure exerted to flatten the longitudinal arch, may force the spring ligament against the nerves in their passage through the abductor hallucis. The role of such pressure on the calcaneal nerves in entities such as pes cavus, "painful heel", and acute foot strain has been suggested by Kopell and Thompson, but this theory has not yet been confirmed. Treatment is directed toward correction of the abnormal foot mechanics. Occasionally, the injection of steroids in the tender area on the medioplantar aspect of the foot may help to relieve the symptomatology. Should conservative therapy fail, then exposure of the spring ligament through a medial plantar incision and transverse sectioning of this structure will relieve the pressure on the nerves and thus the symptomatology.

THE TARSAL TUNNEL SYNDROME

Entrapment neuropathy of the posterior tibial nerve can occur as the nerve passes through the osseofibrous tunnel between the laciniate ligament and the medial malleolus (Fig. 17-5). The most common cause for irritation at this point is a fracture or a dislocation involving the talus, calcaneus or medial malleolus. Persistent edema following trauma in this area or delayed post-traumatic effects, such as tenosynovitis of the adjacent tendons, may exert sufficient pressure on the posterior tibial nerve at this point to produce symptoms. There may occasionally be no history of previous trauma. Burning pain involving the plantar surface of the toes and the sole is characteristic; the pain is also felt at the heel if the calcaneal divisions are involved. In severe

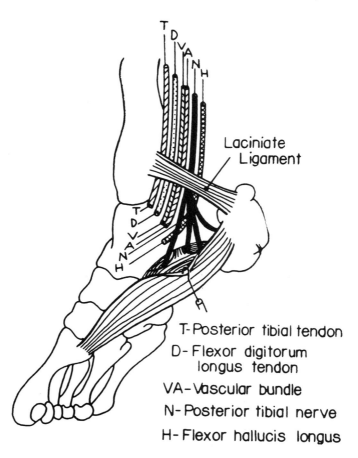

Laciniate Ligament

T - Posterior tibial tendon
D - Flexor digitorum longus tendon
VA - Vascular bundle
N - Posterior tibial nerve
H - Flexor hallucis longus

Fig. 17-5. The "Tarsal Tunnel". Note arrangement of structures beneath the laciniate ligament. The posterior tibial nerve can be easily trapped particularly following an ankle fracture with excess callus formation or any other space-occupying cause in this area.

cases there may be hyperesthesia in the area supplied by these nerves and local pressure over the nerve may reproduce or heighten the symptoms. There may be nerve trunk tenderness, proximal and distal to the point of compression (the Valleix phenomenon). Treatment is directed to correction of abnormal foot mechanics, the injection of steroids in the area below the laciniate ligament, or finally surgical unroofing of the tarsal tunnel.

OTHER NERVE ENTRAPMENT SYNDROMES

The principal site of involvement of the deep peroneal (anterior tibial) nerve (Fig. 17-1B) is primarily the dorsum of the foot in its terminal portion. Because of the subcutaneous position of the nerve where it lies on bone, trauma in this area may result from the mere dropping of an object onto the foot, or the entrapment syndrome of the terminal medial branch may occur as the nerve passes under the tendon of the extensor hallucis brevis and pierces the deep fascia, producing sensory disturbance of the apposing surfaces of the skin between the large and second toes. Evidence of motor involvement of the extensor digitorum brevis indicates injury to the lateral terminal branch.

Involvement of the superficial peroneal nerve (musculocutaneous nerve) (Fig. 17-1A) has been called by Henry "mononeuralgia in the superficial peroneal nerve". The site of entrapment is that point where the two terminal sensory branches of this nerve pass through the deep fascia near the junction of the middle and distal thirds of the leg. The nerve is made more vulnerable by its proximal fixation at the fibular neck and its distal fixation to the subcutaneous tissue. A single or repeated trauma, as from continuous wearing of a high boot, or an inversion and forced plantar flexion injury of the ankle and foot, may be the initiating mechanism producing the injury to the foot. If local infiltration or incision of the deep fascia does not obtain relief, resection of the nerve is the final solution.

The common peroneal nerve (Fig. 17-1A and B) is particularly vulnerable to injury at its point of passage through the peroneus longus muscle around the neck of the fibula. A blow or pressure from a plaster cast may be a source of injury. Quite frequently, such an injury will result in the development of a drop-foot within a matter of six to twelve hours if it is due to a blow. Numbness and inability to extend the toes will develop almost over night if the drop-foot deformity develops after the application of a cast which may inadvertently apply pressure over the head of the fibula and, therefore, the common peroneal nerve as well. The pressure should be relieved immediately; in the former instance by incision and release of the nerve as well as careful inspection; in the latter case by removal of the cast over the afflicted area. In either event, a drop-foot will result. The patient should be fitted with a drop-foot spring brace to prevent the flexion of the foot beyond the neutral position. Nerve function and, concomitantly, muscle power will return within three to six months. If the symptoms due to pressure on the common peroneal nerve are not recognized for forty-eight hours or more after their onset, immediate exploration is indicated. At best, the prognosis for complete recovery in such an instance is guarded or poor.

Kopell and Thompson have presented evidence that a "sudden strong inversion or plantar inversion force applied to the foot and ankle" also is a frequent source of common peroneal neuropathy. The symptoms are pain on the lateral surface of the leg and foot accompanied by typical radiation on pressure over the subcutaneous common peroneal nerve at the neck of the fibula. There may be present motor weakness or paralysis of the musculature supplied by the involved nerve. Usually, measures designed to correct malposition of the foot, such as a lateral sole wedge to maintain eversion, will afford sufficient relief. If conservative measures fail to relieve the symptoms within four to six weeks, surgical exploration and release are indicated for any points of pressure on the nerve in its passage around the neck of the fibula and through the peroneus longus muscle.

The saphenous nerve, the purely sensory termination of the femoral nerve supplying the medial aspect of the foot and longitudinal arch, may be the cause of pain felt over the medial aspect of the knee, calf and medial side of the foot. If local injection does not provide relief, the indication may call for surgical release of the most common point of entrapment at the saphenous opening in the subsartorial fascia.

NEUROTROPHIC ARTHROPATHY (CHARCOT JOINT)

This affliction of the joints is a form of chronic progressive degeneration arthropathy which may involve any joint and primarily the weight-bearing articulations. The relationship between the specific disease of the central nervous system and a destructive lesion of the weight-bearing joint was first described in 1831. It was not until thirty-seven years later, in 1868, that Charcot wrote his classic description of the joint changes associated with tabes dorsalis and hence the name "Charcot Joint". In 1875 Weir Mitchell described a similar condition associated with myelitis. In 1892 the development of neurotrophic joints due to syringomygelia was first described.

The classic paper of Charcot's described two forms of lesions associated with disease of the brain and the spinal cord. The first, seen in locomotor ataxia, consisted of a sudden onset of swelling in the absence of fever, and redness and pain with excessive mobility of the joint. The second form affected the joints of paralyzed limbs in hemiplegia of cerebral origin accompanied by severe pain on movement. Both researchers, Charcot and Weir Mitchell, believed that the destruction of the joint was due to repeated trauma to the insensitive articulation. This view received experimental support in 1917, when Eleosser showed that denervation of the joint alone is not sufficient to produce this effect but must be accompanied by trauma. Cassagrande, Austin, and Indeck demonstrated that not only must there be a loss of pain sensation to produce a Charcot joint, in addition to continued use of the joint, but there must also be a loss of proprioception. What has not yet been explained, however, is why a single joint in an extremity, except for the foot, will develop neuropathic arthropathy, while the other equally insensitive joints (proximal or distal to the involved one) will remain essentially normal. Any spinal cord, posterior root, or peripheral nerve lesion resulting in analgesia with loss of proprioception may lead to the development of neuropathic arthropathy in the foot and ankle. Some of the common causes of the neurotrophic joint are tabes dorsalis, diabetes mellitus, syringomyelia, alcoholism, myelomeningocele, spinal cord compression, peripheral nerve lesions, congenital absence of pain, and leprosy.

In a report of 55 patients seen at the New York Orthopaedic Hospital 15 had involvement of their feet. The disease progresses through three stages: 1) the state of dissolvement with debris formation, fragmentation, dislocation, and disruption; 2) the stage of coalescence with absorption of fine debris and the fusion of larger fragments; 3) the stage of reconstruction with attempt at reformation and increased sclerosis of the bone.

The usual initial complaint is painless swelling of the foot or ankle, but many investigators have stated that the complaint of pain is almost as frequent as the painless swelling. Instability becomes a problem when the joint destruction progresses. The onset of the condition is usually between the ages of thirty-five and sixty-five. Tabes dorsalis has been the most common cause of the development of Charcot joint and the symptoms of the joint involvement begin approximately twenty years after the onset of the infection. Actually, the arthritic symptoms may be the first sign of the neurologic disorder.

In the neuropathy of diabetes, the clinical findings are characterized by varying degrees of loss of the sensations of temperature, touch, vibration and position sense, as well as hyperesthesia or hypesthesia. In

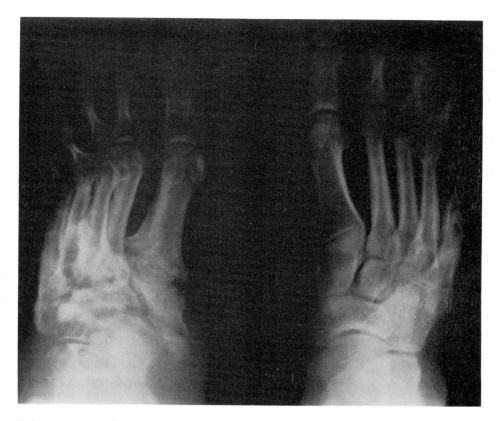

Fig. 17-6.   Charcot Joint — Note fragmentation of midtarsal joints with practically total disappearance of the navicular. Observe opposite foot for comparison.

addition there may be weakness of the musculature of the lower leg, particularly of the quadriceps and extensors of the ankle. Painless trophic ulcers may appear at pressure points, commonly on the plantar surface of the sole opposite the metatarsal heads. Many writers have noted paradoxically that arterial pulsations in the foot are usually present and adequate circulation appears to exist. The diabetes is usually under poor control, but neuropathy may occasionally occur in the patient under good control. Most reports agree that the smaller joints of the feet are those most frequently involved in diabetic neuropathy. It has been reported by Jacobs, that occasionally a milder bony lesion in diabetic neuropathy will undergo spontaneous regression and repair. This is not true of the neuropathic joints associated with tabes dorsalis or syringomyelia.

The roentgenograms of diabetic neuropathy (Fig. 17-6) will commonly reveal exaggerated osteoarthritic changes, with erosion of the joint cartilage, loose bodies, para-articular calcification and sclerosis. The amount of destruction is suprising in view of the lack of clinical symptoms and it furnishes a good clue to the diagnosis of a neurotrophic joint. The tarsal bones reveal a marked disorganization in the midtarsal and subtalar joints. A similar type of disorganization takes place in the metatarsophalangeal joints in diabetes mellitus, but not as much from the standpoint of developing debris as from the standpoint of dislocation of the joints, punched-out areas of destruction, and loss of the normal contours of the bony components of the toes.

Treatment.   The treatment of the Charcot joint, no matter what its etiology, has been far from satisfactory. The disease progresses rapidly to complete destruction of the joint or joints with instability or inability to ambulate. A common occurrence in the Charcot-type foot is the presence of the perforating ulcer, usually called "malum perforans pedis". The ulcer does not necessarily perforate the foot, but it is often associated with neurotrophic arthropathy of the metatarsophalangeal or interphalangeal joints and presents a very difficult problem from the standpoint of therapy. Early surgical treatment has been advised to obtain an arthrodesis of the tarsal and tarsometatarsal joints before the destruction is too marked. Fusion is not easy to obtain, but certainly should be attempted if possible. Infection is a frequent postoperative complication. At times, amputation of the foot may be necessary, but it should be avoided if possible. In all instances of anticipated surgery a careful evaluation of the foot should be performed. The surgical procedure should be conducted without the usual tourniquet and with adequate prophylaxis with broad spectrum antibiotics.

In the metatarsophalangeal area such surgery should consist of removal of the exostosis which may be producing ulcerations due to abnormal pressure, or the amputation of a particular digit if it interferes with ambulation. If the joint disorder is a result of diabetes, it goes without saying that the diabetic patient must be well controlled before, during, and after surgery. If the surgery contemplated is in the tar-

sometatarsal or tarsal area, one must keep in mind that all necrotic bone must be excised in order to procure an arthrodesis. Following this, a compression-type procedure should be attempted (a modification of Charnley's method) in order to gain union. Immobilization of the foot, ankle, and leg should be maintained for a prolonged period of time until fusion occurs. The usual time required for an arthrodesis of the tarsal bones does not apply in the Charcot-type joint.

In the small joints of the foot (the tarsometatarsal and metatarsophalangeal), one finds the destruction frequently associated with diabetes. A number of neurotrophic joints have been reported in this disease. A loss of vibratory sense and of proprioception occurs with decreased reflexes. The earliest sign is the painless swelling of the foot. The foot becomes enlarged and somewhat shortened with a flat everted appearance. The roentgenograms may reveal erosion of the joint surfaces, destruction of the joint, and extra-articular bone formation. Treatment in a mild and early case should consist of good control of the diabetes, administration of vitamin B complex and liver extract, and wearing of corrective shoes. Surgery should be employed only as a last resort.

CONGENITAL ANALGESIA

Charcot joints have been known to develop in an entity known as *Congenital absence of pain.* Ford and Wilkins in 1938 reported three children between the ages of seven and nine years who could not recognize any painful stimulus. The condition dated from birth and seemed to be permanent. The children had analgesia throughout the body with no other sensory loss except pain. In 1953 Petrie reported a woman who had a history of no pain and who, as an infant, had developed a painless swelling of the joints. The joints were similar to a Charcot-type joint and were due to trauma because of the loss of the protective effect of pain. Rose in 1953 also reported a case in a three-year-old child with an osteochondritis of the talus.

Differential Diagnosis. In the differen-

tial diagnosis between the Charcot-type joint and other diseases one must consider rheumatoid arthritis, since marked destruction of the foot may occur in rheumatoid arthritis leading to a severely flattened pronated foot. The destruction is due to synovial invasion of the bone with associated osteoporosis. The talus and the subtalar joints are often involved. The roentgenographic changes resemble a Charcot joint. However, pain sensation and proprioception are normal. At times, chronic osteomyelitis of the tarsal region can also simulate a Charcot joint in appearance. But here again the presence of normal pain sensation and proprioception, as well as the lack of other stigmata associated with the Charcot joint, help in making a differential diagnosis.

FOOT DEFORMITIES SECONDARY TO MUSCULAR IMBALANCE

There is another group of diseases which may be termed neuropathic in origin. They have in common the development of a similar form of foot deformity. The development of so-called pes cavus with a high arch and inversion of the foot may be seen either in its idiopathic variety, without evidence of neurologic disease, or also in Charcot-Marie-Tooth disease, Friedreich's ataxia, and spinal dysraphism (Fig. 17-7).

Charcot-Marie-Tooth disease (peroneal muscular atrophy) (Fig. 17-8) is a familial

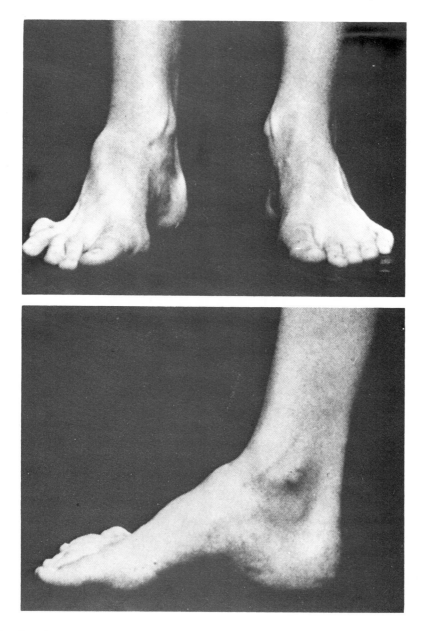

Fig. 17-7.   Pes Cavus — Note the high arch and the mild inversion of the rear foot. The deformity may be idiopathic or due to Charcot-Marie-Tooth disease, Spinal Dysraphism, Friedreich's ataxia, or following poliomyelitis. (Ferguson, Orthopedic Surgery in Infancy and Children, courtesy of Williams and Wilkins Company.)

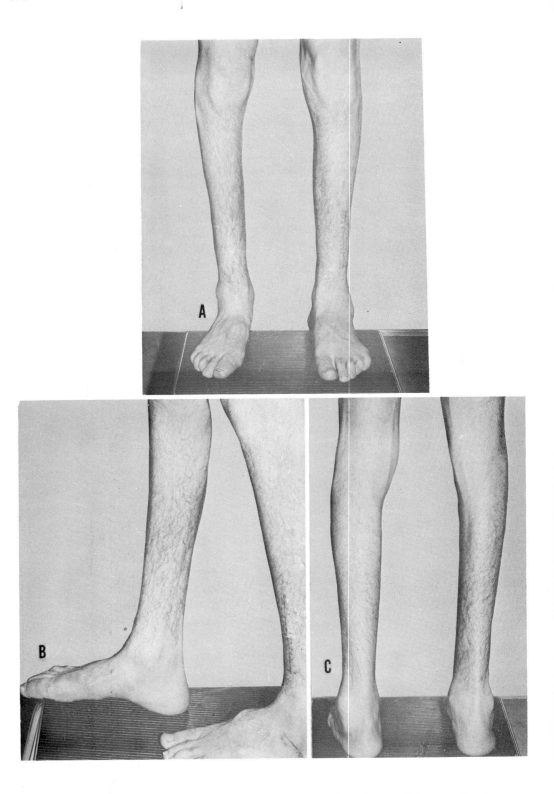

Fig. 17-8.   Charcot-Marie Tooth Disease. Note marked atrophy of musculature of the legs, particularly the triceps surae group. There is a mild cavus deformity of the feet.

disease in which a dominant or recessive hereditary pattern is frequently evident. The condition is understandably confused with other neuropathic and myopathic conditions such as progressive musculature atrophy, amyotrophic lateral sclerosis, and muscular dystrophy. Lucas and Forster have said that "Charcot-Marie-Tooth disease, spinocerebellar ataxia, and possibly muscular dystrophy are variants of a common and hereditary predisposition to neuromuscular degeneration, and mixed pictures, both clinically and pathologically, can be found." According to Dawson and Roberts, electromyographic studies are not characteristic but motor nerve conduction velocity studies are significant. The course of the disease is progressive, with weakness first occurring in the peroneal muscles and progressing distally to the anterior tibial and toe extensor muscles. Later the calf muscles may be affected. These combined muscle weaknesses produce a cavo-varus or a pes cavus deformity. Eventually there follows weakness of the intrinsic hand musculature with further progression proximally.

Another familial and hereditary disease, characterized by demyelination and gliosis of the posterior column of the cord, is *Friedreich's ataxia*. The most common deformity is a symmetrical clawfoot with marked elevation of the longitudinal arch, prominent metatarsal heads, widening of the fore part of the foot, and hyper-extension and clawing of the lesser toes (Fig. 17-9). This foot deformity is secondary to the development of muscle imbalance about the foot. The toes are held in their clawed position by over-active long extensor muscles. There is an associated muscle weakness most commonly of the peronei, either isolated or combined with varying degrees of paresis of the anterior tibial. In the "forme fruste" type of this condition, the one in which there is no progression of the disease, surgery is indicated if the feet are symptomatic. This is necessary because of the inability to fit the patient with comfortable shoes and of the presence of a disturbance in the gait since such a patient will present a mild drop-foot type of gait.

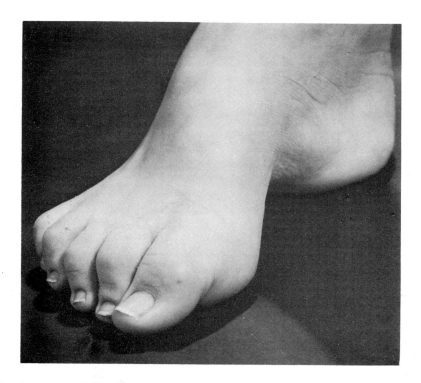

Fig. 17-9. Cavovarus deformity with clawing of toes as seen in Friedreich's ataxia.

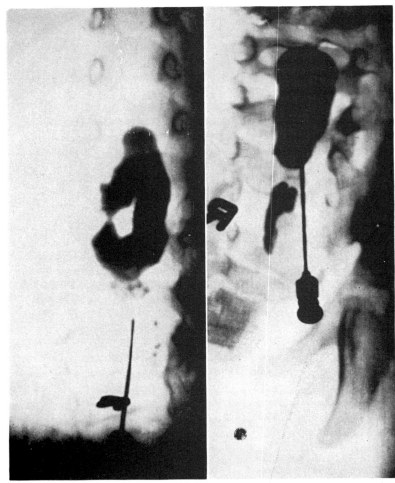

Fig. 17-10.   (Left) Distortion of pantopaque column due to intrathecal mass at the level of L2, L3. (Right) Distortion of pantopaque column due to adhesions on the left side, caudal end of the dural sac. (Giannestras, courtesy of Clinical Orthopedics.)

In patients under the age of twelve to fourteen at the most, the surgical procedure recommended is transplantation of the extensor hallucis longus to the first metatarsal neck with arthrodesis or tenodesis of the interphalangeal joint of the great toe, and transplantation of the lateral four toe extensor tendons to the neck of each of the lateral four metatarsals. Subcutaneous plantar fasciotomy is indicated in most instances. The tendons should be under fairly moderate tension when the foot is in the neutral position at the time of transplantation. The clawing of the lateral four toes will correct spontaneously providing they are placed in a position of complete extension in the cast. The cast should extend from the tips of the toes to the knee with the foot in maximum extension. Not only will there be an improvement in the appearance of the foot, but also in the gait. However, one must not expect an entirely normal gait-pattern to result from this surgery. Cast immobilization should be maintained for six weeks. Following this, active exercises of the extensor muscles should be carried out twice daily for as long as necessary in order to regain the maximum amount of muscle power (which, at best, will be fair to good, but never normal).

In the case of patients over the age of fourteen, tendon transplantation with plantar fasciotomy is insufficient. One must then perform a triple arthrodesis along with a plantar fasciotomy to correct the cavus or the cavo-varus deformity. This procedure is followed six weeks later by the transplantation of the tendons as described, in addition to tenodesis or arthrodesis of the interphalangeal joint of the great toe if the clawing of the toes is not corrected by the triple arthrodesis. Recently, proximal osteotomy of all five metatarsals with extension of the distal portions has been described. It is not recommended since the follow-up period has not been sufficiently long in the cases reported.

Another important cause of the development of pes cavus or cavo-varus deformity of the foot is *spinal dysraphism* or *myelodysplasia*. James and Lassman have emphasized their preference for the former term over that of myelodysplasia, as this latter term is too inclusive. They define spinal dysraphism as indicating a "common origin of the lesions from a failure of development in the mid-dorsal region of the spine and including abnormalities in the cutaneous, muscular, osseous, vascular, and neural tissues which may appear separately or together". The commonest manifestation is that of spina bifida. The commonest clinical picture is a child presenting with a slight cavo-varus deformity of one foot with the affected leg being somewhat shorter. There may be additional reflex changes and possibly trophic ulceration. Pain is rare and sensory changes are difficult to detect. Similar diagnostic problems are seen in cases of overt spina bifida with meningomyelocele, but in the occult form the entire process is slower, the speed of deterioration varying from case to case. The onset of the abnormality of the foot may be at any age, most commonly between four and six.

External cutaneous manifestations such as excess hair, nevus, sacral dimples or sacral lipoma, may help the diagnosis. It is important to note that in the earliest stage the lesion of the spinal cord seems to cause an increased neuromuscular irritability of the inverters of the foot so that they over-act, adducting the forefoot and elevating the arch. On clinical examination there is no detectable loss of power in any of the muscles of the leg and the foot, but as time passes the cavo-varus deformity develops.

The lesions affecting the spinal cord are extrinsic and may be classified as those causing traction or pressure. Traction lesions act by preventing the so called ascent of the spinal cord during the growth in length of the vertebral column. Among the causative factors may be an ectopic posterior nerve root, arachnoid adhesions, or an abnormally developed philum terminale. On the other hand, lesions causing pressure may be transverse bands of ligamentous origin, intrathecal lipomata, dermoid cysts, etc. Lesions may cause both traction and pressure, producing the above combination of equino-cavo-varus foot deformity with diminished or absent sensation.

Sarpyener in 1945 reported on congenital stricture of the spinal canal. In 1953 Giannestras reported a case of right equino-cavo-varus foot due to intrathecal compression and traction which did not respond to conservative therapy. In addition the right lower extremity was insensitive from the level of the supracondylar region of the thigh distalward and anesthetic on most of the dorsal as well as the entire plantar surface of the foot. Lumbar myelogram (Fig. 17-10) revealed the presence of an intrathecal mass at the L-2, L-3 level with adhesions on the left side at the caudal end of the dural sac.

On exploration the neurosurgeon found "a fatty myelinizing tumor measuring approximately 1.5 by 3 cm. and involving the second lumbar root on the right side. The nerve was deficient distal to this point. This small mass had crowded the remainder of the cauda equina to the opposite side of the canal, causing some compression. . . . . The lower end of the spinal canal was explored for other pathology suggested by the myelographic studies. On the left side at the caudal end of the dural sac, the nerve roots were found to adhere to the wall and somewhat to each other. These were freed without injury". Sensory power and temperature discrimination gradually reappeared in the major portion of the leg and foot, permitting subsequent surgical correction of the foot (Fig. 17-11).

One should also consider diastematomyelia in a differential diagnosis of spinal dysraphism. Diastematomyelia is a bifid state of

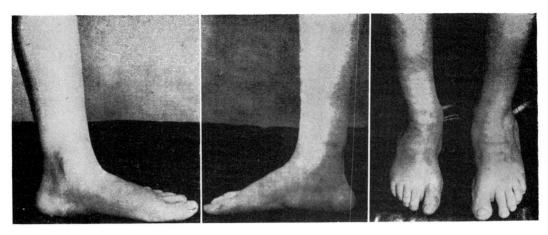

Fig. 17-11. Note appearance of right foot approximately three years after spinal surgery and corrective cast and tendon surgery subsequent to neurosurgical intervention. (Giannestras, courtesy of Clinical Orthop.)

the spinal cord. It is of developmental origin and there may or may not be a bony or cartilagenous septum passing dorsoventrally between the two halves of the spinal cord. This serves to anchor the spinal cord, causing a traction effect. Neurosurgical consultation should always be procured because in many such situations neurosurgical intervention can help to improve the orthopaedic surgeon's subsequent attempt to correct the foot problems.

REFLEX SYMPATHETIC DYSTROPHY

The syndrome of bone atrophy, pain, edema, muscle atrophy, and skin, nail, and hair changes following injury is known as *Sudeck's atrophy or acute reflex bone dystrophy*. Trauma secondary to accidental injury is perhaps the most common cause, there being no relation between the severity of the injury and the intensity, frequency or cause of the condition.

These cases appear to follow most often a minor injury to the areas well supplied with nerve endings, such as the hands and the feet. The upper extremity is involved much more frequently than the lower. Pain is the most prominent and characteristic feature, being at first localized to the site of injury, although with time it spreads and may affect the entire limb. Local hyperesthesia and disturbances of vasomotor function are common. There is an unusual feature common to all cases of acute bone dystrophy (Fig. 17-12); namely, the pain and physical signs usually do not conform to known patterns of nerve distribution, either peripheral or segmental. Further-

more, they have a tendency to spread proximally, involving the entire limb. Other than elimination of the causative factor whenever possible, the consensus is that the preferred treatment for acute bone dystrophy is interruption of the sympathetic nerve transmission by either analgesic block or sympathectomy.

A somewhat similar condition is known as causalgia. However, this is a more disabling potentially neurologic involvement of the foot. This pain syndrome is characterized by constant and usually severe burning pain which follows partial, or less often, complete injury of a peripheral nerve trunk. It is usually associated with parasthesia, hyperalgesia, vasomotor and sudomotor disturbances and trophic changes. The incidence of causalgia following peripheral nerve lesions ranges from 2 to 5 per cent. In the vast majority of cases the sciatic nerve is the one primarily involved in the lower extremity.

Causalgia is pre-eminently a result of penetrating wounds, usually due to high

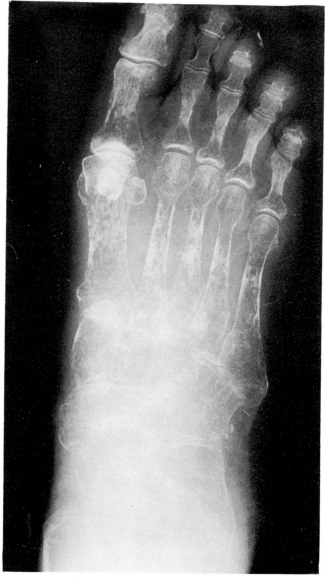

Fig. 17-12. Roentgenogram of foot resulting from severe reflex sympathetic dystrophy (Sudeck's atrophy). There is marked spotty decalcification of the entire foot. There are varying degrees of such spotty decalcification, this represents one of extreme degree following fracture of the ankle. Complete relief of symptoms by sympathectomy.

velocity missiles. It is seen most often during war-time. The onset of pain may immediately follow the injury or may be delayed for weeks or months. The "burning" quality of the pain is the most outstanding characteristic. Nevertheless, the absence of burning should not eliminate the possibility of this diagnosis since cases without this are not uncommon. The burning pain is usually felt superficially in the skin, combined with a deep aching, "tearing", or "crushing" pain. Hyperalgesia and hyperesthesia are almost always present as prominent symptoms. Because of the characteristic nature of the findings, differential diagnosis is not difficult in this instance if one adheres to the above definition. As in the more minor sympathetic dystrophies, treatment, which often proves disappointing, is directed at the sympathetic nervous system either by block therapy or by sympathectomy.

BIBLIOGRAPHY

ANTES, E. H.: Charcot Joint in Diabetes Mellitus, J.A.M.A., *156*:602 (Oct.) 1954.

BAMBERGER, E.: Uber Knochenveraenderungen bei Chronischen Lungen und Herzkrankheiten. Zschr. Klin. Med., *18*:193, 1891.

BETTS, L. O.: Morton's Metatarsalgia Neuritis of Fourth Digital Nerve. Med. J. Austr., *1*:514, 1940.

BURMAN, M. AND PERIS, W.: The Weight Stream in Charcot Disease of the Joints. The Cure of Perforating Ulcer of the Foot. Bull. Hosp. Joint Dis., *19*:31 (April) 1958.

CASSAGRANDE, P. A., AUSTIN, B. P. AND INDECK, W.: Denervation of the Ankle Joint. J. Bone Jt. Surg., *33A*:723, 1951.

CHARCOT, J. M.: Sur Quelques Arthropathies Qui Paressent Dependre D'Une Lesion Du Cereveau Ou De La Moelle Epinier. Arch:hys Norm. Pathol., *1*:161, 379, 1868.

CLASSEN, J. M.: Neurotrophic Arthropathy with Ulceration. Ann. Surg., *159*:891 (June) 1964.

DAWSON, C. W. AND ROBERTS, J: Charcot-Marie Tooth Disease. J.A.M.A., *188*:659, 1964.

DEGENHARDT, D. P. AND GOODWIN, M. A.: Neuropathic Joints in Diabetes. J. Bone Jt. Surg., *42B*:769, 1960.

EICHENHOLTZ, S. N.: Charcot Joints. J. Bone Jt. Surg., *44A*:1485, 1962.

ELOESSER, L.: On the Nature of Neuropathic Affections of the Joint. Ann. Surg., *66*:201, 1917.

FORD, F. R. AND WILKINS, L.: Congenital Universal Indifference to Pain. Bull. Johns Hopkins Hosp., *62*:448, 1938.

GIANNESTRAS, N. J.: Dural & Intradural Compression as a Cause of Club Foot Clin. Orth. *1*: 28-32, 1953.

HENRY, A. K.: *Extensile Exposure*. Baltimore, The Williams & Wilkins Co., 1963.

HURWITZ, D.: Management of Lesions of the Feet in Diabetes. Methods Recommended by the Diabetes Service at the Boston City Hospital. Diabetes, *4*:107 (Mar.-Apr.) 1955.

HURWITZ, D.: Management of Foot Lesions in the Elderly Diabetic. J. Amer. Geriat. Soc., *4*:648 (July) 1956.

JACOBS, J. E.: Observations of Neuropathic (Charcot) Joint Occurring in Diabetes Mellitus. J. Bone Jt. Surg., *54A*:1043, 1958.

JAMES, C. C. M. AND LASSMAN, L. P.: Spinal Dysraphism. The Diagnosis and Treatment of Progressive Lesions in Spina Bifida Occulta. Bone Jt. Surg., *44B*:828, 1962.

KECK, C.: The Tarsal Tunnel Syndrome. J. Bone Jt. Surg., *44A*:180, 1962.

KOPELL, H. P. AND THOMPSON, A. L.: *Peripheral Entrapment Neropathies*. Baltimore, The Williams & Wilkins Co., 1963

LAPIDUS, P. W.: Salicilic Acid Keratolysis in Neurotrophic Diabetic and Circulatory Ulcers of the Foot. Mal Perforant du Pied. Clin. Orth., *37*: 160, 1964.

LOWRIE, W. L., REDFERN, W., AND BRUSH, B. E.: The Diabetic Foot. Clin. Orth., *6*:173, 1955.

LUCAS, G. J. AND FORSTER, F. M.: Charcot-Marie Tooth Disease with Associated Myopathy. Neurology (Minneap) *12*:620, 1962.

MILLER, D. X. AND GILBERT, R. L.: Neurotrophic Ulcer of the Foot. Chicago Med. School Quart., *22*:69, Winter 1962.

MITCHELL, WEIR: Lectures on Diseases of the Nervous System., *19D*:204, 1875.

MORTON, T. G.: A Peculiar Affection of the Fourth Metatarsophalangeal Articulation. Amer. J. Med. Sci., *71*:37, 1876.

NAIDE, M. AND SCHNALL, C.: Bone Changes in Necrosis in Diabetes Mellitus. Differentiation of Neuropathic from Ischemic Necrosis. Arch. Int. Med., *107*:124 (Mar.) 1961.

NISSEN, K. I.: Plantar Digital Neuritis. J. Bone Jt. Surg., *30B*:84, 1948.

OAKLEY, W., CATTERALL, R. C. F., AND MENCER MARTIN, M.: Aetiology and Management of Lesions of the Feet in Diabetes. Brit. Med. J., *2*:953 (Oct.) 1956.

PETRIE, J. F.: A Case of Progressive Joint Disorders Caused by Insensitivity to Pain. J. Bone Jt. Surg., *35B*:299, 1953.

PIPER, C. A. AND MURPHY, T. O.: Care of the Diabetic Foot Rev. Surg., *21*:91 (Mar.-Apr.) 1964.

POST, H. J., GOODMAN, J. I., SILVER, A. G., AND FRANK, I. H.: Management of Diabetic Foot Lesions. Ohio State Med. J., *59*: (May) 1963.

ROBILLARD, R., GAGNON, P. A., AND ALARIE, R.: Diabetic Neuroarthropathy Report of 4 Cases. Canad. Med. Assn. J., *91*:795 (Oct.) 1964.

ROSE, G. K.: Arthropathy of the Ankle in Congenital Indifference to Pain. J. Bone Jt. Surg., *35B*:408, 1953.

SAMILSON, R. L., SANKARAN, B., BERSANI, F. A., AND SMITH, A. D.: Orthopedic Management of Neuropathic Joints. Arch. Surg., *78*:115, 1959.

SARPYENER, M. A.: Congenital Stricture of the Spinal Canal. J. Bone Jt. Surg., *27*:70, 1945.

SHEPPE, W. M.: Neuropathic (Charcot) Joints Occurring in Diabetes Mellitus. Diabetes, *8*:192, 1959.

SPENCER, F. C.: The Leriche Syndrome—Present Concepts of Diagnosis and Treatment. Med. Rec. Ann., *57*:8 (Aug.) 1964.

WHEELOCK, F. C., JR.: Transmetatarsal Amputations and Arterial Surgery in Diabetic Patients. New Engl. J. Med., *264*:316 (Feb.) 1961.

=18=

Fractures of the Foot

ALEXANDER GRACIA, M.D. and JAMES C. PARKES, M.D.

TREATMENT of the fractures of the foot can best be discussed by presenting a logical, thorough, and complete approach to the subject. With some fractures reduction and care do not present any particular problem. In others, such as fractures of the os calcis, no one type of reduction is considered standard. Furthermore, resulting disalignment subsequent to some fractures of the foot can produce a disability of major proportions since many such fractures occur more frequently in the wage earning, laboring class of patients.

Injuries to the foot are not nearly as common as those of the ankle. The most commonly injured bone, the os calcis, is fractured only one-tenth as often as the bones about the ankle. The talus is involved even less frequently; injuries to this bone comprise only 6 per cent of 4000 fractures of the foot, according to Coltart. However, the mechanisms of the injuries of the ankle and foot are related sufficiently to each other so that injury to one should always alert the physician to consider a possible associated injury to the other.

It is important to obtain a good history as to how the injury occurred, for in many instances the way in which the injury took place will give the examiner a lead as to what to look for in the physical and x-ray examinations. This will be brought out further when the various fractures are discussed as individual entities. It is important to question the patient with regard to his general health, since metabolic diseases, such as gout, diabetes, and circulatory insufficiency will affect the management of the fracture.

The physical examination should be carried out carefully and systematically. The foot should be inspected as to color, contour, and breaks in the skin. Palpation should be aimed at picking up points of tenderness, vascular status, crepitus, and conformation deformity noted on inspection. The importance of the circulatory status of the foot cannot be stressed strongly enough and it is, therefore, essential that palpation of the dorsalis pedis and the posterior tibial arteries be carried out in any fracture of any consequence in the foot.

Furthermore, the arterial pulsations of the involved foot should be checked against the normal one, since in an elderly individual absent pulsations do not necessarily mean severe circulatory involvement due to the fracture alone, but may be associated with the age of the patient. A check of the range of motion of the ankle, subtalar, midtarsal, and forefoot joints should also be a routine part of the examination of the injured foot. One should always use the unaffected foot for comparison, and the entire patient should be examined for associated injuries. Only if the examiner routinely carries out the above procedure on even the most obvious injuries will he become skilled at picking up numerous variations from the normal.

After a careful history has been taken and a thorough physical examination carried out, roentgenograms should be ordered. If a fracture is suspected, the involved foot should be splinted before the patient is sent to the Roentgenographic Department. If the examiner has obtained an adequate history and performed a satisfactory physical examination, he is often able to make a tentative diagnosis before the roentgenograms are procured, and he can use the latter as a confirmation of his clinical opinion. This avoids the necessity of unnecessary radiographs and needless manipulation of the injured part.

Certain views, however, should be taken routinely in every injury involving the foot. An anteroposterior view of the ankle mortise gives a good view of the articular surface of the talus and the lateral surface of the os calcis, since the cortex of the latter should not reach the inner surface of the fibula. A lateral view of the foot brings out all the tarsal bones quite satisfactorily. It is particularly helpful in evaluating calcaneal crush fractures and fractures of the head, neck, and body of the talus. Posteroanterior views of the heel are indispensable in fractures of the os calcis of any consequence or of any displacement. The dorsoplantar view or anteroposterior view of the foot brings out the intertarsal joints, i.e., calcanealcuboid, and talonavicular joints, tarsometatarsal joints, the metatarsophalangeal joints, as well as the metatarsals and the phalanges. Oblique views of the foot are particularly useful in visualizing the distal end of the os calcis and the calcaneocuboid joint, as well as separating the metatarsals from a lateral aspect point of view. These various projec-

tions can be further supplemented as necessary. Under the individual sections in this chapter, suggestions will be made when it may be appropriate to obtain these additional views.

For the purpose of clarity, the foot will be arbitrarily divided into three parts: the hindfoot, which includes the talus and the os calcis (calcaneus); the midfoot, which includes the navicular, cuboid, and cuneiform bones; and the forefoot, which includes the metatarsals and the phalanges. Each fracture and dislocation that occur in these areas will be discussed with respect to frequency, mechanism of injury, clinical and roentgenographic examinations, treatment, and prognosis. One must also keep in mind that in severe injuries of the foot, multiple fracture-dislocations can occur, both closed or open. A classification of these fractures is presented for convenience.

FRACTURES OF THE FOOT— CLASSIFICATION

I. Hindfoot (talus and calcaneus)
  A. Fracture of the os calcis
    1. *Extra-articular fractures*
      (a) Fracture of anterior process
      (b) Fracture of posterior process (tubercle)
      (c) Fracture of medial process of the tubercle
      (d) Fracture of lateral process of the tubercle
      (e) Fracture of sustentaculi tali with joint involvement
    2. *Intra-articular fracture*
      (a) Fracture of body with or without depression associated with joint involvement
    3. *Dislocations at talocalcaneal joint*
      (a) Dislocation with fracture of the os calcis
      (b) Dislocation without fracture of the os calcis
  B. Fracture of talus
    (a) Fracture of head
    (b) Fracture of body
    (c) Fracture of neck
    (d) Fracture involving articular surface (osteochondral fractures)
    (e) Fracture of posterior process
  C. Dislocations of talus
    (a) With fracture
    (b) Without fracture
II. Midfoot (navicular, cuboid, cuneiform)
  A. Fracture of navicular
    (a) Fracture of body
    (b) Fracture of tuberosity
    1. Fracture-dislocation of navicular

B. Cuboid
  1. Fracture of the body
  2. Dislocation involving calcaneocuboid and cuboid metatarsal joints
C. Cuneiform
  1. Fracture of body
  2. Dislocation involving the calcaneocuboid joints and metatarsal cuneiform joints
III. Forefoot (metatarsals, phalanges, sesamoids)

A. Metatarsals
  1. Fracture of shaft, neck, and head
  2. Dislocation involving the metatarsophalangeal and tarsometatarsal joints.
B. Phalanges
  1. Fracture of articular surface and/or shaft
  2. Dislocation involving the metatarsophalangeal joints and interphalangeal joints
C. Sesamoids

CALCANEUS (OS CALCIS)

Fractures of the calcaneus (os calcis) will be conveniently divided into the intra- and extra-articular types. (See classification.) The extra-articular fractures are usually accompanied by little, if any, disability, but the intra-articular ones very often require a prolonged convalescence varying from six months to a year. Frequently, in spite of excellent anatomical alignment of the fragments, permanent disability results because of the injury to the surrounding soft tissues, particularly those on the plantar aspect of the os calcis.

Extra-Articular Fractures of Calcaneus

Fractures of the Anterior Process. This is a rather uncommon injury which has no particular sex, age, or group preference. Most investigators feel that the injury is an avulsion-type fracture. As is well known, the bifurcate ligament connects the anterior process to both the cuboid and the navicular bones. When the foot is adducted and plantar-flexed (which is the mechanism responsible for this type of fracture), either the ligament must rupture, or if the ligament does not, then avulsion of the anterior process occurs.

Clinically the patient usually gives a history of having twisted the foot, but as a rule he is unable to recall in exactly which manner. He will complain of pain in the region of the sinus tarsi, at an area usually 1 cm. distal and 1 cm. inferior to the tip of the lateral malleolus. The amount of swelling which will be present over this area on the lateral aspect of the foot will depend upon the severity of the injury. Frequently such injuries are considered sprains of the calcaneocuboid joint and are often misdiagnosed since roentgenograms are not taken. They are only diagnosed when the pain persists, roentgenograms are procured, and the fracture demonstrated.

The roentgenograms, which are necessary to show this lesion, should be taken in the oblique as well as the lateral views. The fracture may or may not be displaced. A high index of suspicion is necessary as the undisplaced variety is often missed (Fig. 18-1).

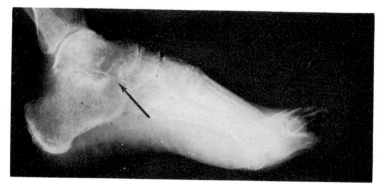

Fig. 18-1. Lateral x-ray of the foot showing fracture anterior process of os calcis.

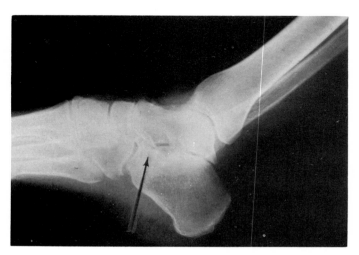

Fig. 18-2.   Lateral x-ray of the foot showing a healed anterior process fracture.

Treatment.   This injury should be treated initially as a sprained calcaneocuboid joint, *i.e.,* ice, elevation, ace bandaging, and crutches. However, the patient should be treated symptomatically, in that weight bearing should be permitted as soon as tolerated by the patient. In some individuals crutches may be required and occasionally, to procure the necessary comfort, a plaster cast can be applied extending from the tips of the toes to the tibial tubercle with the ankle in neutral position.

Prognosis.   In general, the prognosis is good (Fig. 18-2).

Fractures of the Posterior Process of the Tubercle.   The mechanism underlying this injury is the expression of an avulsion force which occurs when a patient falls or jumps from a height with his knees, as well as his feet, held in a position of extension. This results in the application of tension to the tendo achillis and instead of leading to a rupture of the tendo achillis, an avulsion-type fracture occurs. This is an uncommon injury and comprised only 1.02 per cent of the series of fractures reported by Rothberg.

Clinically the patient gives a history of having jumped or fallen from a height, landing with his feet in a flexed position and with the knees extended. The chief complaint is inability to walk and lack of forward thrust on the metatarsal region of the foot as the patient attempts to ambulate. From that standpoint, the limp which is vis-

ible in such a patient is similar to that which is seen with a patient who has suffered a rupture of the tendo achillis. On examination, flexion of the foot is poor and the patient ambulates with a calcaneal gait accompanied with a great deal of pain.

Roentgenographic evidence in the lateral view of the foot will reveal the fracture, which may or may not be displaced (Fig. 18-3).

Treatment.   If displaced, these fractures are best treated by open reduction and fixation of the fragments to the main body of the os calcis with either a screw or a wire

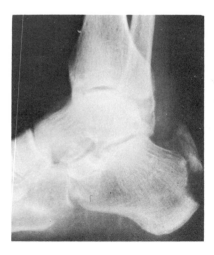

Fig. 18-3.   Lateral x-ray of the hindfoot showing a displaced posterior tuberosity fracture.

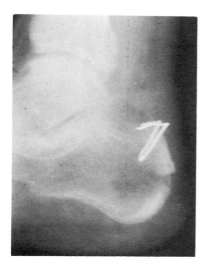

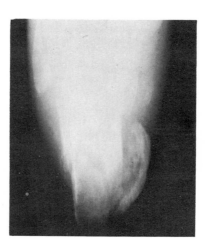

Fig. 18-4. Lateral x-ray of the foot showing a displaced posterior tuberosity fracture that had been wired to main body of the os calcis.

Fig. 18-5. Axial view of the os calcis demonstrating a fracture of the medial process as well as a fracture through the body.

(Fig. 18-4). The foot should be held in an equinus position for approximately four weeks and then for an additional four weeks in a neutral position in a plaster boot. Undisplaced fractures may be treated by immobilizing the foot in neutral position in plaster for a period of six weeks. During the period of immobilization no weight bearing is permitted.

Prognosis. In general the prognosis is excellent. Only 3 of 76 patients did poorly in a series of cases reported by Kleiger.

Fractures of the Medial or Lateral Process of the Tubercle. These injuries are uncommon and are usually secondary to an abduction or adduction force exerted when the patient's heel strikes the ground either in eversion (which will lead to a fracture of the medial process) or in inversion (which will lead to a fracture of the lateral process).

Clinically the patient will give a history of having fallen or jumped from a height, landing directly on his heel. The heel is usually swollen. Ecchymosis may or may not be present, depending upon how soon after the fracture the patient has been examined. Immediately following the injury there is little, if any, ecchymosis present, but within twenty-four hours it is quite prominent. Tenderness is localized usually on either the posteromedial or posterolateral surface of

the heel, depending upon the location of the fracture. There is also tenderness on the plantar aspect of the heel. Ranges of motion of the ankle and of the tarsal and metatarsal joints are within normal limits. There may be some restriction of motion in so far as extension of the foot and ankle is concerned, in view of the tension that is applied to the tendo achillis.

This fracture is best visualized by delineating the posterior aspect of the os calcis through an axial or posteroanterior view (Fig. 18-5).

Treatment. The foot should be elevated, and there should be applied ice and a pressure dressing consisting of the application of one roll of sheet wadding and a snug ace bandage. Motion should be instituted as early as pain will permit. If the fragment is grossly displaced, an attempt should be made to reduce this fracture by compression followed by the application of a well-padded cast firmly molded about the heel. As soon as the swelling has subsided, which usually takes place within seven to ten days, a new cast should be applied, again well molded about the heel. Immobilization should be continued for a total period of six weeks.

Prognosis. The prognosis in these patients is usually good. Non-union rarely, if ever, occurs. Should this take place, the fracture fragment can always be removed.

Linear Fracture of the Body without Involvement of the Talocalcaneal or Calcaneocuboid Joints. Fractures of the body of the os calcis are the most common ones which involve this bone. However, those which do not involve the articular surfaces are less common than those which implicate either the talocalcaneal or the calcaneocuboid articulations. The patient usually falls from a height, landing on his heel. However, the heel is usually in some inversion or eversion and, thus, the compression force of the talus against the calcaneus tends to be less direct, possibly explaining why these fractures are linear and not comminuted. Occasionally, the fracture will extend to the dorsal surface of the os calcis posterior to the articular surface and, even more rarely, there will be dorsal angulation of the posterior portion of the os calcis.

Clinically the patient complains of intense discomfort, pain, and inability to bear weight on the heel, accompanied with a minimal amount of swelling and ecchymosis —if he is evaluated within a matter of thirty minutes to one hour following the accident. After the elapse of an hour to an hour-and-a-half, swelling and extensive ecchymosis take place. There is limitation of extension as well as flexion of the foot due to the pain in the posterior aspect of the foot, and, of course, there is tenderness upon pressure over the heel.

Roentgenographically, this fracture is best visualized in the lateral view. However, it is wisest to procure a posteroanterior (axial view) roentgenograph of the os calcis to make certain that there is no involvement of the talocalcaneal joint. This latter view is of considerable prognostic significance.

Treatment. It is best to treat these patients initially with elevation, ice, and compression if there is no displacement of the fragments. If the fracture should extend to the dorsum of the os calcis posterior to the articular surface, and there should be marked displacement, it is best to insert a Kirschner wire into the posterior fragment and apply downward traction to realign and reduce this fracture. In such instances the Kirschner wire should be incorporated into the cast. The cast should extend from the tips of the toes to midthigh with the knee in 90 degrees flexion in order to relax the triceps surae muscle group. Casting should be carried out after the initial swelling and ecchymosis have subsided with the use of compression dressings, etc. If the fracture is undisplaced, then, of course, active motion is instituted at the end of a week, and although no cast is applied, no weight bearing is permitted. Physical therapy can also be prescribed. Weight bearing is permitted at the end of six to eight weeks, depending upon when the roentgenograms demonstrate healing.

Prognosis. The prognosis in this type of fracture is usually good as compared to those fractures which involve the articular surfaces of the talocalcaneal and calcaneocuboid joints. Even after the fracture is healed, the patient will complain of pain and discomfort of the heel for a period of several months. In addition, there will be a certain amount of swelling. It is considered advisable that the patient wear a heavy type of elastic stocking to control the edema which develops about the ankle and foot. We prefer to prescribe a high-top Bluecher shoe for the patient which fits well about the ankle and heel and supports the foot adequately. Patients who are receiving industrial compensation will, at times, claim to be partially disabled for as long as nine months. However, if the patient is advised that the prognosis in all instances is excellent and is encouraged to use the foot progressively more and more, the period of disability can be shortened.

Fracture of the Sustentaculi Tali. This is an extremely rare injury. The mechanism which produces this type of injury is unclear, but it is felt by some investigators that compression of the calcaneus by the talus, with the foot in extreme inversion, leads to this isolated fracture.

Clinically the patient usually gives a history of a fall in which he strikes his heel or of a twisting injury combined with the fall. On examination, subtalar motion is decreased and painful. The ankle is painless and motion of the ankle is normal. There is point tenderness on the medial aspect of the heel just below and posterior to the tip of the medial malleolus. This is accompanied, of course, with swelling and some ecchymotic discoloration in the area. Another clinical manifestation is that movement of the great toe can cause referred pain to the area of the sustentaculum tali since the flexor hallucis longus tendon passes beneath the sustentaculum to gain entrance into the sole of the foot.

The roentgenograms which best demonstrate this fracture are the axial views. Lateral views will not be of any value, although both views should be procured.

Treatment. The foot should be elevated, and ice bags and compression applied. When the swelling has decreased, a walking boot should be applied for a period of six to eight weeks. If non-union should occur, accompanied by persistent pain on the medial aspect of the os calcis at the level of the sustentaculum, and roentgenograms reveal the presence of non-union, the fragment can be very easily excised.

Prognosis. As in other extra-articular fractures of the os calcis, the prognosis is quite good in those few cases which have been reported.

By and large, therefore, extra-articular fractures of the os calcis do not present any particular difficulties from the standpoint of orthopaedic management. The main problem is that of early diagnosis in order that proper therapy may be instituted. Quite frequently, the symptoms, both objectively and subjectively, are such that one has the tendency to misdiagnose them as a sprain of the talocalcaneal area. It is, hence, advisable to procure roentgenographic evidence to prove or disprove the diagnosis of "sprain." The prognosis is almost invariably excellent when the correct diagnosis and the proper therapeutic regimen are established. The extra-articular fractures of the os calcis comprise only 25 per cent of the total number of fractures implicating this bone.

Intra-Articular Fractures of the Os Calcis

Intra-articular fractures of the os calcis comprise 60 per cent of all tarsal injuries according to Cave and 75 per cent of all fractures of the calcaneus. Thus, the reader can readily surmise that this will be the most common fracture which he will be required to treat. The history of this injury consists of a fall from a height, with the patient landing on his heel or heels in such a manner that the entire body weight is absorbed by the os calcis. Nor does the height of the fall have to be excessive. Patients have given a history of having fallen a distance of only 4 to 5 feet. Hence, it is obvious that the injury depends upon the location of the force of impact. Many of the investigators of this type of fracture hypothesize that the talus, particularly the lateral process, acts as a wedge against the superior articular surface of the os calcis. Superimpose upon this the weight and age of the person, as well as the distance of the fall, and the resulting fracture will present varying degrees of compression, comminution, and widening of the os calcis (Fig. 18-6). If there is sufficient deformity, the "tuber angle" (Fig. 18-7) will be reduced and the effective length of the triceps surae will be decreased. This may cause the patient to walk with a gait with little or no push-off.

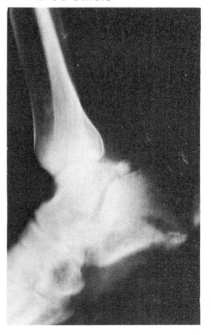

Fig. 18-6.   Lateral laminagram of the foot showing the lateral process of the talus acting as a wedge against the superior aspect of the os calcis. Also, one can see an os trigonum posterior to the talus.

If the comminution of the articular surface is severe, osteoarthritis of the subtalar joint often ensues at a later date. This may neces-

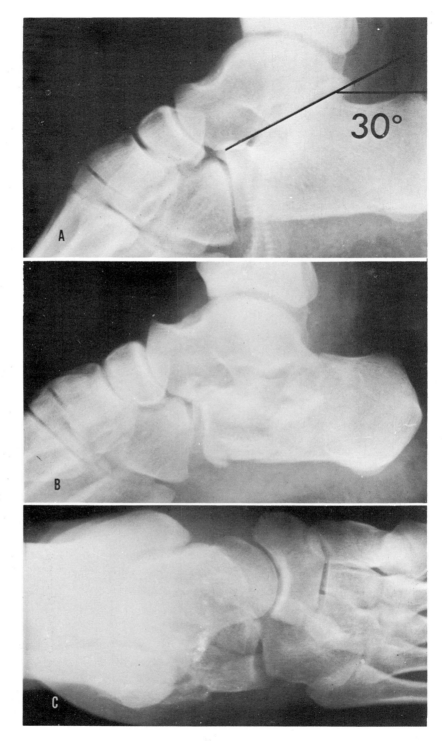

Fig. 18-7.   A.   Note normal "tuber angle".

   B.   Note obliteration of normal "tuber angle" following fracture of the body of the os calcis.

   C.   Note extension of fracture into the calcaneocuboid joint with loss of the normal articular surface of the os calcis.

sitate a triple arthrodesis if the pain is of sufficient intensity to produce disability. Widening of the bone causes lateral impingement of the fibula and consequent entrapping of the peroneal tendons. A stenosing tenosynovitis may supervene and may necessitate release of the peroneal tendons by splitting of the tendon sheaths.

The subjective symptom of such an injury is moderate to severe pain in the heel. Objectively, there is tenderness, swelling, and ecchymosis of the tissues surrounding the os calcis. Subtalar motion is painful and reduced. The normal contour of the hindfoot is usually distorted. Because of the usually violent nature of the injury, one should always look for associated problems. According to Cave, 10 per cent of these fractures are associated with compression fractures of the dorsolumbar spine and 26 per cent present associated injuries of the lower extremity (Fig. 18-8).

Roentgenographic examination should consist of the procurement of anteroposterior, lateral, and axial views of the hindfoot as well as an anteroposterior view of the ankle. These views will demonstrate the

os calcis to the best advantage. The anteroposterior and oblique views delineate the calcaneocuboid joint which is not infrequently disrupted. The lateral view is excellent for demonstrating the tuber angle, and the axial view will indicate whether or not the subtalar joint is involved by the fracture line. The anteroposterior view of the ankle joint is useful because if the lateral border of the os calcis extends to the tip of the lateral malleolus, it implies widening of the heel. Views of the ankle and dorsolumbar spine should always be included since associated injuries of these areas, as previously mentioned, are present in a significant number of cases. The views of the foot taken for the calcaneus are usually sufficient to rule out any associated injuries of other bones of the foot. This type of fracture can well be bilateral, and, therefore, it is always advisable to procure roentgenograms of both feet (Figs. 18-9 and 10).

Treatment. Opinions vary greatly as to how to treat this injury. This great variation of opinion is confusing to the physician who

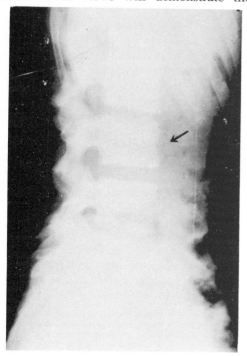

Fig. 18-8. Lateral x-ray of the lumbar spine showing a compression fracture of the 4th lumbar vertebra in association with an os calcis fracture.

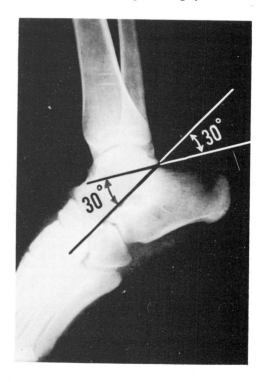

Fig. 18-9. Lateral x-ray of both feet in the same patient. The normal side has a tuber-joint angle of 30 degrees, whereas the fractured side has an angle of only 15 degrees.

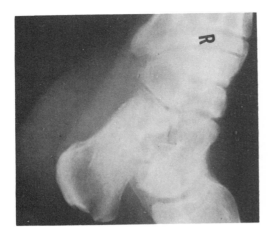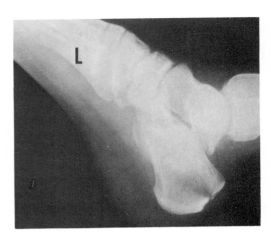

Fig. 18-10.   This patient had bilateral os calcis fractures. Always check the other foot.

must treat his patient. In truth there is no one way to treat these injuries. There are essentially three schools of thought regarding treatment of this disabling fracture. All three will be presented in detail.

Boehler, Herrman, and others feel that the loss of the tuber angle must be regained. If it is not, the patient's gait will be impaired after the fracture is healed, since he will have no push-off power. The first school, therefore, recommends that the tuber angle be re-established and the fracture be reduced by inserting a *threaded* Kirschner wire through the posterior tubercle of the os calcis followed by the application of traction to the os calcis. Counter-traction is procured by insertion of another *threaded* Kirschner wire through the upper end of the tibia below the level of the tibial tubercle. The knee is held in a position of 90 degrees flexion in order to relax the gastrocnemius portion of the triceps surae.

Following the application of traction and counter-traction in order to re-establish the tuber angle, lateral and medial compression are carried out by the application of a Boehler clamp under the medial and lateral melleoli to overcome the calcaneal widening. The use of traction and counter-traction not only re-establishes the tuber angle, but also separates the talocalcaneal surfaces and in a large number of instances

permits adequate reduction of the depressed superior articular surface of the os calcis. A plaster cast is then applied, extending from the tips of the toes to midthigh; the ankle is held in neutral position and the knee in 30 degrees flexion with incorporation of the threaded Kirschner wires in the cast. The cast should be carefully molded under the lateral and medial malleoli to obtain sufficient pressure and to minimize recurrence of the widening of the os calcis. However, the cast should be carefully padded to prevent the development of any pressure areas. This type of immobilization is continued for a period of four weeks. At the end of this time, sufficient organization of the callus has taken place to permit removal of the cast and the Kirschner wires. A new, snug-fitting cast is then applied from the tips of the toes to midthigh with the knee in 25 degrees flexion and the ankle in neutral position. The cast is again well molded under the lateral and the medial malleoli and immobilization is maintained for a period of at least another eight to ten weeks. The cast is then removed, and if the roentgenograms demonstrate adequate healing, active weight bearing is instituted, first with crutches. As the patient's ability to walk improves, the crutches are discarded. It is considered advisable that a steel arch support (preferably the Whitman type) be fitted in the shoe. The shoe should fit snugly to give the patient adequate support. The arch support should be specifically manufactured and fitted to the individual patient. The use of a prefabricated type of arch support is valueless.

On the other hand, the second school of opinion advises that reconstitution of the tuber angle is unnecessary and that therapy should consist of compression dressing along with daily whirlpool baths and active non-weight-bearing exercises. When the fracture demonstrates sufficient organization, partial weight bearing with crutches is instituted and subsequent full weight bearing when the fracture is healed. In fact, within two to three weeks after the injury, some proponents of this method permit the patient to bear weight in a snugly fitted shoe with a specifically and individually designed arch support fitted in the shoe. Proponents of this latter method of therapy claim that the period of temporary disability is appreciably shortened, the patient can return to work much earlier, and the percentage of permanent partial disability is less. Additionally, there is no more impairment of the push-off function of the foot than in the fracture in which the tuber angle has been re-established.

The third group advocates early or immediate open reduction. Palmer, several years ago, reported a series of cases of intra-articular fractures of the os calcis, comminuted in type, in which open reduction of the calcaneus was carried out through the lateral cortex of the os calcis. Reduction of the depressed fracture of the superior articular surface was performed by raising the articular surface into its previous position. A corticocancellous graft from the ilium was procured and this was inserted into the defect which had been created by elevating the articular surface from its original depressed position. Furthermore, by elevating the depressed fragment, Palmer claimed that the widening of the os calcis could be easily corrected. His results, as reported, were much better than either of the two previous methods of therapy. This technique was initially received enthusiastically in this country, but the end-results in the hands of other orthopaedic surgeons were not as good as those of the originator of this method. The period of immobilization in a plaster

cast following Palmer's method of therapy is from eight to ten weeks. Active weight bearing was permitted as soon as the fracture demonstrated adequate healing.

We feel that certain rules should be laid down for the treatment of this type of injury. To some the recommendations may seem dogmatic, but on the other hand, until the individual's experience increases, these precepts will be most helpful.

1) If the fracture is not severely comminuted, but the tuber angle is decreased and marked calcaneal widening is not present, closed reduction should be carried out. This is best achieved by the insertion of threaded Kirschner wires through the upper third of the calcaneal tubercle and through the tibia with the exertion of traction and counter traction. Some orthopaedists still use a Boehler clamp to reduce the widening of the os calcis, and some attempt to correct this widening by the application of medial and lateral compression with their hands. A plaster cast is then applied as previously described for this method of reduction. After the final cast has been removed, the patient should not only be fitted with an arch support as described, but also with a heavy elastic stocking to control the static edema which invariably develops. Active weight bearing and exercises of the foot and ankle are most essential for the early rehabilitation of the patient's foot. Pain will persist for a period of at least one year following the fracture episode. The orthopaedist should not be stampeded into performing any additional surgery during this twelve-month interval but should encourage the patient to continue exercising and walking.

2) If there is severe comminution, widening, and depression of the superior articular surface into the body of the os calcis, the injury is best treated with elevation, ice to both sides of the foot, and a firm compression dressing. After the swelling and ecchymosis have decreased (usually requiring eight to ten days), early active non-weight-bearing motion should be instituted for at least three times daily under the supervision of the physical therapist. Whirlpool baths twice daily should also be prescribed. Weight bearing should be permitted when the symptoms have subsided sufficiently to enable the patient to tolerate the pain —

initially on crutches, subsequently with a cane, and finally with no support. When weight bearing is instituted, the patient should be fitted with a snug, Bluecher-type shoe, an elastic stocking and an individually measured, Whitman steel arch support. The use of an arch support is of paramount importance. Again the patient should be placed under rehabilitative observation for a period of two years. As long as the patient is demonstrating progressive improvement, no matter how slow, triple arthrodesis, or for that matter any type of surgery, should *not* be considered during the first twelve to eighteen months following the injury. If at the end of two years the patient has reached a point of no further improvement, then surgical intervention should be considered.

3) Open reduction by either the Essex-Lopresti method or the Palmer method can be considered for those intra-articular fractures which are not too severely comminuted, with the tuber angle almost within normal limits (25 to 30 degrees), but in which the superior articular surface is depressed with or without comminution. The calcaneocuboid joint should not be involved.

The Palmer technique is as follows: Initially ice, elevation, and pressure are applied for a few days to control the hemorrhage and swelling. Under tourniquet control the lateral surface of the os calcis is exposed through a curvilinear incision beginning at the level of the sinus tarsi and curving inferiorly and posteriorly 2 cm. distal to the tip of the lateral malleolus. The peroneal tendons are retracted dorsally.

Four drill holes are made, outlining an oblong block of bone 1 by 2 cm., and with a fine, *sharp* osteotome the cortex is cut and a window is opened into the cancellous body of the calcaneus. A hemostat is imbedded gently into the cancellous tissue and a lateral roentgenogram is procured to determine the position of the window in relation to the superior articular fragments of the os calcis. A small Key periosteal elevator, 1 cm. wide, or a currette is then inserted and the articular surface is gently and carefully raised to its former position. Another lateral radiograph is procured to determine the position of the fragments. If the operator is satisfied with the position, he views or measures the size of the graft he will need to fill in the defect. A pressure dressing should be inserted into the defect and the tourniquet should be released. Pressure on the dressing should be applied by the assistant while the operator is procuring the proper size bone graft from the outer table of the ilium.

At this point the release of the tourniquet is considered necessary for the enhancement of the soft tissue healing when the incision is closed and the cast applied. Separation of the wound edges has been known to occur due to excessive cancellous bone bleeding. The graft is inserted into position to hold the articular surface in the desired place. The soft tissues are closed and a boot cast, extending up to the knee, is applied with the foot and ankle in neutral position and with the cast well molded under the medial and lateral malleoli. The average period of immobilization is eight weeks. Post-immobilization care is similar to that prescribed with the previous method. However, this same type of fracture can be treated with ice, elevation, and rest followed by early active motion and guarded weight bearing.

The Essex-Lopresti Technique. In order for the reader to understand this method of reduction, it is advisable that the Essex-Lopresti's basic concepts be presented first. He stated that, in essence, there are only two basic patterns of fractures involving the subtalar joint: (a) tongue fractures, and (b) joint depression fractures.

In the tongue type, the mechanism of injury is the result of the talus carrying the deforming force into the subtalar joint thus forcefully everting the posterior facet of the subtalar joint and driving the sharp spur of the talus inferiorly into the crucial angle of the os calcis. Such a force splits the calcaneus at the aforementioned angle, along with the lateral cortex of the body. If the force were minimal, no further deformity developed. With additional force, further deformity occurred, the ultimate being superior and then posterior displacement of the tuberosity with separation from the body of the os calcis as the primary fracture lines opens up inferiorly.

In the joint depression type, the secondary line crosses the body immediately posterior to the joint carrying with it the lateral half of the subtalar joint. This frag-

ment is forced into the cancellous bone of
the calcaneal body immediately inside the
lateral cortex producing broadening of the
body of the os calcis commonly found with
crushing injuries of the subtalar joint.
When severe, the tuberosity is driven superiorly with loss of the tuber angle and
spreading of the primary fracture site.

Treatment, therefore, should consist of
reduction and internal fixation in as nearly
normal position as possible and with early
mobilization of the surrounding joints.
The reduction is as follows:

(1) Place the patient prone on the table.

(2) Make a small incision over the calcaneal tuberosity just lateral to the attachment of the tendo achillis.

(3) Introduce a heavy Steinman pin into the tongue fragment in a longitudinal
direction, angling slightly to the lateral
side.

(4) After roentgenographic determination of the position of the pin, flex the
knee, reduce the fracture by lifting upward
on the pin until the knee clears the table,
thus elevating the tongue fragment from
its depressed position.

(5) Reduce the lateral spreading by
compressing the os calcis with the heels of
the clasped hands and simultaneously rock-
ing the calcaneus in order to settle the
small comminuted fragments into position.

(6) Drive the pin across the fracture
into the anterior fragment of the os calcis.

(7) Apply a slipper type cast incorporating the protruding portion of the pin.

For the first two weeks, elevation and
supervised active exercises of the toes and
ankle, as well as the subtalar joint, is the
standard regimen of treatment. The cast
and pin are removed at the end of four
weeks and a short leg cast is applied extending from the tips of the toes to the
tibial tubercle with the foot in neutral
position. Usually, at the end of eight to
ten weeks, guarded weight bearing is permitted following roentgenographic confirmation of union.

Prognosis. Most people have found that
no matter how one treats these patients
initially, if there is significant comminution,
widening, and compression, only 50 per
cent eventually end up with either a good

or excellent result. Other investigators feel
that the percentage of good results is even
higher. This applies to any intra-articular
fracture, no matter how comminuted. Those
fractures which do not have significant comminution and widening, even though they
are intra-articular, tend to have a much better prognosis. Early motion and guarded
weight-bearing for the comminuted variety
give no better long-term results than those
treated by traction and casting. They do
tend, however, to allow the patient to leave
the hospital sooner, have fewer complications, and begin effective weight bearing at
an earlier date than with other methods of
treatment. In general, when possible, it is
better to avoid plaster immobilization in
patients over the age of fifty-five since
midfoot stiffness in these patients tends to
outweigh the anatomical results one might
get with the more vigorous and prolonged
methods of therapy.

If at the end of two years' time the patient
still complains of pain in the region of the
os calcis, the physician should determine
whether or not this pain is located in the
subtalar joint or whether it is due to entrapment of the peroneal tendons. Occasionally
excessive bone formation on the plantar
aspect of the os calcis may be the cause of
the symptomatology, or the pain can also be
due to injured septa in the heel pad. These
septa are ruptured at the time of impact
and are tender for a long period of time.
Occasionally, only one of the above reasons
are the cause for the pain. On the other
hand, there are times when more than one
of the areas are involved in the same patient.

If the cause of the symptomatology is due
to subtalar joint osteoarthrosis, the injection
into this articulation of 1 cc. of one of the
intra-articular steroids with 1 cc. of a 1 per
cent solution of a local anesthetic should
give temporary relief for a period of several
hours to several days. Triple arthrodesis is
the best method of coping with this problem. The subtalar arthrodesis as advocated
by Gallie and others may alleviate symptoms for a period of time, but the midtarsal
(talonavicular, and calcaneocuboid joints)
joints deteriorate due to the extra strain to
which they are subjected with the loss of
subtalar motion. Indeed, it is a rare calcaneal fracture in which the articular sur-

face, if involved, has full subtalar motion. The most satisfactory results are those in which spontaneous ankylosis occurs. The contributors of this chapter and the author do *not* recommend early subtalar anthrodesis.

If the pain is caused by stenosing tenosynovitis of the peroneal tendons due to compression by the lateral fragments, then it should be relieved temporarily by the instillation of a 1 per cent local anesthetic into the tendon sheath. When this occurs, permanent relief can then be obtained by splitting the tendon sheath, and removing any of the bone which impinges against the peroneal tendon.

Occasionally, the cause of pain resulting from a fracture of the os calcis is due to excessive bone formation on the plantar aspect of the heel. In such a situation, again, the tender area should be initially treated with the use of 1 cc. of one of the intraarticular steroids. If the injection should give only temporary relief, then excision of the excessive bone or exostosis should be performed.

A fourth cause of pain is due to injury of the septa in the heel pad. These are ruptured at the time of impact and remain tender for a long period of time. Such a problem is best managed by the manufacture and insertion of a heel pad similar to that used in the relief of symptomatology due to a calcaneal plantar spur.

Occasionally, in spite of all of these methods of therapy to solve the problem of pain in the heel, the symptoms will persist and the patient will continue to remain totally disabled. In such instances the use of selective sensory denervation of the painful heel may be considered. This consists of sectioning the sural nerve just above the level of the os calcis and of the three sensory branches from the posterior tibial nerve which constitute the sensory source of the skin of the heel and the medial aspect of the sole of the foot.

TALUS

The talus is the second most commonly injured tarsal bone. The mechanism of injury is usually the application to the foot of a sudden, forceful, extensive, dorsiflexion force, as when slamming on a brake to prevent an accident. These fractures were common during World War II when combat pilots would crash land with their planes.

Fracture of the Head. According to Pennal, this injury comprises approximately 10 per cent of the fractures and dislocations involving the talus. It is usually due to the effect of the impact of a fall on a completely extended (dorsi-flexed) foot. The talar head is compressed by the force transmitted from the forefoot to the navicular.

The patient gives a history of a fall and complains of pain over the talonavicular joint. Objectively, upon pressure, there is tenderness over the head of the talus and there is usually swelling and ecchymosis of the overlying soft tissues. Eversion and inversion provoke definite pain which is referred to the talonavicular area. Ankle motion is usually well preserved.

Roentgenographically, the fracture is best seen on the anteroposterior and lateral views of the foot. It is often comminuted, but seldom displaced since the fragments are held in place by the strong intertarsal ligaments of the foot.

Treatment. Initially the patient should be treated with ice, elevation, a firm compression-dressing of the foot, and rest, as well as the application of a posterior molded plaster splint. Several days after the swelling has decreased, a snug, below-the-knee, plaster walking-boot is applied. The fracture is immobilized for a period of from six to eight weeks, depending upon the severity of the comminution.

Prognosis. These fractures heal well and in general the prognosis is good. However, if the comminution is severe, there is pain subsequently due to the development of either an extensive chondromalacia involving the head of the talus, or osteoarthrosis involving the talonavicular joint. Should this occur, and should the symptoms be relieved by the use of intra-articular steroids injected into the talonavicular joint, then arthrodesis of this articulation can be carried out. Some orthopaedists prefer to perform a triple arthrodesis.

Fracture of the Body. These fractures comprise 20 per cent of the injuries involving the talus. The mechanism, if the fracture is linear, is similar to that encountered in the talar neck-fractures — namely, excessive extension of the foot and ankle. Comminution also implies that, in addition to extension, a significant compression force was exerted.

On examination the patient will usually give a history of an accident in which the foot was acutely extended. He complains of pain in the region of the ankle-joint and unless the joint capsule surrounding the talus is ruptured, there is intense pain present. On examination there is marked tenderness and swelling (most noticeable over the anterior aspect of the ankle mortise). Ankle motion will be extremely painful, and since this fracture involves the subtalar joint, inversion and eversion will also provoke pain. The force required to produce such an injury is great and, therefore, it is not uncommon to find subtalar dislocation and open wounds communicating with the fracture.

Treatment. The undisplaced linear fractures are best treated with non-weight bearing with a snug below-the-knee cast for a period of six to eight weeks. However, in the displaced fractures where closed reduction is unsuccessful, open reduction should be performed. Following reduction, the foot should be placed in a position of acute flexion in a cast extending from the toes to above the knee, with the knee in 25 degrees of flexion for a period of four weeks. A new cast is then applied with the foot in neutral position for an additional four weeks. No weight bearing is permitted. When the second cast is removed, roentgenographs should be procured to establish whether or not avascular necrosis is present. If avascular necrosis is radiographically apparent, and the fracture is in a patient under the age of sixteen, continued non-weight bearing should be carried out until the body of the talus revascularizes itself. On the average this usually requires nine to twelve months. In an adult, however, the period of revascularization is much longer and usually, in spite of revascularization, the patient will continue to complain of pain and disability of

the ankle joint. In such instances, quite frequently a pantalar arthrodesis is necessary.

In the severely comminuted fractures of the body of the talus in the adult, pantalar arthrodesis should be considered as a primary treatment if the patient's condition is sufficiently stable, the injury is fresh, and the fracture is closed. If the fracture is open, then after reduction, the wound should be left open to heal by secondary intention. Tetanus toxoid and antibiotics should be administered. A posterior plaster of paris splint should be applied extending from the toes to the midthigh with the ankle at neutral position and the knee in 25 degrees flexion.

When the problem of infection has been well controlled and there is no evidence of any drainage for a period of at least six months, surgery consisting of pantalar arthrodesis can then be carried out. In old injuries in which the soft parts are swollen and devitalized, the ideal therapy consists of elevation, and application of splint for several days to determine the extent of the soft tissue damage before surgery is considered. To operate on devitalized tissues, not knowing the exact amount of involvement, invites disaster anywhere, particularly about the foot.

The development of avascular necrosis is due to several facts. The blood supply to the body of the talus is derived primarily from the medial capsule of the ankle where it attaches beneath the articular surface, as well as from the anterior capsule where it attaches to the superior surface of the neck and in the area of the sinus tarsi. According to Coltart, if more than two-thirds of the blood supply is interrupted, avascular necrosis is likely to occur. Therefore, the more posterior the fracture line is from the level of the head, the greater the hazard of avascular necrosis. Likewise, if the fracture is associated with subtalar dislocation, more than 80 per cent of such patients will develop an avascular necrosis of the talus. Comminution or displacement that is not accurately reduced will lead to mechanical incongruity of the ankle and the subtalar joint, thus inducing traumatic osteoarthrosis and resulting in pantalar arthrodesis as well. Therefore, it is necessary that anatomical

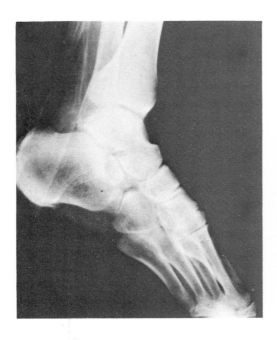

Fig. 18-11. This lateral x-ray of the foot reveals an undisplaced fracture of the talar neck.

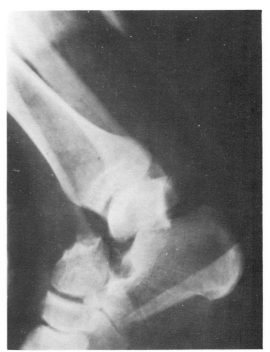

Fig. 18-12. This lateral of the hindfoot demonstrates a displaced fracture of the talar neck associated with posterior subluxation of the body.

alignment of the fragments be procured in all instances. At best the prognosis of such a fracture is only fair.

Fracture of the Neck. In Pennal's series of fractures of the talus, the fracture of the neck comprised approximately 30 per cent. The basic cause is excessive extension, that is, when the ankle joint reaches its maximum range of extension, the talar neck is brought into contact with the anterior lip of the tibia. Further motion in this direction leads to fracture of the talar neck. If the force stops at this level, the fracture will remain undisplaced. However, if the extension force continues, separation of the fracture fragments takes place. Upon cessation of the extension force, there is posterior displacement of body of the talus due to spasm of the strong plantar flexors, secondary to the injury.

On examination the patient usually gives a history of a serious accident. He will complain of pain in the foot and in the ankle. There is swelling and loss of the normal bony contours of the foot at the level of the ankle joint. Frequently, the injury

is open in type, and occasionally, the proximal talar fragment may be lost from the wound. If the proximal fragment is dislocated, it may be felt posterior to the lateral malleolus and the skin in this area will either be broken or will be under great tension. Motion of the foot in any direction produces pain.

Lateral roentgenographic views of the foot delineate the fracture line quite satisfactorily. The fracture may be displaced or undisplaced. The proximal fragment is often subluxated or occasionally, dislocated posteromedially (Figs. 18-11, 12 and 13).

Treatment. If the fracture is undisplaced, the foot is immobilized in a below-the-knee cast with the ankle in neutral position for eight weeks. At the end of this time the cast is removed and roentgenograms are procured. If there is no sign of avascular necrosis, and the fracture is healed, weight bearing is permitted as tolerated.

However, the presence of avascular necrosis will necessitate the continuation of non-weight bearing until the talus shows signs of reconstitution. In the adult this may take as long as two years. In patients under the age of sixteen, the period of reconstitution is shorter. The general consensus is that in order to avoid this long period of disability, treatment in the adult should consist of pantalar arthrodesis as soon as a diagnosis of avascular necrosis is made. It is well recognized that with a pantalar arthrodesis one will lose almost 90 per cent of the motion in the ankle and foot. On the other hand, there is no guarantee that there will be a normally functioning ankle or subtalar joint after the body of the talus reconstitutes and revascularizes itself. If the fracture is displaced, closed reduction should, of course, be attempted under general anesthesia with complete relaxation. If the reduction is successful, the foot should be held in a position of flexion for four weeks, with the cast extending from the toes to above the knee. The cast should then be removed and a new one applied for a period of another eight weeks, with the ankle in neutral position extending from the toes to the knee. Following this period of immobilization in the neutral position, the cast should be removed, and roentgenograms procured to determine what future therapy will be necessary.

Failure of closed reduction necessitates open reduction and fixation of the fracture fragments with the use of crossed, thread-ed, Kirschner wires. The foot is then held in a neutral position for a period of eight to twelve weeks and thereafter treated in a manner similar to that employed with the undisplaced type of fracture. If the proximal fragment is dislocated, prompt, accurate reduction is indicated, followed by the same management as for the undisplaced fracture.

This is one type of fracture in which delay should not be permitted. If the fracture is seen soon after the initial injury, usually closed reduction can be performed. If a delay of from three to five hours ensues, then it is well nigh impossible to effect a closed reduction. When displacement and dislocation occur, open reduction is necessary. If an open injury takes place and the talus is contaminated, debridement must, of necessity, be carefully carried out. The talus should be reduced and left *in situ*. After primary healing of the soft tissues has taken place, pantalar arthrodesis will almost invariably be required.

Coltart advocates removal of the talus when it is contaminated and potentially infected, thus requiring its total excision. He found that 30 per cent of his patients did well without the talus, and the remainder required a talocalcaneal fusion for relief of the pain. It is our considered opinion that pantalar arthrodesis offers a better long-term functional result than astragalectomy. If possible, the talus should

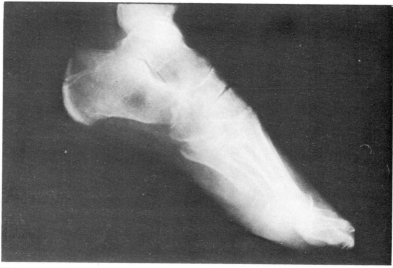

Fig. 18-13. This x-ray shows avascular necrosis of the body of the talus following a displaced talar neck fracture which had been reduced.

be retained and following thorough debridement and cleansing, the osseous structures and the soft tissues should be given the opportunity to heal under an adequate antibiotic "umbrella."

Prognosis. The prognosis for the undisplaced fracture is quite good. The displaced linear fracture without dislocation or subluxation of the proximal fragment carries a good prognosis in a considerable number of patients, if reduced accurately, held in proper position, and reduced practically immediately. However, if the proximal fragment is subluxated or dislocated, avascular necrosis results in between 80 to 100 per cent of the cases in whom such a complication occurs. The bulk of these require pantalar arthrodesis.

Fracture of the Articular Surface (Flake). Twenty-two per cent of the injuries in Pennal's series represented this type of fracture. In Coltart's series it was the most common fracture involving the talus. The mechanism involved is considered to be a compression of the articular surface of the talus against the contiguous surface of the ankle mortise. It occurs most commonly when the foot is inverted in either the flexed or extended position. This injury has often been misdiagnosed as an osteochondritis dissecans. However, it is currently felt that it is a traumatic injury, in other words, an osteochondral-type fracture.

The patient usually gives a history of twisting the ankle and, if seen initially, may demonstrate tenderness, swelling, and discoloration over the lateral collateral ligament of the ankle joint. However, in many patients, there may be a minimal amount of symptomatology suggestive of a sprain of the lateral collateral ligament. If the diagnosis is not made at the time of injury, the patient will continue complaining of ankle pain which increases with activity and diminishes with rest. Displacement of the fragment may lead to locking of the ankle-joint. The patient will also demonstrate the presence of tenderness over the ankle mortise anteromedially or anterolaterally, depending upon the location of the fracture site. The fragment may at times be palpable; usually it is not. Crepitus is occasionally palpable upon motion of the ankle joint.

For roentgenographic examination, multiple views are necessary in order to bring out the fracture which may be displaced or undisplaced and which roentgenographically usually appears smaller than it actually is. The best projection to bring out the fracture is that of an anteroposterior view of the ankle with 15 degrees of internal rotation.

Treatment. The treatment of choice in this instance is excision of the loose fragment and saucerization of the underlying bone. Usually this defect fills in with fibrocartilage. Failure to remove the fragment almost invariably leads to mechanical incongruity of the joint and subsequent development of osteoarthrosis and additional disability.

Fracture of the Posterior Facet. This is not a common injury and the mechanism is not well understood. Kleiger believes that extreme flexion of the ankle leads to compression of the posterior facet between the posterior lip of the tibia and the os calcis (Fig. 18-14). However, there are other investigators who feel that excessive extension of the ankle leads to increased tension on the posterior talofibular ligament which avulses the lateral aspect of the posterior facet. The latter believe that this is the most common pattern of injury.

On examination the patient usually gives a history of a twisting injury involving the foot and ankle. He complains of pain over the posterior aspect of the ankle joint and tenderness can usually be localized posterior to the lateral malleolus over the region of the ankle mortise. Extension or flexion of the ankle will evoke pain whereas eversion or inversion of the foot are symptomless.

On roentgenographic examination, the anteroposterior and oblique views of the ankle will bring out the fracture line satisfactorily. It is located posteriorly and inferiorly to the lateral malleolus as it tends to implicate the lateral aspect of the facet. Of course, care must be taken to rule out the presence of an accessory ossification center, the os trigonum (better known as a sesamoid bone). The presence of an os

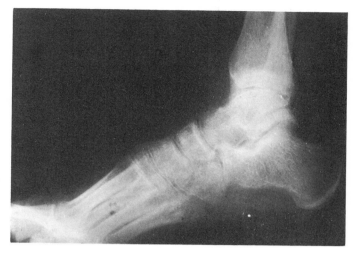

Fig. 18-14. Lateral x-ray of the foot showing a fracture of the posterior process of the talus.

trigonum can frequently be confused with the fracture. In differentiating between the two, it is important to remember that the adjoining surfaces between the talus and the os trigonum are smooth and there is evidence of bone condensation along the edge of the talus, as well as along the edge of the os trigonum. On the other hand, if a fracture of the posterior facet is suspected and the injury is a fresh one, the edges will be found to be jagged rather than smooth and rounded. Roentgenograms of the opposite ankle may be of help.

Treatment. It is the consensus of most investigators that this injury should be treated similarly to a sprained ankle, *i.e.*, elevation, ice, and compression. As the pain subsides, gradual increase in weight bearing is permitted particularly when the symptoms and the swelling have decreased. If the fragment should continue to cause symptomatology after several weeks, it can be excised without any postoperative sequelae.

Dislocation of the Talus with or without Fracture. *Subtalar Dislocation.* Subtalar dislocation alone, without fracture, accounted for 15 per cent of the injuries to the talus in Pennal's series. However, it is not infrequently associated with fracture of the talus. The mechanism of the dislocation alone is usually due to a force in flexion combined with inversion of the foot leading to rupture of the talocalcaneal lig-

aments and displacement of the other tarsal bones as well as the forefoot medially. This type of dislocation is also known as peritalar dislocation (Fig. 18-15).

On examination the patient gives a history of severe trauma to the foot and the injury may or may not be open. The entire foot is swollen. Motion of the ankle, as well as subtalar motion, is quite painful. There is total loss of the normal bony contours of the foot in the region of the ankle joint. One can frequently palpate the talar head on the plantar surface of the foot, and the contour of the foot is so deformed that the forefoot and the calcaneus are displaced medially.

On roentgenographic examination, anteroposterior and lateral views of the foot will reveal the talus to be in a flexed position and the forefoot plus the os calcis to be displaced medially in relation to the talus. One should always be on the alert for associated fractures of the other tarsal bones, and especially of the talus, since occasionally these will occur.

Treatment of Subtalar Dislocation. Closed reduction should be carried out with the patient under general anesthesia, followed by immobilization in a cast extending from the toes to the knee with the foot in neutral position for a period of two weeks. This followed by active *non-weight-bearing* exercises. If at the end of eight weeks there is no evidence of avascular

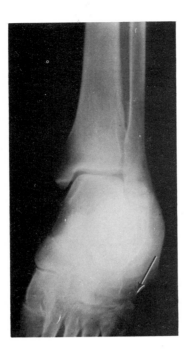

Fig. 18-15. This x-ray reveals a subtalar dislocation with medial displacement of the os calcis and foot with respect to the talus.

necrosis, active weight bearing is instituted. If there is a fracture of the talus associated with this dislocation, the foot should be treated for that fracture after the subtalar dislocation has been reduced.

Prognosis in Subtalar Dislocation. Isolated subtalar dislocations almost invariably progress quite satisfactorily, and few, if any, develop avascular necrosis. However, if the dislocation is associated with fractures of the neck or of the body of the talus, then the chances of developing an avascular necrosis are quite good, and the prognosis is extremely poor.

Total Dislocation of the Talus. Total dislocation of the talus comprised approximately 3 per cent of the total number of injuries in Pennal's series. The mechanism for producing this type of dislocation is one of severe flexion of the foot leading to total dislocation of the talus dorsolaterally, while the remainder of the foot becomes displaced medially.

As with subtalar dislocations, these injuries are due to rather severe trauma. In fact, they are frequently compounded and the talus is often extruded from the wound. The entire foot is swollen and motion of the subtalar or ankle joint produces severe pain. One may palpate or observe the talus protruding from the dorsolateral aspect of the ankle.

For roentgenographic examination, anteroposterior, lateral, and oblique views of the ankle and foot are necessary to evaluate this injury adequately. As previously mentioned, the talus lies dorsolaterally while the remainder of the foot is displaced medially.

Treatment of Total Dislocation of the Talus. If the injury is closed, then one should attempt open reduction as soon as possible and seek to replace the talus in the mortise and the os calcis beneath the talus. Following reduction, immobilization should be carried out in a long leg-cast for a period of three weeks. Following removal of the cast active exercises with no weight bearing should be instituted. If avascular necrosis of the talus occurs, then a pantalar arthrodesis will be necessary. Open injuries are most favorably treated by debridement and the application of the best surgical judgment possible as to whether or not the talus should be preserved. Some recommend removal of the talus followed by talocalcaneal fusion. We feel that a pantalar arthrodesis presents, by far, a better long-term functional result than astragalectomy. If possible, the talus should be retained unless it is severely contaminated, and even then an attempt should be made to preserve it.

Prognosis in Dislocation of the Talus. Prognosis, in so far as function of the ankle and the subtalar joint are concerned, is poor. Almost invariably there is avascular necrosis of the talus which leads to osteoarthrosis of the subtalar and the tibiotalar joints and, of course, makes a pantalar arthrodesis mandatory.

MIDFOOT

This area consists of the navicular, cuboid, and cuneiform bones. Isolated injuries of the midfoot are in most cases secondary to direct trauma and do not occur too frequently. When injuries to the midfoot do occur, there is usually a combination of multiple fractures. Quite often these are associated with either subluxation or dislocation of the midtarsal joints. The midfoot region is the least frequently injured area of the foot.

Navicular

Fractures of the Body. This is a rare injury. The cause is often direct trauma. In such a case the body of the navicular is comminuted, but the fragments are not displaced since this osseous structure is well endowed with strong intertarsal ligaments which hold the fragments together. Extension of the foot plus compression can lead to an isolated fracture of the dorsal lip of the body with displacement in that direction. In other instances, a patient may give a history of a heavy object having dropped on his foot or of a severe twisting injury coupled with a fall.

On examination the patient complains of pain localized over the area of the navicular. Upon inversion or eversion of the foot there is pain referred to the involved area. Adduction or abduction of the forefoot also evokes pain. One must keep in mind that there are often other associated tarsal and ankle injuries and these should be carefully excluded.

Roentgenographic examination will best bring out this fracture through anteroposterior and lateral views.

Treatment. The comminuted and/or displaced fracture should be treated with a snug, below-the-knee walking-cast extending from the toes to the tibial tubercle, with the ankle at neutral position for a period of six to eight weeks. The patient should then be fitted with a well-molded arch support and active weight bearing should be permitted. If the fracture is displaced, an attempt should be made to reduce it by closed methods. Usually, this will fail. Open reduction is frequently required and once the fragment is reduced, all that is necessary to hold the fragments in place is immobilization with one or two threaded Kirschner wires. On the other hand, if extensive damage to the articular cartilage is evident at the time that open reduction is carried out, it may be necessary to consider immediate arthrodesis either of the talonavicular or the naviculocuneiform joint, since almost invariably articular changes of these joints do take place at a later date.

Fracture of the Navicular Tuberosity. Fracture of the navicular tuberosity is not uncommon. The responsible mechanism involves eversion of the foot, leading to sudden increased tension on the posterior tibial tendon which, in turn, places an avulsion pull on the navicular tuberosity and subsequently leads to fracture. The major insertion of the tibialis posterior tendon is in the navicular tuberosity. The fracture is not commonly displaced to any degree since the other insertions of the posterior tibialis tendon in the forefoot prevent it from such displacement.

The patient usually gives a history of having twisted his foot and on weight bearing complains of pain over the navicular tuberosity. This area is swollen and tender. Moreover, pain is referred to the involved area upon attempted eversion which increases the tension on the posterior tibial tendon and thus on the fracture site.

Oblique roentgenograms of the foot best delineate this fracture. At the same time, one should be careful to rule out the possible presence of an accessory scaphoid (os tibialae externum) which is not uncommonly found in this region, and which can be confused with a fracture. However, the os tibialae externum is a congenital anomaly. It is usually bilateral and the edges of the articulation between the os tibialae externum and the navicular are smooth and well-outlined, whereas the edges of a fracture of the navicular are jagged, sharp, and not as well delineated.

Treatment. Most orthopaedists treat this injury in a manner similar to that employed with a sprained ankle. A Gibney adhesive tape dressing with a superimposed ace bandage or an elastoplast dressing is applied. Occasionally, however, if the symptomatology is severe enough, it is better to apply a plaster of paris walking-cast extending from the toes to the knee and to immobilize the area for a period of approximately four weeks. By this time the fracture is usually healed and active weight bearing can be instituted. In this type of fracture it is considered best not to generalize the therapy but to treat each instance individually. If the patient concerned is one who will not participate in any strenuous activities and who will not be forced to

perform a great deal of walking or manual labor, then his fracture can be treated as a sprained ankle with strapping and ace bandage. On the other hand, should the fracture occur in an active individual, such as a football player or one who is likely to place a great deal of strain on the foot, as in the case of a construction worker, then a walking-cast is the better method of therapy by far. Occasionally, non-union does ensue and should the fracture remain symptomatic due to non-union, excision of the loose fragment can be performed. When this is carried out, it is advisable to resuture the tibialis posterior to the raw surface of the bone and to support the foot for a period of three weeks in a cast or on crutches without weight bearing until this portion of the posterior tibialis tendon has reattached itself to the navicular.

Cuboid and Cuneiform

Since fractures of either the cuboid or any of the cuneiforms individually are uncommon, they are grouped as one. Such fractures are usually caused by direct violence. As with the body of the tarsonavicular fractures in this area are usually comminuted but undisplaced due to the maintenance of the position by the strong intertarsal ligaments. Again, however, one should be warned that fractures of these bones are often associated with tarsometatarsal as well as midtarsal dislocations and that the cuboid is often involved in a calcaneal fracture.

The patient may give a history of having had a heavy object dropped on his foot or of his having fallen from a height, landing on his foot and twisting it. He complains of pain in the region of the forefoot, which is tender and swollen directly over the involved bones. Adduction and abduction of the forefoot, as well as inversion or eversion, will provoke pain, particularly if the cuboid is involved.

Anteroposterior, oblique, and lateral roentgenograms are necessary in order to demonstrate these fractures. As previously stated, they are usually comminuted but not displaced unless they are associated with a dislocation.

Treatment. The foot should be immobilized in a snug below-the-knee, plaster of paris walking-cast for a period of from six to eight weeks, following which gradual ambulation may be permitted as tolerated. Again, a well-fitted, arch support is necessary for these patients to use for a period of several months until all subjective and objective symptoms have subsided. The patient usually progresses quite satisfactorily. The fractures heal without difficulty, and since there is little motion in these joints to begin with, there is no impairment of function of this portion of the foot.

One last word of caution: As mentioned previously, the most common type of injury to this portion of the foot is a fracture-dislocation of the midtarsal area due to a rather severe injury. Since this injury is usually the result of a heavy object falling on this portion of the foot, associated with twisting, excessive amount of soft tissue damage does occur. It is, therefore, extremely important that the patient be very carefully observed for two or three days following reduction of the fracture. This is crucial since, in some instances, permanent soft tissue damage will present itself in the form of necrosis of the skin and the underlying soft tissues forty-eight to seventy-two hours after the injury. It is recommended, therefore, that after reduction of such a fracture and the application of a cast, the patient be carefully observed either by reporting to the office daily, or preferably by hospitalization and daily observation until after this period of danger to the soft tissues passes. If necessary, a window can be cut on the dorsum of the cast to permit inspection of the underlying foot. On the other hand, if there is any suspicion of soft tissue damage, we prefer that the cast be removed at the end of three days, the foot carefully examined, and a new cast applied to immobilize the foot and leg.

FOREFOOT

The forefoot consists of all of the metatarsal bones as well as the phalanges of the five digits. Injuries to the forefoot are quite common and are usually the result of direct trauma. Frequently, particularly in the case of the second, third, and fourth metatarsals, and the corresponding toes, the cause of the injury is a crushing-type blow on the dorsum of the foot. One will usually find some abrasions on the dorsum of the foot, and a moderate amount of underlying hematoma of the soft tissues. Roentgenographically multiple fractures are evident.

Frequently, the surgeon or orthopaedist will mistakenly feel that this injury is not one of great consequence and proceed with the reduction of the fractures without carefully investigating the intensity of the blow which produced this injury. As a result, he will frequently reduce the fractures, place the foot in a cast, and permit the patient to go home. Within three to four days the patient will return with necrosis of the soft tissues on the dorsum of the foot, with resulting slough. The inevitable consequence is a prolonged period of disability and ultimately permanent disability of the forefoot. It is our recommendation that as long as there is evidence of soft tissue damage, a patient be hospitalized if he has an injury involving the metatarsal or metatarsophalangeal region of the foot and in which a direct blow of any consequence has been suffered, irrespective of how minimal the displacement of the bones may be. After reduction the foot should be elevated, ice should be applied to the area, as well as a firm, Shantz-type, pressure-dressing, and the foot should be observed for a period of forty-eight to seventy-two hours. If there is no evidence of any soft tissue necrosis, the fractures can be immobilized and the patient discharged from the hospital.

Fractures of the Metatarsal Shaft. This is a fairly common injury that is usually the result of direct trauma to the forefoot. The March fracture, which is a fatigue-type fracture of the metatarsal shaft, involves a different mechanism and will be discussed separately.

The patient usually gives a history of having dropped a heavy object on his foot or of having had some machine run over it. He will complain of pain in the forefoot which is usually swollen—most markedly on the dorsum of the foot. Upward pressure on the plantar surface of the involved metatarsal head will produce pain and, possibly, crepitus of the shaft or shafts. Axial pressure, (using the toe at the end of each metatarsal) will also lead to pain over the involved bone.

In order to visualize the fractures adequately, oblique, lateral, and anteroposterior views of the foot are necessary. These fractures can be oblique, transverse, or comminuted in type. They may also be displaced or undisplaced. As mentioned, more than one metatarsal is involved. If displaced, the distal fragment is usually projecting plantarward due to the secondary pull of the strong toe-flexors.

Treatment. The undisplaced fractures are best treated with a below-the-knee cast for a period of two to three weeks with non-weight bearing followed by a walking-cast for a period of another three weeks. This type of therapy should be instituted when either the first metatarsal is fractured or when more than one of the remaining four metatarsals are involved. On the other hand, if the fracture is a solitary one (either the second, third, fourth, or fifth metatarsal shafts), the treatment consists of the application of a comma-shaped, felt pad on the plantar aspect of the foot, with

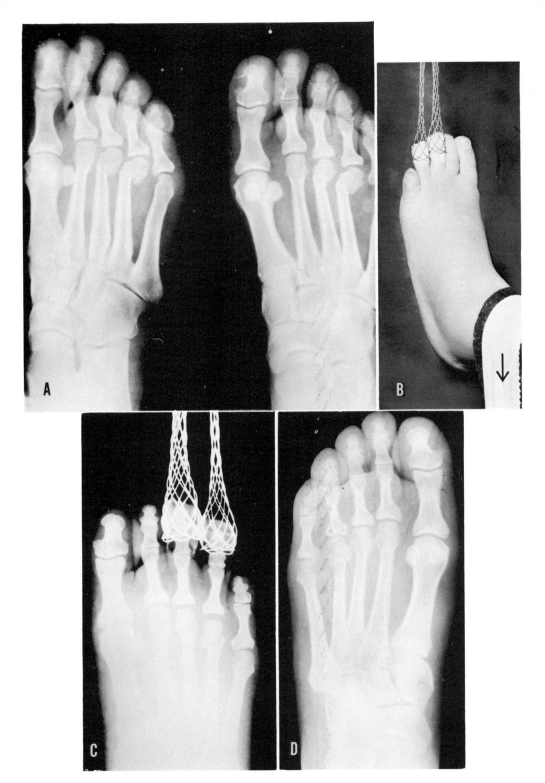

Fig. 18-16. A. Displaced fracture of metatarsals — closed method of reduction — chinese finger trap to each toe.

B and C. Early attempt at reduction with manipulation and use of chinese finger traps on toes and countertraction on ankle will result in satisfactory alignment. Roentgenographic appearance of same metatarsals with traction applied.

D. Fractures reduced and healed.

strapping of the pad to the foot and permission to bear weight guardedly. In such a situation the pad and the strapping should be changed weekly, since the pad does thin down, and the adhesive strapping does become loose. The metatarsal is supported in this fashion for a period of three weeks, at the end of which time all support can be discarded. Some investigators recommend the use of a longitudinal arch. It should be inserted in the shoe following removal of the cast. Weight bearing is then permitted. We feel that if active weight-bearing is permitted too early, exuberant callus formation will result at the site of the fracture. It is believed by many others, however, that this contingency is more academic than real.

With displaced fractures of the metatarsals an attempt should be made to achieve their reduction by closed method. This is best carried out by the use of a Chinese finger trap to each of the toes as soon as possible after the fracture is seen (Fig. 18-16A). Early attempt at reduction with manipulation with the use of Chinese finger trap traction to the toes and countertraction at the ankle will result in very satisfactory alignment (Fig. 18-16B). If this fails, then open reduction is necessary via a dorsal incision and reduction of the fragments in anatomical position with the insertion of a transfixing Kirschner wire to hold the fragments in position. The ends of the Kirschner wire are cut close to the bone. The soft tissues are closed and the fracture is then treated in the same manner as with the undisplaced type. Some surgeons prefer the use of a wire loop with stainless steel wire to tie the two fragments together. If open reduction is performed, and it should be carried out only as a last resort, the soft tissues must be handled gently, since there is a great deal of soft tissue damage. If the tissues are roughly handled, necrosis can develop and can complicate the situation.

Comminuted fractures of the metatarsal shaft can present a rather difficult problem. DePalma suggests that these can be treated with a banjo-splint to exert traction and maintain alignment and length for three weeks. Removal of the traction can take

place at the end of this time and a cast can be applied. Others feel that this type of therapy is unnecessary, since one can accept axial shortening as long as the weight-bearing points are maintained in anatomical relation. Another method of therapy involves the drilling of an 18-gauge needle through the proximal phalanx of the corresponding digit. The needle is then cut off close to the skin permitting only 1/4 of a cm. to protrude from the skin edge on either side. Stainless steel wire is then passed through the needle and looped in order to permit the application of traction to the digit and, therefore, secondarily to the involved metatarsal. A plaster boot extending from the metatarsophalangeal joint to the midleg is then applied with the ankle in neutral position. An outrigger is prepared by the use of a wire coat-hanger and rubber-band traction is applied from the end of the wire to the outrigger. The rubber band recommended is the cuff end of a surgical glove, since this rubber is of excellent quality and will not stretch as will an ordinary rubber band after applying traction for a period of time. The distance should be 10 cm. between the end of the wire loop to which the rubber band is attached to the end of the outrigger. The amount of traction exerted is 5 to 6 pounds if the rubber band is doubled around the wire loop and then attached to the wire outrigger. Usually, this amount of traction is sufficient to line up the shaft of the metatarsal and overcome any overriding. If the fracture occurs at the neck of the second, third, or fourth metatarsals and the surgeon finds it difficult to effect and maintain reduction, then open surgery is necessary. If the operator finds reduction can be effected, which occasionally does happen, it should be carried out. If, on the other hand, the operator finds that the distal fragment is too small to align adequately with the proximal fragment, then resection of the head should be performed. Usually these cases respond quite well to either the open or the closed method of therapy unless the fracture should heal with marked displacement or with exuberant callus formation. In such instances the patient will complain of pain upon ambulation, and it may be necessary at a later date to intervene surgically to remove the plantar bony irregularity.

March Fracture of Metatarsal Shaft.
This fracture has been given the term *March* fracture since it occurs most frequently in military personnel. It is a fatigue-type fracture which most frequently involves the second and, occasionally, the third metatarsal shaft. The patient will begin to complain of pain in the involved shaft much earlier than the fracture can be demonstrated by x-ray.

On examination the patient will often give a history of having been involved in a long march or, if he is an athlete, of having participated in a long, cross-country run. There will be tenderness which will be located over either the second or the third metatarsal. There will be no crepitation and no abnormal mobility. There will be practically little or no swelling. If the symptoms have been present less than a week to ten days, there will be no additional findings. After ten days, on examination one will find a certain amount of swelling of the involved shaft.

Roentgenographically, if the x-rays are procured within a week after the onset of symptoms, the fracture is frequently missed, since it is almost invisible. If one keeps the possibility of this diagnosis in mind, he may frequently find on the anteroposterior and the oblique views the presence of a very fine line transsecting the shaft of the metatarsal. After approximately ten days, roentgenographic examination will disclose the transverse line more distinctly, but there will be evidence of early callus formation in a fusiform fashion surrounding the fracture site. No displacement has been found in this type of fracture (Fig. 18-17).

Treatment. In the service, unless the patient had an extreme amount of pain, treatment consisted of the application of a felt, comma-shaped, metatarsal pad on the plantar aspect of the metatarsal region of the foot, extending from just proximal to the first metatarsal head to that of the fifth metatarsal. The pad was fixed with adhesive strapping and the patient was permitted to return to duty. Within a matter

of a few days, his symptomatology would usually subside. The pad was changed weekly and the patient was restricted from participating in any strenuous activities, such as combat training and/or drilling or marching. In civilian life the same type of therapy is indicated. There is no need for the application of a plaster cast to support this type of fracture. If the patient is cooperative, with a transverse, comma-shaped, metatarsal pad strapped to the foot, his symptoms will subside within a matter of a few days. At the end of three weeks there is sufficient callus formation to warrant removal of all support and permission may be given to the patient to participate in all activities. Although the amount of callus formation may initially appear to be excessive, with the lapse of time, a considerable amount of callus is spontaneously absorbed, and there is no resulting disability.

Fracture of the Base of the Fifth Metatarsal. This is probably the most common of all metatarsal fractures. The underlying

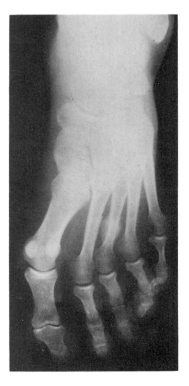

Fig. 18-17. This A-P view of the foot shows a classical March fracture of the third metatarsal shaft.

mechanism is believed to be one of inversion stress leading to sudden increase in tension to the peroneus brevis tendon. With this force there will be avulsion of the styloid process of the fifth metatarsal. In other instances a direct blow is responsible for this type of fracture, and in such cases the fracture is a transverse one at the base of the fifth metatarsal, usually within 1 to 1.5 cm. from the articular surface.

The patient will usually state that either someone stepped on his foot, or an object fell on it, or that he twisted his foot under him. He complains of pain directly over the lateral and dorsolateral aspects of the foot over the base of the fifth metatarsal. On examination marked tenderness and some swelling are apparent. If the patient has delayed reporting to the physician for several days, there will be some ecchymosis of the surrounding soft tissues. Because of the absence of displacement and the moderate amount of discomfort, many patients frequently feel that the injury is nothing more than a sprain. However, because of the persistence of the symptoms, they will finally report to the physician for further care. On examination, active inversion of the foot or attempted forced eversion increases the tension on the peroneus brevis leading to pain in the involved area.

Roentgenographic evaluation can best be carried out with the anteroposterior and oblique views of the fifth metatarsal base (Fig. 18-18).

Treatment. If there is displacement of the fracture, as illustrated, then with the ankle in neutral position the foot should be immobilized in a walking boot-cast extending from the toes to the tibial tubercle. This reduction can be effected by the infiltration of a local anesthetic (making sure to select one to which the patient is not allergic) at the fracture site and manipulation can then be performed. The fracture is usually immobilized for a period of four weeks, by the end of which time it is healed and weight bearing can be tolerated. On the other hand, if there is no displacement, then the treatment should consist of nothing more than strapping of the foot as one would with a sprained ankle, using the Gibney basket-weave adhesive strapping

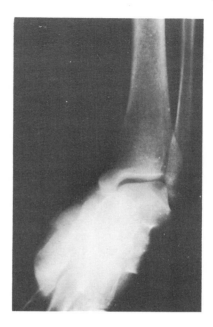

Fig. 18-18. The x-ray shows a typical undisplaced fracture of the base of the fifth metatarsal.

with 1-inch-wide adhesive tape, and an Elastoplast dressing over the adhesive. The patient is then requested to report to the office weekly so that the dressing can be snugged up. The patient who is treated with this ambulatory method of treatment may or may not require crutches or a cane for the first twenty-four to forty-eight hours. The end results from this type of fracture are invariably excellent.

Dislocation of the Tarsometatarsal Joints with or without Fracture. This is an uncommon injury. It is usually due to a combination of a twisting and crushing force. If the patient's forefoot is fixed and he forcibly pronates the hindfoot, the metatarsals will tend to dislocate dorsolaterally. Conversely, supination of the hindfoot will tend to lead to plantar dislocation particularly of the first tarsometatarsal joint. With this type of dislocation there is frequently an accompanying fracture of the base of the second metatarsal since this structure is recessed between the medial and the lateral cuneiform bones.

On examination the patient gives a history of a cracking injury of the foot, accompanied by a twisting component. The foot is swollen, extremely painful, and the normal anatomical landmarks are lost. The dorsalis pedis pulsation is frequently not palpable either because of the dislocation or because of the surrounding swelling. Any attempt to manipulate the forefoot is strongly resisted by the patient.

From the roentgenographic standpoint it is necessary to procure x-rays in the anteroposterior, lateral, and oblique views in order to evaluate the fracture adequately. It is better to anesthetize the patient and procure additional x-rays to gather all the information possible before any attempt is made to manipulate the fracture. The key point is to evaluate the anteroposterior roentgenogram of the foot for displacement between the first and second metatarsals which are normally apposed to one another. Separation of these two metatarsals at their base indicates that dislocation has taken place. It is also important to evaluate the roentgenograms for associated fractures at the base of the second metatarsal. On the lateral view of the foot, the first metatarsal will not be aligned with the medial cuneiform, the navicular, and the talar head as it normally should be (Fig. 18-19).

Treatment. Closed reduction should initially be attempted under general anesthesia. Local anesthesia is inadequate in this situation. If one successfully reduces the dislocation and there is stability of the reduction, a below-the-knee plaster cast should be applied for a minimum of six weeks. No weight bearing should be permitted. Again, in view of damage to the soft tissues because of the type of injury, it is important that the patient be hospitalized and observed for at least forty-eight to seventy-two hours following reduction to make certain that necrosis does not take place in the soft tissues on the dorsum of the foot. The patient's toes should be observed carefully. Upon the slightest evidence of congestion or of circulatory impairment of the toes, the cast should be immediately bivalved, its anterior portion removed, and the skin carefully evaluated. In spite of every precaution, there are times when skin necrosis will occur and, therefore, the patient or the family should be warned of this possibility at the time of initial evaluation.

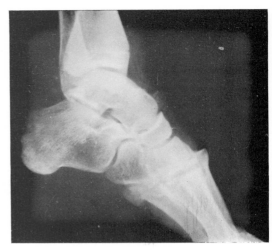

Fig. 18-19. These x-rays demonstrate a dorsolateral dislocation of four lateral metatarsals on the tarsal bones. In this case, the first metatarsal was not involved nor was there a fracture of the second metatarsal bone.

Should the fracture-dislocation prove unstable and should it be impossible to reduce it by closed reduction, then open reduction is necessary. This is done by the insertion of Kirschner wires across the tarsometatarsal joints for fixation. The soft tissues must be handled carefully to avoid any more trauma than absolutely necessary. Occasionally, in spite of adequate reduction by either the closed or open method, sufficient damage to the tarsometatarsal joints has taken place to require an arthrodesis of these joints in order to relieve the symptoms. The patient usually has a long period of convalescence. According to Jeffrey, 20 per cent of patients who suffered this type of injury developed tarsometatarsal arthritis with pain. Failure to recognize this injury or its poor reduction can lead to prolonged disability.

Fractures of the Phalanges. This is a common injury that is usually caused by direct trauma or indirect compression-force applied to the toe. The first digit is more frequently involved than the lateral four.

The patient gives a history of either stubbing the toe or a heavy object dropping on it. The involved toe is swollen, tender to palpation, and may or may not present crepitus. There is often an associated subungual hematoma. If the patient is seen within a matter of an hour or two following the injury, there will be no ecchymosis of the soft tissues. However, within twenty-four hours ecchymosis and marked swelling of the involved digit do take place.

Anteroposterior, oblique, and lateral view roentgenograms of the toe should be procured in order to evaluate the amount of displacement present. Comminution is frequently found, but unlike fractures of the phalanges of the fingers, this injury rarely has any marked degree of displacement, except for the proximal phalanx of the great toe.

Treatment. One should relieve any subungual hematoma by drilling the nail and releasing the pressure. If an open fracture is present, the wound should be cleansed and debrided as with any other fracture. If, on the other hand, the fracture is closed, treatment will depend upon which digit is involved. If it is the second, third, fourth, or fifth, a single layer of sheet-wadding should be placed between the adjacent two digits. The three toes should be strapped with adhesive tape fairly snugly but not so tightly as to impair the circulation of the involved digit. Within forty-eight hours, the dressing should be changed and another strapping applied. Ambulation is permitted in a stiff-soled shoe in which the toe has been cut. If the fracture involves the first toe, with or without displacement, it is advisable that a plaster boot be applied, extending from the tips of the toes to the midleg. The boot should have a walking heel. If there is any displacement of either the proximal or distal phalanges of the great toe, every attempt should be made to reduce it.

A minimal amount of angulation or displacement of the phalanges of the lateral four toes is of no great consequence. Reduction should be attempted but if it is not anatomical, one need not be too concerned as long as the general alignment of the toe is satisfactory. Immobilization is maintained for a period of three weeks.

Dislocation of the Metatarsophalangeal Joint. This type of injury most frequently involves the first metatarsophalangeal articulation.

The patient gives a history of having stubbed his toe with consequent compression of the proximal phalanx against the metatarsal head. This force, if excessive, leads to disruption of the joint capsule and dorsal dislocation of the proximal phalanx on the first metatarsal. On examination the patient will present complete loss of the normal anatomical contour of the first metatarsophalangeal joint, as well as swelling, tenderness and a great deal of pain. The metatarsal head is, of course, displaced and prominent on the plantar aspect of the foot.

This fracture is best visualized roentgenographically in the lateral and oblique views, with the proximal phalanx situated dorsally in relation to the first metatarsal head (Fig. 18-20).

Treatment. This fracture can usually be reduced by the injection of a local anesthetic in the region of the metatarsophalan-

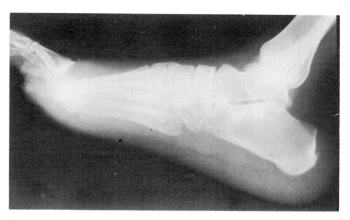

Fig. 18-20. This lateral roentgenogram of the foot demonstrates the dorsal dislocation of the great toe at the metatarsophalangeal joint.

geal joint. After the anesthetic has become effective, the dislocation can be reduced by exerting traction upward and distally with the use of a Chinese finger-trap on the great toe. At the same time, pressure on the plantar aspect of the first metatarsal head is carried out and this is followed by flexion of the great toe as reduction occurs. Immobilization is maintained for a period of two to three weeks by the application of a dorsal metallic splint to prevent extension of the first metatarsophalangeal joint. Following this the patient may be permitted to begin weight bearing to the point of tolerance. In the majority of instances, there is no disability due to this type of injury. However, occasionally the patient may return in four to five years with symptoms indicative of early osteoarthrosis of the first metatarsophalangeal joint with restriction of motion typically found in hallux rigidus.

Fracture of the Sesamoids. This injury is infrequent. Most commonly involved are the sesamoids under the first metatarsal head and, more frequently, the medial than the lateral. The basic cause is usually a fall, with the patient landing directly on the ball of his foot with most of the weight borne on the head of the first metatarsal, thus compressing the sesamoids on the first metatarsal head. This type of fracture has also been known to occur as a stress fracture in pregnant women and in dancers.

The patient gives a history of having fallen from a height, landing on the ball of his foot. On examination there is tenderness, swelling and pain on the plantar aspect of the first metatarsophalangeal joint, particularly directly under the first metatarsal head. Manipulation of the great toe, either passively or actively, produces pain on the plantar aspect of the first metatarsal head because of the increased amount of tension that is placed on the flexor brevis tendons.

Roentgenographic examination of this type of fracture requires not only an anteroposterior view of the first metatarsophalangeal joint centered directly on this articulation, but in addition, a tangential view of the plantar aspect of the first metatarsal head. The fracture lines are irregular and usually comminuted. Occasionally, the fracture of the sesamoid may be confused with a bipartite sesamoid, but usually the bipartite sesamoid is bilateral and additionally, its lines are smooth and well delineated, whereas in the fracture, the lines are jagged and sharp.

Treatment. This injury is best treated by the insertion of a comma-shaped metatarsal pad in the shoe to relieve the pressure on the plantar aspect of the first metatarsal head, or by the use of a transverse metatarsal bar for a period of six to eight weeks. Occasionally, symptoms may persist because of non-union which can take place in this type of fracture, or because of the chondromalacia which can develop on the articular surface of the sesamoid due to the type of injury sustained. When such a disability develops, excision of the involved sesamoid is necessary.

BIBLIOGRAPHY

AITKEN, A.: Fractures of the Os Calcis Treated With Closed Reduction. Clin. Orth., *30*:67, 1963.

BOHLER, L.: *Treatment of Fractures.* 5th Ed., 3 vols, New York, Grune & Stratton, Inc., 1956.

CASSEBAUM, W.: Fracture of Lisfranc's joint. Clin. Orth., *30*:116, 1963.

CAROTHERS, RALPH G.: Personal Communication.

CAVE, E.: Fractures of the Os Calcis, The General Problem. Clin. Orth, *30*:64, 1963.

COLTART, W.: Fractures of the Talus. J. Bone Jt. Surg., *34B*:545, 1952.

CONWELL, H. E. AND REYNOLDS, F. C.: *Key and Conwell's Management of Fractures, Dislocations and Sprains.* 7th Ed., St. Louis, The C. V. Mosby Co., 1961, pp. 1068-1129.

CRENSHAW, A. H.: *Campbell's Operative Orthopaedics.* 4th Ed., St. Louis, C. V. Mosby Co., 1963, pp. 399-404.

DE PALMA, A.: *The Management of Fractures and Dislocations.* Vol. II, Philadelphia, W. B. Saunders Company, 1959, pp. 902-958.

ESSEX-LOPRESTI, P.: The Mechanism, Reduction, Technique, and Results in Fractures of the Os Calcis. Brit. J. Surg., *39*:395, 1952.

GELLMAN, M.: Fracture of the Anterior Process of the Os Calcis. J. Bone Jt. Surg., *33A*:382, 1951.

HERRMAN, OTTO J.: Conservative Therapy for Fracture of the Os Calcis. J. Bone Jt. Surg., *19*: 709, 1937.

JEFFERYS, T. E.: Lisfranc's Fracture Dislocation. J. Bone Jt. Surg., *45B*:546, 1963.

KLEIGER, B.: Fractures of the Talus. J. Bone Jt. Surg., *30A*:735, 1948.

X-Ray Evaluation of Calcaneus. J. Bone Jt. Surg., *43A*:961, 1961.

Fracture of the Tarsal Bones, Their Mechanism and Evaluation. Clin. Orth., *30*:10, 1963.

LAPIDUS, P.: Mechanical Anatomy of the Tarsal Joints. Clin. Orth., *30*:20, 1963.

LENONARD, A.: Treatment of Fracture of the Os Calcis. Arch. Surg., *141*:890, 1955.

LINDSAY, W.: Fractures of the Os Calcis. Amer. J. Surg., *95*:555, 1958.

McLAUGHLIN, H. L.: Trauma. Philadelphia, W. B. Saunders Co., 1959, pp. 299-332.

Treatment of Late Complications After Fractures of the Os Calcis. Clin. Orth., *30*:111, 1963.

MAXFIELD, J.: Fractures of the Os Calcis Treated by Open Reduction. Clin. Orth., *30*:91, 1963.

PALMER, IVAR: The Mechanism and Treatment of Fractures of the Os Calcis. Open Reduction With Use of Cancellous Grafts. J. Bone Jt. Surg., *30A*:2, 1948.

PENNAL, G.: Fractures of the Talus. Clin. Orth., *30*:53, 1963

ROTHBERG, A.: Avulsion Fracture of the Os Calcis. J. Bone Jt. Surg., *21*:218, 1939.

WATSON-JONES, R.: *Fracture and Joint Injuries.* 4th Ed., Baltimore, The Williams and Wilkins Co., 1955, pp. 862-906.

=19=

Problems of the Tarsal Portion of the Foot

in the Adolescent and the Adult

THERE are a number of conditions of the foot that occur either during adolescence and/or adulthood which merit discussion in the same chapter. No one of these problems is of itself so extensive in its total clinical picture as to require a separate chapter. Yet, each of them leads to sufficient dis- ability for the patient to warrant presentation. Some of these clinical problems involve only one specific bony structure. Others involve the foot as a whole. The more common problems are included in this section.

ADOLESCENT CALCANEODYNIA (CALCANEAL APOPHYSITIS)

Sever in 1912 first described pain and fragmentation of the apophysis of the os calcis during adolescence and suggested the term apophysitis. Other writers since that original description have blithely followed in his tracks. Even to the present day, they state that there is increased density and fragmentation of the calcaneal apophysis along with condensation and have likened the condition to Legg-Calvé-Perthes disease of the hip and to Osgood-Schlatter disease of the tibial tubercle. I am in complete disagreement with the premise of fragmentation and increased density.

In a five-year period we have observed an average of 400 to 450 children annually for various foot problems. Although the exact number of adolescents complaining of painful heels has not been recorded, at least an average of 15 per year have been treated. In none of these patients was calcaneal apophysitis (*i.e.*, fragmentation and condensation) found radiographically. In approximately 50 per cent of these youngsters the symptoms were unilateral, yet the roentgenograms presented a similar picture bilaterally (Fig. 19-1). In not a single instance were there any changes found in the os calcis which could be even inferentially interpreted as indicative of any avascular necrosis of the calcaneal apophysis. My findings are in complete agreement with

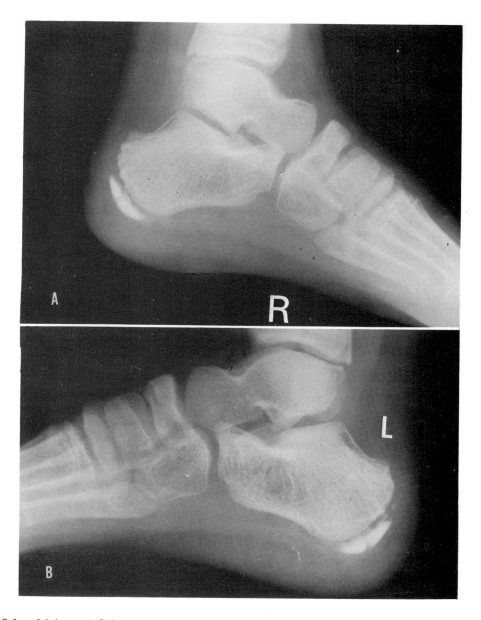

Fig. 19-1.   Adolescent Calcaneodynia (Calcaneal Apophysitis). Right heel is painful and presents all symptoms which were previously related with apophysitis of the os calcis. It was generally accepted that in such instances the apophysis was fragmented. These illustrations of the symptomatic right foot and the asymptomatic left foot certainly do not demonstrate such fragmentation. Refer to text for additional information.

those of Ferguson and Gingrich who have suggested that the cause may be a prominence of the posterosuperior angle of the os calcis or a synovitis of the Achilles tendon. There is no question that there is a clinical entity of painful heel or heels in the adolescent. I would humbly suggest, therefore, that the misnomer, calcaneal apophysitis, be replaced by the more accurate descriptive term *adolescent calcaneodynia* since the latter clearly denotes adolescent painful heel. As to the cause of the symptomatology, I feel that it is in some manner involved with the rapid growth spurt which takes place during this period, superimposed upon strenuous activity. This, in turn, produces a tenosynovitis of the Achilles tendon at the level of its insertion into the os calcis.

Clinical Findings. The subjective findings consist of nothing other than the complaint of pain in the heel upon weight bearing. The pain is localized to the posterosuperior portion of the os calcis. No patient has been seen presenting this symptomatology who has been under the age of eight or over fourteen. The average age is ten years.

Objectively, there is definite tenderness upon both lateral and direct pressure over the posterosuperior surface of the heel.

There is no sign of swelling. The skin may or may not be callused and/or reddened. Quite frequently, particularly if the lesion is unilateral so that comparison can be made, there is slight thickening of the Achilles tendon and the surrounding soft tissues adjacent to the point of insertion of the tendon into the os calcis. Upon compression of the tendo achillis between the thumb and index finger, the patient complains of tenderness. Not infrequently the examiner will find a tight heel cord when testing for true passive extension.

Treatment. The treatment consists merely of elevating the entire heel of the shoe 1/2 an inch. This increase should be maintained for a period of six months even though the symptoms usually subside within two to four weeks.

CALCANEAL SPUR

A spur on the os calcis may be found either on the plantar surface at the area of the attachment of the plantar fascia to the calcaneal tuberosity, or on the superior surface at the site of insertion of the tendo achillis into the os calcis. It is primarily an osteophytic proliferation of bone found most frequently on the plantar aspect of the os calcis just in front of the calcaneal tuberosity. Frequently, but not always, when it is on the plantar surface, it extends across the entire width of the calcaneus (Fig. 19-2).

Etiology. The conditions presumed to be the factors responsible for the development of this type of spur are so numerous and so varied as to border on the ridiculous. A few of the more far-fetched etiologic diseases reported in some texts as its cause are "metabolic disturbances especially of gallbladder and gastrointestinal origin"; "a subacute inflammatory process"; "foci of infection due to ordinary cocci or other bacteria". It is, therefore, obvious that no one has as yet found its true etiology. Many theories have been suggested, but so far none of them has been completely tenable. Furthermore, no specific factor or factors will be conclusively proved as the cause for the development of a calcaneal spur. Suffice to say, a spur on the plantar aspect

of the os calcis appears to be an osteophytic bone formation as a response to ordinary wear and tear. I have not seen a plantar calcaneal spur in a child or a young adult. It is usually observed during middle age and later, except when it results from a severely comminuted fracture of the os calcis. Furthermore, not all plantar calcaneal spurs are painful. In many instances they have been observed as an incidental roentgenographic finding when roentgenograms have been procured for some other foot problem. On some occasions one will find bilateral spurs of the os calcis with unilateral pain. Conversely, on numerous occasions, patients have been examined because of pain on the plantar aspect of the heel and the roentgenograms have failed to reveal any plantar spur. Thus, the spur, per se, is not the cause of pain on the plantar aspect of the heel. It is only an incidental finding. In our opinion the cause of pain is still an enigma.

Symptoms. On the average, the patient with a painful heel complains of discomfort which is present only upon standing or walking. As soon as the patient sits down or assumes a non-weight-bearing position as far as the feet are concerned, the pain subsides until he again assumes the plantigrade position. The intensity of the symp-

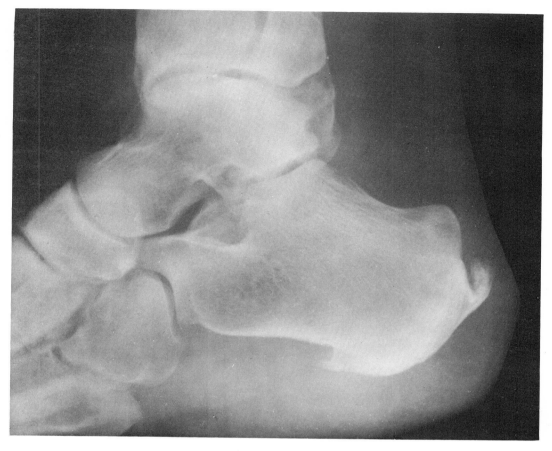

Fig. 19-2. Calcaneal spurs. Note presence of spurs not only on the plantar aspect of the os calcis but also on the superior surface at the site of insertion of tendo achillis.

toms varies with the individual as well as with the length of time the patient has been ambulatory. In some, the pain is intense—almost to the point of being unbearable. In others, it is a dull ache. In all cases, however, the discomfort is sufficiently bothersome to cause the concerned individual to seek help.

Objectively, there are no findings other than acute tenderness upon pressure on the plantar aspect of the os calcis at the point of insertion of the plantar fascia into this bony structure. This tender area or trigger point is well localized to the aforementioned location. In addition some patients will also complain of associated pain along the peripheral soft tissues of the heel. The spur, even if present, cannot be palpated

except in instances where the bony protuberance is a result of a comminuted calcaneal fracture. There is no evidence of any inflammatory reaction. In fact, on observation, the heel appears to be normal.

Therapy. Whether a plantar spur is or is not demonstrable, the treatment is the same. It consists of the construction of a heel pad with a depression at exactly the location where the tender spot is found (Fig. 19-3). The tender spot may be slightly off center in any direction and if the depression is not properly located in the pad, this remedial measure will fail to bring relief. When the pad is properly constructed and correctly inserted in the shoe, the patient will notice immediate relief of the symptoms upon weight bearing. Occa-

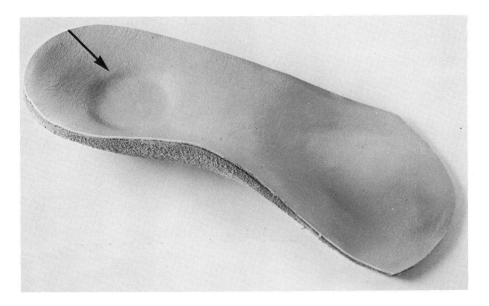

Fig. 19-3.   Pad for calcaneal spur. Note that it is not exactly in the center, but is located to relieve pressure in area of tenderness on plantar aspect of the foot.

sionally a patient will not experience complete relief with the pad alone. In such situations the injection of 1 cc. of one of the steroid preparations into the trigger area, once weekly for two or three times, will relieve the remaining symptoms. The patient should be advised that he will need to wear the pad in the shoe for at least one year and possibly longer. He should be requested to return one month after the initial fitting of the pad in order to evaluate the results. Once the foot has become asymptomatic, the patient should report for a check-up every three months for a period of one year. There are some patients who, upon removing the pad at the end of the year, will experience a recurrence of the symptoms. Such individuals should be advised that they will have to wear the pad indefinitely, and must return annually to be fitted with a new pad. Additionally, patients with continued symptoms should be examined for subclinical gout. Should the blood uricase be found to be in excess of the average values or in the high normal range, one half gram of Benemid twice daily or the equivalent dose of allopurinol

twice daily should be prescribed. In some patients the response to this medication is gratifying.

What about surgical intervention in painful heels which have not responded to conservative therapy? The term "never" is not considered a part of the physician's medical vocabulary. Therefore, let it be said that I have yet to find it necessary to recommend surgical intervention for the relief of pain in the heel except when the pain results from the development of a spur following a comminuted calcaneal fracture. There are some physicians who advocate surgery and/or roentgenotherapy. Fortunately, they are in the minority. Radiation therapy should not be used for this condition. If and when surgery is necessary in order to remove a painful exostosis as a result of a comminuted calcaneal fracture, the bony prominence should be adequately exposed through one of the plantar incisions illustrated in Chapter 21. The exostosis or spur should be adequately removed and the soft tissues meticulously closed. Weight bearing should not be permitted for at least three weeks.

BURSITIS OF THE TENDO ACHILLIS ("PUMP BUMP")

Ordinarily there is a bursa overlying the tendo achillis at the level of the insertion of this tendon into the os calcis. Occasionally, this may become irritated and inflamed if the heel counter of the shoe presses against the underlying bony prominence. Usually the symptoms are eliminated when the patient changes to another type shoe or wears a 1/2-inch piece of felt inside the heel of the shoe to raise the tender area away from the edge of the heel counter.

There is another clinical condition in association with this problem which Dickinson, Coutts, Woodward, and Handler have aptly termed "pump bumps." This is characterized by a bony enlargement on the posterolateral surface of the os calcis at the area of insertion of the tendo achillis (Fig. 19-4). These bumps are almost invariably found in women's feet and are associated with the wearing of high-heeled shoes. In the great majority of women, these prominences are asymptomatic and except for their ugly appearance are of no consequence. Occasionally, however, a patient will complain of almost disabling pain and of inability to wear shoes of any type other than a sling-

heel pump. Although these patients comprise a small segment of the orthopaedist's practice, they represent a serious problem since they are quite incapacitated by this defect.

Etiology. This bony protuberance is found both in males and females and is almost invariably bilateral. Under ordinary circumstances it is asymptomatic and not particularly prominent. However, among the symptomatic cases, there is an appreciable preponderance of females. In a small number of females this bump, as well as its overlying bursa, becomes gradually but progressively more pronounced and more symptomatic because of the type of shoe worn by the individual. In our considered opinion, these prominences become symptomatic because the patient has worn an improperly-fitted (usually short) shoe. Furthermore, once the symptoms become firmly established, they are difficult to correct by conservative means. Of course, one can advise the patient to wear a sandal with no heel counter or to go barefoot. Dickinson and co-workers have suggested

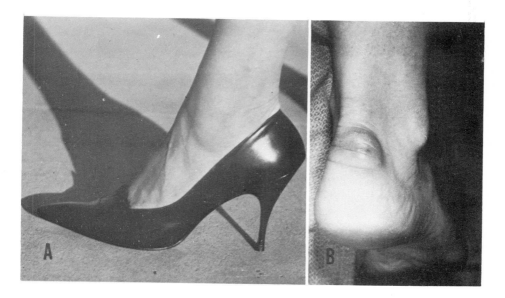

Fig. 19-4.   A.   A high-heeled pump, showing the close contouring of the shoe counter to the heel that is thought to be one of the factors in the development of pump bumps.

B.   Prominence on the calcaneus in the region of the attachment of the tendo achillis referred to as a pump bump. (Dickinson et al, courtesy of J. Bone & Joint Surg.)

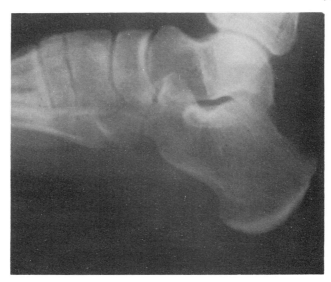

Fig. 19-5. Roentgenogram of foot with a pump bump, showing the hatchet shape of the calcaneus. (Dickinson **et al,** courtesy of J. Bone & Joint Surg.)

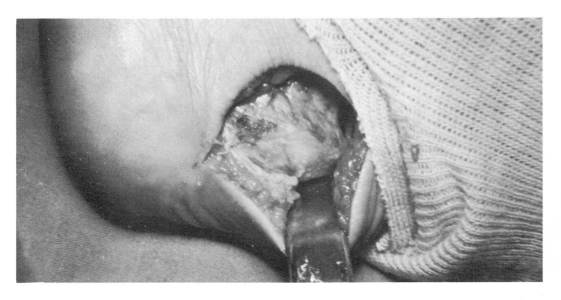

Fig. 19-6, 7 and 8. Exposure of the calcaneus through medial incision. Note size of bone fragment excised and the postoperative roentgenographic appearance of the calcaneus after removal of the bone prominence. (Dickinson **et al,** courtesy of J. Bone & Joint Surg.) (Author recommends transverse incision.)

that there may be an underlying congenital factor since in these patients the os calcis is more hatchet-shaped than usual (Fig. 19-5). In their series of 21 patients, 20 were female.

Treatment. Conservative therapy should be given a thorough trial. This consists of the insertion of an elevation inside the heel of the shoe. In addition, sling-heel pumps or sandals should be worn and steroids should be injected in the region of the tender area in order to relieve the symptoms. With this regimen in most instances the symptoms will disappear. However, in the occasional case where conservative therapy has failed, surgical intervention is indicated.

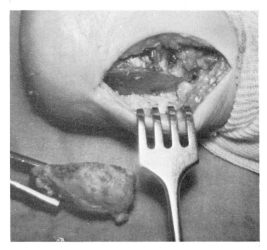

Fig. 19-7.

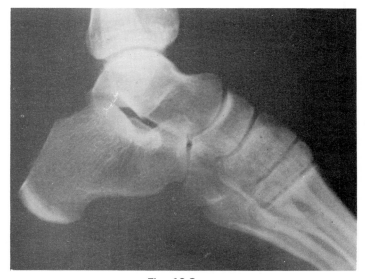

Fig. 19-8.

Operative Procedure. Under tourniquet control the incision should be made on the medial aspect of the heel just forward of the tendo achillis. It should begin 1 cm. above the upper border of the os calcis and curve slightly forward. The incision need not be more than 4 cm. in length. The reader may wonder why I recommend placing of the incision on the medial aspect of the heel when the prominence is on the posterolateral aspect. The answer is simple: for cosmetic reasons. A scar is less visible on the inner aspect of the heel. In a few patients I have used a transverse incision, parallel with the calcaneal creases, to ex-

pose this area. Cosmetically, the resulting scar has been virtually invisible.

The medial plantar branch of the posterior tibial nerve is located just forward of the incision and, therefore, care should be exercised as the incision is carried down to the bone. Subperiosteal dissection is then carried out and, if necessary, the superior portion of the tendo achillis is partially dissected free in order to expose the bony prominence. A 1-cm. wide bunion retractor is then slid around the os calcis to the lateral surface (Fig. 19-6). With a broad, thin, sharp osteotome the posterosuperior prominence of the os calcis is removed.

The osteotome should be directed in an oblique manner from a superior to inferior direction, as well as from medial to lateral, thus insuring complete removal of the posterolateral prominence (Fig. 19-7 and 8). When this procedure is attempted for the first time, the operator tends to be a little hesitant about the amount of bone to be excised. Sufficient bone should be removed so that the previously palpable prominence will be entirely absent after completion of the operative procedure. Insufficient bone resection will lead to operative failure. The incision is closed in a routine manner except that the skin is closed with a sub-cuticular monofilament wire suture. A plaster boot is applied with the foot in complete flexion (equinus) position. Immobilization is maintained for four weeks. Following removal of the cast, active weight bearing with crutches is instituted initially. Full, unsupported weight bearing is permitted two weeks later. The patient should be advised that some discomfort will be experienced for at least three to six months after surgery.

I performed this operation initially in 1944 using the incision described above. The end-results are similar to that of Dickinson and his co-workers.

PERONEAL SPASTIC FLATFOOT

This clinical entity is characterized by spasticity of the peroneal muscles, particularly the peroneus longus. Associated with the spasm is a valgus position of the rearfoot of varying degree, thus producing, minimally, a pronation of the foot and, maximally, complete loss of the longitudinal arch. The condition may or may not be symptomatic and bilateral.

Etiology. The exact cause of this condition is as yet unknown. There are several bony anomalies of the talocalcaneal, calcaneonavicular, and talonavicular joints which account for the major portion of this deformity, but they are not the sole cause of the peroneal spastic flatfoot.

Prior to 1921 this deformity was thought to be due to spasm of the peroneal muscles. It was the concensus that this spasticity was due to such conditions as an infectious synovitis of the peroneal tendons, a manifestation of early rheumatoid arthritis in the foot, or an irritation of unknown etiology of the sinus tarsi, to name a few.

In 1921 Sloman suggested that one of the causes of peroneal spastic flatfoot was the presence of a calcaneonavicular bar. His work was further confirmed by Badgley's observations on this same problem in 1927. However, not much attention was paid to these two reports until 1948 when Harris and Beath demonstrated that a high percentage of cases of peroneal spastic flatfoot was due to the presence of a medial talocalcaneal bridge. These three publications established, to a great extent, the current opinion that peroneal spastic flatfoot is, in most instances, the clinical manifestation of a congenital syndesmosis or a synchondrosis or fusion of the tarsal bones of the hindfoot associated with spasticity of the peroneal muscles.

Outland and Murphy reported bony bridging of the talosustentacular joint as a cause of peroneal spastic flatfoot. They also listed 8 additional conditions, infectious and/or traumatic, as causes of the same deformity. I have observed a fourteen-year-old female who first presented herself with a symptomatic peroneal spastic flatfoot. The initial roentgenograms (Fig. 19-9A) were negative. However, over a period of one year, she developed roentgenographically demonstrable arthritic changes in the talocalcaneal joint (Fig. 19-9B). We have also observed the presence of peroneal spasm in several patients who have undergone surgical correction of flatfeet upon initiation of active weight bearing following removal of the casts. In these latter instances, the situation has gradually subsided spontaneously with active exercise to stretch the peroneal muscles, as well as physical therapy.

Wray and Herndon suggested a possible hereditary transmission of calcaneonavicular coalition. They proposed that "at least some, and perhaps all, cases of calcaneonavicular bar are caused by a specific gene mutation which behaves as an autosomal

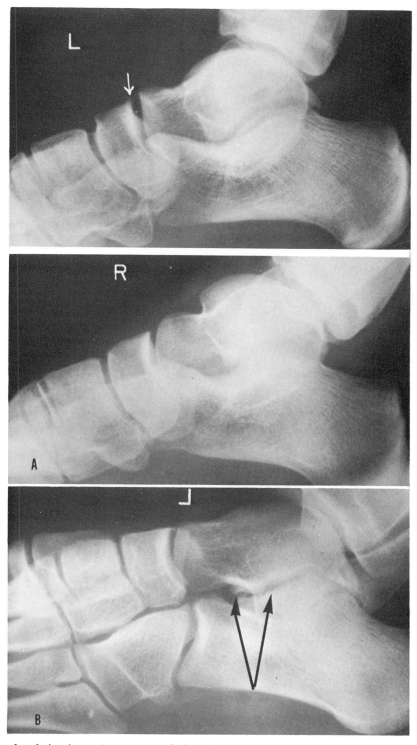

Fig. 19-9.   A.   Lateral roentgenogram of the right and left feet essentially the same except for minimal spurring of the talonavicular joint. There is no evidence of any arthritic changes or spurring of either talocalcaneal joint. Left foot, however, demonstrated peroneal spasm.

B.   Oblique roentgenogram of left foot one year later demonstrating early but definite arthritic changes.

dominant, probably with reduced penetrance."

In summary the etiology of peroneal spastic flatfoot is due in most instances to one of a number of tarsal coalitions. The most frequent of these are: 1) medial talocalcaneal bridge, and 2) calcaneonavicular bar; those of less frequency are: 3) talosustentacular fusion, 4) posterior talocalcaneal bridge, 5) talonavicular fusion, 6) calcaneocuboid fusion, and 7) cubonavicular fusion. Occasionally, multiple intertarsal fusion may occur. When such tarsal coalitions are not found, peroneal spastic flatfoot can be due to 1) a localized arthritic process (Fig. 19-9A and B), 2) trauma, 3) following surgical correction of a flatfoot deformity, and 4) in association with congenital flatfeet.

The cause for the spasticity of the peroneal muscle still remains unknown and unsolved. In their original article Harris and Beath felt that there was no peroneal spasm and that the tightness of the peroneal tendons was "thought to be an adaptive shortening of the peroneal muscles related to the valgus position of the foot". In his most recent article Harris unqualifiedly agrees that spasm of the peroneal muscles occurs in practically every patient sometime during the course of the disease. Furthermore, he feels that in the severe cases the extensor digitorum longus group of muscles can also develop spasticity. Dr. George Phalen of Cleveland, Ohio, in a personal communication stated that in a series of patients in whom he found clinical evidence of spasticity of the peroneal muscles, a certain number, on exploration, demonstrated the presence of a synovitis of the tendon sheaths of the peroneus longus and brevis muscles.

Subjective Symptoms. The primary subjective symptom is pain in the foot, particularly the rear portion. This appears spontaneously, is not severe, and is usually observed after an episode of excessive hiking, or possibly after a twisting injury following sport participation, or in some patients following the wearing of a new pair of shoes which are stiff and unyielding. The pain is relieved with rest, but reappears upon the initiation of weight bearing.

Most of the patients are adolescents. Occasionally, the condition may first manifest itself during young adulthood. It is interesting to observe that even when synostosis is the cause and it is a congenital lesion, almost invariably subjective symptoms do not appear until adolescence.

Objective Symptoms. When examined in a standing position, the rearfoot presents a valgus deformity and automatically pronation of the entire foot of varying degree. On the other hand, if the subjectives symptoms do not manifest themselves before adulthood, the foot may be perfectly normal in appearance. The pronation may be severe or it may be slight. If the valgus deformity is pronounced, there is a greater likelihood of a medial talocalcaneal bridge. The patient's gait is stiff: he ambulates "flatfootedly", i.e., he does not present a normal heel-toe gait, but picks up each foot and places it down as a completely rigid unit.

Examination of the foot or feet at rest will reveal marked limitation of motion with almost, if not complete, loss of adduction of the heel and inversion of the foot. Usually, the entire foot is held rigidly in a valgus position. Furthermore, when passive inversion of the foot is attempted, the patient complains of pain, and the peroneal tendons stand out quite prominent and taut. Again, if there is a talocalcaneal bridge present, there will be almost total absence of motion in the subtalar joint. If the deformity is due to a calcaneonavicular bar, motion may be markedly restricted in both joints, but not completely eliminated. Extension and flexion motions of the ankle and of the foot are full and painless.

Roentgenographic Findings. In order to demonstrate these various intertarsal coalitions special views are necessary in addition to the standing anteroposterior and lateral views. Furthermore, there are certain changes demonstrable in the routine views which, according to Harris, are of as much diagnostic importance as is the demonstration of the congenital coalition. Therefore, in addition to the standard standing views, the following views should be procured:

A roentgenogram is taken with the patient standing on the cassette and the tube

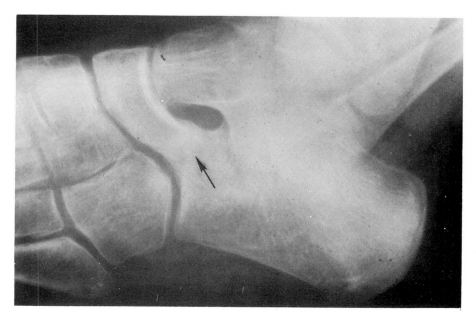

Fig. 19-10.   Calcaneonavicular bar is demonstrable only in the oblique view.

tilted so that the x-ray beam will pass in an oblique manner at an angle of 45 degrees from lateral to medial through the midportion of the foot. At least one other view should be obtained, preferably a routine oblique view at rest. These two views will demonstrate the presence of a calcaneonavicular bar (Fig. 19-10). The other view which demonstrates the talocalcaneal bridge is the posterior oblique one which is used to show the sustentaculotalar joint. It can be taken either in a standing position with the tube placed so that the x-ray beam will be directed from behind downward and forward, or at rest in the usual posteroanterior os calcis position. In either position care must be taken to delineate the talocalcaneal joint very clearly, particularly the sustentaculotalar portion (Fig. 19-11).

The secondary changes, which Harris and Beath have especially emphasized and which they feel are important diagnostic aids, are best visualized in the standing lateral view. These changes are: 1) beaking of the head of the talus which is found invariably with a talocalcaneal bar and frequently with a calcaneonavicular bar, and 2) obliteration of the joint space between the bodies of the talus and the os calcis,

as well as between the sustentaculum and the neck of the talus which is found only with the talocalcaneal bridge.

Treatment. The type of therapy to be instituted will depend upon the severity of the symptomatology as well as the amount of deformity of the foot. If there is no evidence of any tarsal coalition, treatment should consist of injection of the tendon sheaths and/or the sinus tarsi with steroids. In at least 50 per cent of this group of patients the use of steroids has proved quite beneficial and has overcome the subjective, as well as the objective symptomatology. Conservative therapy should first be attempted in all patients whose symptomatology is due to a calcaneonavicular bar, particularly if the deformity of the foot is mild to moderate. Conservative treatment is also indicated in those patients who have a talocalcaneal bridge but who have little or no deformity of the foot and minimal pain and muscle spasm. The best therapeutic measure is a well-fitted monel steel Whitman plate. In addition, the injection of 1 cc. of one of the steroid solutions into the soft tissues surrounding the calcaneonavicular bar will also prove beneficial. If the conservative measures should fail or if at least the deformity *and the symptoms*

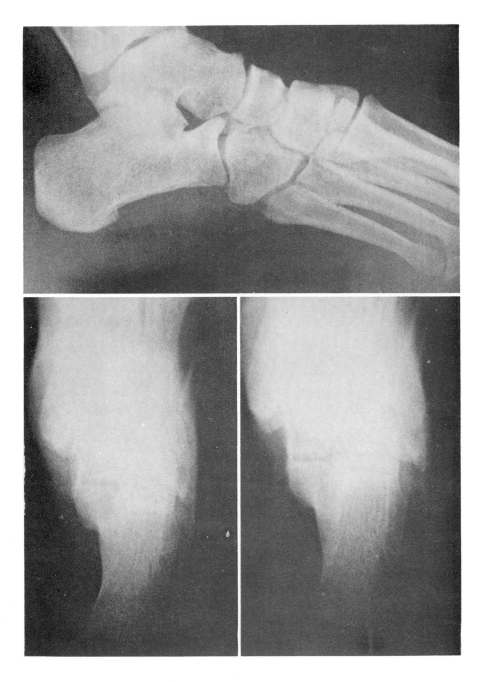

Fig. 19-11. (Top) There are molding changes at the talonavicular joint. No bar is seen. (Bottom, left) The joint fissures are normal. There is a thin plaque of bone bridging the talosustentacular joint. (Bottom, right) Changing the position of the x-ray tube alters the shape of the plaque but does not eliminate it. (Outland and Murphy, courtesy of Clinical Ortho.)

are moderately disabling, surgical intervention is indicated. One must keep in mind that many patients with this type of a problem go through life with remarkably slight, if any, disability. Furthermore, surgery is not the cure-all of this problem. It should be recommended only as a last resort.

I have encountered too few cases which have required surgical procedures and, therefore, cannot speak with authority regarding the end-results. However, Harris' recent conclusions are pertinent:

1. "Late childhood or adolescence (eight to sixteen years) is a good age to operate."

2. "I have not been impressed by my own results after resection of the calcaneonavicular bar and consequently prefer triple arthrodesis as a more reliable method of obtaining a stable, painless foot without deformity."

Consequently, when surgery is indicated in a patient, who has not responded to conservative measures and whose foot symptomatology is due to a calcaneonavicular bar, the procedure of choice is a triple arthrodesis through the standard lateral Kocher incision. If the roentgenograms reveal a talocalcaneal bridge, a medial approach is used to expose both the talocalcaneal and the talonavicular joints, providing there is no severe valgus deformity of the foot. The incision begins just posterior and below the medial malleolus and extends forward with a slight curve dorsally to the distal articular edge of the navicular.

Should the talocalcaneal bridge be solid, then only arthrodesis of the talonavicular joint is necessary. If there is evidence of motion present at the talocalcaneal joint because of incomplete fusion, then the talocalcaneal joint, in addition to the talonavicular joint, requires fusion. It is not necessary to fuse the calcaneocuboid joint. If, on the other hand, there is a valgus deformity of the foot of moderate to major proportion associated with a talocalcaneal bridge, I prefer to approach the foot through the lateral Kocher incision. The bridge between the talus and the os calcis is carefully osteotomized, care being taken not to injure the medial structures of the foot. A Grice procedure is performed and the talocalcaneal joint is thus fused in the corrected position. The talonavicular joint should also be arthrodesed. One word of caution: When performing the talocalcaneal arthrodesis in a still growing foot, *do not place the os calcis in the neutral position.* Placing it in the neutral, or even in the slightest varus position in the adolescent will result in the development of a varus deformity of the heel. It is best to leave the os calcis in a minimal amount of valgus. Cast immobilization is carried out for six weeks with no weight bearing, followed by a walking cast for another six weeks.

Mitchell, of Edinburg, Scotland, recommends excision of the calcaneonavicular bar accompanied by removal of adequate portions of the adjoining surfaces of the os calcis and the navicular.

SNAPPING PERONEAL TENDON

This condition is mentioned simply for the sake of completeness with reference to the various symptomatic problems involving the tarsal region of the foot. It is nothing more than slipping of the peroneal tendon from its natural groove. As it slips back into position, there is an audible snap. The tendon most frequently involved is the peroneus longus. The condition is seldom disabling, but the audible snapping is annoying to the patient. In some instances pain develops. Occasionally, the same symptoms are found over the medial aspect of the foot due to subluxation of the tibialis posterior tendon.

Treatment. Usually no therapy is re-

quired since almost invariably there is no pain associated with the snapping. Should there develop pain and disability of the ankle, surgical intervention may be required. This consists merely of lengthening of the involved tendon just distal to the lateral malleolus in the case of the peroneus longus, and distal to the medial malleolus when the tibialis posterior is involved. The foot is immobilized in a plaster boot for a period of three weeks. There are several complicated and extensive bone-block procedures which have been described for the surgical correction of this type of condition, but one can liken these to the individual who "runs a mile to jump a foot ditch."

RUPTURE OF THE TENDO ACHILLIS

Loss of continuity of the Achilles tendon may be due to direct trauma, as in a laceration, or to a tear of the tendinous tissues as a result of an abnormal stress superimposed on attritional changes.

Clinical Evaluation and Therapy. When direct laceration occurs, immediate repair is indicated. This should be carried out within the first four to six hours following the injury. The tendon ends are usually sharply severed and healthy. Therefore, after thorough cleansing of the wound under tourniquet control, repair should be carried out. The *sine qua non* for the achievement of a secure repair is the use of meticulously applied mattress sutures to gain anatomical approximation of the tendon ends. Following closure of the soft tissues, immobilization of the extremity is instituted by the application of a plaster cast which extends from the level of the tibial tubercle to the toes with the foot in complete flexion (plantar flexion). The cast is removed in six weeks and active weight bearing is instituted. I have not found it necessary to extend the cast above the knee.

When rupture of the tendo achillis occurs, it is due to the application of an abnormal amount of strain or stress on a preexisting intrinsically degenerated tendon due either to disease (which is rare), or more commonly to attrition. Loss of continuity takes place through the degenerated portion of the tendon as the result of sudden contraction of the calf muscle against resistance. It occurs almost invariably in males who are over thirty years of age and who sporadically engage in sports. The tear occurs most frequently near the level of the insertion of the tendon. However, it can occur at higher levels up to the musculotendinous junction.

The patient gives a history of sudden onset of pain in the calf of the leg. He will frequently state that he experienced a sensation similar to that of being struck in the calf with a baseball bat.

On examination the patient lacks the heel-toe gait. He is unable to stand on the toes of the afflicted foot. If the rupture is low, a definite sulcus is palpable in the contour of the Achilles tendon as compared to the opposite side. On the other hand, should the tear be at a higher level, one will be unable to detect such a loss in continuity. Furthermore, with a higher level tear, the patient will demonstrate only partial loss of active flexion (plantar flexion) of the foot against resistance, suggesting an incomplete rupture. This is only wishful thinking on the examiner's part. The persisting muscle power is due to the presence of an intact tendon sheath within which the tendon has been torn.

The Thompson Test. Dr. T. Campbell Thompson has devised a highly accurate clinical test to determine loss of continuity of the tendo achillis. Although he first presented this diagnostic test in 1955, he did not report it in the literature until 1962. When rupture of the Achilles tendon is suspected, the patient is asked to kneel on a chair with his feet hanging over the edge or to lie prone on the examining table with the feet hanging over the edge of the table. The calf muscle of the unaffected leg is first squeezed just below the widest segment of the posterior portion of the leg (in the middle third of the calf). Normally this causes extension (plantar flexion) of the foot. The same procedure is carried out on the suspected leg. If there is a rupture of the Achilles tendon, there will be no response of the foot, *i.e.*, extension will not take place. According to Thompson, the squeeze test has been found to be extremely accurate.

Treatment. The only therapy is surgical repair unless the patient wishes to walk with an impaired gait for the remainder of his life. Operative repair is difficult because of the poor quality of the tissues. Upon exposure of the tendon one will find a segment of this structure at least 3 or 4 cm. in length to consist of nothing more than shreds of tissue. The tendon appears as though a vegetable shredder had been applied in an effort to destroy its continuity. Any attempt to repair the tendon ends is, as Dr. Harrison L. McLaughlin aptly described it, "like attempting to sew the ends of two paint brushes together, and is about as effective." Several procedures for repair

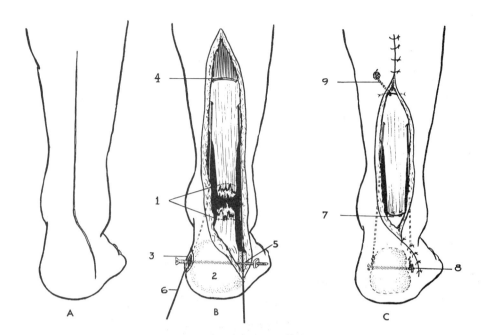

Fig. 19-12.   Repair of ruptured tendo achillis by removable suture.

A.   A midline incision is made which curves laterally in its distal portion to avoid shoe pressure upon the scar.

B.   The tendon ends are not only separated, but frayed and fragile. Each must be trimmed back to reasonably healthy tissue (1). A drill hole is made through the calcaneus (2), and a stab wound made at its point of emergence (3). A long heavy wire mattress suture is placed at the musculotendinous junction (4). A long screw is passed through the drill hole in the os calcis (5) and the proximal tendon fragment is pulled down into position by the two ends of the wire suture (6), which are then fastened to the projecting ends of the screw.

C.   With retraction thus counteracted, the trimmed tendon ends may then be sutured (7). The superfluous portion of the screw is cut free and removed (8). A twisted wire (9) with a split lead shot (for palpable localization of the mattress suture at the time of renewal, is attached to the proximal portion of the wire suture. A and B, McLaughlin, Trauma, courtesy of W. B. Saunders Co.; C, McLaughlin, in Cole's Operative Technic in General Surgery. (Courtesy of Appleton-Century-Crofts, Inc.)

of this tendon have been described in the past. The following techniques have proved most effective.

If the rupture involves the proximal half of the tendo achillis, McLaughlin's procedure is the preferred one (Fig. 19-12 A, B, and C). He recommends excision of the diseased tendon ends. Although a defect will be created which may measure as much as 10 cm. in length, this can be overcome by flexion of the knee and of the ankle. In addition, special repair with wire suture is necessary to obviate the pull of the calf muscle group. This is clearly described in Figure 19-12. Immobilization is

maintained for eight weeks at which time the screw, washer, and wire sutures are removed and active weight bearing is instituted. This method is also quite useful for late repairs.

Should the rupture be located in the distal half of the Achilles tendon, then Lynn's method of repair is applicable (Fig. 19-13 A and B). In this procedure, following exposure of the rupture site and loose approximation of the tendon shreds into a reasonable facsimile of a tendon, Lynn detaches and/or sections a good portion of the adjacent plantaris tendon. This structure is then gently spread out to form a

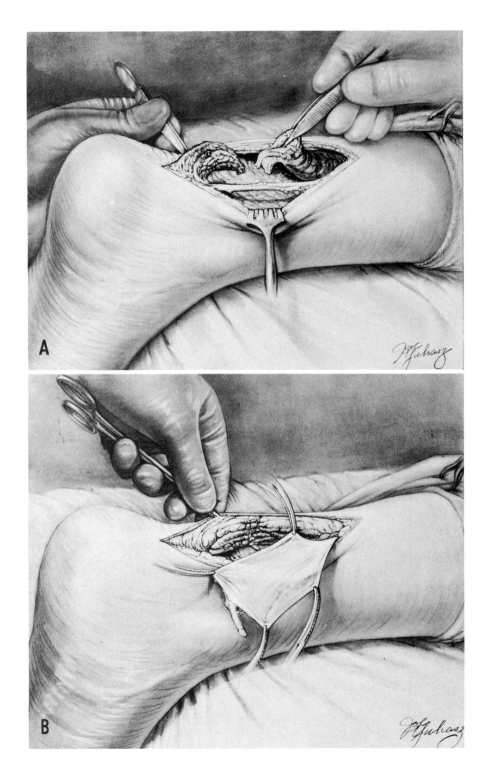

Fig. 19-13.   A.   Torn ends of fresh rupture of Achilles tendon and intact plantaris tendon.

   B.   Ragged ends have been apposed and sutured. The plantaris tendon has been freed at its distal attachment and is being fanned out into a membrane.

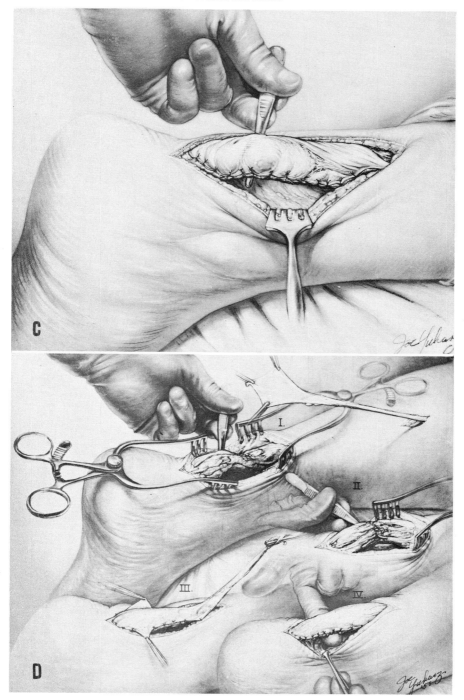

Fig. 19-13.   Continued.

C.   The fanned-out plantaris has been wrapped about the anastomosed Achilles tendon for about two-thirds of its circumference and has been sutured to that structure by the edges. The repair is complete.

D.   I. A ten-day-old rupture of the Achilles tendon bridged by a slender bit of fibrous tissue. The ruptured plantaris is brought out through an incision in the calf.   II. The fibrous band has been excised and the ends of the Achilles tendon sutured.   III. Free graft of the plantaris fanned out and sutured by edges. The redundant portion is discarded.   IV. The complete repair. (Lynn, courtesy of J. Bone & Joint Surg.)

thin, but firm sheet of tissue which is placed around the tendon in a tube-like fashion. The proximal and distal edges of this tube are sutured to the healthy tendon above and below the point of attritional rupture and the free edges of this graft are sutured to each other, thus encasing the entire area of the rupture of the tendo achillis. Immobilization with the foot in a position of flexion (equinus) is maintained for eight weeks. Active weight bearing is then instituted. It is unnecessary to extend the cast above the knee as has been done in the past.

KÖHLER'S DISEASE
(Avascular Necrosis of the Tarsal Navicular)

This condition, although relatively infrequent, is seen in children between three-and-one-half and eight years of age, rarely, up to the age of ten. It is considered to be an avascular necrosis of the tarsal navicular. The same disorder has been reported in adults. However, I have not seen an adult with this condition.

Clinical Findings. Subjectively the child will complain of vague pain over the dorso-medial aspect of the foot and will present a slight limp. The parents are invariably at a loss to account for the onset of the pain since there is no history of injury. An objective evaluation will disclose a limp of the involved foot. The gait is one of attempted protection of the medial side of the foot and the youngster thus walks along the lateral aspect of the involved foot. On palpation there is definite tenderness directly over the tarsal navicular. There is limitation of inversion due to pain. Because of this limitation of inversion, one gains the impression that there is peroneal spasm. In reality the peroneal muscles are not spastic. The limitation of inversion is simply a protective mechanism. Should there be pronation of the foot in the standing posi-

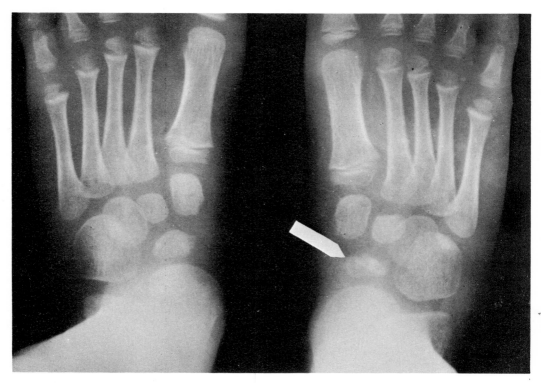

Fig. 19-14.   Kohler's Disease. Note narrowing of navicular, fragmentation, and increased density as compared to opposite side.

tion, one should not misinterpret this as due to the Köhler's disease. It is an incidental finding. There may or may not be swelling of the tissues in the vicinity of the navicular, depending upon the acuteness of the process.

Roentgenographic Findings. Roentgenographically the navicular appears much thinner in width than the opposite normal navicular. There is increased density of the entire bony structure. One must exert some care in interpreting the roentgenographic findings since occasionally the navicular ossifies from multiple centers rather than a single one. At times this apparent fragmentation can be misinterpreted as an avascular necrosis. Therefore, comparative roentgenograms should be procured (Fig. 19-14).

Treatment. Therapy consists primarily of support and rest. The patient should be fitted with a steel shank shoe plus some support under the longitudinal arch, preferably this should be a rubber cookie. If the process is acute, one may consider placing the patient on crutches for a few days. Usually within three to nine months, revascularization of the navicular takes place.

ACCESSORY NAVICULAR (OS TIBIALAE EXTERNUM)

The os tibialae externum which is more commonly known as the accessory navicular, is a sesamoid bone found in approximately 12 per cent of patients. It is located on the medial aspect of the foot and articulates with the navicular tuberosity, although at times the articulation may be difficult to delineate because of fibrous union and thus the navicular may appear to be a single bony structure. There has been a misconception that it is associated with pronated feet. This, however, is incorrect (Fig. 19-15). Clinically, one does get the impression that there is pronation of the foot because of the prominence of the navicular tubercle on the medial aspect. However, if standing x-rays are procured (Fig. 19-16), one will find that there is no evidence of foot pronation either on the lateral or the anteroposterior position. In my experience only occasionally does one find foot pronation associated with this clinical entity.

Symptoms. The majority of such feet are asymptomatic. Occasionally, one may find the patient, usually an adolescent, who will complain of pain directly over the prominence of the medial aspect of the navicular. This is usually due to the pressure of the shoe on the prominence. When it is symptomatic, it occurs usually in the adolescent. It is seldom found as a symptomatic entity in the adult. Occasionally the adult female will complain of the presence of this prominence because of inability to be fitted comfortably with shoes. The symptoms are localized directly over the accessory process itself.

Treatment. Kidner has recommended removal of the accessory navicular and transposition of the tibialis posterior to the plantar aspect of the navicular. He felt that by transposing the tibialis posterior to the plantar aspect of the tarsal navicular, improvement of the longitudinal arch would take place since he had observed that in his cases, pronation of the foot was commonly associated with the presence of an os tibialae externum. In my experience, transposition of the tibialis posterior is unnecessary providing the tendon has not been detached from its insertion during the process of removal of the accessory bone. I recommend the procedure that has been used at the New York Orthopaedic Hospital over the past thirty years. This consists of exposing the tibialis posterior tendon over the navicular tubercle through a 5-cm. curvilinear incision and gently and carefully pealing out the accessory navicular from its insertion in the tibialis posterior. After this has been completed, the tendon is sutured to the surrounding soft tissue structures from which it has been partially dissected free with interrupted number 00 chromic sutures. A firm pressure dressing is applied postoperatively and guarded weight bearing with crutches is permitted at the end of ten days. Full weight-bearing is per-

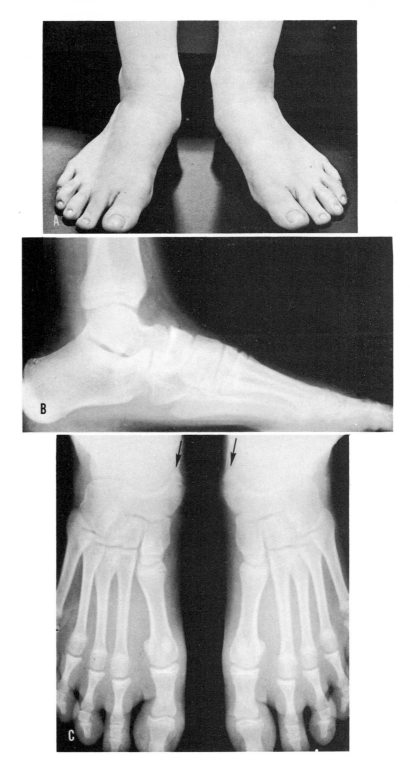

Fig. 19-15. ACCESSORY NAVICULAR. (Os Tibialae Externum)

A. Note apparent pronation of both feet whereas in reality the longitudinal arch is within normal limits and the presence of the accessory navicular causes the medial tarsal portion of the foot to protrude causing the appearance of pronation.

B. Standing roentgenogram of the right foot demonstrating normal longitudinal arch.

C. Anteroposterior view of both feet demonstrating presence of accessory navicular bones bilaterally and producing the apparent clinical pronation of the feet.

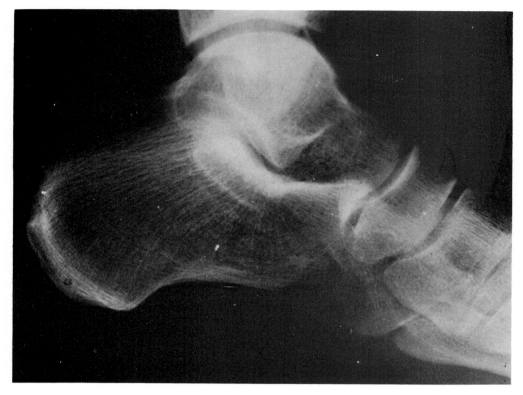

Fig. 19-16.   Asymptomatic calcaneocuboid synostosis. (Courtesy of Veteran's Hospital Roentgeno-graphic Department, Cincinnati, Ohio.)

mitted at the end of three weeks. On the other hand, should the posterior tibial tendon be accidentally dissected free, it is then reattached to the plantar medial aspect of the tarsonavicular with interrupted number 00 chromic sutures, and a firm pressure dressing is applied. Weight bearing is not permitted for a least four weeks and preferably six.

TARSAL SYNOSTOSES

This condition is mentioned only for the sake of completeness of the chapter. Almost invariably such synostoses are asymptomatic and are found incidentally. These may be single synostoses between two bones such as the calcaneocuboid (Fig. 19-16) or may be multiple as in one patient in whom all the cuneiform bones were synostosed in one mass of bone (Fig. 19-17).

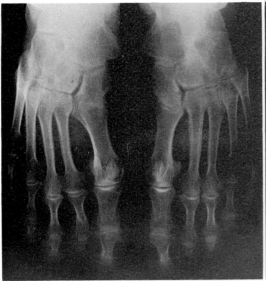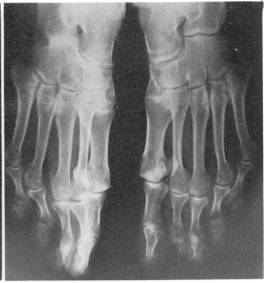

Fig. 19-17. Multitarsal synostosis as well as synostosis of proximal and middle phalanges of the lateral four toes. The patient has similar multiple synostoses of the carpus and of the phalanges of the fingers. (Courtesy of the Veteran's Hospital, Department of Roentgenology, Cincinnati, Ohio.)

DORSAL EXOSTOSES OF THE MIDTARSAL REGION

Exostoses on the dorsal or dorsomedial aspect of the naviculocuneiform or cuneiform metatarsal joints are seen fairly frequently (Fig. 19-18). However, these exostoses seldom require anything more than conservative therapy unless they become exceptionaly large or painful.

Etiology. There are several conditions of the foot which are contributory factors to the development of this bony prominence and its symptoms. It is most frequently found in an arthritic pronated type foot. In many patients, particularly men, this exostosis has been found to become symptomatic and enlarged because the shoe laces have been tied too tightly across the dorsum of the foot. An exceptionally high-arched foot which has been improperly shod will also present a similar appearance.

Symptoms. The patient frequently complains of pain on the exostosis after having worn a tie-shoe as well as difficulty in wearing any oxford-type shoe. The area is slightly reddened and tender to touch. There may or may not be some thickening of the overlying tibialis anterior tendon sheath.

Treatment. Conservative therapy is the procedure of choice. This consists of pre-scribing the type of shoe which will not place any pressure over this region. This measure can be carried out easily in the female by the use of a pump-style shoe. In the male it is much simpler to relieve the pressure by placing a properly-fitted half-donut-shaped pad on the under surface of the tongue of the shoe to relieve the pressure on the exostosis.

Should conservative measures fail, then removal of the exostosis is indicated. A roentgenogram should be procured prior to surgical excision to determine the exact position of the exostosis. Frequently, the examiner will be surprised to find that roentgenographically the prominence, as in a bunion, is much less discernible than it is clinically. The incision should be slightly curved toward the medial surface of the foot. The overlying soft tissue structures should be reflected by careful sharp dissection. The tibialis anterior tendon should be retracted gently. Not only should the exostosis be removed, but the base should be so excised with a curved osteotome that a portion of the surrounding cortex is "scooped out" as well. In other words, the operator should be conservatively liberal

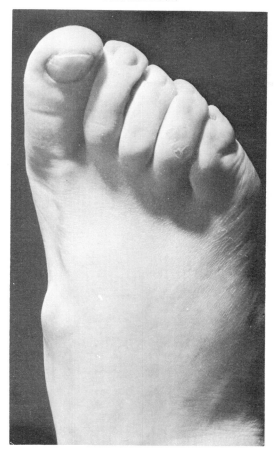

Fig. 19-18. Dorsomedial exostosis of the naviculocuneiform joint.

in the amount of bone to be removed in addition to the exostosis. If the tibialis anterior tendon sheath is hypertrophied in this area, it should be excised as well. Following closure of the soft tissues, partial weight bearing is permitted after the fifth postoperative day.

SPRAINS OF THE INTERTARSAL AND TARSOMETATARSAL REGIONS OF THE FOOT

Although minor to moderate ligamentous injuries (sprains) are seen most frequently in the region of the ankle (involving specifically the fibulocalcaneal and the deltoid ligaments), injuries of the intertarsal and tarsometatarsal ligaments occur with sufficient frequency to warrant discussion.

Etiology. The cause, of course, is a twisting motion placing undue strain on the ligamentous structure, thus producing incomplete tear of the capsuloligamentous tissues.

Symptoms. The principal subjective complaints are immediate onset of pain and inability to bear weight on the foot because of the discomfort. Objectively there is marked tenderness localized in the area of the injury. The amount of swelling of the overlying subcutaneous tissues depends upon the amount of hemorrhage which takes place at the site of the injury. Occasionally, in spite of a minimal twist, ruptures of the surrounding venous structures may take place resulting in the formation of a fair-sized hematoma associated with few subjective complaints.

In addition to the soft tissue swelling there is tenderness over the injured area and there is pain upon motion of the foot particularly on inversion or eversion. At no time is there any abnormal mobility or any restriction of motion. The presence of either of these aforementioned objective symptoms is indicative of greater damage than a sprain to the foot.

Treatment. Therapy consists of the application of a supportive dressing. In the past, a basket-weave adhesive dressing using 2.5 cm. wide tape was considered the standard procedure. At present our method of treatment consists of the injection of 5 to 10 cc. of a local anesthetic solution (providing the patient has no allergy to any of the local anesthetics) into the area of tenderness followed by the application of a snug adherent elastic-like dressing (elastoplast) and the institution of immediate weight bearing. We have not found it necessary to restrict weight bearing or to apply a walking cast which is, at times, indicated in a severe ankle sprain. A supportive dressing is usually necessary for approximately ten days. Occasionally a tender trigger point may remain at the site of the previous ligamentous injury. This can be relieved by the injection of 1 cc. of one of the steroid preparations.

BIBLIOGRAPHY

BADGLEY, C. E.: Coalition of the Calcaneus and the Navicular. Arch. Surg., 15:75, 1927.

DICKINSON, P. H., COUTTS, M. B., WOODWARD, P. E., AND HANDLER, D.: Tendo Achillis Bursitis. J. Bone Jt. Surg., 48-A:77 (Jan.) 1966.

FERGUSON, A. H., JR., AND GINGRICH, R. M.: The Normal and Abnormal Calcaneal Apophysis and Tarsal Navicular. Clin. Orth., 10:87-95, 1957.

HARRIS, R. J. AND BEATH, F.: Etiology of Peroneal Spastic Flat Foot. J. Bone Jt. Surg., 30-B:624 (Nov.) 1948.

HARRIS, R. J.: Retrospect—Peroneal Spastic Flat Foot (Rigid Valgus Foot). J. Bone Jt. Surg., 47-A:1657 (Dec.) 1965.
  Rigid Valgus Foot Due to Talocalcaneal Bridge. J. Bone Jt. Surg., 37-A:169 (Jan.) 1955.

KIDNER, F. C.: The Prehallux (accessory scaphoid) in its relation to flatfoot, J. Bone Jt. Surg., 11: 831, 1929.
  The prehallux in relation to flatfoot, J.A.M.A., 101:1539, 1933.

LYNN, R. A.: Repair of Torn Achilles Tendon, Using the Plantaris Tendon as a Reinforcing Membrane. J. Bone J. Surg., 48-A:268 (March) 1966.

McLAUGHLIN, HARRISON, L.: *Trauma.* Philadelphia, W. B. Saunders Co., 1959, p. 367.

OUTLAND, F. AND MURPHY, J. D.: The Pathomechanics of Peroneal Spastic Flatfoot. Clin. Orth., 16:64, 1960.

PHALEN, GEORGE: Personal Communication.

SLOMAN, N.: On Calitio Calcaneonavicularis. J. Orth. Surg., 3:586 (Nov.) 1921.

SEVER, J. W.: Apophysitis of the Os Calcis. New York J. Med., 95:1025, 1912.

THOMPSON, T. CAMPBELL: Spontaneous Rupture of Tendon of Achilles: A New Clinical Diagnostic Test. J. Trauma., 2:126 (March) 1962.
  A Test for Rupture of the Tendo Achillis. Acta. Orth. Scandinavica, XXXII, Fasc., 3-4, 1962.

WRAY, J. B. AND HERNDON, C. N.: Hereditary Transmission of Congenital Coalition of the Calcaneus to the Navicular. J. Bone Jt. Surg., 45-A: 365 (March) 1963.

= 20 =

The More Common Dermatologic Disorders of the Feet

LEON GOLDMAN, M.D.

THE dermatologic disorders of the foot are similar to those which may occur elsewhere on the body. However, on the foot an eruption is often complicated by the results of stasis. This intensifies the vascular aspect of the skin lesion and may even affect prognosis. Moreover, the continuous wearing of shoes leads to increased perspiration and constant trauma, thus further aggravating the lesions.

NEVI

Various types of cellular nevi may occur on the foot. Because of the high incidence of melanoma on the lower extremities, junctional and mixed nevi are of some special concern. The junctional nevi are characterized by flat, dark-brown spots. Mixed nevi are usually elevated pigmented lesions. Some may have dark, thick nevus hairs. Pigmented nevi on the dorsum of the toes, in the intertoe areas and even in the plantar areas of the feet are common, especially in children.

Essentially, the differential diagnosis of nevi must take into account chronic subcutaneous hemorrhage and melanoma. At times, an old hemorrhage may be difficult to diagnose even with clearing of the skin with oil or xylone and the use of a bright light and a magnifier. With skin microscopy (microscopy with magnifications to 20X of living skin), the isolated foci of the pigment in the nevi can often be distinguished from the homogeneous color of freckling and the diffuse reddish-brown coloration of the subcutaneous hemorrhage. Examination of the nevi under moderate magnification and with a good light may often show the peripheral ring of redness around the areas of the nevi, indicating early evidence of irritation or even of cancerous changes.

Melanomas may start as melanomas or develop from pre-existing junctional or mixed nevi. The appearance of irritation about the periphery is important since most of the other signs of ulceration and growth are those of late cancer. Melanotic whitlow or melanoma about or under the nail also must be differentiated from benign nevi and hemorrhage. The diagnosis of hemorrhage may be confirmed by nail drilling and the use of peroxide. Otherwise, a biopsy must be done. The hereditary tendency to melanomas should also be considered. Occasionally, in children or young adults, a bluish-red lesion (the so-called juvenile melanoma), may be found on the foot. This is not malignant and simple excision is effective as treatment.

The therapy of nevi is excision. The scar should be arranged so that it is not painful and that closure can be effected with a minimal amount of tension. This may be difficult in the excision of deep nevi on the plantar surface. Here, grafting may be necessary.

The problem of elective excision is a difficult one in patients with many nevi on the feet. Unless the lesions are actually traumatized, elective surgery is not indicated in most instances, especially in children or young people. The nevus which is frequently traumatized and which is irritated, especially in the adult, should be excised. Moreover, the sections from the entire lesion should be examined in detail. Excision of nevi in young children may be associated with recurrence of pigment foci in the scars. This does not indicate any tendency to melanoma or even juvenile melanoma but merely emphasizes the multicentric activity of the junctional nevi.

The therapy of melanoma is surgical excision. For melanotic whitlow, amputation of the toe is to be done. Radical excision, lymph node dissection, and deep and extensive "skinning operations" may be necessary for melanomas of the foot and leg. Perfusion techniques with cancer chemotherapeutic agents may be done pre- or postoperatively. The choice of therapy of the melanoma of the foot and leg depends upon the individual patient, type of lesion, age of the patient, results of lymph node biopsies, degree of melanuria, and presence or absence of evident visceral metastases.

Often, at birth or shortly thereafter, or even after many years, a linear, warty-type of growth may develop (Fig. 20-1). This is an epidermal nevus, so-called nevus unius lateris. At times, it may be localized to the foot or spread extensively over the body. These are benign epidermal nevi. If severe pruritus develops at the site of the lesions, a localized neurodermatitis may result. The treatment of epidermal nevi, if treatment is desired, is surgical excision since incomplete removal by cauterization, dermabrasion or cryotherapy often leads to recurrences.

Connective tissue nevi may also occur as small nodules in various parts of the foot. The diagnosis is made chiefly by biopsy.

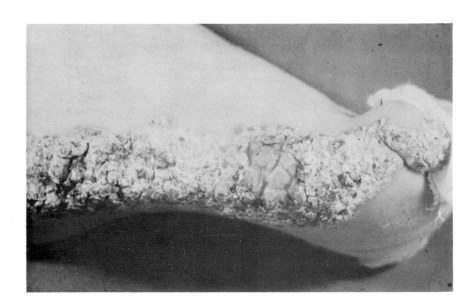

Fig. 20-1. Linear psoriasis looking like linear epidermal nevus.

ANGIOMAS

Angiomas present particular problems especially when they are deep and enlarging progressively. The superficial type can be observed and checked for signs of spontaneous disappearance. Cryotherapy, laser radiation and Grenz-ray radiation may be used on the cavernous types. Neither laser nor Grenz-ray radiation affect the epiphyseal lines. However, if the cavernous types of angiomas grow rapidly, these should be excised surgically. For routine care of static angiomas, careful records should be kept of the lesion with frequent photographs and measurements to determine the progress and growth. Deep angiomas may be associated with changes in growth patterns of the foot, with hypertrophy not only of soft tissue but of the bones as well, and if these are progressive, extensive plastic surgery may be necessary.

Mixed hemangiomas and lymphangiomas may occur also on the foot and lower legs and even produce changes in the size of the foot. Granulomas acquired about the nails are called pyogenic granulomas. They may grow rapidly and therefore require early diagnosis and treatment. Destruction by electrosurgery or cauterization, or even controlled radiation, may be effective in the therapy of these paronychial lesions. In the adult, this condition must be differentiated especially from the amelanotic melanoma.

It is well to remember that with congenital abnormalities or genodermatoses of the foot, a skin lesion may occur as part of a generalized condition. Of interest to the orthopaedic physician are such uncommon congenital disorders as the bullous types, epidermolysis bullosa and pachyonychia congenita associated with leukoplakia of the tongue. Ichthyosis may also be found on the foot and may be severe during the wintertime. Here, dryness and scaling of the skin of various degrees may be found. Less frequent bathing and application of hydrophilic creams are of value both in the prevention and management of this disorder.

REACTIONS OF HYPERSENSITIVITY

There are a number of types of hypersensitivity reactions of the foot that are of interest to the clinician. These reactions include primary irritant dermatitis from simple dryness and irritation of the skin, eczematous contact dermatitis from a delayed type of allergic response to contact irritants, eczematous reactions to local infections, either pyogenic or fungal, and finally, the drug eruptions.

The specific problems that relate to primary irritation occur chiefly in people with dry skin. One common cause is dryness from excessive bathing in cold months. The skin of the lower leg and foot can become pruritic, and itching is aggravated by bathing. The simple treatment for this condition is the avoidance of soap or the use of waterless cleansers, hydrophilic salves or salves which take up moisture, and the reduction or even temporary cessation of bathing.

Contact dermatitis may occur from the finish or dye in stockings or socks and from various chemicals in shoes (Fig. 20-2). Contact dermatitis is recognized by the appearance of dermatitis over the dorsum of the toes and foot as opposed to the intertoe and plantar lesions of the sweating disturbances and fungal infections of the foot. Sometimes, as in the dermatitis from thongs, the characteristic streak of dermatitis is recognizable. Othertimes, detailed patch testing with various types of materials used in shoes must be done to identify the agent. In the meantime, sandal shoes or some open type shoes may be worn. In extreme conditions, vegetable tanned leather or even canvas shoes may be substituted.

Occasionally, there is a dermatitis due to the use of topical agents for the treatment of various kinds of infections (Fig. 20-3). This is recognized as a causative factor by

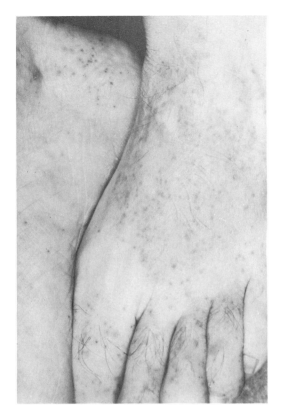

Fig. 20.2 Dermatitis of foot — photodermatitis induced by finishes on socks. Thong protected portion of skin.

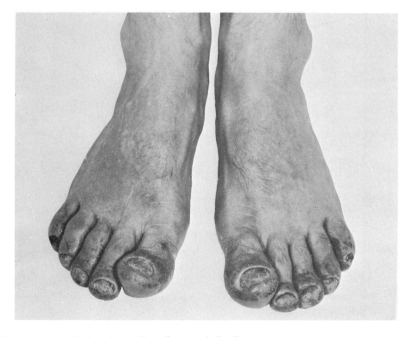

Fig. 20-3. Pustular psoriasis simulating fungus infection.

the severe flare from the use of such substances.

Drug induced eruptions may spread on the foot and become purpuric due to the presence of stasis. Such eruptions cannot be recognized solely from examination of the skin of the foot. The entire skin must be scrutinized. Occasionally, a fixed drug eruption with a localized lesion on the foot or on the ankle may be associated with those drugs which commonly give such drug eruptions. These include phenolphthalein, sulfonamides, antipyrine, etc. In the case of drugs causing photodermatitis, such as some of the antibiotics and tranquilizers, exposure of the dorsum of the foot to the sun may produce localization of the lesions at that site.

FUNGUS INFECTIONS OF THE FOOT

Every instance of intertoe scaling is not necessarily caused by a fungus infection. Some are just excoriations, intertrigo from excessive sweating. Some lesions may even be due to pyogenic or monilial types of infection. Often, scrapings and cultures are needed to determine the exact nature of the causative agent. The characteristic moccasin type of scaling, scaling on plantar areas up on the sides of feet, of Trichophyton rubrum infections may be recognized by simple inspection. In other cases, detailed examination of the scales for fungal elements and cultures may be necessary. Indolent paronychial infections associated with excessive sweating, especially in a diabetic, may indicate a monilial rather than a pyogenic type of infection. Here the monilial antibiotics, such as Nystatin and Amphotericin-B may be used topically.

It is impossible to look at a toenail and make a diagnosis by simple inspection and conclude that the nail changes are due to fungus infection, to dryness, circulatory disturbances in the nail or to trauma from pressure. In the absence of any infection of the contiguous skin, it is impossible to be certain about a diagnosis of this type.

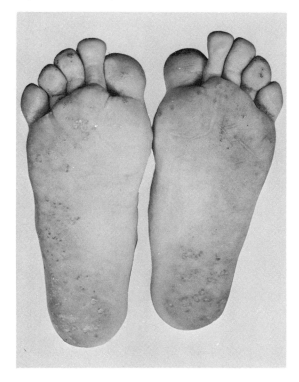

Fig. 20-4. Bilateral plantar psoriasis simulating fungus. Note heavy white dry scaling and absence of blisters.

Nail scrapings may be examined, especially nail biopsy. Any nail biopsy showing fungus elements deep in the nail plate points to a diagnosis of fungus infection, even though saprophytes are obtained repeatedly on cultures. If the diagnosis of fungus infection is established, then specific therapy may be indicated. The anti-fungal-antibiotic griseofulvin is effective only in infections caused by superficial pathogenic fungi. Such factors as sweating and infection make even this type of so-called specific therapy impractical because of the number of recurrences which may ensue (Fig. 20-4). Even confirmed nail infections are particularly resistant. Oral griseofulvin therapy for fungal invasion of nails, especially toenails, may require years of treatment with all the hazards associated with such prolonged drug therapy. The removal of the nail plate in toto by menostats under anesthesia, or by grinding with high-speed drills, sometimes does accelerate improvement after systemic griseofulvin therapy. The permanent removal of the nails may sometimes be necessary in severe recurrences. Topical chemotherapy for fungus infections of the intertoe and plantar varieties is often effective (Fig. 20-5). Tolnaftate (Tinactin) is used extensively at present for such infections. However, topical fungicides are ineffective in confirmed fungus infections of the nail.

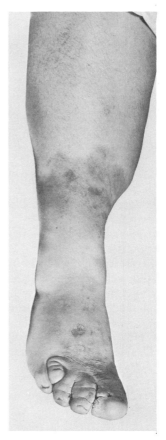

Fig. 20-5. Chills and fever associated with recurrent streptococcal intertoe infection with cellulitis. This is often secondary to an intertoe fungus infection and is called erysipeloid epidermophytide. Chronic lymphedema may result.

VIRAL INFECTIONS

Molluscum contagiosum may occur and spread on the feet, especially the toes. The diagnosis is based on the presence of the characteristic whitish or whitish-red papule with central umbilication. This lesion can be opened and the small pearly mass examined. A typical honey-combed appearance of the cellular mass under the microscope is diagnostically significant. Simple currettage or electrocoagulation will clear these types of lesions.

WART PROBLEM

Unfortunately, the problem is not so simple with warts (Fig. 20-6). These infections are becoming more frequent and perhaps even more in urban groups. Warts are common, not only the plantar types, but also the intertoe warts associated with corns and even the warts on the dorsum of the foot. Their differential diagnosis is often not difficult except in the case of that which is called the miliary corn. This lesion is, in reality, a wart. It is a small cornified or waxy area which spreads rap-

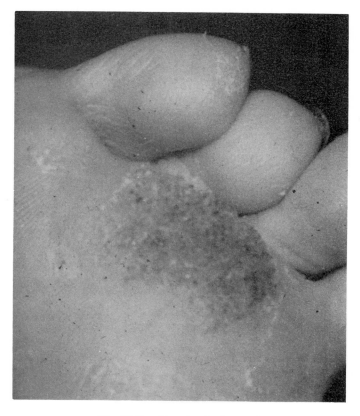

Fig. 20-6.   Mosaic plantar wart.

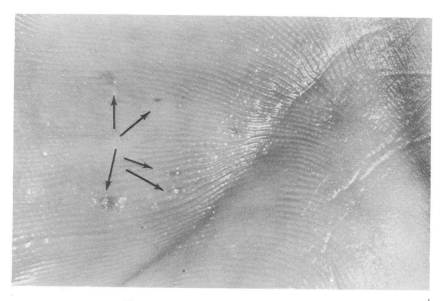

Fig. 20-7.   Miliary type of plantar wart.

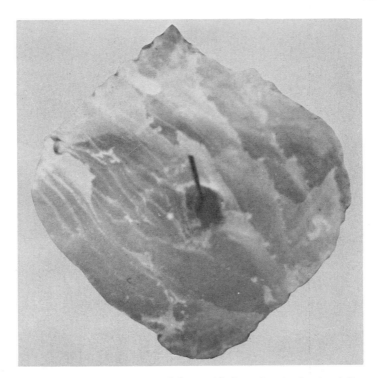

Fig. 20-8. Hair penetrating plantar area of foot with hyperkeratosis simulating corn or wart.

idly, sometimes on areas of pressure, sometimes not. These may occur not only on the feet but also on the hands (Fig. 20-7). The ordinary plantar wart can be differentiated from callosities and clavi by removal of hyperkeratotic elements, cleaning the skin with xylol or mineral oil, then examining the lesion in a strong light with moderate magnification. Under a small skin microscope or sometimes even with a magnifier, plugs characteristic of this condition can be readily seen (Fig. 20-8). Black spots of old dried hemorrhages are not of diagnostic value. It is important to make a differential diagnosis since the corn is the result of pressure, the wart of viral parasitism. Occasionally the two may combine and complicate the problem of therapy.

The differential diagnosis of the intertoe soft corn and the plantar keratosis depends upon the findings of the presence of bone deformity in the background of the soft corn, the presence of plugs in the center of the corn eye area, and the existence of infectious warts elsewhere.

The orthopaedist plays a very important role in the management of plantar keratoses. Unless the pressure is relieved and the structural difficulty is corrected in the area of keratosis, treatment is tedious and often unsuccesful.

There is no single satisfactory treatment for keratosis. The fact that everyone has his own favorite treatment is indicative of the lack of specific and completely effective therapy.

True plantar warts (verruca plantaris) are contagious; at the same time it is necessary to consider them infectious for the individual, himself, and for the community. Therefore, whatever the therapy, it necessitates covering the wart, preferably with some type of adhesive dressing, and bandaging of it during the period of soreness.

The commonest type of topical therapy is still the old faithful salicylic acid 5 to 20 per cent in plaster itself, in collodion, in alcohol or in salve. If this therapy is not successful, then various other materials may be added to it, as in cryotherapy by the use of liquid nitrogen or carbon dioxide. The subsequent procedure is electrosurgery

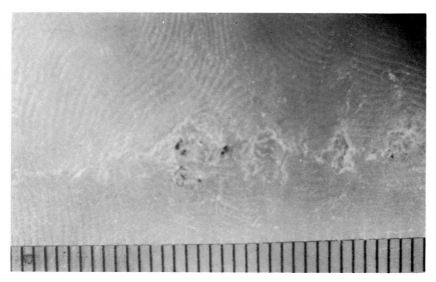

Fig. 20-9.   Plantar keratoses recurrent after extensive excision.

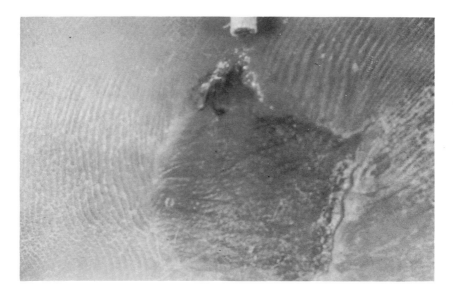

Fig. 20-10.   Plantar keratosis recurrent years after full thickness skin graft.

(Fig. 20-9) usually with local anesthetic and currettage. The lesion is then allowed to heal.

At this stage, vigorous cytotoxic agents, such as podophyllin, may also be used. These should be employed with due precautions because of possible severity of reaction. Topical 5-fluoraurcil is still under investigation as a possible anti-viral agent which can be absorbed intracellularly with specific action on the wart particles.

If all the treatment at this stage is still unsuccessful, the entire situation should be re-appraised. The possibility of surgical intervention (excision, with or without full thickness graft, removal of toes, etc.) should be given careful consideration (Fig. 20-10). In the presence of multiple lesions, an autogenous extract may be used. This is prepared under sterile conditions in a Berkefeld filter, activated and given over a period of time. Due controls with placebo are necessary for the evaluation of an autogenous extract. Little is known as yet about the immunobiology of warts. Although the presence of non-specific antibodies has been suspected, there is still no proof to explain resistance to infection, spontaneous clearing, etc.

With warts occurring in the family-epidemics and in institutional epidemics, vigorous measures should be taken to control spread, controls should be used as regards bathing, swimming and gymnasium facilities. This necessitates the isolation of the infected individual or individuals from public facilities, the continued inspection of those who use public places and continued therapy of everybody with any form of plantar or digital warts.

PYOGENIC INFECTIONS

The pyogenic infection (Fig. 20-11) (impetigo, pustule, furuncle, ecthyma, carbuncle and cellulitis) is important because the trauma of the foot often predisposes to spreading of such conditions until deeper types of infections develop. For example, impetigo may lead to an ulcerated condition, so-called ecthyma. Pyogenic lesions are infectious, spread rapidly in the foot area and the important feature of therapy is rest, removal of shoes, stockings, and rest and elevation of the lower extremity to secure complete healing.

The topical therapy of pyogenic infections include such agents as wet dressings, aluminum acetate fortified with antiseptics, or a solution of Alibour, copper sulfate, and zinc sulfate. Where there is a possibility of secondary infection of tinea pedis, systemic therapy includes the use of broad spectrum antibiotics or penicillin.

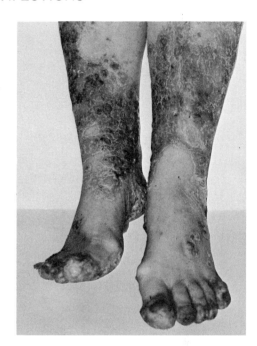

Fig. 20-11. A resistant type of chronic pyogenic infection aggravated by stasis, a dermatitis vegetans.

PARASITIC INFECTIONS

Various types of bites of arthropods may occur on the foot. It is often impossible to tell the type of arthropod by mere inspection of the bite. A common characteristic of the bite reaction is the nodular pruritic lesion. A bullous reaction is found in those areas of the country where the chigger-mite is prevalent. In flea bites there is often a number of small tense pruritic papules. In tropical areas the chigoe-flea may infest the intertoe areas. Myiasis may also be found in the intertoe areas. The local necrotic reaction of spider bites can be suspected but not proved unless direct evidence of the spider is found. The Portuguese Man-of-War irritation may lead to severe burning and pruritus associated with papular and urticarial reactions. If severe enough, shock may develop. The irritating caterpillars may also produce sever reactions even through the thick plantar skin. Sometimes the systemic reaction is severe enough to produce death.

A characteristic parasitic reaction, which can be diagnosed by inspection, is the tunnel of larva migrans (Fig. 20-12). This

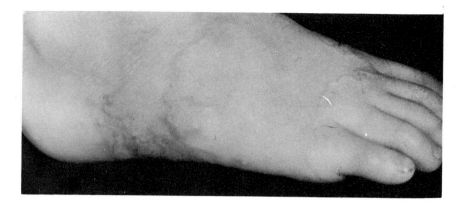

Fig. 20-12. Larva migrans in young uncomfortable child.

worm infestation occurs in endemic areas in the southern states and the causative agent is usually the *Ancylostoma brasiliense*. This reaction begins with intense pruritus any place on the foot and in the intertoe area. If confined to the intertoe area, the oozing and desquamation may be confused with tinea pedis.

PSYCHOSOMATIC REACTIONS

Psychosomatic disorders of the foot occur in the form of excessive sweating, with its concomitants of bromidrosis and the appearance of intertoe and plantar clear blisters (so-called dyshidrosis). Occasionally, neurotic excoriation may be produced. These are bizarre lesions which have an artificial appearance from the first glance. Occasionally these have patches of thickened pruritic lesions which are called neurodermatitis. This is not an etiologic diagnosis but merely a designation for the type of thickened pruritic skin produced by scratching and rubbing. Therapy of chronic neurodermatitis is difficult without complete and prolonged bandaging. Plastic surgery may be necessary for excision of any heavy infiltrated masses. Before plastic surgery is undertaken, an effort should be made to determine whether there is central fixation or internal origin of the pain and discomfort. Otherwise, the patient will get little relief and may sometimes even excoriate the skin graft. Occasionally, psychosomatic factors may aggravate a severe intertoe fungus infection and secondary infection (Fig. 20-13) even to severe cellulitis and sepsis.

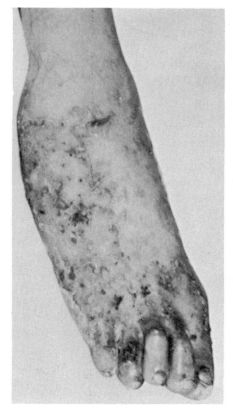

Fig. 20-13. Pemphigus vulgaris resembling a pyogenic infection.

GENERAL ASPECTS OF PREVENTION OF DERMATITIS OF THE FEET

Very early in the course of the development of an individual, it is soon apparent what type of skin the individual has—whether it is the normal, or dry type, or greasy type, ichthyotic or greasy type, seborrheic or hyperreactive type or atopic. With the inheritance of the dry type of skin, early efforts should be made to prevent irritation, increased rubbing or increased sweating of the skin. This indicates the cautious use of mild soaps, such as waterless cleansers, frequent greasing with hydrophilic salves, the wearing of loose-type shoes, and a preference for cotton stocking, and similar measures. Secondary infection, especially of the pyogenic group, should be prevented by attempting to contain or bandage the individual primary lesion. Systemic therapy should be used as a means of helping to clear up the infection. Rest and elevation of the foot should be advocated as much as possible.

The allergic or hyperreactive secretions of the foot should be diagnosed from the etiologic standpoint, not from the response to corticosteroid therapy. A prevention program should be set up. Efforts should be made to try to teach the patient the skin-patch testing technique if the reactions are of the eczematous contact type.

In regard to other infectious lesions, the earliest appearance of a wart is a sign for immediate vigorous surgery and the bandaging of the lesion to prevent the spread. In those who are subject to recurrences of tinea pedis after effective therapy, efforts should be made to prevent flare-ups by use of powder or a daily application of Tinactin or Tolnaftate even after the skin is cleared. Sandals, or open-type shoes should be worn especially in the hot seasons of the year.

TROPHIC DISTURBANCES OF THE FOOT AS RELATED TO THE SKIN

For the clinician, it is important to recognize various types of trophic disturbances of the foot. The most significant is scleroderma. This may be either generalized, as

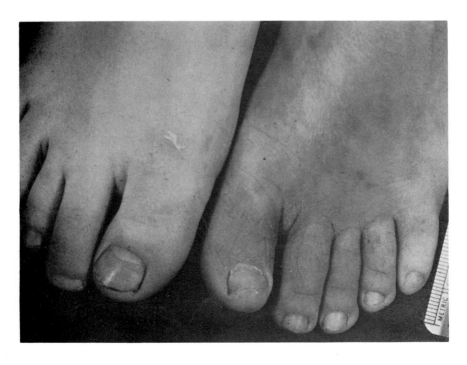

Fig. 20-14.   Linear scleroderma of left foot in young boy with permanent deformity of foot.

part of a systemic sclerosis, or it may be localized. In generalized sclerosis, especially the type associated with Raynaud's syndrome, there may develop acrosclerosis, the typical atrophic foot, similar to that of the hands. The atrophic areas may extend up along the leg.

In localized scleroderma, linear atrophic bands may be present along the top of the foot. These may become progressive, cause ulceration and even necrosis. If these bands occur early in life and the progress is not checked, deformity of the bone actually may result.

The generalized scleroderma involving the foot is treated as scleroderma elsewhere, systemically with corticosteroids; locally with topical fluocinolene creams. The linear or localized band forms of scleroderma are treated topically with the same measures including mecholyl iontophoresis. Plastic surgery has also been done in localized scleroderma (Fig. 20-14). In spite of the poor vascularity of the area, full thickness grafts do take and are of considerable value in relieving the deformity and the inactivity that may be associated with the severe localized scleroderma.

The hypertrophies of the foot occur with varying degrees of lymphedema, with the secondary infection of the skin surface giving rise to severe vegetating areas, so-called dermatitis vegetans. Sometimes these may be the result of deep fungus infections, such as Maduramycosis or chromoblastomycosis. The prognosis of these types of hypertrophies of the foot, associated with an infectious origin and lymphstasis, depends upon the degree of infection of the skin surface and also to considerable extent on the degree of dermal fibrosis. Special soft-tissue x-ray studies will often disclose the intensity of the subepidermal fibrosis and aid in determining the prognosis as to relief or continued obstruction. They may also sometimes be of value in gauging the merits of extensive Kondoleon operations and extensive removal of the tissue down to the muscle.

Various types of infectious granuloma

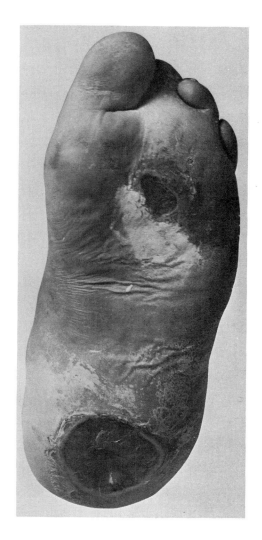

Fig. 20-15.   Mal perforans ulcers of foot.

may involve the foot, producing neurologic deformities. Chief of these are leprosy or Hansen's disease, with characteristic trophic disturbances of the foot in the forms of ulcerations similar to the mal perforans of Tabes, (Fig. 20-15) and with absorption of the bones, leaving only small bits of the toes, commonly so-called "podalic leprosy" with its characteristic x-ray picture.

In addition to the trophic changes in syphilis, there may be actual gummatous changes in the form of deep ulcerations, syphilitic osteitis or osteoperiostitis.

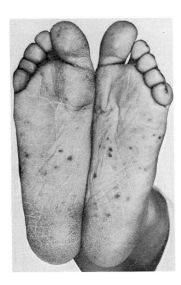

Fig. 20-16.   Acute disseminated lupus erythematosus with hemorrhagic plantar lesions.

Tuberculosis may produce superficial skin lesions in the form of warty types of growths, (Fig. 20-16) so-called tuberculosis verrucosa cutis or tuberculous osteitis with draining sinuses. Sarcoidosis may involve the foot with the development of nodules and occasionally toe lesions similar to the sarcoidal osteitis of the fingers. Blastomycotic osteitis with draining sinuses has also been observed in the feet and ankle areas.

Occasionally, metabolic disorders may involve the foot, occurring as downward extensions of leg lesions. These may appear with localized myxedema involving the foot with such uncommon disorders as lipoid proteinosis with deep nodules and hardness of the skin. These xanthomas may involve the skin with the yellow streakings of the plantar surfaces and may be associated with large nodules about the toes, about the ankles, and about the heels. There is an obvious characteristic, yellowish appearance of these lesions.

In addition to pure stasis dermatitis with all its concomitants of the dilated intercommunicating veins about the malleolus, the hemosiderotic tattooing of the foot, peculiar punched-out whitish lesions representing the atrophic phase of a vasculitis, so-called "atrophie blanche" also may occur around the ankle and foot area. This must be differentiated from serious malignant papulosis or small anemic infarcts with alabaster-like spots on the skin. These are associated with profound visceral disturbances especially gastrointestinal and occasionally cerebral and are often fatal. They represent a type of anemic infarct in the

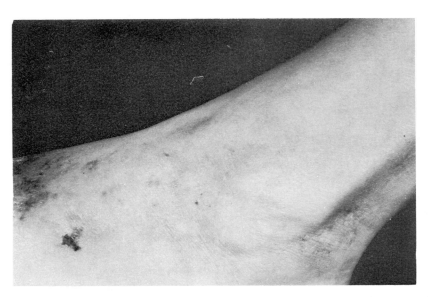

Fig. 20-17.   Ten-year duration of an allergic necrotizing vasculitis with atrophic, hemorrhagic and hemosiderotic lesions.

skin. In addition, various types of allergic vasculitis (Fig. 20-17) may appear on the skin. These occur as petechiae, as deep hemorrhagic areas or as ulcerated areas. A biopsy will show characteristic endothelial changes with hyalinization of the blood vessel wall and thrombosis and hemorrhage. Such lesions must be differentiated from the microangiitis of diabetes.

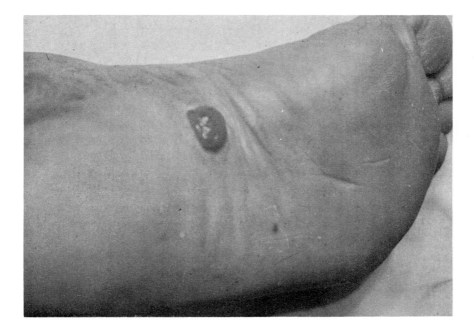

Fig. 20-18.   Benign granuloma pyogenicum — exuberant granulation tissue — simulating amelanotic melanoma.

TUMORS

Benign tumors of the feet include tumors of practically every structure on the foot, from the skin and subcutaneous tissues down to the bone areas. Perhaps the commonest types of lesions in this category are the epidermal cysts, the fibromas, the inflammatory lesions, simulated fibromas around so-called "skin buttons," or subepidermal nodular fibrosis, the cartilaginous tumors of the skin and osteomas. Occasionally, foreign bodies, such as hairs, may produce clavi (heloma durum) or fibrous tumors.

The commonest malignant tumors of the skin, of course, (Fig. 20-18) are the melanomas and the hemorrhagic sarcomas of Kaposi. The melanomas, as indicated previously, may occur in pre-existing nevi, may occur as ulcerative lesions in the form of pigmented melanomas or as amelanotic melanomas. They also may occur in the form of the melanotic whitlow.

The hemorrhagic sarcoma of Kaposi (Fig. 20-19) commonly involves the foot. At first, in the angiomatous phase, there is a reddish diffuse edema. At this stage the nature of the disease may not be suspected. Then, in the intertoe and toe area, nodular red lesions develop which become diffuse, confluent or large. Biopsies will show the characteristic phases of the early angiomatous or late phase of the sarcomatous lesion. The lesions are responsive to radiation or to perfusion therapy with nitrogen mustard or radioisotopes. Laser radiation effectively destroys small tumors but has little effect on the large ones. Kaposi's hemorrhagic sarcoma is long lasting. Only rarely does it give rise to metastatic lesions (Fig. 20-20). This form of malignancy should be differ-

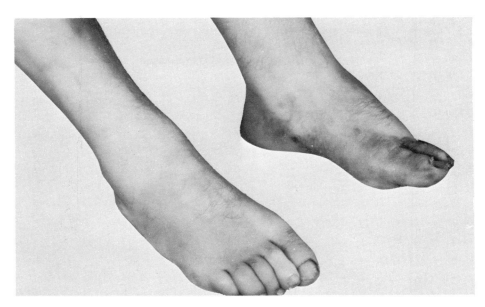

Fig. 20-19.   Hemorrhagic sarcoma of Kaposi — infrared photograph — demonstrating diffuse involvement.

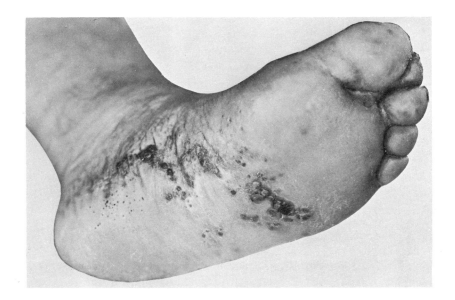

Fig. 20-20.   Hemorrhagic sarcoma of Kaposi with nodular lesions. These cleared spontaneously at a later date.

entiated from the malignant angiosarcomas which rapidly spread, involving the feet. Various types of malignant lymphomas also involve the feet, producing diffuse thickness of the skin or heavy nodules with characteristic pictures. A cytological tissue press will often help to arrive rapidly at a diagnosis by ascertaining the nature of the significant cellular types that are present.

Squamous carcinoma may occur on the foot about the ankles, toes or even plantar areas. Basal cell carcinoma is uncommon on the foot. A tumor related to the basal cell carcinoma, the eccrine poroma, may be found on the lower leg and foot, appearing as a vegetative type of lesion. Metastatic lesions of visceral malignancies may also occur on the foot. There may be a reddish cast to the lesions due to the development of stasis.

= 21 =

Tumors and Infections of the Foot

KENNETH C. FRANCIS, M.D.

TUMORS

TUMORS of the foot are rare. This is particularly evident when primary malignant bone and soft tissue tumors are considered. Nevertheless, an intelligent and enlightened approach to the management of this problem is mandatory for successful treatment. The majority of tumors arising in the foot are benign and of soft tissue origin. One should not be lulled into a false sense of security, however, since malignant tumors do occur at this site, are often subtle in their presentation, and can be devastating in potential. *Metastatic cancer of bone distal to the knee and elbow is unusual.* Nevertheless, it can occur, and the clinician must be aware of this possibility.

Clinical Considerations

The foot is concerned primarily with locomotion and weight bearing. Any lesion that interferes with the functional integrity of its components will naturally produce some degree of disability or pain, or both. Since the foot is the most important weight-bearing unit of the lower extremity, any lesion interfering with this function may be noted sooner by the patient in this site than in many others.

The most common initial symptom in a patient suffering from a tumor of the foot is swelling or a mass, or pain, or both. Tumors located on the dorsum of the foot can interfere with the normal fit of the shoe, thus becoming evident to the patient early in the course of their progress.

The symptom and degree of pain must be accurately evaluated. Is it only present with weight bearing or is it constant and keeping the patient awake at night? The former history is more compatible with benign tumors, while the latter is typical of most malignant bone tumors. Do salicylates

452

completely or partially relieve the discomfort? The pain of osteoid osteoma can be totally eliminated by aspirin (acetylsalicylic acid). An accurate history relative to the course of pain should be obtained. Has it been static, decreased, or increased, and if so, to what extent?

Some benign lesions are subjectively asymptomatic and diagnosed incidentally if a roentgenogram is obtained for some other problem, such as trauma. A pathological fracture can be the initial symptom of a tumor, and a history of trauma is often obtained. This is not surprising when one considers the potential trauma to which a foot may be subjected in this day and age of buses, subways, crowds, and other so-called modern conveniences. A patient may suffer a minimal injury to the foot and subsequently discover a mass. Trauma has no relation whatever as an etiological factor to the occurrence of a true neoplasm. Ewing has described the relationship of trauma to malignancy as "traumatic determinism", specifically, *the trauma serves to call the attention of the patient to a tumor which was already present.*

A thorough physical examination is imperative. The patient should be disrobed so that *both* lower extremities and feet can be examined. It is important to observe the gait. It is essential always to compare *both* feet. A subtle malignant tumor, for example, one involving the os calcis and producing minimal swelling, may easily be missed if only the suspected foot is examined. When palpating a tumor of the foot, the examiner must be thorough and gentle. It is important to note the tenderness of a mass, its consistency (cystic, firm, bone hard), and its mobility (fixed, movable). Is the mass discrete, or ill-defined and elusive? The color of the overlying skin, dilatation of superficial veins, temperature of the area, and induration should also be noted. Whether a mass pulsates or not is of obvious importance. I place no reliability on transillumination of a tumor. Finally, the entire extremity should be examined including local lymph-node-bearing areas, such as the popliteal space and the groin. Some bone and soft tissue lesions can actually be multiple and the lesion involving the foot may be the only symptomatic area. If the foot alone were to be examined in such an instance, sound diagnosis of the basic problem could be seriously impaired.

Biochemical determinations are of minimal clinical value in the management of tumors of the foot. Serum calcium, phosphorous, alkaline phosphatase, and protein determinations should be obtained if indicated. Obviously, it would be superfluous to determine the foregoing if the problem is a typical ganglion swelling. Conversely, the patient with an osteoblastic or lytic lesion in bone should have the benefit of such studies. Hyperparathyroidism can be associated with destructive osseous disease and the serum calcium level is of basic diagnostic importance. The serum alkaline phosphatase may be increased with osteogenic sarcoma.

Although there is seldom involvement of the bones of the foot in multiple myeloma, diagnostic protein and electrophoretic studies should be performed if indicated. A tumor of the foot can present an elusive problem, and the clinician must always exercise judgment relating to the specific laboratory determinations indicated. Roentgenograms should be obtained routinely. Although this may seem unnecessary in some instances, it is conceivable that a serious malignant tumor, detectable only by a roentgenogram, could be missed. Bone tumors in any location are notoriously difficult to diagnose by roentgenograms alone. Nevertheless, adequate roentgenographic study is a valuable adjunct for the accurate and thorough evaluation of this clinical problem. Satisfactory treatment of bone and soft tissue tumors demands close cooperation between the surgeon and radiologist.

It should be axiomatic that an accurate histologic diagnosis must be made before definitive treatment is undertaken. Tumors of bone in any location best exemplify this concept. Again, close cooperation of surgeon, radiologist, and pathologist is basic. All clinical and roentgenographic data must be made available. It is grossly unfair to expect an intelligent histologic or roentgenographic evaluation to be made if the pathologist or roentgenologist has not been supplied with pertinent clinical information. Obviously, the purpose of a biopsy is to obtain a representative specimen of the tumor for microscopic examination. Ideally, as noted previously, an accurate histologic diagnosis should be obtained before definitive therapy is begun.

Benign soft tissue tumors of the foot are occasionally encountered which can be surgically resected, the procedure thus serving both as a biopsy and definitive therapy. In such a situation the surgeon's judgment is paramount. The "blithe" local resection of a tumor of the foot, which clinically was benign, would create consternation if it were an unsuspected synovial sarcoma. If there is even the most remote clinical suspicion of malignancy, it is preferable to perform a gentle and atraumatic biopsy prior to resection. A frozen-section technique can be of immense value. If there is any suspicion that the lesion is malignant, a frozen section would provide a rapid diagnosis, and more radical surgery could be performed immediately if necessary. In my opinion, bone tumors do not lend themselves to sound histologic diagnosis by frozen section. Again, the surgeon's judg-

ment is paramount, since there are certain benign bone lesions which can be treated definitively at the time of biopsy. If there is any suspicion whatever clinically or roentgenographically that a bone lesion in the foot is malignant, only a biopsy should be performed and definitive treatment delayed until the diagnosis has been confirmed.

There have been instances when a tumor of low-grade malignancy could have been adequately resected later and amputation avoided, had the diagnosis been made first and the entire surgical field not "contaminated" with malignant disease from an inadequate and injudicious "resectional biopsy". The use of x-ray therapy as a "test", or for treatment, before biopsy should be decried. Even small amounts of x-ray treatment can so distort the histologic condition of some tumors that accurate diagnosis may be impossible. This is particularly true of Ewing's sarcoma and reticulum cell sarcoma, both highly radiosensitive lesions. Giant cell tumors of bone can also be extremely difficult to interpret histologically after irradiation.

Soft Tissue Tumors

The vast majority of soft tissue tumors that occur in the foot are benign. Few have any tendency to undergo malignant transformation and local surgical excision is the treatment of choice. Since the foot is an important weight-bearing unit, an occasional large and deep lesion can present a perplexing problem. Some malignant soft tissue tumors are amenable to radical local resection; however, appropriate amputation is usually indicated. The management of soft tissue sarcomas arising in the foot will be considered in more detail later in the chapter.

Benign Soft Tissue Tumors. *Ganglion.* The simple ganglion occurs in the foot and is identical to that encountered in the hand and wrist. The etiology of these lesions is unknown. Classically, the dorsum of the foot in the midtarsal area is the most frequent site of origin. The cyst is thin walled and contains clear gelatinous fluid. It is interesting that, in my experience, the lesion always has communication with a joint via

a thin-walled stalk. The latter may be tortuous and its course difficult to identify.

The treatment of choice is surgical excision if the mass is painful or interfering with normal fit of the shoe. A careful surgical dissection is necessary, and the stalk must be followed to the joint and excised. Recurrence is frequent if only the ganglion itself is excised. General anesthesia is recommended and the procedure should be performed in the operating room. Inadequate excision can result when local anesthesia is used and the operation performed in the office. In a small percentage of instances a small ganglion may be successfully treated with injection of hydrocortisone. Traumatic bursting or aspiration of a ganglion is inadequate and eventual recurrence is the rule with these measures.

Xanthoma. Another term for this lesion is giant cell tumor of tendon sheath origin. The reader should not confuse this benign, and completely innocuous, soft tissue tumor with giant cell tumor of bone, a completely

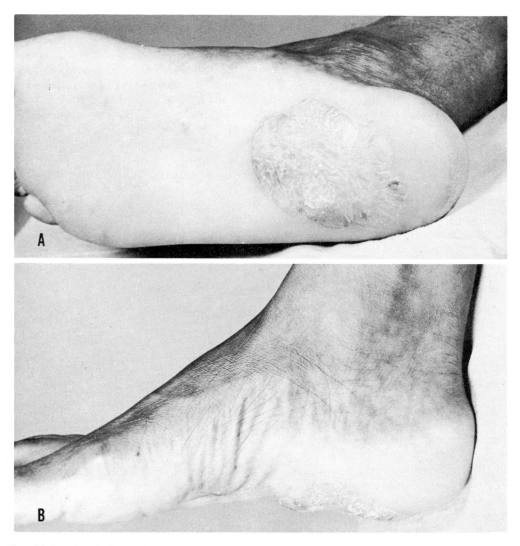

Fig. 21-1.   A.   Solitary fibroma plantar surface right foot.   B.   Lateral view of same lesion.

unrelated entity. Xanthomas can appear anywhere in the foot. As noted they are of tendon sheath origin and most frequently encountered on the dorsum. They are generally asymptomatic unless pressure from a shoe produces pain. Clinically, the tumor is firm, solid, and discretely movable. Tenderness is rare. Histologically, there are whorls of xanthoma cells interspersed with a varying amount of fibrous stroma. Surgical excision is indicated if the lesion is painful due to shoe pressure or if it causes a disturbance in normal function of the foot.

Hemangioma. Hemangiomas are most frequently of the cavernous type. The foot can be the primary site of small, solitary lesions, or it may be secondarily involved when there are multiple lesions involving the extremity. Solitary and discrete hemangiomas of the foot are best treated by surgical excision. If the patient is very young, *i.e.,* a baby, it is advisable to observe the lesion until the foot is of sufficient size to permit an adequate surgical resection. Systemic hemangiomatosis, involving an entire limb, can be a serious problem. The anlage of these tumors is present in the embryonic state, and as the limb bud grows, the arteriovenous communciations also proliferate to intimately involve and infiltrate the adjacent muscles and nerves. Adequate surgical resection can be a difficult and time-consuming procedure. Any area of the foot may be involved including the plantar surface. As noted previously, meticulous surgery is the treatment of choice. X-ray therapy is not indicated, since telangiectasis and scarring results. In addition, the patients are usually young children. Cryotherapy may occasionally be valuable for a small localized lesion in the foot. Systemic hemangiomatosis can produce overgrowth of an extremity and the foot. These patients should be closely followed clinically since growth arrest of one or more epiphyses may be required at the appropriate time.

Lymphangioma. Lymphatic tumors of the non-malignant type are unusual in general. Occasionally one encounters the so-called "lymphangioma" in the foot. Simple surgical excision is the treatment of choice and may be indicated for functional or symptomatic reasons.

Neurofibroma. Von Recklinghausen's neurofibromatosis is a congenital abnormality of considerable orthopaedic importance. The lower extremity can be the site of extensive involvement with resultant deformity and cosmetic calamity. McCarroll has contributed greatly to the fundamental management of these difficult problems. Treatment of each individual patient is "that of the whole," and the foot itself is usually the least important single anatomic unit involved. Surgical resection of as many lesions as possible should be performed. Occasionally, this is a virtual impossibility.

Fibroma and Fibromatosis. Solitary fibromas (Fig. 21-1 A and B) are rare and the treatment of choice is surgical excision. Stout has defined the fibromatoses as so-called "desmoblastic" and "benign" lesions which do not metastasize. However, patients have died because of inadequate treatment and local extension. Microscopic diagnosis is not the total answer to this problem, *i.e.*, it is benign as far as histologic diagnosis is concerned and yet, recurrence may occur and the problem in the foot became locally inoperable. It is probable

that amputation should be performed earlier, before the disease infiltrates proximally into the leg or even higher.

Fibrosis of the plantar fascia is similar to Dupuytren's contracture in the hand. Indeed, every patient with the latter condition in the hand should be examined for a similar process in the foot, since both sites are frequently involved simultaneously. Plantar fibrosis may produce pain with weight bearing. Pathologically, the process may be diffuse or locally nodular within the plantar fascia (Fig. 21-2). Surgical excision is indicated if symptomatic, and recurrence is infrequent.

Should the tumor be located in the plantar fascia, total excision of the plantar

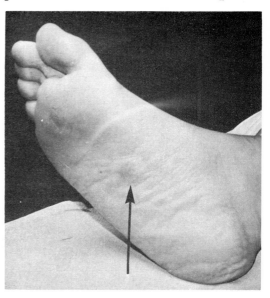

Fig. 21-2. Fibrosis of the plantar fascia. This lesion may be single or multiple and occasionally involves the entire plantar fascia. This may be unilateral or bilateral.

fascia is indicated. The surgical dissection is not difficult but if the skin incision is not properly placed, loss of a portion of the dermis will almost inevitably result. Therefore, one should follow specific incisional lines on the plantar aspect of the foot just as carefully as one does on the palmar aspect of the hand. Properly placed scars on the plantar aspect of the foot are no more symptomatic or disabling, once they heal by primary intention, than they are on the palmar aspect of the hand.

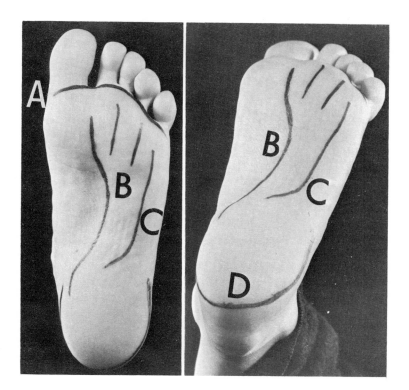

Fig. 21-3. PLANTAR INCISIONS.
Diagrammatic plan illustrating the incisional lines best suited for the plantar aspect of the foot.
   A. Transverse incision to expose plantar aspect of metatarsophalangeal joints as well as the proper digital nerves.
   B. Plantar incision to expose the medial plantar and plantar portion of the fascia.
   C. Line of incision to approach the lateral plantar aspect of the foot.
   D. Horseshoe-shaped incision to expose plantar aspect of the os calcis.

The diagrammatic plan (Fig. 21-3) illustrates the incisional lines best suited for the plantar aspect of the foot. Line A illustrates the transverse incision which can be safely made just proximal to the transverse flexion crease to expose the plantar aspect of the metatarsophalangeal joints. The weight-bearing portion of the forepart of the foot is quite proximal to it. Line B, or any part of it, is the direction of the incision which should be used to expose the medioplantar and the plantar aspect of the foot to expose and resect the plantar fascia. Line A can be utilized for plantar exposure of the digital neuromas. We have excised a plantar keratosis through a longitudinal elliptical incision on the plantar aspect of the foot in at least 50 patients in the past fifteen years. As long as closure of the tissues is meticulously performed and weight bearing is not permitted for three weeks, not a single incident of a painful scar has been reported or seen. Nothing is foolproof nor perfect and possibly tomorrow a patient may report a painful scar or a keloid in one of these plantar incisions, but up to the present time, such a complication has not arisen. Line C is the line of incision used to approach the plantar lateral aspect of the foot, and Line D, which is a horseshoe-shaped incision, can be used to expose the plantar aspect of the os calcis.

Lipoma. Abnormal deposits of adipose tissue are occasionally encountered in the region of the foot and ankle. These are not specifically abnormal and usually not neoplasms. The true, encapsulated and asymptomatic lipoma is rarely encountered in the foot. The author (Francis) has treated one patient with such a lesion arising lateral to the Achilles tendon which had slowly increased in size over a number of years. Surgical excision is indicated as the treatment of choice.

Malignant Soft Tissue Tumors. *Skin.* Squamous cell carcinoma and malignant melanoma account for the majority of malignant soft tissue tumors. The former is more common in the hands, presumably due to external irritants from which the foot is protected. The treatment of squamous cell carcinoma is dictated by the specific clinical situation; however, wide surgical excision with or without inguinal node dissection is the usual treatment indicated. If there are palpable inguinal nodes, node dissection is mandatory.

The astute clinician should be ever mindful that the foot can be the site of origin of malignant melanoma. Booher and Pack reported 122 melanomas of the foot and ankle during a sixteen-year period, from a total of 917 patients, or an incidence of 13.3 per cent. These authors found melanoma located on the dorsum of the foot in 55.7 per cent and on the plantar surface in 44.3 per cent. It is interesting that of these 122 patients, only 4 lesions involved the ankle, while 118 were located on the foot itself. When the lesion arises in a toe or the distal foot, the treatment of choice is local amputation: *i.e.*, toe or "ray" amputation. In other locations in the foot, wide surgical excision with a split thickness skin graft is indicated. The indications for therapeutic inguinal node dissection are distinct: specifically, enlarged and palpable inguinal nodes. The value of prophylactic inguinal node dissection is open to debate. It is my opinion that it should be performed if there is any clinical suspicion of inguinal node involvement. During excision of a melanoma of the foot, isolated perfusion of the extremity with an alkylating agent, such as phenylalanine mustard, may prove to be a valuable technique. If an inguinal node dissection is indicated, I prefer to perform this procedure first. Isolation of the limb and perfusion can then be carried out during excision of the primary lesion in the

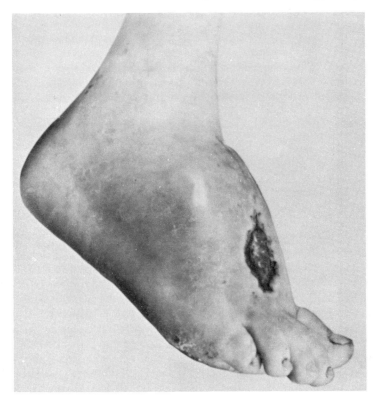

Fig. 21-4. SYNOVIAL SARCOMA.
Note marked swelling of the soft tissue localized to the dorsum of the foot.

foot. The purpose, of course, would be to destroy circulating tumor cells possibly released concommittantly from excision of the primary melanoma in the foot. Booher and Pack report the following results in the treatment of malignant melanoma of the foot:

1. The five-year cure rate for melanoma of the foot treated by local excision alone was 34.4 per cent.
2. Elective groin dissection in the absence of clinical node involvement resulted in a 33 per cent five-year cure rate.
3. Elective groin dissection with histologic evidence of node involvement resulted in 20 per cent five-year cure rate.
4. The overall five-year cure without recurrence for melanoma was 25.3 per cent.

Synovial Sarcoma. Although most frequently encountered in the region of the knee, this tumor can involve the foot. Since synovial sarcomata do not arise from joints per se, they can be easily mistaken in their early stages of proliferation for innocuous ganglia, etc. Pain is infrequent and an enlarging painless mass is usually the initial complaint. These tumors are firm, more or less fixed, and non-tender. Radiographically, a soft tissue mass may be noted, depending upon the size of the tumor. Actual bone involvement is unusual. This may occur more easily in the foot, however, as the tumor proliferates to involve the closely adjacent bone (Fig. 21-4). In the absence of demonstrable metastases, the treatment of synovial sarcoma of the foot is amputation below the knee. The incidence of regional lymph node involvement has been found to be approximately 20 per cent. Inguinal node dissection is indicated in addition to treatment of the primary lesion in the foot, even in the absence of palpable glands. X-ray therapy can be of palliative value for pulmonary or other metastases; however, it is of no value as definitive treatment.

Other Soft Tissue Sarcomas. Fibrosarcoma, liposarcoma, neurogenic sarcoma, rhabdomyosarcoma and angiosarcoma are rare in the foot (Fig. 21-5). Needless to say, accurate diagnosis is mandatory and

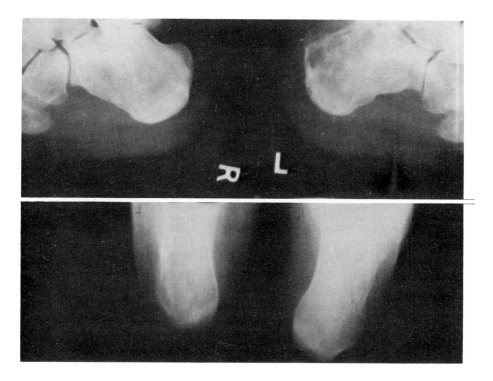

Fig. 21-5. SOFT TISSUE SARCOMA. Fibrosarcoma of left foot involving os calcis.

the subsequent treatment of these unusual problems must, of necessity, be individualized. Conceivably a small, histologically low-grade fibrosarcoma or liposarcoma could be amenable to wide local excision in the foot. Amputation would be indicated in the majority of these cases, with the level of amputation dictated by the specific situation under consideration.

Bone Tumors

Tumors of the bones of the foot are infrequently encountered by the clinician. Nevertheless, these lesions can be of significance since the foot is the principal unit of locomotion and supports the entire body weight. As a result, small lesions which would be relatively insignificant in large bones may be of devastating magnitude when situated in the bones of the foot. Since these bones are essentially small and strong, and they function as a complex unit, any abnormality in their structure can be magnified early and their symptom aggravated with weight bearing. In addition, the clinician must consider that little superfluous soft tissue, except perhaps on the plantar aspect, is present in the normal foot. Therefore, an expanding neoplasm primarily involving the bones of the foot produces a mass, or causes abnormalities in the contour of a specific bone. This can often be readily apparent and leads to earlier diagnosis and treatment. This is particularly evident when one compares the vagaries of palpable clinical examination in the vicinity of the buttock and low back. Since foot pain is a frequent and often distressing problem, both to the patient and physician, in my opinion, the importance of an intensive and thorough investigation of any foot problem, insignificant though it may seem, cannot be emphasized too much. A serious neoplasm may be easily overlooked unless a thorough history is taken and a complete examination performed. As mentioned at the beginning of the chapter, it is now being repeated to reemphasize and reimpress upon the reader the thought that one should not be lulled into a false sense of security, since the foot is by no means immune to the ravages and often tragic results of malignant disease.

Benign Bone Tumors. *Cartilage Tumors.* Osteochondromas and enchondromas are occasionally encountered in the

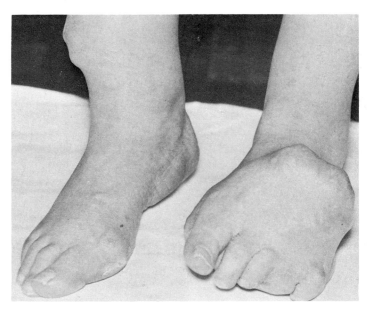

Fig. 21-6.   CARTILAGE TUMORS. Note marked swelling and deformity of left foot.

foot. The former, arising from the distal tibia, can affect the adjacent epiphysis and produce growth disturbances resulting in deformity of the ankle and foot. These lesions are uncommon in the bone of the foot per se. Patients suffering from multiple hereditary osteochondromas may have concurrent involvement of the hands and feet (Figs. 21-6, 7, 8 and 9). Enchondromas occur in the phalanges, and are extremely

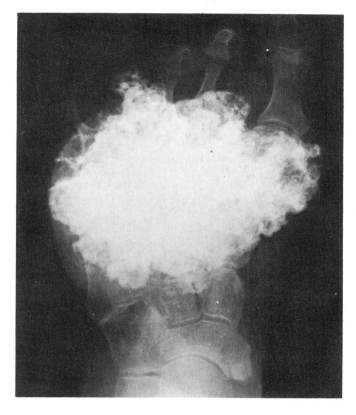

Fig. 21-7.   Roentgenographic appearance of tumor illustrated in Figure 21-6.

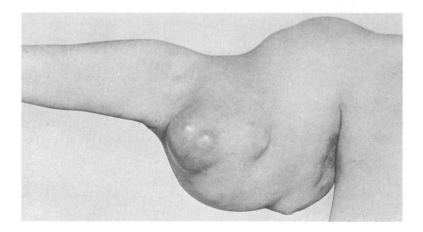

Fig. 21-8.   Cartilagenous tumor involving the right humerus of the same patient.

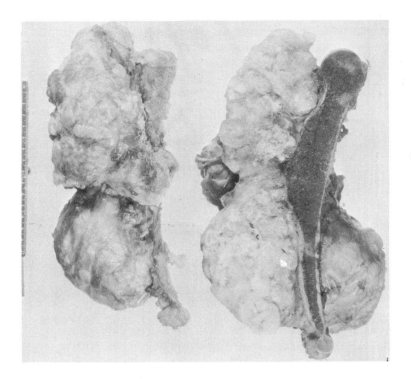

Fig. 21-9.   Gross pathological specimen of same tumor as in Fig. 21-8.

unusual in any other location of the foot. Histologically, these tumors are composed of benign cartilage. Clinically, they more frequently manifest themselves to the patient by deformity, or, as in the case of an enchondroma, a pathological fracture may be the presenting symptom. Surgical excision of an osteochondroma is occasionally indicated for cosmetic reasons. Interference with normal function or shoe wear would provide another indication for excision. As mentioned previously, occasional growth disturbances occur and this possibility might indicate surgery to prevent deformity or alter progression of the lesion. Curettage of an enchondroma with insertion of a bone graft would be indicated to prevent pathological fracture and possible resulting deformity.

Osteoid Osteoma. This interesting lesion was first described by Jaffe in 1935. Since that time a considerable number of examples have been recorded in the medical literature. Osteoid osteoma has been observed in many different bones. However, it is unusual in the foot. In a series of

80 cases reported by Freiberger, 6 lesions were located in a bone of the foot. The cardinal initial symptom of this condition is low-grade pain, which typically is completely relieved by salicylates. The reason for this specific salicylate response is unknown, but it can be an important differential feature in diagnosis. The roentgenographic characteristic of osteoid osteoma is the intense cortical and periosteal new bone formation induced by the usually lucent nidus within the cortex or subcortical layers. Since the bones of the foot are small and of varying arthitecture, the roentgenographic appearance may not be as typical as that observed when the lesion is located in a long bone. This has been noted with osteoid osteomas located in the neck of the femur and spine. The most important differential diagnosis is that of infection, since the roentgenographic findings may be almost identical. Demonstration of a nidus is of fundamental importance. Tomograms have been of definite value in demonstrating a nidus not visible on routine films. The indicated treatment of osteoid

osteoma is surgical excision of the entire nidus. Roentgenographic control in the operating room can be of benefit to locate an elusive nidus and to document its complete removal. Unless the nidus is totally removed, symptoms persist and reoperation is required.

Unicameral Bone Cyst. The foot can be the primary site of a unicameral bone cyst. Symptoms are usually absent and the diagnosis is made incidentally or because of a pathological fracture. In a recent study of a large number of these lesions, the os calcis was found to be the most frequently involved bone in the foot, specifically, 5 in a series of 175 patients. Characteristically, the cyst is located in the anterior inferior potion of the os calcis. The reason for its predilection for this area of the bone is unknown. The indicated treatment, if the cyst is of sufficient size, is curettage and filling the cavity with a bone graft.

Benign Giant Cell Tumor. Giant cell tumors are rare lesions. They are even more rare in the bones of the feet. Coley describes two giant cell tumors located in the foot, one in the os calcis and the other in a metatarsal. In a series of 96 patients reported by him from the Memorial Hospital in New York City there was none located in any bones of the foot. Dahlin has reported one in the foot. Giant cell tumors of bone are potentially dangerous in any location. Surgery is the treatment of choice. The specific operation performed must be predicated upon absolute and total removal of the tumor. It may be possible to perform radical resection and leave the patient with a functional foot. However, if there is any question that the lesion may not be adequately excised, amputation would be necessary, its level depending upon the area of the foot involved.

Paget's Disease. Paget's disease may exist in the foot. The condition may be either monostotic or polyostotic. When the foot is involved, the first symptom is usually an increase in the size of the foot and difficulty in wearing shoes. There may be pain from this mechanical problem, and it is well known that this condition can also produce low-grade pain. Roentgenographically there is usually enlargement of the affected bone with thickened and coarsened trabeculae intermingled with areas of resorption. In this condition both processes progress simultaneously. The treatment of symptomatic Paget's disease involving bones of the foot should be conservative. It consists mainly of obtaining the correct shoes. Small doses of x-ray may occasionally be of benefit in reducing the pain.

Miscellaneous Benign Tumors. Other benign bone tumors are extremely rare in the foot. Isolated examples of aneurysmal bone cyst, chondroblastoma, fibrous dysplasia, non-osteogenic fibroma, and hemangiomas have been described.

Malignant Bone Tumors. *Primary Tumors.* Malignant bone tumors are relatively uncommon when one considers the cancer problem as a whole. They are infrequent distal to the elbow and knee. The most important initial symptom of a primary malignant bone tumor is pain. Since the bones of the foot are small and have a minimum of overlying soft tissue, the presence of a tumor may be detected earlier than with a similar lesion located in an area such as the pelvis where abundant soft tissue frequently masks the tumor. In addition, the clinician must realize that since the foot is a weight-bearing unit, it is constantly being traumatized. Any disturbance in this normal function may be noted earlier by the patient than in other areas of involvement. The author (Francis) prefers to follow the classification of Jaffe and consider osteosarcoma, chondrosarcoma, intramedullary fibrosarcoma, and angiosarcoma as distinctly separate entities. The inclusion of all these lesions under the broad definition of osteogenic sarcoma seems confusing and ambiguous. Under the designation of osteogenic sarcoma, I include osteosarcoma, juxtacortical low-grade osteogenic sarcoma, irradiation osteogenic sarcoma, and Paget's osteogenic sarcoma.

The importance of an early roentgenogram cannot be overemphasized. It is basic procedure to obtain a roentgenograph when any patient complains of persistent pain in the foot. This is particularly true in children, since their mild complaints are often disregarded as "growing pains" or signs of other ethereal conditions.

Thorough clinical examination of the patient is of fundamental importance. It must be emphasized again that both feet should be compared, the gait observed, and palpation thorough and unhurried. The patient should be disrobed.

Osteogenic Sarcoma. OSTEOSARCOMA. This neoplasm is the most common of the primary malignant bone tumors. It is most frequent in the distal femur and proximal tibia, these two sites accounting for approximately 75 per cent of these tumors. Osteosarcoma can also occur in the foot. In a recent report McKenna *et al.* noted 3 osteosarcomas in the bones of the foot, 2 in the metatarsal and 1 in the os calcis. Dahlin reported 490 osteogenic sarcomas and 5 arose in a bone of the foot. It is obvious, therefore, that this tumor is exceedingly rare in the foot.

Pain is the most important initial symptom concurrent with progressive disability. The roentgenogram is characterized by bone destruction with varying degrees of associated osteoblastic change. The tumor may be completely lytic, densely osteoblastic, or usually a combination of both. The differential diagnosis must include infection, metastatic disease, and other primary malignant tumors. Some authorities have had the impression that the more distal the site of origin of an osteosarcoma from the axial skeleton, ·the better the prognosis. My personal experience in the treatment of this disease does not support this concept. McKenna *et al.* reported 3 osteosarcomas arising in the foot and none of these patients survived five years. The treatment of osteosarcoma in any location is surgical, specifically, amputation. Roentgen therapy alone is not satisfactory definitive treatment and must be reserved for the inoperable tumor in the spine and elsewhere. The value of preoperative x-ray therapy is controversial at the present time. My experience further reveals that the five-year-survival rate without disease is essentially the same whether x-ray therapy was administered before amputation or whether amputation alone was performed. Coventry and Dahlin report a 20 per cent five-year survival without disease with amputation alone. Therefore, an *osteosarcoma arising in the foot should be treated with a below-the-knee amputation, with or without preoperative x-ray therapy. Any lesser amputation is contraindicated* (regardless which bone in the foot is involved) since there would be an excellent possibility of local recurrence from an inadequate margin of resection. It should be obvious that the foregoing remarks pertain to the patient who has been thoroughly investigated clinically and found to have no evidence of metastatic disease. Investigation should include thorough clinical and laboratory examination, roentgenograms of the affected part, chest, and a skeletal survey. The latter are obtained routinely since the incidence of metastases to other bones is higher than generally considered, namely 10 to 15 per cent in my experience.

Treatment of the patient who presents with metastatic osteosarcoma to the lungs or other bones can be a very difficult problem. Amputation of the primary site is usually contraindicated in such circumstances. A palliative amputation may be indicated if the tumor is fungating, producing agonizing pain, or has failed to respond symptomatically to x-ray therapy. It is our practice to treat the primary tumor with x-ray therapy. It is our practice to treat the primary tumor with x-ray therapy *when metastases are present elsewhere.* The primary tumor may be controlled for a short period of time and amputation avoided; symptomatic sites of metastatic disease are similarly treated as necessary. Pulmonary metastases should be treated with x-ray therapy if there are symptoms such as spontaneous pneumothorax, hemothorax, or severe pain. It is obvious that each of these problems must be individualized.

JUXTACORTICAL LOW-GRADE OSTEOGENIC SARCOMA. This tumor is exceedingly rare. The definition (juxtacortical) refers to the position of the tumor in relation to the cortex. It is important to emphasize that the basic significance of this tumor is its histology. It may be of low-grade malignancy throughout. One must realize, however, that one area of a specific tumor may be histologically low-grade, while anaplastic osteosarcoma may be noted in other

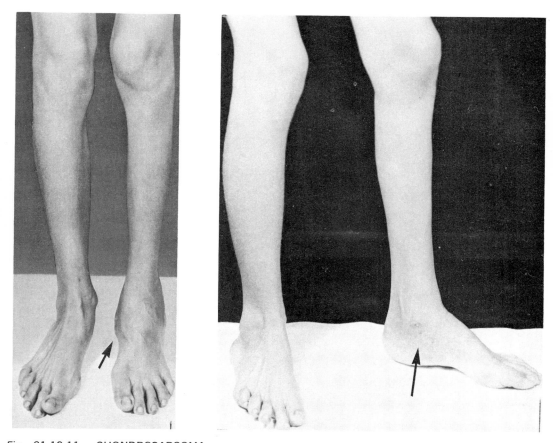

Fig. 21-10-11. CHONDROSARCOMA.
  Symptomless mass of the rear foot which upon investigation proved to be a chondrosarcoma of the os calcis.

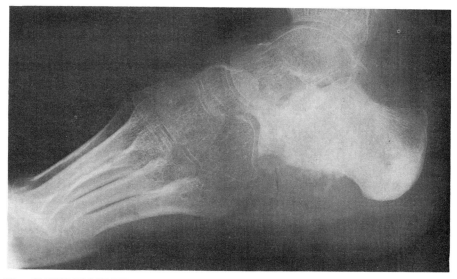

Fig. 21-12. CHONDROSARCOMA OF THE OS CALCIS.
  Roentgenographic appearance of the foot illustrated in Figures 21-10 and 11. Roentgengraphically a chondrosarcoma is a destructive lesion with varying degrees of stippled calcification within the tumor.

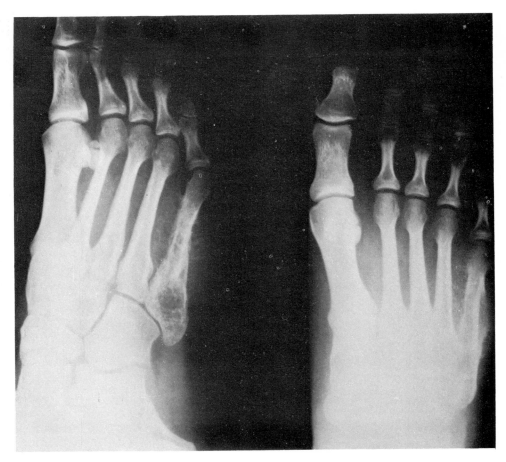

Figs. 21-13-14. EWING'S SARCOMA.
Destructive lesion of the fifth metatarsal roentgenographically diagnostic of a Ewing's sarcoma.

areas. Such a tumor must be considered a fully malignant osteosarcoma despite the radiographic appearance. McKenna *et al.* reported 22 of these tumors, none located in the foot. The author of this chapter has recently observed a low-grade juxtacortical osteogenic sarcoma arising in the fourth metatarsal. A local excision had been done in another institution four years previously. The patient first noted recurrence when she found it difficult to wear her shoe due to increased width of the foot. There was no pain. The tumor was treated surgically, with radical resection of the fourth metatarsal and toe, shifting the fifth metatarsal medially. The patient has done well, walks without symptoms and wears a normal shoe. It should be emphasized that such procedures should be performed only when the entire tumor can be adequately resect-

ed. If there is any possibility that the surgical procedure could not provide an adequate margin of resection, amputation would be indicated.

Chondrosarcoma. This primary bone sarcoma is rare in the foot. Coley and Higinbotham in 1954 reported 52 secondary chondrosarcomas, none located in the foot. Dahlin noted 2 tumors in the foot. McKenna *et al.* recently reported the experience of Memorial Hospital from 1925 to 1955. There were 139 chondrosarcomas and 2 of these were located in the foot, specifically, the os calcis. The most frequent symptom of chondrosarcoma is a mass with or without pain (Fig. 21-10 and 11). It can arise in a child or an adult. Since many chondrosarcomas are initially of low-grade histologic malignancy, the history may be of considerable duration. In the foot, the

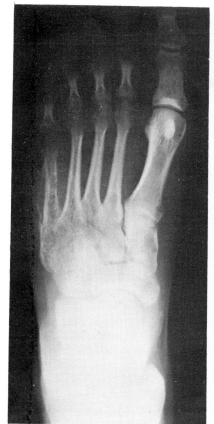
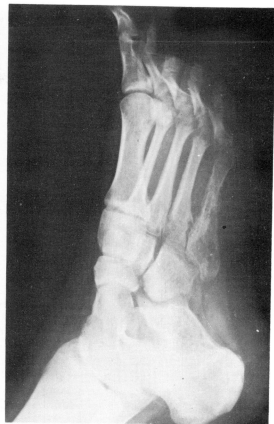

Fig. 21-14.

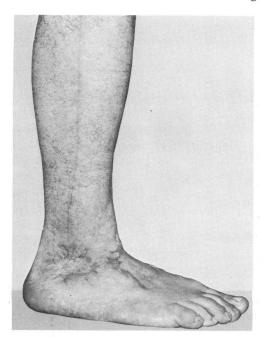
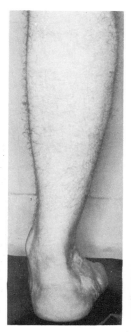
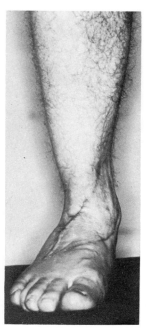

Figs. 21-15-16-17. Postoperative photographs of patient who had undergone radical resection of the entire fibula because of a Ewing's sarcoma. The lateral aspect of his ankle joint has stabilized with scar tissue and he is able to walk normally.

most frequent initial symptom, again, is interference with normal fit of the shoe. Roentgenographically, chondrosarcoma is a destructive lesion with varying degrees of stippled calcification within the tumor (Fig. 21-12). The treatment of chondrosarcoma, only if the tumor is of low-grade malignancy, may consist of radical local resection to preserve a functioning extremity. This may be possible in the foot. However, the choice of a specific surgical procedure must be highly selective, based upon the individual circumstances and predicated upon adequate and total removal of the tumor. If the tumor is histologically fully malignant or anaplastic, amputation is mandatory. Below-the-knee amputation would be indicated for such a tumor arising in the foot. The importance of the margin of resection cannot be overemphasized. We have observed numerous recurrences of chondrosarcomas in various locations which had been treated initially with an inadequate resection (when the tumor was still low-grade) only to have the tumor recur subsequently with greater malignancy. Suffice to say, had adequate surgery been performed initially, local recurrence and possible subsequent metastases would probably have been avoided.

Ewing's Sarcoma. Ewing's sarcoma is an enigma. This tumor most frequently affects younger children under ten years of age. However, it can be encountered up to the age of twenty-five. The most frequent initial symptom of this neoplasm is pain. Not infrequently a mass is noted by the patient or his parents. Any bone may be the site of origin. Clinically the patient may be febrile with a leukocytosis and increased sedimentation rate. Since a soft tissue mass is one of the characteristics of this tumor, the unsuspecting physician may consider the lesion to be an abscess and injudicious incision and drainage may be performed. The roentgenographic appearance of Ewing's sarcoma is quite variable. However, a fusiform area of "moth-eaten" destruction with periosteal new bone formation is usually present. Again, the roentgenogram can certainly be confused with acute inflammatory disease of bone. It is obvious, therefore, that an accurate his-

tologic diagnosis must be made by biopsy prior to the institution of any definitive therapy.

A thorough clinical evaluation of the patient should be performed, including roentgenographic examination of the chest and all other bones. The serum alkaline phosphatase is rarely elevated unless there is extensive metastatic disease. Most authorities are in agreement that there is a definite entity labeled Ewing's sarcoma. On the other hand, a difficulty is encountered when attempting to histologically differentiate Ewing's sarcoma from reticulum cell sarcoma and metastatic neuroblastoma. Ewing's sarcoma metastasizes invariably to other bones and frequently to the lungs. We have never seen a patient suffering from Ewing's sarcoma with metastases who did not have other bone involvement. Metastatic disease may also be widespread to the soft tissue and viscera. The question of the preferred treatment of a patient suffering from Ewing's sarcoma in the absence of demonstrable metastases is completely unsettled. While the tumor is radiosensitive, it is rarely radiocurable, in my experience. Coley reported 4.1 per cent cure utilizing radiation therapy in the treatment of the primary lesion. Dahlin reported 141 patients (the foot was the site of origin in 6) and advised amputation as probably the best treatment. I have personally treated 30 patients in the past ten years, and none has survived five years after treatment with x-ray therapy alone. Two patients are alive and well, one and two years, respectively, since surgical treatment without x-ray therapy. It is, therefore, obvious that a new approach to this problem is mandatory. I have treated 4 patients with Ewing's sarcoma arising in a bone of the foot. Two of the lesions were located in the lateral malleolus, one in the first metatarsal and one in the fifth metatarsal (Figs. 21-13 and 14). Both patients with tumors in the metatarsal who were treated with x-ray therapy developed documented recurrent lesions in the original tumor. One patient subsequently underwent leg amputation. However, both have died. Two patients with tumors arising in the lateral malleolus were treated

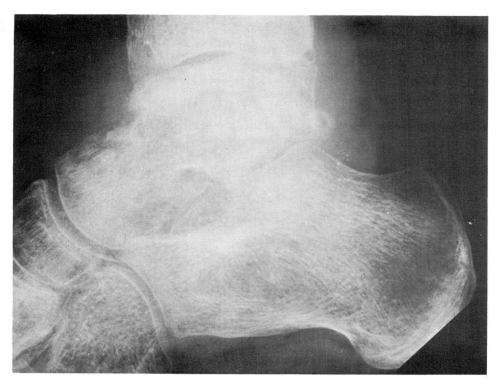

Fig. 21-18. RETICULUM CELL SARCOMA.
This is a rare, isolated reticulum cell sarcoma of the talus. Symptoms were minimal. X-ray therapy is the indicated treatment.

surgically by radical resection of the entire fibula together with the tumor and lateral cortex of the distal tibia. One was alive and well one-and-one-half years after treatment, and the other expired with widespread disease three months postoperatively. Radical resection of the entire fibula can be performed and accomplish the same purpose as an amputation, namely, removal of the entire bone in which the tumor is situated. The surviving patient noted above is able to walk normally with no instability, and the lateral aspect of his ankle joint has stabilized with scar tissue (Figs. 21-15, 16 and 17). It should be emphasized that the resectional surgery for these tumors is not generally advocated, unless the lesion arises in a location where such a procedure can be performed. At the present time it is our considered opinion that amputation with or without preoperative x-ray therapy is the treatment of choice.

Reticulum Cell Sarcoma. Reticulum cell sarcoma can arise as an isolated lesion in bone (Fig. 21-18). It can occur at any age, symptoms are frequently minimal, and x-ray therapy is the indicated treatment. The foot is rarely involved. If systemic disease is present, chemotherapy should be instituted. Local recurrence following x-ray therapy is extremely unusual. The five-year-survival rate following x-ray therapy for a local osseous lesion with no evidence of disease is 55 per cent and the ten-year-survival rate is 35 per cent.

Intramedullary Fibrosarcoma. This tumor is unusual and few cases have been reported in the foot (Figs. 21-19 and 20). It can occur at any age and it can involve any area. McKenna *et al.* report 60 tumors, 2 arising in the bones of the foot, 1 in the os calcis, and 1 in a metatarsal. In one of these the patient survived five years. Surgery is the treatment of choice, namely below-the-knee amputation.

Paget's Osteogenic Sarcoma. As discussed previously, Paget's disease may be encountered in the foot. Osteogenic sar-

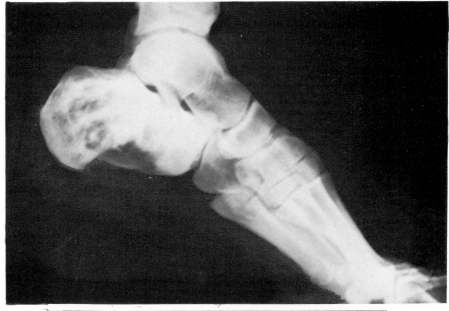

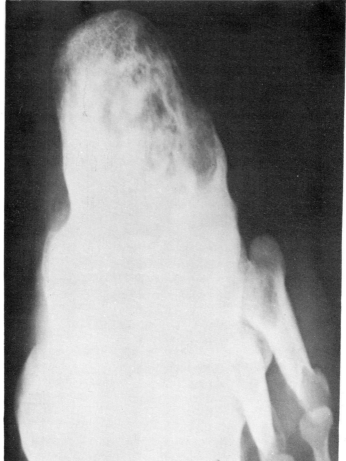

Figs. 21-19-20. INTRAMEDULLARY FIBROSARCOMA.
Lesion arising in the os calcis. Treatment of choice is below the knee amputation.

coma complicating Paget's disease is rare (Fig. 21-21). In the past ten years I have treated 5 patients suffering from Paget's osteogenic sarcoma, with 1 case involving the os calcis. None of these patients has survived after amputation. The tumor is highly malignant and the prognosis is essentially hopeless despite any type of therapy. The patients are usually in the older age group, the disease is rapidly progressive and pain can be severe. Amputation is occasionally necessary as a palliative procedure since the tumor is highly radioresistant. Metastases occur rapidly, almost invariably to the lungs, and most patients succumb to the disease within one year.

Multiple Myeloma. This is a systemic disease and frequently must be considered in the differential diagnosis of primary malignant bone tumors. Although the disease may initially present as a solitary bone lesion, it will always eventually become systemic. The bones of the feet are rarely involved unless there is widespread disease. The most efficacious treatment for symptomatic lesions is x-ray therapy and appropriate systemic chemotherapy. The most effective agent at present is Alkeran (phenylalanine nitrogen mustard) administered orally. There is as yet no curative agent for this condition.

Secondary (Metastatic) Bone Tumors. Any malignant tumor can metastasize to bone. It is true that the majority of metastatic lesions in bone are proximal to the elbow and knee. Nevertheless, they can occur distally and the foot can be involved. One should always be cognizant of this fact when a patient who has been treated for a malignant tumor complains of pain in the foot. The first evidence of metastatic disease can be an osseous metastasis. I have observed metastatic disease in the bones of the foot from breast carcinoma, adenocarcinoma of the colon, renal carcinoma, lung and prostate carcinoma. The treatment of metastatic disease in the bones of the foot depends upon the specific situation. Generally, x-ray therapy is indicated for symptomatic relief.

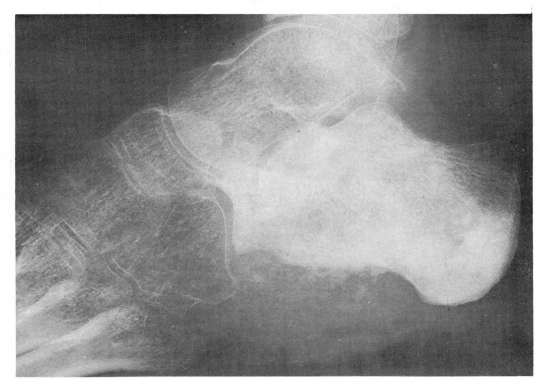

Fig. 21-21. OSTEOGENIC SARCOMA COMPLICATING PAGET'S DISEASE.
 Paget's osteogenic sarcoma involving the os calcis. This type of tumor is highly malignant and prognosis essentially hopeless.

Summary

Although unusual, bone and soft tissue neoplasms of the foot can pose an important and difficult problem for the orthopaedic surgeon. Tumors of the foot have been discussed in regard to their classification, symptoms, diagnosis, and treatment. Specific tumors have been discussed in detail. The foot is the most important weight-bearing unit of the lower extremity; a thorough knowledge and appreciation of the neoplasms that can arise in the foot are fundamental to the intelligent management of the patient.

INFECTIONS OF THE FOOT

Infections of the foot are included in this chapter since occasions do arise wherein the differential diagnosis between tumor and chronic low-grade infection must be made (Fig. 21-22).

The infectious processes in the foot can be divided essentially into 1) the more common coccal (staphylococcus, pnemococcus, and streptococcus), 2) the bacillary (tubercle and leprosy acid-fast bacilli), 3) the pathogenic fungi (blastomyces, actinomyces, and coccidiodes), and 4) the spirochetal (*Treponema pallidum* of syphilis and the *Treponema pertnue* of yaws). There are also several rare tropical diseases which affect the foot, but not much information is available on these at the present time. However, with the United States Armed Forces spread all over the globe, it is anticipated that more reports will be coming in relative to the nature of Madura Foot, Ainhum disease, cutaneous Leishmaniasis (Delhi or Aleppo boil or Oriental sore) and other rare diseases, as well as to known methods of treating them.

Soft Tissue Infections. Acute cellulitis of the foot and localized soft tissue infections do not occur as frequently as they once did. This is due, in all probability, to the fact that the greatest portion of the population now walks about with some foot covering. Furthermore, since the advent of antibiotics, an infection is controlled at an early stage and thus, in many instances, it is prevented from progressing to the development of systemic symptoms. In soft tissue infections, the therapeutic regimen consists of rest, the administration of the antibiotic or antibiotics which the physician may feel will best control the infection, and the application of moist warm dressings and/or heat. Should fluctuation appear, incision and drainage should be carried out. The basic principles of good surgical care also apply.

Osteomyelitis of the Foot. The surgical principles which have been propounded in

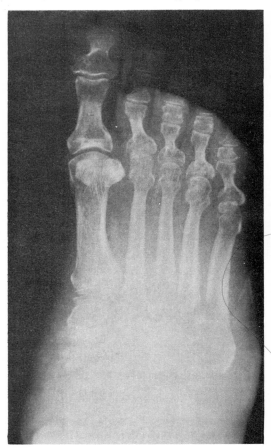

Fig. 21-22. Differential diagnosis between tumor and infection is sometimes difficult. Is this midtarsal destruction due to tumor or infection? Biopsy proved it to be an infectious lesion, namely, tuberculosis.

the treatment of acute osteomyelitis of other portions of the upper and lower extremities also apply to the foot. Initially, of course, the diagnosis must be made. Hematogenous osteomyelitis of the foot is extremely rare and is seen almost exclusively in children, particularly infants. In the majority of instances osteomyelitis of the foot arises as a direct extension of injuries to the soft tissues of the toes, or occurs following open fractures of the foot, or as extension of an infection through a trophic ulcer (as in diabetes), or following insertion of Kirschner wires or pins through the os calcis.

Only rarely is the classical systemic symptomatology of an acute toxic disease manifested in acute osteomyelitis of the foot. The patient usually demonstrates a mild-to-moderate temperature elevation, no toxic manifestations, and only a moderate elevation of the white blood count. In fact, except in infants, the systemic reaction is usually mild.

Locally, the patient complains of intense pain in the foot, inability or unwillingness to bear weight on the foot due to the pain, and limitation of motion. If the infection should be limited to one of the toes or the metatarsophalangeal joints in an adult, the examiner may be hard put at times to differentiate this condition from acute gout since the symptoms are only local. In fact, this holds true for the entire foot and not only for the digits.

Roentgenographically, the diagnosis cannot be made for at least ten days after the onset of the symptoms. Then the classical picture of osteomyelitis is demonstrable.

Again, treatment differs somewhat from that in other portions of the extremities. Immediate incision and drainage without a specific area of localization is not indicated. The patient should be placed at absolute bed rest with the foot elevated as well as wrapped in constant warm, but not necessarily wet dressings. A blood culture should be routinely procured although it will not be positive too frequently. A wide spectrum antibiotic (to which the patient is not, of course, allergic) should be given in large doses either intravenously or intramuscularly, preferably the former.

In my experience, oral antibiotics, even in massive doses, when given alone have not been as effective as when given by either of the other routes of administration. Once the infection has localized, incision and drainage should be carried out, the organism should be identified, and the proper antibiotic prescribed. In the toes and the metatarsophalangeal area localization will take place even before roentgenographic changes will be demonstrable. In the tarsometatarsal structures, as well as the posterior tarsal bones, such early localization is seen only in an acute pin infection in the os calcis. Otherwise, the treating physician is required to wait until roentgenographic changes have taken place.

In children, when incision and drainage is contemplated, it is not wise to enter the involved bone or bones with vigor. To do so will result in destruction of the growth centers and lead to deformity of the foot. At most, only one or two small drill holes should be made in the involved bone to establish drainage. The essential regimen is antibiotic therapy, as well as general supportive treatment. The foot and leg should be immobilized in a well-molded posterior or anterior plaster splint to permit dressing of the foot. Do not use a windowed cast since window edema inevitably results. In many instances the involved tarsal bone or bones may apparently disappear roentgenographically. However, with carefully supervised immobilization of the foot and leg, in time the bones reconstitute themselves and reappear with, at most, a minimum amount of deformity. Usually no deformity occurs as long as the foot is properly immobilized.

In the adult, a trap-door type of opening should be made in the involved tarsal bone. This should be not more than 1 cm. square to insure adequate drainage. In the metatarsal shafts a portion of the dorsal cortex may be unroofed. If any of the intertarsal joints or the tarsometatarsal joints should be involved, the only procedure indicated is establishment of drainage by sectioning the capsular structures. The insertion of a drain between the articular surfaces is against all tenets of good orthopaedic surgery. Here, again, adequate supportive antibiotic therapy and immobilization are necessary. Every attempt should be made to preserve the bony structures of the foot.

In chronic osteomyelitis the problem is an entirely different one and the philosophy of treatment is radically different. In the first place chronic suppurative osteomyelitis seldom, if ever, develops in a child. In the adult an acute osteomyelitic process may progress to a chronic one, no matter what the cause of the acute process may be. However, even in the chronic stage the

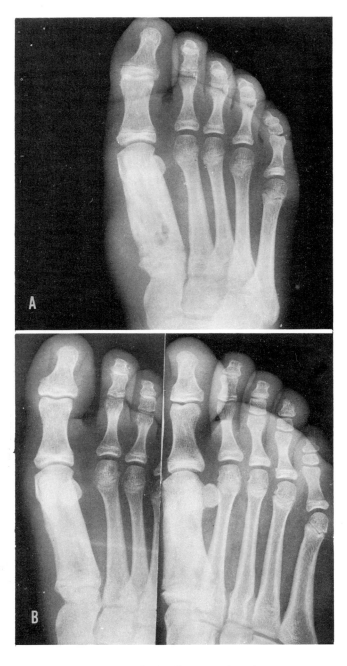

Fig. 21-23.   A.   Chronic osteomyelitis of the first metatarsal.
    B.   Postoperative films indicating healed lesion one year following sequestrectomy and closed system irrigation with the appropriate antibiotics.

treatment of the foot differs appreciably from that of the long bones and of the hand. The therapeutic regimen is, of course, sequestrectomy of the involved bone followed by closure with minimally scarred tissue, if at all possible, as well as the establishment of constant local irrigation with antibiotic solutions and suction. The use of a Snyder Hemovac perforated tube has been quite helpful. After irrigation through a closed system for ten days, cultures should be taken of the solution which has irrigated the area and when five consecutive negative cultures are obtained, irrigation is discontinued. If the cultures are not negative, then additional sensitivity studies should be made and the medication changed to another antibiotic should the sensitivity test show that the organism concerned has become insensitive to the drug that had been administered. Such continued irrigation may be maintained for a period of as long as three weeks to a month without any detriment to the patient. If, by the end of this time, negative cultures have not been obtained, then other means of therapy should be considered.

For example: A patient appeared at my office complaining of foot pain and swelling of several weeks duration. She had been treated by her family physician with oral and intramuscular antibiotics followed by a local incision and drainage of the medial aspect of the foot by the surgeon in the town in which she was living. Drainage had ceased within a week. The patient became ambulatory and was relatively comfortable until two weeks prior to consulting me. The foot presented a hot, swollen, tender appearance over the first metatarsal shaft. Roentgenograms (Fig. 21-23 A) demonstrated the presence of a sequestrum in the first metatarsal shaft. Surgery consisted of unroofing the metatarsal shaft, along with culturing of the purulent material and sensitivity studies, as well as currettement of the medullary canal and sequestrectomy. Two perforated Hemovac tubes were inserted with the points of entry of one and exit of the other well away from the incision. The incision was closed tightly and irrigation with a broad spectrum antibiotic (1 gm. per 1000 cc. at

15 drops per minute) was instituted. Systemic antibiotic therapy was also established with the dosage at three times the average (in other words, 3 gm. daily), such as chloromycetin for 3 days. Sensitivity studies did not warrant changing the antibiotic. Serial cultures taken daily for five days, beginning on the tenth day following surgery, were all reported as negative. Irrigation was discontinued, the tubes were removed and the foot immobilized in a cast. At the end of eight weeks the cast was removed and weight bearing permitted. The patient remained asymptomatic and was discharged one year later (Fig. 21-23 B).

Of course, such an ideal solution does not always occur. In many instances, particularly in those patients in whom a chronic osteomyelitis has developed following an open fracture with loss of tissue and extensive scar formation, the situation is entirely different. If the process should involve a toe, a metatarsophalangeal joint or a metatarsal, amputation of the toe or excision of the metatarsophalangeal joint should be performed. If the metatarsal shaft is involved, amputation of the entire ray may, at times, be indicated if all other therapy has failed. This does not apply to the first metatarsal ray. Every attempt possible should be made to preserve it, since this is a portion of the weight-bearing surface of the foot.

When the anterior tarsal bones are involved, one cannot resort to treatment as radical as with the forefoot. The surgeon should make at least one attempt to eradicate the disease by thorough currettage of the bone or bones, followed by local antibiotic irrigation and suction through a closed system along with primary closure of the wound. In a large number of instances he will be successful. Immobilization should be maintained for at least three months in order to permit healing and reconstitution of the bony structures. Usually spontaneous fusion of these bones results. If all else fails, then the involved tarsal bones will require total excision followed at a later date by attempted fusion between the remaining tarsal and metatarsal bones. Excision of the talus can be performed with or without fusion of the tibia to the adjacent talar bones.

Chronic osteomyelitis of the os calcis poses a difficult problem even in this age of the so-called wonder drugs. Once a chronic osteomyelitic process of the os calcis is established it is difficult to eradicate. When sequestrectomy is indicated, two methods of approach may be used. Gaenslen in 1931 recommended the split-heel incision (Fig. 21-24). In this procedure, the patient is in a prone position with a sand bag placed under the ankle. Under tourniquet control, a longitudinal incision is carried out at exactly the midline beginning 4 cm. above the level of the insertion of the tendo achillis into the os calcis and extending exactly in the midline to a point opposite the level of the styloid process of the fifth metatarsal. The plantar fascia is split in the plane between the short toe flexors and the abductor digiti quinti, care being taken not to injure the lateral plantar artery and nerve. These two structures will be found at the distal portion of the exposure. The quadratus plan-

tae muscle is then identified and split longitudinally along with the long plantar ligament. The calcaneus is split in two with a broad osteotome from a posteroinferior to an anterosuperior direction just short of the articular surface. The os calcis is spread apart exposing the entire cancellous portion. All of the diseased bone is curretted out preserving only the cortex and any healthy appearing cancellous bone. It is then preferable to insert a constant irrigation suction apparatus to irrigate the defect with the properly-indicated antibiotic as described earlier in this section, followed by complete closure of the incision. A plaster splint is then applied along the medial, anterior, and lateral sides of the foot, ankle, and leg, after application of a firm pressure dressing. Cultures of the draining solution are taken for five consecutive days after the tenth postoperative day. If all five cultures are reported negative, irrigation is discontinued. If the cultures continue to remain positive, additional sensitivity studies are performed and if indicated, the antibiotic is changed until five consecutive

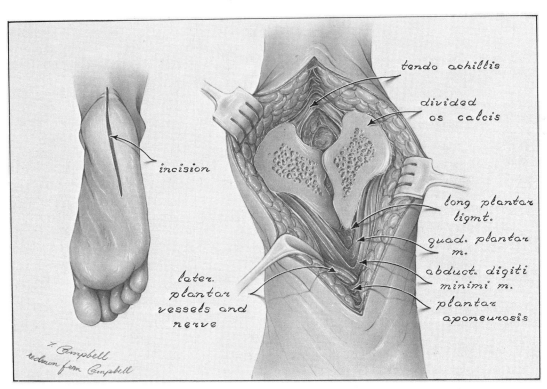

Fig. 21-24. Gaenslen split heel incision. Refer to text for details of this procedure.

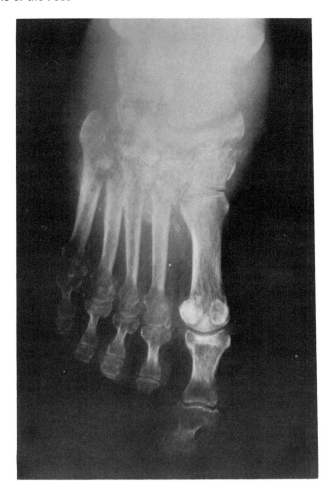

Fig. 21-25. Tuberculosis of the midtarsal region of the foot. The diagnosis was established through biopsy. (Courtesy of the Department of Roentgenography, Veterans Administration Hospital, Cincinnati, Ohio.)

sterile cultures are reported *even if irrigation must be carried out for one month.* The incision must not be disturbed for at least thirty days. Weight bearing is not permitted for at least six months or until the roentgenograms reveal adequate bony reconstitution. Another type of skin incision for an approach to the os calcis is the horseshoe-shaped one (previously described in this chapter) with transverse sectioning of the tuberosity of the os calcis, and currettage of the contents of the os calcis. I have had no experience with this approach.

Tuberculosis of the Foot. Tuberculosis is, of course, an infectious disease affecting any or all parts of the soft tissues and/or the osseous structures of the human body. As is well known, it is caused by the tubercle bacillus, a gram-negative rod. There are three types of bacilli, namely, the human, bovine, and avian. Until approximately the last fifteen years, the most common type of tuberculous infection in the human was the bovine type. Gradually, however, because of the constant careful supervision of the cattle herds, as well as the improved living and dietary standards, bone tuberculosis today is much less frequent than it was in 1935. It was a common occurrence thirty years ago to see case after case of bone tuberculosis on the wards of such orthopaedic centers as the New York Orthopaedic Dispensary and

Hospital, Boston Children's Hospital, as well as many other outstanding institutions. Today bone tuberculosis is considered a relatively infrequent disease. In addition to the improved hygienic and dietary conditions, the introduction of arthrodesis of the involved tuberculous joints, initially of the knee and spine, by Dr. Russell A. Hibbs in 1911, led the way to gradual and almost total arrest of joint tuberculosis.

Tuberculous involvement of the tarsal bones and of the toes is very rare. In fact, because of its rarity, it is often difficult to distinguish this disease from other forms of infectious or suppurative arthritis of the tarsal bones. However, it must be kept in mind (Fig. 21-25).

The symptomatology is so indefinite that other than the presence of chronic low grade pain in the foot, associated with some swelling and a slight increase in temperature locally, there are no symptoms which can be considered diagnostic. If and when chronic draining sinuses appear, it is a sign that the disease is well established.

Treatment of this condition has changed quite appreciably with the advent of specific chemotherapy. Although even today some textbooks recommend amputation as the procedure of choice, I do not recommend it. With the judicious use of antibiotics, as well as arthrodesis of the involved tarsal or tarsometatarsal joints, followed by prolonged cast immobilization, the disease can be arrested.

The established and recommended therapeutic routine consists of the use of various antibacterial agents in combination as soon as the diagnosis is established. These are streptomycin, para-aminosalicylic acid, and isonicotinic acid hydrazide. Establishment of the diagnosis is best carried out by biopsy. Upon receiving a positive report, the patient should be placed on a daily regimen of 1 gm. of streptomycin in two divided doses, 10 gm. of para-aminosalicylic acid four times daily, and 3.5 mg. per kg. of body weight of isonicotinic acid hydrazide (INH). Bosworth recommends the use of iproniazide (isonicotinyl-isopropylhydrazine) alone. He reports excellent response. The patient should be placed on absolute bed rest. A chest plate should be

procured and the kidneys should also be checked as a possible source of infection. In the presence of tuberculous involvement the sedimentation rate is elevated and on evaluation of the differential white count, there is frequently an increase in the number of monocytes. A tuberculin test should be performed routinely and if the #1 tuberculin test is negative, the #2 should be performed. The absence of a positive tuberculin test does not indicate the absence of a tuberculous infection. On the other hand, biopsy is the only true criterion of the presence of bone tuberculosis.

The treatment of the local involvement consists of arthrodesis of the involved bone or bones. If the talus is involved, a pantalar arthrodesis is the procedure of choice. Cancellous bone chips procured from the ilium should be used to pack any bony cavities or defects which result from the surgery. This is especially indicated when the os calcis is involved. Many texts recommend total excision of the os calcis. Such a procedure produces a rather severely deformed and disabled foot. With the adjuvant chemotherapeutic regimen, thorough currettage of the os calcis, followed by packing of the defect with autogenous cancellous bone chips procured from the ilium and closure of the wound, will result in an arrest of the disease. Cast immobilization is maintained until the bone is thoroughly reconstituted. If all else fails, then excision of the os calcis may be considered.

When the other tarsal bones are involved, fusion should extend from the apparently adjacent healthy bones proximally to healthy bone distally. Cast immobilization should be maintained until it is evident by roentgenographic evaluation that fusion has occurred and the disease is arrested—no matter how long a period of time is required.

Occasionaly, one may find a mixed infection involving the tarsal bones. Aerobic and anaerobic cultures should be procured. If any anaerobic organisms are found, the sinus or sinuses should be packed with zinc peroxide. The release of the oxygen from the zinc peroxide will inhibit the growth and thus indirectly destroy the anaerobic organisms. The aerobic ones are destroyed or controlled by the subsequent irrigation of the sinus with an antibiotic to which the organisms are sensitive. Following eradication of the infection, arthrodesis is carried out. Miltner and Fanz reported that the os calcis is the most frequently involved bone in the foot, followed in order of involvement by the talus, first metatarsal, navicular, and first and second cuneiforms.

The treatment of tuberculosis of the metatarsals varies from that of the tarsal bones. If the shaft of the second, third, fourth, or fifth metatarsals is involved, treatment consists of excision of the entire ray followed by primary closure of the soft tissues, along with the administration of the combined chemotherapeutic agents. If the first metatarsal is involved, it should not be sacrificed since this is an important portion of the weight-bearing surface of the foot. As with the os calcis, it should be thoroughly curretted, packed with cancellous bone chips, and the soft tissues closed. Cast immobilization then follows. The treatment for phalangeal involvement is amputation of the involved toe.

One must also keep in mind that the chemotherapeutic agents already mentioned as anti-tuberculous drugs do exhibit toxic effects. Therefore, any evidence of eighth nerve deafness or visual impairment warrants immediate cessation of administration of the specific drug, at least temporarily. This is particularly true with children.

Fungal Infections. Fungal infections of the tarsal bones should always be kept in mind when a patient presents himself because of a chronic indolent draining ulcer associated with little, if any, pain. Usually, there is a localized inflammatory reaction but no other clinical findings referable to the foot. This is particularly true in an infection due to *actinomyces*. When the involvement is due to *coccidioides immitis*, the process can be either acute or chronic.

Actinomycotic osteomyelitis of the tarsal bones is rare. The causative organism is a gram-positive one which is nonmotile. Although it is related to true bacteria, it is primarily a fungus-like filamentous non-acid-fast organism which, on microscopic section, presents branching mycelia. It can best be identified microscopically by the presence of the so-called "sulfur granules." These consist of masses of filamentous mycelia contained within the purulent detritus which exudes from the abscess. Although the infection is found to affect primarily the mandible, it can occasionally involve the tarsal bones as the primary area of infection. Early in the disease, it affects one tarsal bone only, but as the condition progresses, the disease may extend to the adjacent structures.

Clinically, the findings are those of a chronically inflamed indolent ulcer. The patient usually will give a history of undiagnosed pain in the foot for a period of several months with negative roentgenographic findings when the discomfort first manifested itself. After several months of continued pain, a small furuncle-like lesion appears and begins to drain, bringing initial relief of the pain. When the drainage fails to cease, the patient invariably decides to seek further medical aid.

Roentgenographic examination of the involved bone will usually reveal a single punched-out lesion affecting one of the tarsal bones, with little or no surrounding reaction. There are no characteristic features roentgenographically which will distinguish this lesion. If it is polyostotic in its involvement, there is destruction of the articular surfaces.

Therapy of this lesion, according to Altemeier, consists of the administration of massive doses of penicillin and sulfadiazine (2-sulfanilylamidopyrimidine) for a period of at least eight months. The patient should be hospitalized. Initially the patient is placed on a regimen of one-half-million units of penicillin every four hours for four months. In addition, sufficient sulfadiazine should be administered to establish a blood concentration of 6 to 10 mg. per cent. Such a blood concentration requires the administration of at least 1 gm. every four hours. This blood level is maintained for one month. At the end of the one-month period, the sulfadiazine is tapered to 1 gm. three times daily for the next three months. At the end of four months, penicillin-V (phenoxymethyl penicillin) 250 mg. four times daily is substituted for the penicillin.

The sulfadiazine dosage is cut down to 1/2 gm. three times daily. The patient is maintained on this regimen for another four months.

If the roentgenograms demonstrate bony sequestration, thorough currettage of the involved tarsal bone should be performed without closure of the incision and permission of the incision to close by secondary intention. Although in the past, amputation of the foot was the procedure of choice, with this regimen, it has seldom been found necessary.

In *coccidioidomycosis* the cause of the infection is the *Coccidioides immitis*. The organism is endemic to the San Joaquin Valley of California and is also known as San Joaquin Valley Fever. Prior to World War II, the disease was localized to residents of that area. But, when troops were brought into that portion of California for training, cases subsequently appeared sporadically over the country. The initial focus of involvement is usually pulmonary and the osseous lesions are what may be termed metastatic abscesses. Occasionally, however, the initial lesion is found in the tarsal bones.

The subjective and objective lesions do not present any oustanding recognizable characteristic. If there is a chronic pulmonary involvement, there are systemic manifestations of low grade fever, malaise, fatigue, bone pain, and chronic cough. The local bony lesions do not demonstrate any particular findings roentgenographically. The prognosis in the disease is guarded. The acute pulmonary process presents all the signs of an acute pneumonitis. If the acute process should be a fulminating one and remain undiagnosed, the patient becomes progressively more ill and death ensues in approximately 50 per cent of such cases. The coccidiodin skin test is, of course, a valuable adjunct in the diagnosis of this disease.

Treatment consists of the administration of amphotericin B. This is a toxic drug and caution should be used during its administration. The requisite dosage varies. Generally one begins with the administration of 1/4 mg. per kg. of body weight. The dosage is gradually increased until the patient is receiving 1 mg. per kg. of body weight. If daily blood urea nitrogen and nonprotein nitrogen evaluations should exceed 20 and 40 mg. per cent respectively, administration of the drug should be interrupted until normal blood levels are reached. If, because of the toxic reaction, therapy has been interrupted more than seven days, resumption of treatment should begin with 1/4 mg. per kg. of body weight.

Locally, curettage of the involved tarsal bone or bones is indicated with adequate support and non-weight bearing. According to McMaster, such a plan of therapy, particularly if there are no pulmonary manifestations, usually brings about an arrest of the disease. However, therapy must be continued for several months.

Blastomycotic infections of the foot have not been reported in the recent literature. I have seen roentgenograms of a case of blastomycosis of the knee, but have had no experience with any therapeutic regimen for this.

Spirochetal Osteomyelitis. Osteomyelitis, due either to syphilis or to yaws, is mentioned only for the sake of completeness of the chapter. I have had no experience with either of these diseases, nor is there very much information available about either condition in the medical literature. Suffice to state, should such a diagnosis be made, the use of antibiotics and other antispirochetal drugs will control the situation quite rapidly without the necessity of any surgery.

BIBLIOGRAPHY

ALTEMEIER, WM. A.: Personal Communication.

BOOHER, R. J. AND PACK, G. T.: Malignant Melanoma of the Feet and Hands, Surgery, 42:1084, 1957.

BOOHER, R. J.: Personal Communication.

BOSWORTH, D. M.: The Treatment of Tuberculous Lesions of Bones and Joints with Iproniazid (Marsilid). New York J. Med., 56:1281, 1956.

BOSWORTH, D. M., WRIGHT, H. A., FIELDING, J. W., and WILSON, H. J., JR.: The Use of Iproniazid in the Treatment of Bone and Joint Tuberculosis, J. Bone Jt. Surg., 35-A:577, 1953.

COLEY, B. L.: Neoplasms of Bone, 2nd Ed., New York, Paul B. Hoeber Inc., 1960.

COLEY, B. L. AND HIGINBOTHAM, N. L.: Secondary Chondrosarcoma. Ann. Surg., 139:547, 1954.

COVENTRY, M. B. AND DAHLIN, D. C.: Osteogenic Sarcoma; Critical Analysis of 430 Cases. J. Bone Jt. Surg. 39-A:741, 1957.

DAHLIN, D. C.: Bone Tumors. Springfield, CHARLES C THOMAS, 1957.

EWING, J.: Neoplastic Diseases, 4th Ed., Philadelphia, W. B. Saunders Co., 1942.

FREIBERGER, R. H., LOITMAN, B. S., HELPERN, M., AND THOMPSON, T. C.: Osteoid Osteoma. Amer. J. Roentgen., 82:194, 1959.

GAENSLEN, F. J.: The Split Heel Incision. J. Bone Jt. Surg., 13:759, 1931.

HIBBS, RUSSELL A.: An Operation For Progressive Spinal Deformities. New York J. Med., 93:1013, 1911.
An Operation for Stiffening the Knee Joint. Ann. Surg., 53:404, 1911.

HUTTER, R. V. P., WORCESTER, J. N., FRANCIS, K. C., FOOTE, F. W., AND STEWART, F. W.: Giant Cell Tumors of Bone, Benign and Malignant: Clinicopathological Analysis of the Natural History of the Disease. Cancer, 5:653, 1962.

JAFFE, H. L.: "Osteoid Osteoma": A Benign Osteoblastic Tumor Composed of Osteoid and Atypical Bone. Arch. Surg., 31:709, 1935.
Tumors and Tumorous Conditions of the Bones and Joints. Philadelphia, Lea and Febiger, 1958.

McCARROLL, H. R.: Clinical Manifestations of Congenital Neurofibromatosis J. Bone Jt. Surg. 32-A:601, 1950.

McKENNA, R. J., SCHWINN, C. P., SOONG, K. Y., AND HIGINBOTHAM, N. L.: Sarcomatoma of the Osteogenic Series (Osteosarcoma, Fibrosarcoma, Chondrosarcoma, Parosteal Osteogenic Sarcoma and Sarcomata Arising in Abnormal Bone). An Analysis of 552 Cases. J. Bone Jt. Surg. 48-A:1, 1966.

McMASTER, P. E.: Personal Communication.

McMASTER, P. E., AND GILFILLAN, C.: Coccidioidal osteomyelitis. J.A.M.A., 112:1235, 1939.

MILTNER, LEO J., AND FANZ, H. C.: Prognosis and Treatment of Tuberculosis of the Bones of the Foot, J. Bone Jt. Surg. 18:287, 1936.

NEER, C. S., FRANCIS, K. C., MARCOVE, R. C., TERZ, J., AND CARBONAVA, P. N.: Treatment of Unicameral Bone Cyst: A Follow-up Study of 175 Cases. J. Bone Jt. Surg. In press.

STOUT, A. P.: Fibrosarcoma, The Malignant Tumor of Fibroblasts, Cancer, 1:30, 1948.

= 22 =

Circulatory Disturbances of the Foot

ALTON OCHSNER, JR., M.D.

THIS chapter has been written for the physician who is faced with a diagnostic circulatory foot problem complicating the orthopaedic complaints. A limited number of the more common circulatory problems are illustrated in color since many of the circulatory diagnostic signs are based on the color of the skin as well as the general appearance of the foot. Therefore, black and white illustrations would be of no value to the reader. The indicated therapeutic regimen is presented for some of the more common conditions only. It is not our intent that this chapter serve as a complete text regarding circulatory problems of the foot. It was written more as a guide to the more common circulatory diseases and problems encountered in orthopaedics along with the indicated basic therapeutic principles.

The circulation of the foot consists of an inflow system (the arteries) and an outflow system (veins and lymphatics). The circulatory system maintains life of the tissues by bringing oxygen and nutriments to them and removing the products of metabolism.

GENERAL TYPES OF CIRCULATORY DISTURBANCES

Circulatory disturbances may be hemodynamic, involving either the inflow or outflow systems or structural in nature. The adequacy of blood flow into the foot is dependent upon the absolute volume flow, or blood flow per unit mass of tissue, and is modified by the quality of the blood and the tissue requirements. The absolute blood flow is dependent upon (1) the amount of blood available during any period of time for perfusion through the leg and foot, (2) the arterial perfusion pressure, and (3) the vascular resistance to flow. The blood available for perfusion is basically determined by the cardiac output, which is related to the total blood volume (particularly the venous return) and the efficiency of the heart. The percentage of this cardiac

482

output that will enter the leg or foot, assuming no proximal blood loss from arterial injury, is dependent upon the relationship between the total (body) and local (leg) vascular resistances. The pressure available for perfusion is also generated by the heart (*i.e.*, central aortic pressure), but is reduced a variable amount, dependent upon the vascular resistance proximal to the foot. Loss of pressure occurs physiologically as blood flows through the arteries to the lower extremity but may also occur pathologically if there is a proximal arteriovenous fistula or arterial stenosis. In addition, the flow into the foot is influenced by the vascular resistance which is set by the degree and extent of vasomotor tone and organic occlusive disease of the small arteries, capillaries and veins. The effectiveness of the blood flow is determined by the oxygen and nutriment (especially glucose) content and the needs of the tissues for these substances as established by their metabolic rates.

Theoretically at least, inflow vascular disturbance can be (1) too much inflow (arterial plethora) or (2) too little inflow (arterial insufficiency).

The outflow of fluid from the leg is adequate if there is no retention of fluid in the leg. The volume flow of fluid out of the leg and foot is dependent upon (1) the fluid volume available for removal, (2) the expulsion pressures, and (3) the resistance to flow in the venous and lymphatic systems. The volume of fluid that requires removal from the leg and foot at any one time depends on the capillary blood flow the tissue volume flow (*i.e.*, water turnover). The force for removing this fluid from the foot is generated by the vis-a-tergo (*i.e.*, what remains of arterial pressure on the venous side of the capillary bed), the contracting "muscle pumps," the tissue pressure and is opposed by the central venous and lymphatic pressures. The resistance to outflow depends on the cross-sectional area of the veins and lymphatics, which, of course, is related to the amount of vascular obstruction and the effectiveness of the collateral circulation.

Outflow vascular disturbances can therefore be problems of (1) venous insufficiency, (2) lymphatic insufficiency, or (3) a combination of both.

Structural abnormalities of the vascular system are pathologic conditions of the arterial, capillary, venous and/or lymphatic system without hemodynamic disturbances. These can be abnormalities of number, size, shape or connection of neoplasms.

SYMPTOMS AND SIGNS OF CIRCULATORY DISTURBANCE

Complaints relative to vascular disturbances of the foot will be discussed below under the headings of pain, skin color, skin temperature, skin moisture, size of leg, trophic changes, associated dermatologic conditions, structural vascular changes and functional impairment.

Pain

There are different patterns of pain seen in vascular disease. They vary according to the type of pain, the intensity of the pain, the duration, extent, location, the effect of position and of temperature, and associated sensations. It is possible for different types of pain patterns to coexist. The general types of pain patterns seen in vascular disturbances of the feet are ischemic pain, congestive pain, inflammatory pain, neuritic pain and paresthesia. In addition, there are special types of pain patterns including claudication, nocturnal cramps, restless legs, erythermalgia, phlebodynia, causalgia and glomic pain.

Ischemic pain is only seen in vascular disturbances, although it may be precipitated by nonvascular conditions, such as infection. When associated with organic occlusive arterial disease, it is usually severe in type, often described as agonizing. When associated with vasospastic occlusive disease, it is moderate in nature and described as aching. In organic occlusive arterial disease, the pain is constant. In vasospastic occlusive disease, it is usually intermittent. The pain may be localized or diffuse. It is usually peripheral in nature, sometimes limited to one or more digits, to an area of an ulcer, or to a muscle compartment. Ischemic pain is increased by elevation of the extremity. Conversely, it is decreased when the extremity is in a dependent position, and it is not uncommon for a patient with ischemic pain to sleep with his leg dangling over the side of the bed. Application of heat tends to decrease the pain of ischemia. The application of cold will increase it.

Congestive pain is entirely due to vascular causes. It is described as a dull, aching or "bursting" pain, moderate to severe in nature. It is an intermittent pain depending on the dependency of the leg. It is usually a diffuse type of pain except when associated with varicose veins or perforating veins when it is located to the veins themselves, more often in the lower leg and the proximal foot. The pain is decreased by elevation of the extremity.

Inflammatory pain is seen in vascular and nonvascular conditions, usually mild to moderate, persistent and localized to the area of inflammation, which in the case of arteritis or phlebitis may be very small, or in the case of erysipeloid cellulitis, very large. There may be some relief of inflammatory pain with elevation, as there is often associated congestion. There is some relief by heat application. There is usually associated tenderness.

Neuritic pain also may have a vascular or nonvascular etiology. It is usually described as "shooting," "burning," "tearing," or "throbbing," and is frequently associated with paresthesia. The pain is usually severe and constant with spasmodic accentuation. It is more frequently seen in the proximal portion of the foot than the distal portion, and sometimes slight relief is obtained with dependency of the extremity but not to the degree seen in ischemic pain.

Paresthesias. Patients with arterial insufficiency complain of numbness and tingling ("pins and needles"), apparently related to ischemia of nerve endings. Patients with venous insufficiency complain of itching, prickly sensation and formication, apparently related to congestion of nerve endings.

Special Types of Pain Patterns

Claudication is an ischemic muscular pain, precipitated by exercise (walking), but relieved within a few minutes by cessation of the exercise. The pain may be a mild discomfort expressed as "muscle tiredness" or a "muscle tightness" or cramp of increasing severity as exercise is continued. The pain may be located in the muscles of the foot or just above the ankle. It is usually located at a higher level, such as the calf or thigh. The claudication associated with an arteriovenous fistula is atypical in that it is not rapidly relieved by cessation of walking.

Nocturnal cramp is a severe muscle (primarily calf) cramp, which comes after stretching of the leg in bed. These usually follow an active day of leg exercise. *Restless legs* is an unpleasant, pulling and drawing sensation of both legs at rest, which produce an irresistible urge to move the legs. This type of pain may not be definitely related to vascular disease. *Erythermalgia* is a pain in the ball of the foot and the tips of the toes, precipitated by heat. The pain may begin as a prickly sensation but becomes an intense, burning pain with increased heat. The skin is hot and red. The pain is decreased by a cold application and elevation of the extremity, and is increased by dependency of the extremity. *Causalgia* is a burning pain in the hyperesthetic and usually sweaty foot. *Phlebodynia* is pain along normal veins without evidence of thrombophlebitis, and the pain of a *glomic tumor* is excruciating, usually in a digit, precipitated by pressure.

In evaluating pain in the foot one must, of course, consider the many nonvascular causes for such discomfort (Table 22-1).

PLATE 22—1

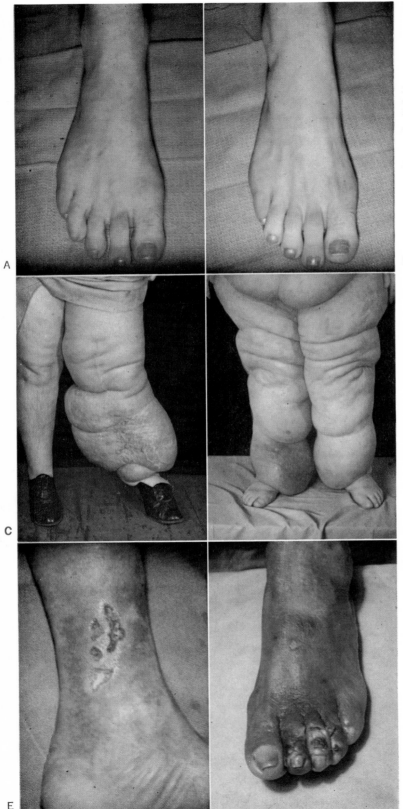

A, Appearance of foot in Raynaud's disease. Note that the toes appear slightly congested.

B, Same foot after exposure to cold. Note blanching of skin on the toes.

C, Elephantiasis. Due to extreme lymphatic insufficiency resulting in excessive fibroplastic reaction.

D, Venous stasis. Due to obesity with resultant stasis dermatitis. Note that lesion is bilateral in contrast to the unilateral elephantitic condition.

E, Post-thrombophlebitic ulcer. The skin is pigmented. The ulcer is usually found on the medial supramalleolar region of the leg.

F, Diabetic gangrene. This is the wet type of gangrenous involvement of the toes.

TABLE 22-1.   NONVASCULAR CAUSES OF FOOT PAIN

Spinal Cord
Ruptured disc, degenerative processes, tumors, tables, arachnoidism
Nerves
Neuritis (diabetes, macrocytic anemia, vitamin B deficiency, lead and arsenic poisoning), compression and entrapment neuropathies (peroneal nerve from fat or cast, posterior tibial nerve in tarsal-tunnel syndrome), plantar neuroma.
Bones and Joints
Arthritis (including gout), osteoporosis, osteochondritis (Freiberg's disease, Kohler's disease),

osteo-arthropathy, spur, Paget's disease, flat feet.
Muscles and Tendons
Myositis, tendinitis, fasciitis, bursitis, ligamentous strain, ruptured muscle or tendon, muscle hernia, low calcium syndrome, low salt syndrome, myoglobinuria.
Skin and Subcutaneous Tissue
Cellulitis, panniculitis
Shoes
Tight shoes, changing height of heel.
Hysteria

Skin Color

Skin color reflects only the circulation of blood through and in the region of the skin itself. Frequently, however, this is representative of the total blood flow to the foot. Skin color is dependent on the amount of blood flowing through the skin (volume flow) and the color of the blood (oxygen saturation). The oxygen saturation of blood is dependent both on the rate of flow and on temperature. The slower the flow and higher the temperature, the greater the oxygen dissociation and the deeper the cyanosis. Skin color is best reflected in the nail beds.

Variations in skin blood flow are reflected by three types of skin color, namely, cyanosis, erythema and pallor. In addition, there are special color phenomena seen in vascular disturbances of the foot that should be recognized. These include acrocyanosis, erythermalgia, livedo reticularis, Raynaud's phenomena, purpura, ecchymosis and petechia, and pigmentation.

Cyanosis is a frequent sign of vascular disturbance indicating sluggish blood flow. It is a dark bluish to purple discoloration. The skin is usually cool to cold, depending on the extent of blood flow reduction. If heat has been applied to the extremity, however, the skin may be warm. It can be seen in both inflow and outflow types of vascular disturbance. In venous insufficiency the cyanotic color will deepen when the extremity is dependent but this maneuver may lighten the cyanosis in arterial insufficiency. In fact, such a foot may become red (see next paragraph).

Erythema (rubor) presents as varying degrees of skin redness. There is usually increased blood flow causing the skin to be warm. Erythema results from inflammation or vasodilatation that may or may not be a sign of vascular disturbance. When the erythematous skin is cold, it is a sign of vascular disease. There has been ischemic vascular damage, resulting in marked vasodilatation and possible vessel disruption with intercutaneous and subcutaneous hemorrhage. It is seen in severe arterial insufficiency when the foot is dependent after elevation. When seen at rest this type of erythema may not blanch with elevation of the extremity, although there is usually pallor of the surrounding skin at this time.

Pallor is a white, usually waxy, appearance of the foot which represents an almost virtual arrest of skin blood flow. This is always a sign of some vascular disturbance. In severe arterial insufficiency it can be seen by elevation of the extremity with extension(dorsiflexion)movements of the foot.
Special Color Phenomena

Acrocyanosis is a painless condition of constant, symmetrical peripheral cyanosis which exists without underlying organic vascular disease. *Erythermalgia* has been described in the preceding section on pain. *Livedo reticularis* is a mottled, blotchy, or reticular reddish-blue pattern of skin discoloration. It is most noticeable when the extremity is cold. It is seen with or without vascular disease.

Raynaud's phenomena (Plate 22-1, A and B) are variable skin colors reflecting changes in vasomotor tone. These consist of pallor from vasoconstriction and/or cyanosis from capillary stagnation, depending, of course, on the degree of vascular occlusion and, finally rubor from reactive hyperemia after the vasoconstriction is released. These color changes are precipitated by cold or emotional disturbances. They may represent a primary disease (Raynaud's disease), but are frequently seen secondary to other vascular diseases. If they are unilateral in nature, they are probably secondary phenomena. *Purpura, ecchymosis* and *petechia* are "spontaneous" intracutaneous and subcutaneous hemorrhages and are not uncommon in vascular disturbances, either as a result of increased capillary fragility or increased capillary pressure. However, when these lesions are scattered about the body, other causes must be considered (thrombocytopenia, hypoprothrominemia, scurvy, toxic states, allergic states).

Pigmentation. In chronic arterial insufficiency, there are frequently small irregular areas of reddish-brown discoloration. These are due to hemosiderin deposition following intracutaneous or subcutaneous hemorrhage. In chronic venous insufficiency, there is frequently diffuse light brown to almost black discoloration in the supramalleolar region. This results from melanin deposition associated with atrophy and inflammation. There is also a specific condition called "acro-angiodermatitis" in which there are purplish lesions formed by proliferation of small blood vessels, fibroblasts, purpura and hemosiderin on the extensor surface of toes, the dorsum of the foot and sometimes beneath the malleoli.

Skin Temperature

The temperature of the skin reflects the blood flow through the skin. The greater the flow, the higher the temperature. As with skin color, skin temperature does not absolutely reflect the total blood flow through the foot, depending, of course, on the degree of vasodilatation in the skin and subcutaneous tissue and functional status of the arteriovenous anastomoses. Among other things, these are controlled by this ambient temperature and humidity of the room, so skin temperature cannot be adequately evaluated when the surrounding area is either hot or cold. In arterial insufficiency, the level of temperature change is at least one-third of the extremity distance below where the artery is actually occluded. A subjectively cold foot in the presence of objective warmth suggests a peripheral nerve or thalamic disturbance, rather than a vascular one.

Skin Moisture

Patients may complain of excessive sweating or dry skin. Hyperhidrosis is a symptom of reflex dystrophy and localized anhidrosis is seen after sympathectomy and in some chronic arteriovascular diseases, especially diabetes. However, problems of perspiration may be of cutaneous, central nervous system, or thyroid origin.

Size of Leg

Increased Leg Size. Increased size of the leg and foot may result from swelling, hypertrophy or elongation.

The types of *swelling* seen in vascular disturbances are edema, brawny induration, and elephantiasis. *Edema* represents fluid retention which can result from venous hypertension, sodium retention, increased capillary permeability or decreased intravascular oncotic pressure. Characteristically, it pits (that is, leaves an indentation) on pressure. In vascular disturbances it is usually due to venous insufficiency but may be seen in arterial insufficiency when the foot has been left in a dependent position for a long period of time. Swelling due to edema can be reduced by elevation of the extremity. *Brawny induration* results from protein retention with fibroplastic reaction. It is due to lymphatic insufficiency.

It does not pit on pressure. *Elephantiasis* (Plate 22-1 C and D) is due to extreme lymphatic insufficiency resulting in excessive fibroplastic reaction. This causes hypertrophy of the hypodermal and dermal connective tissue and can result in the development of a huge, grotesque leg.

An additional vascular cause of foot swelling is a local arteriovenous fistula where the regional veins are dilated and tense.

Hypertrophy of the foot is the result of long-standing lymphedema. *Clubbing* of the toes may result from cyanosis (local or generalized) that persists for several years. *Elongation* of the foot is seen when there is an arteriovenous fistula appearing before the closure of the epiphyses of the bones.

There are, of course, numerous causes other than vascular disturbances which can produce leg swelling. These would include congestive heart failure, nephritis and nephrosis, sodium retention due to mineral corticoid administration or hyperaldosteronism. There is some evidence that the problem of any persistent edema may be compounded by secondary hyperaldosteronism. Edema of the foot from increased capillary permeability may be caused by injury, inflammation (*i.e.*, cellulitis, bursitis, arthritis) and allergy (angioneurotic edema). Hypoproteinemia by reducing the intravascular oncotic pressure can cause edema. Even a tumor must sometimes be considered in the differential diagnosis of leg swelling. Finally, two conditions, lipedema and localized myxedema, deserve special consideration. *Lipedema* is a nonpitting, generalized, symmetrical swelling of the lower extremities seen in women with obesity of the legs and buttocks. The skin and subcutaneous tissue is soft and pliable. The swelling goes down very little at night. *Localized myxedema* is a non-pitting, swelling most often seen on the dorsum of the foot or in the pretibial area but may involve the entire lower leg. It may resemble brawny induration or even elephantiasis. It is almost always associated with exophthalmus. Biopsy confirms the diagnosis.

Decreased Leg Size. Decreased size of the leg or foot can result from poor nutrition (chronic arterial insufficiency) or disuse (immobilization or paralysis).

Trophic Changes

Trophic changes due to vascular disturbances may be reflected in the skin (and subcutaneous tissue) and its appendages.

In chronic arterial insufficiency these consist of *atrophy* of the skin and subcutaneous tissue (sometimes a parchment appearance) of the lower leg and dorsum of the foot with *excessive callus* formation on the sole of the foot, *decreased hair growth* and *nail changes*. The nails are frequently thin and brittle with longitudinal ridging and splitting at the free edge. There may also be onycholysis and discoloration. With acute and chronic arterial insufficiency there may be *necrosis* and *gangrene*. It is sometimes limited to punctate areas (usually on the lower leg and side of the foot) but most frequently involves the toes, dorsum of the foot, or the heel. The gangrene may be "dry" (*i.e.*, the tissue mummified) or "wet" (*i.e.*, associated inflammation, usually infection). With slough or debridement of this tissue an ulcer may result.

With chronic congestion of the tissue (*i.e.*, outflow insufficiency) the trophic changes seen are *skin and subcutaneous tissue hypertrophy and thickening*, in the foot but in the lower leg there is frequently atrophy and hair loss in chronic venous insufficiency. Subcutaneous *calcification* and even *ossification* may be seen in the lower leg. *Nail changes* (thickening and abnormal shape) are also present. Nail infections are more common in this group of patients. Cutaneous ulceration is a very common trophic disturbance associated with chronic congestion of the legs.

Leg Ulcers. The genesis of a leg or foot ulcer is usually a minor trauma to an abnormal tissue, although even "normal" tissue in the lower leg region may be slow in healing and a chronic ulcer can easily develop here. In most such ulcers there is an underlying vascular disturbance. It is usually venous insufficiency due to deep vein thrombosis (the post-thrombophlebitic syndrome) and is less commonly due to varicose veins (especially incompetent perforator veins). These ulcers occur in the supramalleolar region most commonly on the medial side. (Plate 22-1, E.) They are usually small in size in the beginning but can become very large and irregular. They are not extremely painful unless secondarily infected. The tissue about these ulcers is usually edematous and indurated and the skin pigmented. Ischemia is the second most common cause of leg and foot ulcers. If it is due to an occlusion of large and medium sized arteries, the ulcer is usually distal at the tip of the toes. If the ischemia results from occlusion of small arterioles, the ulcer may be located more proximal in the foot or in the lower leg. Ischemic ulcers are round ("punched out") and very painful. Leg ulcers occur in numerous non-vascular conditions, which can be classified as neurotrophic, infectious, traumatic, metabolic and nutritional, neoplastic and miscellaneous dermatologic diseases. Of course, these must always be given some consideration even in the patient with obvious vascular disease. Particularly is this true of the neurotrophic ulcer since neuropathy so frequently accompanies vascular disease. Neurotrophic ulcers are usually seen on the sole of the foot in diabetics. They are painless, usually deep and undermining. Infectious and traumatic ulcers are usually identified by history and appearance. Neoplasia must always be suspected in any leg ulcer that fails to heal.

Dermatologic Conditions

The extremity with vascular disturbances, either ischemic or congestive, is particularly vulnerable to infection. There are also other dermatologic conditions which seem to occur with increased frequency in these limbs.

These include stasic dermatitis, chronic eczematous dermatitis, lichen simplex chronicus, erythema nodosum and necrobiosis lipoidica diabeticorum.

Structural Changes of Vessels

Some vascular conditions do not present as hemodynamic abnormalities, but as distended vessels, tender vessels and masses. Distended (and invariably tortuous vessels) may be varicose veins or lymphatics. Intracutaneous vascular abnormalities are telangiectatic lesions and venous stars. The latter are frequent on the dorsum of the foot. Blood flows in them from the periphery to the center.

The tender areas may be inflamed arteries, veins or lumphatics. There may not be any erythema associated with a tender artery but there usually is with the veins or lymphatics.

A pulsatile mass may represent an aneurysm or an arteriovenous fistula. With the latter there should be distended veins. A non-pulsatile mass could be a thrombosed vein, thrombosed arterial aneurysm, hemangioma or venous aneurysm.

It is obvious that the above conditions must be differentiated from non-vascular inflammatory lesions, cysts, tumors, hematomas and a muscle hernia.

Functional Impairment

Sometimes the presenting difficulty is one of locomotion. Difficulty in walking may be the result of pain (especially with reflex dystrophy), stiffness and heaviness, associated with edema and elephantiasis, weakness from muscle atrophy or, as a manifestation of claudication or limitation of joint motion because of an adjacent congenital vascular malformation.

EVALUATION AND MANAGEMENT OF CIRCULATORY DISTURBANCES

The mere presence of some of the above symptoms or signs is an indication of circulatory disturbance. Evaluation of the patient determines the type of disturbance, and need for and urgency of treatment.

The examiner must decide whether there is an hemodynamic disturbance or a structural abnormality. Is the hemodynamic disturbance of the inflow or the outflow type? Does it involve arteries, veins and/or lymphatics? Remember that the vascular system of the foot is the most peripheral extension of the total body circulatory system so that vascular disturbances in the foot need not be due to local blood vessel pathology but may reflect pathologic processes involving the circulatory system at a higher level in the extremity and sometimes within the abdomen or even the chest.

A reasonably accurate diagnosis can be made by an office examination which carefully assesses the history and utilizes the visual, palpatory and auscultatory senses. An angiogram is needed for an accurate anatomic diagnosis. An accurate etiological diagnosis will frequently require confirmatory laboratory tests.

Management of vascular disturbances of the foot should be planned to correct or improve, and to prevent the progression or recurrence of these conditions. The selection of optimum treatment for any individual requires a careful assessment of the degree of disability (amount of discomfort or incapacity, the socio-economic handicap of the disturbance and the threat it imposes on life or limb). The general health of the patient as it may influence the operative risk must also be assessed. The choice of therapeutic modalities must weigh the chance of curing or relieving the patient against the disability the patient will continue to have without treatment, the potential dangers of treatment (especially complications, disability or chance of death) against the prognosis of the disease without treatment, and the fears the patient may have about the treatment regarding disfigurement, dismemberment or death, against the patient's desires and socio-economic need for relief of his symptoms.

Inflow Disturbances

Arterial Plethora. There are few conditions which cause enough accentuation of local blood flow to produce symptoms. The two that are most commonly seen in the feet are *erythermalgia* and a local *arteriovenous fistula*. Phlebarteriectasia is a less common cause.

Erythermalgia (*erythromelalgia*) is a functional vascular disturbance seen primarily in middle aged men. There may be systemic symptoms (palpitation, vertigo, headache), but the prominent feature is the painful itching and burning (see Signs and Symptoms for full description). Aspirin may provide dramatic relief. Cooling and elevation of the feet produces some amelioration. Desensitization to heat has been used for definitive treatment.

Local arteriovenous fistula following penetrating injury to the foot may cause increased temperature and hypertrophy of the part (*i.e.*, a toe). A thrill and murmur are apparent. Arteriography confirms the diagnosis. The specific therapy is wide excision. Occasionally, if the lesion is very extensive, amputation may be necessary.

Phlebarteriectasia is a congenital anomaly in which there is dilatation and lengthening of the arteries and veins, suggesting an arteriovenous fistula, but no such fistula can be demonstrated. The circulation time is normal. The foot will be enlarged and warm with prominent varicosities and increased arterial pulsations. Arteriography and phlebography reveal the dilated tortuous vessels with no evidence of an arteriovenous fistula. The treatment is to ligate the large branches of the main arteries and to excise as many of the dilated veins as possible.

Arterial Insufficiency. *Etiology.* Since the effective blood flow into the foot is dependent not only upon the absolute volume flow, but also upon the life sustaining qualities of the blood and the metabolic demands of the tissues, then arterial insufficiency can result, in a qualitative sense, from a decrease in the oxygen content in the blood, in an absolute quantitative sense from the decrease in blood flow, and in a relative quantitative sense from an increase in tissue oxygen requirements beyond which the blood can provide.

Actually, the quality of the blood will not, per se, produce any significant symptoms in the foot without injury to more vital organs first. However, in the presence of mild arterial occlusive disease, a decrease in blood oxygen may precipitate symptoms that would not have been present otherwise. The blood oxygen content is important, but the ease with which the hemoglobin gives up the oxygen is equally important.

Qualitative arterial insufficiency can exist, therefore, with either a decrease in blood oxygen content or a reduction in the oxygen hemoglobin dissociation. The blood oxygen content may be reduced by an inability of the lungs to completely oxygenate the blood because of a central right-to-left, shunt, as can occur with certain intracardiac septal defects and with pulmonary arteriovenous fistulas, or because of an alveolar capillary block in the lungs. Decreased blood oxygenation may also result from a decrease in oxygen carrying capacity, resulting from a decrease in the amount of hemoglobin (as in anemia) or from a decrease in affinity of hemoglobin for oxygen. A decreased dissociation of oxygen from the hemoglobin can be seen in acidosis and cold blood.

An absolutely quantitative type of arterial insufficiency can occur if there is a decrease in blood available for perfusion, a reduction in perfusion pressure, or an increase in resistance to flow into or from the foot. Decreased availability of blood may exist if there is a decreased cardiac output or if there is a diversion of blood away from the foot or leg into other parts of the circulatory system, or extravascular loss of blood as occurs with hemorrhage.

A decrease in arterial perfusion pressure for the foot results when there is a decrease in central aortic pressure or when some of the pressure is lost through a proximal arteriovenous fistula or is consumed in overcoming a proximally located organic arterial occlusive lesion (Table 22-2). Such an obstruction to blood flow could be located anywhere from the aorta through the popliteal artery. It is not likely that obstruction of either one or two of the branches of the popliteal trifurcation will have much physiologic effect on the foot as long as the other branch is unobstructed. The condition which would most commonly cause such proximal arterial obstruction is atherosclerosis, although not uncommonly it results from thromboangiitis obliterans (Buerger's disease), arterial embolism, or arterial injury.

Atherosclerosis is a generalized disease, but obstructing atheromata are often limited to localized areas of the arterial system. It is a progressive disease beginning in youth, but becoming symptomatic in later life. Although atherosclerosis involving the legs may result in loss of limb, it is not a threat to life. The symptoms produced by atherosclerosis are usually not symmetrical.

Thromboangiitis obliterans is a progressive arterial disease related to smoking. There has been recent debate as to whether this really is a separate entity or a form of atherosclerosis. The disease has its onset at a very young age. The symptoms are usually bilateral and symmetrical. The upper extremities are more frequently in-

TABLE 22-2.   PROXIMAL ARTERIAL OCCLUSIVE DISEASE

Atherosclerosis
Thromboangiitis obliterans (Buerger's disease)
Arterial embolism
Arterial injury
Arterial compression
    Tourniquet, cast, ligature, fibrosis
Aneurysm
Dissecting, ruptured, clotted
Abdominal coarctation
Retroperitoneal fibrosis
Congenital dysplasia
    Absence, atresia, abnormal position
Fibromuscular hyperplasia
Intimal hyperplasia

PLATE 22—2

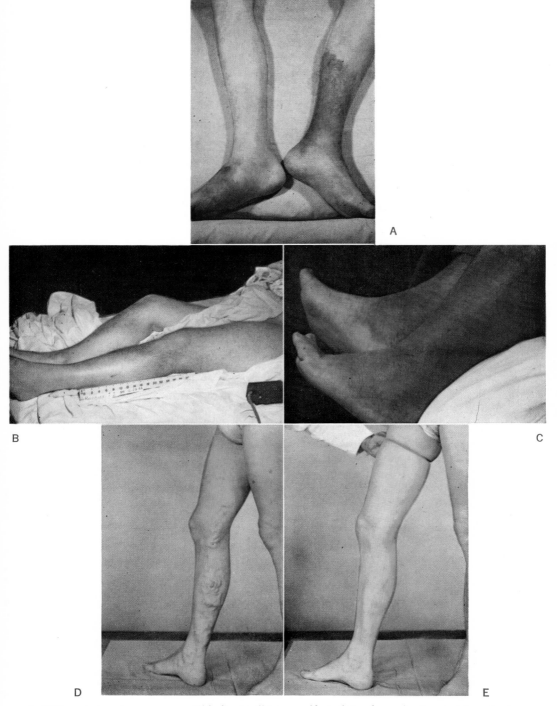

A, Diffuse ischemic gangrene. This is usually a manifestation of proximal arterial occlusion.
B, Phlegmasia cerulea dolens. The leg is swollen, cyanotic, and cold. The arterial pulsations are reduced because of the extensive venous thrombosis which interferes with arterial inflow.
C, Post-thrombophlebitic syndrome. This is due to thrombosis of the major veins of the lower leg resulting in chronic congestion and its subsequent complications.
D, Superficial varicosities of the lower extremity.
E, Tourniquet test. Used to determine the efficacy of the deep venous system. (Same patient as in *D.*)

TABLE 22-3. DISTAL ARTERIAL OCCLUSIVE DISEASE (VASOSPASTIC)

Acrocyanosis	Livedo reticularis
Chronic pernio	Raynaud's disease
Ergot poisoning	Sympathetic reflex dystrophy
Hypersecretion of catecholamines	Vasoconstrictor drugs (Levarterenol)

volved than in atherosclerosis. Frequently, there is an associated migratory superficial thrombophlebitis.

Arterial emboli most often originate from the left atrium (chonic atrial fibrillation), the left ventricle (infarct), or from an aortic aneurysm. Actually, only one-half of the cases show a sudden onset of symptoms.

Arterial injury may produce only transient symptoms of arterial insufficiency. It can result in chronic arterial insufficiency. Arterial injuries are usually associated with injuries of other organ systems.

Increased resistance to flow through the foot can be caused by occlusive disease of the small arteries or even the veins in the case of extensive venous thrombosis (phlegmasia cerulea dolens). It may also be caused by those conditions which alter the viscosity of the blood. The arterial occlusive diseases offering such resistance can be classified as vasospastic (Table 22-3) and organic (Table 22-4).

Although acrocyanosis and livedo reticularis are more common in the foot than anywhere else, they are not of great importance and, whereas Raynaud's disease is the most frequently occuring vasospastic condition on this list (Table 22-3), it is seldom recognized as a problem in the foot, partly because the feet are not as exposed as the hands. The most significant vasospastic condition involving the foot is probably *sympathetic reflex dystrophy*. This distressful and usually disabling condition follows minor trauma, usually to the posterior tibial nerve. The patient complains of a causalgic pain (described under Signs and Symptoms), the foot is swollen, the skin is shiny, and there is usually hyperhidrosis. Lumbar sympathetic nerve block provides dramatic relief. After this, the patient must be encouraged to exercise to regain function.

Diabetes is certainly the most important organic occlusive arterial disease directly affecting the foot. More than half of the patients with diabetes have clinical evidence of arterial insufficiency of the foot. Occlusive arterial disease is eleven times more common in the rest of the population. (Gangrene is forty times more common.) It has been fairly well established that in diabetes there is a specific small vessel angiopathy which consists primarily of endothelial proliferation. It is true that atherosclerotic occlusive disease may be more advanced in diabetes (as it apparently is in the presence of gout and hypertension, as well), but the severe arterial insufficiency seen in these patients is a combination of the large (atherosclerotic) and the small (diabetic) occlusive arterial disease. What appears to be the effect of arterial insufficiency in the diabetic patient is not always that, however, since two other major complications of diabetes, *i.e.*, neuropathy and infection, can also lead to gangrene and ulceration. The combination of all three complications produces the clinical picture of the "diabetic foot" and the relative role of each must be assessed in properly treating these patients. (Plate 22-2A)

The collagen diseases are also of some importance in the evaluation of arterial insufficiency in the foot, particularly in the absence of occlusive disease in the more

TABLE 22-4. DISTAL ARTERIAL OCCLUSIVE DISEASE (ORGANIC)

Diabetes	Hypertensive ischemia
Collagen diseases	Gout
Dermatomyositis	Arteritis
Felty's syndrome	Hypersensitivity arteritis
Nodular vasculitis	Disseminated arteritis
Periarteritis nodosa	Infectious arteritis
Rheumatoid arthritis	Thrombocytopenic purpura
Systemic lupus erythematosus	Psoriasis
Systemic sclerosis (scleroderma)	Osteoarthritis

TABLE 22-5.   CONDITIONS INCREASING BLOOD VISCOSITY

Polycythemias	Cold antibody hemolytic anemia
Polycythemia vera	Dysproteinemia
Secondary polycythemia	Macroglobulinemia
Erythrocythemia	Cryoglobulinemia
Anemias	Hypercholesterolemia
Sickle cell anemia	Severe dehydration
Thalassemia	Intra-arterial thrombosis
Congenital hemolytic anemia	

TABLE 22-6.   FACTORS CAUSING HYPERCOAGULABILITY OF BLOOD

Physiologic
  Bed rest and lack of exercise, stress, pregnancy, fat ingestion, rapid weight reduction, surgical procedures.
Pathologic
  Trauma, hemorrhage, carcinoma, acute infections, diabetes, Buerger's disease, hemolytic anemias, paroxysmal nocturnal hemoglobinemia, thrombotic thrombocytopenic purpura, collagen disease, cryoglobulinemia, amniotic fluid embolism, abruptio placenta.
Drugs
  Barbiturates, narcotics (morphine sulfate, Demerol, procaine), Sparine, corticosteroids, progestional agents, Adrenalin, tobacco, methylxanthines (caffeine, theobromine, theophylline, aminophylline), cardiac glycosides,? antibiotics.

proximal artery. These conditions are often difficult to diagnose, but certainly should be considered where there are persistent and recurrent foot and lower leg ulcerations.

Without structural changes in the vessels, primary intravascular clotting and agglutination of the cellular elements may affect the plasticity of the blood and increase the viscosity to flow. Hematopoietic and other conditions listed (Table 22-5) are believed to act primarily in this fashion. A number of physiologic and pathologic conditions, as well as drugs, have been incriminated as causing hypercoagulability of the blood to a degree that is capable of producing intravascular clotting (Table 22-6).

Significant arterial insufficiency may be precipitated by increased tissue needs for oxygen. This will happen in hyperthyroidism, but the effect is counteracted to a certain extent by the increased cardiac action. Increased tissue metabolism is most commonly the result of active disease in the tissues, especially infection or inflammation from other causes.

Evaluation. In the evaluation of these patients it is desirable to establish a concept of the amount of absolute blood flow (*i.e.,* normal, increased, slightly decreased or markedly reduced), as well as the quality of the blood (*i.e.,* hemoglobin concentration) and degree of tissue metabolism (any evidence of infection).

Many sophisticated diagnostic procedures, such as phlethysmography, isotope clearance from the tissues, isotope (macroaggregated albumin) distribution, indicator dilution, and ultrasonic echography are available in certain medical centers but no patient will suffer because of the lack of them. All the information that is needed to handle these patients properly can be obtained from the history, the physical examination and the arteriogram. The patient's description of his symptoms and the history of the onset, duration and progression of symptoms, of injuries, of previous medical problems and their treatment is extremely important. In the case of injury, the history of even transient symptoms of arterial insufficiency is significant. A careful clinical examination of the foot is absolutely essential, but to be definitely certain of the diagnosis, the entire lower one-half of the body, with a comparison of both extremities is necessary. Particular attention must be paid to the color, especially position color changes, trophic changes, skin temperature, moisture and arterial pulsations. The abdominal aortic, femoral, popliteal, posterior tibial and dorsalis pedis pulses should be checked. Additional information can be secured by feeling the peroneal pulse anterior to the lateral malleolus. The volume of the pulse is important. The absence of the pulse suggests, but does not definitely indicate occlusive arterial disease, since the artery may be congenitally absent or in an anomalous position. The dorsalis pedis pulse cannot be felt in 5 per cent of young people. Conversely, a very good pulse volume (3+ on the scale of 4) can sometimes be palpated in the presence of even complete proximal arterial occlusion, indicating, of course, a very good collateral circulation. Such a pulse may disappear following exercise, however. Oscillometry is helpful in establishing objective values of pulse flow, particularly when pulses cannot be palpated. For proper interpretation, oscillometric excursions must be measured in the arm as well. Auscultatory murmur over an artery indicates stenosis, the degree of which is directly related to the intensity and duration of the murmur, assuming a good proximal flow. Of course, no murmur will be heard in the presence of complete occlusion. Vasomotor tone in the foot can be evaluated by the presence of sweating, the response to temperature and the response to lumbar sympathetic or posterior tibial nerve block. Arteriography is necessary to establish a definitive diagnosis regarding location and extent of occlusive arterial disease.

Even though the symptoms are only in the foot, it is important to visualize the circulatory system from the abdominal aorta to at least beyond the popliteal artery, demonstrating the three major branches of this vessel. Translumbar aortography is safe and simple. For best concentration of the radiopaque material and protection of the kidneys, the injection should be made below the renal arteries, unless there is diastolic hypertension. With this condition, the injection should be high enough in the aorta to visualize the kidneys and rule out renal artery stenosis. One bolus of "dye" with serial x-ray films is usually sufficient to visualize the major arterial system of both lower extremities. A femoral arteriogram should be done in the special situation where detained visualization of the arteries in the foot is desired. Interpretation of the arteriogram is critical and the failure to visualize a major distal vessel does not definitely rule out its patency, unless there is distal filling.

The demonstration of either proximal or distal occlusive arterial disease does not rule out the coexistence of the other. The extent of ischemia or gangrene can also be misleading. When it is quite localized, as to one toe, it may be due to digital artery occlusion or it may be related to occlusive disease at a much higher level but in this situation, to be so localized, one must assume that there has been a local increase in oxygen requirement, as could occur with infection or trauma. Diffuse ischemia or gangrene (Plate 22-2B) is usually the manifestation of a proximal arterial occlusion but also may be the result of multiple small vessel occlusions as seen in frostbite, prolonged vasospasm and phlegmasia cerulea dolens. Diffuse ischemia is rarely seen in atherosclerosis, diabetes or collagen disease.

The recognition of the underlying etiologic disease will usually require selective laboratory determinations, including fasting blood sugar, cholesterol, studies of accelerated clotting ("sensitized clotting time," platelet adhesiveness, thromboplastin generation), LE preparation, cold agglutination test, cryoglobulins, serum electrophoresis, urinalysis, urinary catecholamines, hemoglobin concentration, blood oxygen tension, and dermal biopsy.

Management. Basically the management of patients with arterial insufficiency is to increase the blood flow if at all possible,

TABLE 22-7.   TREATMENT OF ARTERIAL INSUFFICIENCY—IMPROVE QUALITY OF BLOOD

I. Increase available oxygen
  A. Increase blood oxygen content
    1. Correct cardiopulmonary disturbance
      a. Close intracardiac shunts
      b. Eliminate pulmonary AV shunts
      c. Decrease "alveolar-capillary block"
    2. Increase oxygen carrying capacity
      a. Correct anemia
      b. Increase hemoglobin affinity for oxygen
    3. Increase oxygen in solution
      a. Hyperbaric oxygen
      b. Hydrogen peroxide arterial infusion
  B. Increase oxygen hemoglobin dissociation
    1. Treat acidosis
    2. Maintain warm body temperature
II. Increase available nutriments
  A. Good diet

TABLE 22-8.   TREATMENT OF ARTERIAL INSUFFICIENCY—INCREASE BLOOD FLOW

I. Increase blood available for perfusion
   A. Increase cardiac output
      1. Increase stroke volume
      2. Increase heart rate
   B. Decrease proximal diversion of blood
      1. Control hemorrhage
      2. Close arteriovenous fistula
II. Increase perfusion pressure
   A. Increase central aortic pressure
      1. Increase myocardial contractile force
      2. Vasopressor drugs
      3. Mechanical systolic pressure augmentation
   B. Decrease proximal pressure loss
      1. Control hemorrhage
      2. Close proximal arteriovenous fistula
      3. Open proximal arterial occlusion
         a. Mechanical dilatation (Dotter)
         b. Embolectomy
         c. Thrombo-endarterectomy
      4. Bypass of proximal arterial occlusion
      5. Develop normal collateral circulation
         a. Walking
         b. Buerger's exercises
   C. Increase local perfusion pressure
      1. Dependent position of foot
      2. Intermittent compression of dependent leg
III. Decrease resistance to blood flow
   A. Vasodilatation
      1. Stop smoking
      2. Retain local heat
      3. Apply systemic heat
      4. Vasodilator drugs
      5. Sympathectomy
   B. Eliminate distal acute arterial obstruction
      1. Clot lysis — heparinize
      2. Thrombectomy in phlegmasia cerulea dolens
   C. Decrease blood viscosity
      1. Hydrate
      2. Low molecular Dextran
      3. Decrease cholesterol
      4. Decrease stress
      5. Exercise
      6. Treat hematopoietic causes

to improve oxygen content in the blood, if that seems necessary, to decrease the oxygen requirements of the tissue if they are abnormally high, and to treat the underlying etiologic process. Tables 22-7, 8, and 9 list the measures available for correcting arterial insufficiency. Some of the procedures are obviously most applicable to the treatment of chronic arterial insufficiency but the principles for management are the same for acute arterial insufficiency, except that one must frequently treat the acute form as an emergency in order to save the extremity. In either the acute or chronic forms of arterial insufficiency, it is important to be sure that a normal blood volume, especially circulating red cell mass, is maintained. Some anemic patients with arterial insufficiency become asymptomatic with only correction of the anemia. Treatment of cardiopulmonary problems may allow for additional blood oxygenation. The use of hyperbaric oxygen and of hydrogen peroxide arterial infusions is still in the experimental stage, but they give some promise for an additional modality one may be able to use in the future for special acute ischemic problems.

Exercise seems to be the best means to increase the cardiac output and the central aortic systolic pressure. Of course, maximum cardiac tone should be maintained. This will require digitalization of some patients. Vasopressor drugs are to be avoided, except when there is neurogenic shock.

For vasospastic disorders lumbar sympathectomy will provide the greatest benefit, but it also has a place in the treatment of organic occlusive arterial disease. It should not be done, however, without preliminary demonstration of effectiveness by sympathetic or posterior tibial nerve block. Sympathectomy cannot be expected to improve claudication. For the localized organic occlusive process, thromboendarterectomy is the procedure of choice if the arteriograms have demonstrated good arterial inflow and outflow segments and the patient is not considered a poor operative risk. The arteriotomy incision is best closed with an autogenous vein patch. In the abdomen synthetic bypass graft seems to be very acceptable but only a vein bypass should be used in the leg. Such a bypass can be brought down as far as the arteries at the ankle level. In the poor risk patients, Dot-

TABLE 22-9.   TREATMENT OF ARTERIAL INSUFFICIENCY REDUCE OXYGEN REQUIREMENTS OF TISSUE

Local cooling   Treat hyperthyroidism
Control infection

ter has been able to salvage limbs by mechanical dilatation of the stenotic artery. Embolectomy is best performed with the balloon catheter of Fogarty. The presence of limited gangrene should not discourage one from reconstructive surgery if a successful outcome will allow for a more constructive amputation.

When reconstructive surgery is not possible, some improvement in circulation can be obtained by walking to tolerance and Buerger's exercises. The latter consists of elevating the foot for about one minute (or until it blanches), hanging it dependent for approximately two minutes (or until color returns) and then putting it back on the horizontal for three to five minutes. To provide optimum help, this should be done in a repetitive fashion on a set schedule throughout the day. Abstinence from tobacco, good hydration, administration of low molecular dextran and reduction in blood cholesterol have all proved beneficial in the relief of symptoms. Vasodilator drugs are highly unpredictable. We favor whiskey for patients with organic occlusive process and dibenzyline for arteriospastic conditions. Long-term anticoagulants do not seem justified, except when it has been demonstrated that the patient has an accelerated coagulation mechanism.

The control of infection is the best way to reduce tissue oxygen requirements. Local cooling is only used as a preliminary to amputation.

Specific complications of arterial insufficiency require attention, quite separate from the problem of improving circulation. *Gangrene* is irrevocable death of tissue. If it is confined to the terminal part of the toe and is painless, spontaneous separation will occur and an expectant policy is, therefore, justified. If there is no evidence of infection, the patient can be kept ambulatory. If gangrene extends as far as the interphalangeal joint, amputation is necessary. If there is no infection but clear cut demarcation, which is evidence of good local circulation, then local amputation can be considered. If the gangrene is localized to the distal one-half of the toe, local amputation of the toe should be performed, leaving a vertical wound with a long plantar extension for drainage. The bone section should

be through cancellous bone and the wound edges approximated with Steristrips. The same principles apply to gangrene that has extended to the proximal part of the toe, but a "wedge" amputation removing the metatarsal head is necessary. With gangrene involving the forefoot, a transmetatarsal amputation should be considered only when one of the pedal pulses is present. This will seldom be the case in gangrene associated with atherosclerosis. This situation may be found in diabetic patients and, indeed, the tissue death in these patients may not be related to arterial insufficiency as much as it is to the neurotrophic changes. For gangrene of the forefoot without pedal pulses a below-the-knee amputation is the lowest level that should be considered and then it should be attempted *only* when the skin at this level is healthy, warm but uninflamed, and bleeds when sectioned. For gangrene spread beyond the foot *only* a supracondylar amputation should be done. Oschner adheres to the following principles regarding amputation for circulatory problems: No tourniquet, small lateral skin flaps (to allow better posterior drainage), meticulous hemostasis, loose approximation of tissue over bone in the tibia, loose approximation of skin edges with small stainless steel wire, loose dressing. When the foot is infected, a primary delayed closure of the skin is performed in five days. It is preferable not to amputate until the infection is localized and stable and the patient is afebrile. In massive gangrene with infection, refrigeration of the foot (*i.e.*, packing in ice) is helpful in controlling infection and relieving pain. Cooling should not extend to the level of the proposed amputation. It should be maintained until that time.

Pain in arterial insufficiency is of varying types. Sometimes it is relieved by analgesics or mild narcotics. Often it is severe and, unless the circulation can be improved, amputation will have to be done for pain alone. In selected incapacitated patients crushing of all sensory nerves at the level of the mid calf can be tried in lieu of amputation. Vitamin B_6 and B_{12} may help the neuritic pain. Sometimes this pain and especially causalgia responds to sympathetic blocks. Anti-inflammatory drugs are used to relieve inflammatory pain.

Ischemic ulcers may heal spontaneously if the arterial circulation can be improved. Skin grafting is sometimes necessary. Split thickness skin grafts can be used in the lower leg. They are most successful when placed directly on muscle after some granulation tissue has formed. Ulcers of the heel present a special problem. When they are large, a full thickness skin graft, as a pedicle or cross-leg flap, must be used. For the elderly patient amputation is often the wisest choice. Small ulcers of the back of the heel can sometimes be closed with small rotation flaps from above.

The treatment of *neuropathy* is primarily the control of diabetes. Vitamin B complex, thiamine and intramuscular procaine may be tried for sensory symptoms.

Outflow Disturbances

Etiology. Venous and lymphatic insufficiency is basically a result of obstruction, either functional or organic, to flow through these two systems. The general pathologic situations that can cause this are listed in Table 22-10.

Evaluation. As with inflow, evaluation of fluid outflow from the foot requires assessment of the presenting symptoms and a careful history establishing the duration and progression of symptoms, the types of previous illnesses, particularly "phlebitis" or "milk leg," injuries and operations.

Some form of fluid retention has to be or has been present to diagnose "outflow insufficiency." However, obstruction to smaller veins (as in thrombophlebitis of the calf) may only produce local venous insufficiency and, although the calf may be tense, this will not be recognized as edema. Usually, the patient will present with edema or a history of this, brawny induration or elephantiasis. Of course, some patients do not appreciate that they have or have had edema. Questioning regarding the effect of leg position is important, since edema and pain patterns of outflow insufficiency are characteristically relieved by leg elevation. In some patients, walking pain will be present, but there will not be quick relief of discomfort with cessation of walking, as occurs with claudication. Skin trophic changes in the lower leg "garter area" are highly suggestive of chronic venous insufficiency. Distention of the veins with leg in the horizontal position suggests increased venous pressure. This can, of course, be measured directly with a needle and a manometer, but in those individuals in which this information is most needed (*i.e.*, where the clinical diagnosis of venous insufficiency is questionable), the resting supine and erect venous pressure may not be significantly abnormal. Only exercise or ambulatory venous pressure will provide an accurate assessment of the venous hemodynamics. Normally, the venous pressure in the foot drops markedly and suddenly with walking. With valvular incompetency, the decrease in pressure will be much reduced. With deep vein obstruction, it may actually increase with ambulation.

Distention of the lymphatics is sometimes seen and measurement of lymphatic pressure can be made. However, it is simpler to measure tissue pressure.

Valuable information regarding the size, patency, and valvular competency of the veins and lymphatics can be obtained by phlebography and lymphangiography.

TABLE 22-10.   VENOUS AND LYMPHATIC INSUFFICIENCY
PATHOLOGY

Increased central and lymphatic pressure
  Congestive heart failure
  Hypopnea
  Central arteriovenous shunt
Extravascular compression
  Obesity
  Abdominal distention—ileus, ascites
  Distended bladder
  Tourniquet effect—tight garter, panty girdle
  Arterial aneurysm
  Fibrosis—retroperitoneal, postirradiation, post-
    infectious
  Ligature
Intravascular obstruction
  Inferior vena caval membrane
  Venospasm
  Thrombosis
  Tumor
  Filariasis
  Congenital dysplasia
  Surgical absence

As is the case with arterial insufficiency, the cause of venous and lymphatic insufficiency may not be in the leg, but at a higher level in the abdomen or chest, so in puzzling cases, the manometric and angiographic studies should be carried to those levels.

Management. The problems of outflow disturbances are basically those of venous insufficiency, lymphatic insufficiency, or a combination of these. Although such pa-

tients do not all have venous insufficiency, perhaps each one does have some lymphatic insufficiency, if only in a relative sense, since in situations of venous insufficiency, there would, theoretically, be no fluid retention if the lymphatics could handle the excess tissue fluid formed. The specific vascular disturbances will be discussed under deep vein thrombosis, post-thrombophlebitic syndrome, lymphedema, and diffuse angiodysplastic syndromes.

Deep Vein Thrombosis

Deep vein thrombosis is seen most frequently in the spring and fall. Post-mortem examinations indicate that it occurs in more than half the patients who have had prolonged bed rest. The thrombus most frequently forms in the veins of the calf muscles, especially the soleus, although it sometimes starts in the plantar and in the iliofemoral veins. There may be progression of the thrombus from its site of origin. Clinically, it is seen most frequently in the left lower extremity. This is apparently related to the fact that the left iliac artery can produce significant compression where it crosses the left iliac vein. Post-mortem studies indicate that there are usually thrombi in both legs, however.

Basically, there are two forms of deep vein thrombosis, phlebothrombosis and thrombophlebitis, which present as at least three different clinical syndromes: Bland thrombosis, phlegmasia cerulea dolens and deep thrombophlebitis (phlegmasia alba dolens).

Phlebothrombosis is intravenous clotting without inflammation of the veins. Venous stasis and hypercoagulability of the blood seem to be major etiologic factors. Thrombophlebitis is intravenous clotting with inflammation of the veins. The phlebitis caused by vascular injury or perivenous lymphangitis usually precedes the throm-

bosis, but sometimes it is the end result of phlebothrombosis.

The diagnosis of deep vein thrombosis can be difficult or easy, depending on the clinical picture. There is no universal agreement as to how these problems should be handled. This is primarily because many physicians seem to be completely confused about it and fail to recognize the significance of the variations in this disease. Many modalities of therapy have been suggested and all are probably useful in a selective sense (Table 22-11).

Bland Thrombosis. This is phlebothrombosis. It is the type of deep vein thrombosis to be feared because not only is it the major source of pulmonary emboli, but usually there are no clinical symptoms, except for tachycardia and apprehension (a sense of something being wrong) prior to the time of embolization. It may even be difficult to recognize the pulmonary embolus, for the patient may only express a feeling of "weakness" or slight tachypnea and not the classic signs of sudden chest pain, which becomes pleuritic associated with hemoptysis. As soon as the pulmonary embolus is recognized or only with a strong suspicion of it, the inferior vena cava should be ligated. Anticoagulants will not prevent further pulmonary emboli. Of course, the only answer to this problem is

TABLE 22-11.   TREATMENT OF DEEP VEIN THROMBOSIS

Relieve symptoms
  Leg elevation
  Sympathetic nerve block
Prevent progression
  Elastic compression
  Exercise—ambulation

Dextran infusion
Anticoagulants
Eliminate thrombus
  Thrombolytic drugs
  Thrombectomy

TABLE 22-12.   PREVENTION OF VENOUS THROMBOSIS

Prevent venous stasis
Treat obesity, treat congestive heart failure, deep breathing, active leg exercise, avoid kinking of veins, avoid constricting clothing and dressings, keep warm, elevate legs, avoid abdominal and bladder distention, elastic compression of legs, early postoperative ambulation, dextran infusion.

Reduce hypercoaguability of blood
Stop smoking, anticoagulants, tranquilizers,? vitamin E.

Prevent venous injury
Avoid interavenous infusions into legs, avoid vein compression and retention during surgery.

---

one of prevention (Table 22-12). Prophylactic angiocoagulants are recommended only for the high risk patients, especially when immobilized for a long period of time.

Phlegmasia Cerulea Dolens. Phlegmasia cerulea dolens is probably phlebothrombosis primarily. In this condition, the leg is swollen, markedly cyanotic, and cold. (Plate 22-2 C). The arterial pulsations are reduced. There may be bullae formation and impending gangrene of the distal part of the foot. This is due to extensive venous thrombosis in the entire leg, severe enough to interfere with arterial inflow. This condition is frequently associated with malignancy and the incidence of pulmonary emboli is high. Some patients improve significantly with sympathetic nerve block, but the best treatment is to give a lumbar anesthetic, perform a venous thrombectomy through a femoral venotomy, give the patient heparin, elevate the extremity, give Dextran, and encourage active exercise of the foot. With the development of gangrene, an amputation may be necessary.

Deep Vein Thrombophlebitis. This is not a life-threatening condition, as the thrombus is attached to the vein by the inflammatory process and pulmonary emboli are rare, except when it is a suppurative process. The sequelae in the legs can be significant, however. There is usually an associated reflex arterial and venous spasm, accounting for some of the symptoms, such as the white leg in phlegmasia alba dolens. When the thrombus is restricted to the plantar veins, the only symptom may be pain on squeezing the foot. When restricted to the veins of the calf, there will be tenseness of the calf muscles and pain on squeezing the calf (when done with the sphygomanometer, it is the "cuff test"), and pain on extension of the foot (Homan's sign.) Edema may or may not be present, depending to a certain extent on the amount of reflex venous and arterial spasm. With involvement of the femoral and iliac veins, there is edema, sometimes of tremendous proportions. The leg may be cool because of the reflex arteriospasm. This is a good confirmatory sign of thrombophlebitis.

The patient is best treated by elastic bandages to *both* legs and ambulated. If there is severe pain, relief is usually obtained with the performance of a lumbar sympathetic block. If the leg is markedly swollen and tense, the patient is kept in bed for one or two days until the edema begins to subside. The foot of the bed is elevated 4 to 6 inches. The legs are wrapped and active (not passive) exercise of the foot, calf and thigh muscles is encouraged. The administration of Dextran solution may be of some additional benefit. The patient is given laxatives and every effort is made to avoid straining at stool. The patient is permitted to have bathroom privileges. The bedpan is not used. Thrombectomy is theoretically of value in these patients, but there has been no conclusive proof that the leg sequelae are significantly less when this operative regimen has been carried out. Even the patients with the most massive edema initially may end up with insignificant residual edema. One cannot argue with the reasoning of using anticoagulants to limit extension of the thrombotic process, but this does not seem to be necessary. Anticoagulants should not be used for the reason of preventing pulmonary emboli. In the rare situation where a pulmonary embolus does occur in deep thrombophlebitis, it is recommended that a partial occlusion clip, rather than ligation, be used on the inferior vena cava to minimize the venous stasis already existing.

Sequelae, if only slight edema, are found in most of the legs following deep thrombophlebitis. When the iliac through popliteal veins are involved, the post-thrombophlebitic syndrome may develop (see next section). When only the veins of the calf muscles are involved, the syndrome of "chronic mural phlebitis" may result (see phlebitis).

Post-Thrombophlebitic Syndrome

Following thrombosis of the major veins of the lower leg, there will be recanalization of a portion of them. This results in deep vein sufficiency from venous obstruction and/or valvular incompetency. A number of complications develop which together are known as the post-thrombophlebitic syndrome. (Plate 22-2 D). The superficial veins may dilate to compensate for the reduction of flow through the deep veins. They may overdistend, develop incompetent valves, and become varicose, at which time they compound the problem of venous insufficiency. The chronic congestion of the lower leg interferes with the nutrition of the subcutaneous tissues and skin resulting in a large number of complications including ulceration, induration, and elephantiasis, recurrent phlebitis, recurrent cellulitis, stasis dermatitis and several different types of pain patterns. To manage this condition, one must control the tissue congestion and treat the individual complications. The patient can be promised considerable relief, but never a complete cure. The patient must be reassured to avoid a "post-phlebitic neurosis." The patient should return to the physician at regular intervals, for the education process is a continuous one.

To *control edema,* the patient should wear elastic compression dressings (bandages are better than stockings) as long as there is any tendency to swelling. This increases the tissue pressure thus minimizing the loss of fluid from the veins and increases lymphatic flow. He should be advised to become an enthusiastic walker, taking advantage of his "muscle pumps." He should learn to breathe deeply, since by performing this activity and by exercising he will decrease the central venous and lymphatic pressures. At no time should the legs be in a still, dependent position. When standing in one position, the patient should keep his legs in motion. When sitting, he should elevate his legs and, if he has any edema when in bed, he should elevate the foot of his bed. If he is obese, he should reduce! Diuretics will help mobilize fluid. Spironolactone is especially valuable for the management of persistent edema.

Varicose veins should be excised, but only after it is determined that the patient is not depending on them for the removal of fluid from his leg. If the patient is more uncomfortable wearing an elastic support which, of course, compresses the superficial veins, an ambulatory venous pressure evaluation should be performed in order to determine the significance of this venous pathway.

Stasic ulcers appear to be formidable problems, but respond well to careful conservative management. If the ulcer is infected, it must be cleansed with intermittent compresses of a bland solution such as Dakin's. Antibiotics are used only for a severe infection. Enzymatic debridement may be helpful. Surrounding skin eczema should be controlled. When infection has subsided, the patient is placed in an ambulatory "boot" constructed with zinc oxide, foam rubber and Elastoplast. A stasic ulcer should always heal with this treatment unless there is underlying arterial insufficiency. The patient must not become discouraged, as it may take several weeks and frequent "boot" changes to effect healing. The status of the arterial circulation may be difficult to assess, as the pedal pulses are sometimes difficult to feel in the presence of edema and brawny induration. An arteriogram is sometimes necessary. If the ulcer recurs because of marked induration of surrounding tissue, the area should be excised and skin grafted.

Elephantiasis is treated by resection of the soft tissue and fascia in the same fashion as lymphedema, but these operations are not as successful in this situation because of the poor condition of the skin.

Recurrent superficial thrombophlebitis is treated with moist heat applications and anti-inflammatory drugs. Sympathetic block, heparin, and Dextran solutions are considered to be of some help but seem unnecessary.

Cellulitis is usually an erysipeloid infection due to a streptococcus. It is treated with antibiotics and if it becomes a recurrent problem, prophylactic sulfonamides or antibiotics should be used. The portal of entry for this infection is usually a break in the skin. Therefore, the feet should be kept clean and epidermophytosis vigorously treated. If hyperhidrosis makes the control of epidermophytosis difficult, a lumbar sympathectomy is indicated. *Furunculosis* is also more frequently seen in the post-thrombophlebitic syndrome.

Stasic dermatitis, if exudative, requires wet compresses to cleanse the area, followed by 1 per cent hydrocortisone lotion. An ointment is used when the area becomes dry. The skin of these patients is sensitive to allergens, so every effort must be made to eliminate these. The patient should bathe without soap, adding Aveeno or Alpha-Keri to the water. Emollients should be used on the skin. *Heat and actinic rays should be avoided.*

Pain. There are many forms of discomfort from many different causes in the post-thrombophlebitic syndrome. The individual types of pain seem to respond to different forms of therapy. The *congestive* type of *pain* which can be localized about a perforating vein or can be diffuse over the entire lower leg is best controlled, of course, by treatment of the varicosities and control of the edema. *Neuritic pains* may respond to thiamine chloride or sympathetic blocks. Superficial discomfort manifested by *itching and formication* is best treated with antihistaminics, calamine lotion and Temaril. *Nocturnal cramps* can be relieved by muscle exercise but are best prevented by taking a hot bath with muscle massage, or by prescribing 5 grains of quinine sulfate just prior to retiring for the night. *Restless legs* respond to exercise, particularly walking. It is important that anemia, which is common in these patients, be corrected.

If residual pain does not seem to respond to any of the above measures, contrast baths, trypsin injections, ultrasonic wave application or steroid injection (prednisolone) along the posterior tibial vein can be tried.

Lymphedema

Lymphedema may be functional (increased lymphatic flow) or organic (abnormalities of the lymphatic vessels). The latter can be classified as primary in which there is congenital dysplasia of the lymphatic vessels, or secondary in which the lymphatics are blocked or destroyed by infection, parasites (filariasis), neoplasm, irradiation or surgical intervention. The primary forms of lymphedema are present at birth (*e.g.,* lymphedema from "amniotic bands") or become apparent about the time of puberty. The secondary forms usually do not appear until later in life (after forty years of age). Some forms of lymphedema are familial due to a genetic disorder. These are known as Nonne-Milroy's disease when the onset is at birth and Meige's disease when the onset is at puberty. Sudden onset of unilateral lymphedema in the adult may be the heralding sign of malignancy, usually carcinoma of the prostate or lymphoma.

The leg with lymphedema is firm and non-tender. The swelling does not recede with elevation. In the primary form there may be associated chylous complications—chylothorax, chylous ascites, and even discharge of chyle through the skin of the legs. Lymphangiography is useful in distinguishing the various types of lymphedema. Except in some rare instances of lymphedema in premature infants, the condition progresses. With increasing fibroplastic reaction, elephantiasis may develop. Lymphosarcoma sometimes arises in the lymphedematous extremity.

Treatment of lymphedema is not entirely satisfactory. The legs should be kept as soft and as pliable as possible. Use of an intermittent compressor unit and the continuous use of elastic stockings help. The most definitive treatment is the total resection of the skin, subcutaneous tissue and fascia with replacement of the skin. There may be a role for the use of full-thickness dermal flap grafts from the abdomen to the groin to bridge defects in the lymphatic system.

Diffuse Angiodysplastic Syndromes

These congenital conditions include phlebectasia, phlebangiomatosis, angiodysplasia with arteriovenous fistulae and hemolymphatic dysplasia. Anatomically, they may involve veins only, arteries and veins, or arteries, veins and lymphatics. Clinically, most of the patients have a combination of angiectasia, angiomatous nevi and hypertrophy of the extremity. The foot is swollen and may contain angiomatous masses. Angiography is important in defining the true nature of these conditions. These syndromes are usually recognized during infancy but the appearance of symptoms late in life has been reported. The treatment consists of excising as much of the vascular malformation as possible and replacing the angiomatous cutis with a skin graft. In some cases of phlebectasia, there is hypoplasia or absence of the deep veins. This should be evaluated by phlebography before the superficial veins are sacrificed. Epiphysiodesis should be considered in order to control the increasing length of the involved extremity, but only after careful evaluation of the overall problem.

STRUCTURAL CHANGES

Many vascular abnormalities of a morphologic nature, without hemodynamic disturbance, may be found in the foot. These can be grouped as inflammations, dilated veins, arterial aneurysms and vascular tumors.

Inflammations

Vascular inflammations include phlebitis and lymphangitis, which are common, and arteritis, which is rare. *Phlebitis* may be superficial or deep. When deep, there may be only tenderness. When superficial (superficial thrombophlebitis), there is associated redness, sometimes extending a considerable distance along the vein. Phlebitis may arise spontaneously, particularly in a varicose vein, or be induced by the trauma of injury or an intravenous catheter. There are rarely any systemic symptoms. The condition is best treated by bed rest, moist heat and anti-inflammatory drugs. When there is obvious progression of the thrombophlebitis, a ligature should be placed at the upper end of the vein. Regular Dextran is also helpful. Antibiotics are of no benefit and should not be used. When the phlebitic process is a recurrent problem, the blood coagulation mechanism should be evaluated and a malignant tumor, particularly of the pancreas, should be considered. Recurrent phlebitis can often be controlled by the cessation of smoking and by the daily administration of a therapeutic dosage of vitamin E. "Chronic mural phlebitis" is an important sequela of deep thrombophlebitis. It is seen in the leg veins below the popliteal vein and represents the reactional inflammation in the vein wall and perivenous tissue resulting from thrombosis and recanalization. It occurs most often in the posterior tibial vein. This condition is persistent, precipitating recurrent inflammatory reactions and symptoms. It probably accounts for much of the discomfort in the post-thrombophlebitic syndrome. It does not respond readily to the treatment. Anti-inflammatory drugs and other measures, including prednisolone injections along the posterior tibial vein, should be continued until there is no pain on digital pressure over the vein or on compression of the calf.

In *lymphangitis* there are also tender red areas with streaks but, in addition, there is usually tender lymphadenopathy. The foot may be swollen and there are systemic symptoms (chills, fever, malaise). This is a bacterial infection, the portal of entry being a break in the skin, such as seen in epidermophytosis. The treatment of lymphangitis is rest, elevation of the extremity, moist heat and antibiotics. Epidermophytosis should be vigorously treated to prevent recurrence.

Arteritis presents as tenderness and pain with little signs of inflammation. It is best treated with steroids.

Arterial Aneurysms

Aneurysms in the foot are rare but have been seen in the posterior tibial and dorsalis pedis arteries. They have been congenital, traumatic, mycotic and secondary to arteritis. They may present as a mass or discomfort on walking. They are best excised.

Vascular Tumors

Vascular tumors may be hamartomas or neoplasms. They may arise from vascular tissue in general or, specifically, from the lymphatic system or veins. The general benign tumors are hemangiomas, glomus tumors and telangiectasis. Malignant tumors are hemangio-endotheliomas, hemangiosarcomas, and Kaposi's sarcoma. Specific lymphatic tumors are the benign lymphangiomas and cavernous lymphangiomas and the malignant lymphangiosarcomas. Benign tumors of the veins have been endotheliomas and leiomyomas. The malignant tumor of the vein is a leiomyosarcoma.

Hemangiomas, which are vascular sinuses supported by various amounts of fibrous stroma, are clinically classified as cavernous, capillary, plexiform, and sclerosing hemangioma. Cavernous hemangiomas are formed of dilated thin-walled vessels and may lie deep in the foot but usually present near the surface as a soft, circumscribed purplish red mass, which must be differentiated from varicose veins. There will be a decrease in size of this tumor with elevation of the extremity. These tumors progressively enlarge, but usually show spontaneous thrombosis and resolution in due time. Expectant treatment can be used unless they are causing great discomfort. If extensive, they may be difficult to excise. Sclerosing agents may then be helpful. *Capillary hemangioma,* or "birthmark," consists of many dilated cutaneous capillaries. It is usually flat and extensive ("port wine stain"), but is occasionally localized and tuberous ("strawberry nevus"). It does not require specific treatment. *Plexiform hemangioma* is a penetrating form of vascular tumor. It seems to represent a combination of the cavernous and capillary hemangiomas. *Sclerosing hemangioma* resembles a fibroma and represents the end result of an occluded hemangioma.

Glomus tumor represents neoplastic change of the normal glomus body. It is usually located in the nail bed of a digit but can be found anywhere in the skin of the foot. The chief symptom is pain initiated by trauma and not helped by posture or temperature changes. The area of tenderness on pressure may be localized and often there is little to see. This tumor can produce erosion of bone. The treatment is excision.

Telangiectasis indicates dilatation of arterioles, venules or capillaries. It may be congenital or acquired. *Hereditary hemorrhagic telangiectasis* (Rendu-Osler-Weber syndrome) is a generalized condition with lesions in the mucous membranes and gastrointestinal tract. This usually represents dilated capillaries beneath the epidermis which blanch on pressure. *Spider nevi* are dilated cutaneous arterioles which form a star. They can be obliterated by pressure on a central point as blood flows from the center. They are frequently associated with liver disease and are rarely seen in the feet. *Venous stars* are dilated venules which are much more commonly found on the feet. The blood in them flows from the periphery to the center. *Senile ectasis* are small bright, reddish, purple areas of dilated capillaries and have no particular significance.

Hemangioendotheliomas are solid, elevated, non-compressible purple red tumors, 1.0 to 5.0 cm. in diameter. They are low grade malignancies and can be locally excised. *Hemangiosarcomas* present as a soft bluish, red nodule, which may pulsate and have a thrill. These are highly malignant tumors which metastasize early, and should be widely excised.

Kaposi's sarcoma presents as multiple bluish or red nodules often along the course of the veins. Itching, pain and tenderness are common. The tumors metastasize early and treatment is difficult. X-ray therapy is sometimes beneficial with local lesions. Hopefully chemotherapy may prove of some benefit in the future.

Lymphangiomas are rare tumors in the foot. They present as small circumscribed nodules filled with lymph. *Cavernous lymphangioma* appear at birth. It is often associated with hemangiomas. There are 1.0 to 2.0 cm. nodules in the subcutaneous tissue or thick-walled vesicles. The treatment is excision.

Vein neoplasms previously mentioned are solid lesions that present as painless masses.

Dilated Veins

Phlebectasia which is a congenital form of dilated and elongated veins may be restricted to the foot. However, the most common cause of such vein abnormality is *varicose veins*. They may be primary or secondary, the latter being seen with the post-thrombophlebitic syndrome and the arteriovenous fistula. There are multiple theories as to why primary varicose veins develop. The fundamental difficulty is the incompetency of the valves, particularly at the saphenofemoral junction and the communicating veins between the superficial and the deep venous systems.

The "primary" varicosities are more prominent in the proximal portion of the extremity and the "secondary" varicosities are most common distally. Therefore, any "primary" varicosities of the foot would be overshadowed by varicose veins in the rest of the leg. Varicose veins are tortuous and frequently large. They can be most easily visualized with the patient standing. (Plate 22-2 E and F.) It is important that the examination be made in this position. In fat legs, they are often best evaluated by palpation. They may be asymptomatic or cause an "aching" or "bursting" pain, the latter is associated with an incompetent communicating vein. Also, with incompetent communicating or perforating veins, there is frequently pigmentation of the overlying skin. Injury to this area may result in profuse hemorrhage or ulceration. There is no relation between the severity of the varicose veins and the severity of the symptoms.

In evaluating varicosities it is important to determine whether the veins are tributaries of the greater or lesser saphenous system or the result of an incompetent communicating vein. This evaluation is easily done with the multiple tourniquet test, by vein percussion and by palpation of the fascial defects caused by the perforator veins.

Treatment of varicose veins is recommended only when they are symptomatic or when the patient desires it for cosmetic reasons. Mild symptoms of varicosities can even be controlled by elastic stocking. An ulcer should be healed with an ambulatory "boot" prior to operation to reduce the chances of wound infection or deep thrombophlebitis. In a woman, the operation is best delayed until she has had her last pregnancy, since a new crop of varicosities can develop with each pregnancy. The principle of the operation is to ligate the superficial varicose veins at their junction with the deep veins ("high ligation") making certain that all the tributaries at that level are divided and to remove as many of the superficial varicose veins as possible ("stripping"). It is by design a destructive operation. Vertical incisions provide the best exposure. Multiple incisions are usually necessary but these should be small to avoid necrosis of the skin edges as the result of extensive undermining. Any residual veins can be treated by sclerosing injections if they seem significant to the patient.

TABLE 22-13.   PREVENTION OF TRAUMA

Toughening of tender skin—daily alcohol sponging.
Softening of brittle nails—soaks and oil.
Careful pedicure of nails, corns and calluses.
Avoid application of strong antiseptics.
Avoid application of allergenic drugs.

Avoid application of direct heat when arterial insufficiency exists.
Protective foot covering—properly fitted (not too
  loose or too tight).

TABLE 22-14.   PREVENTION OF INFECTION

Skin cleanliness
  Daily wash with Hexachlorophene G soap
Prevent maceration of skin
  Careful drying
  Powder
  Dry socks
  Sympathectomy when severe hyperhidrosis

Prevent dryness and cracking of skin
  Keep soft and supple with lanolin ointment
Treat minor injuries
Treat infections vigorously
  Bacterial
  Epidermophytosis

PREVENTION OF PROGRESSION AND RECURRENCE
OF VASCULAR DISTURBANCES

It is obvious from the previous discussions that most of the vascular disturbances involving the foot are chronic and persistent problems. The treatment that has been outlined is primarily symptomatic. Most of the etiologic conditions cannot be cured. However, they can be controlled and complications prevented.

Continued care of the patient cannot be overemphasized. He must be specifically instructed regarding the care of his feet. The patient should be told that there are certain things he can or must do and certain things he cannot do. If he wishes to prevent further foot trouble, he may have to readjust his way of life. He may have to change his manner of dress, his eating habits, recreational habits or even his job. In most cases, he will be allowed to keep his wife and children, although with such changes they may want to get rid of him.

The preventive measures which are listed in Tables 22-12, 13, 14, 15, 16 and 17, include prevention of trauma to and infection of the foot, the prevention of interference with the circulation through the foot and measures designed to increase this circulation, particularly exercise. It is also important to control the underlying etiologic conditions.

TABLE 22-15.   PREVENT INTERFERENCE WITH CIRCULATION

Stop smoking
Avoid garters and girdles
Avoid crossing legs

Avoid cold
Avoid stress

TABLE 22-16.   INCREASE CIRCULATION

Exercise—walking
If chronic arterial insufficiency:
  correct anemia
  whiskey

If chronic venous insufficiency:
  elastic support
  leg elevation
  avoid still dependency of legs

TABLE 22-17.   CONTROL ETIOLOGIC CONDITIONS

Control atherosclerosis:
  Treat obesity
  Low cholesterol diet
Treat hypertension, diabetes, gout, collagen dis-

orders and hematopoietic diseases
Treat hypercoagulability states:
  Anticoagulants
Treat auricular fibrillation

BIBLIOGRAPHY

BAFFES, THOMAS G. AND AUGSTSSON, MAGNUS, H.: Changing Concepts in Hyperbaric Oxygen Therapy: Dis. Chest, 49:83 (Jan.) 1966.

BALLA, G. A., FINNEY, J. W., ARONOFF, B. L., BYRD, D. L. (D.D.S.), RACE, G. J.: MALLAMS. J. T., AND DAVIS, G. (R.N.): Use of Intra-arterial Hydrogen Peroxide to Promote Wound Healing. Part I—Regional Intra-arterial Therapy-technical Surgical Aspects. Amer. J. Surg. 108, 621 (Nov.) 1964.

BURCH, G. E. AND SODEMAN, W. A.: The Estimation of Subcutaneous Tissue Pressure by a Direct Method. J. Clin. Invest., 16, 845, 1937.

CALLOWAY, J. L.: Chronic Leg Ulcers. J.A.M.A., 186, 1080 (Dec.) 1963.

DE CAMP, P. T., WARD, J. A. AND OCHSNER, A.: Ambulatory Venous Pressure Studies in Postphlebitic and Other Disease States. Surgery, 29, 35, 1957.

DEGNI, M., TOTH, V., LANFRANCHI, W., AND MAIA, A. C.: Chronic Mural Phlebitis. J. Cardiovascular Surg., 6, 495, (Nov.-Dec.) 1965.

DETERLING, R. A.: Is there a Place for Peripheral Nerve Crush. J. Cardiovascular Surg., 3, 329, 1962.

DOTTER, CHAS. T., et al: Transluminal Recanalization and Dilatation in Atherosclerotic Obstruction of Femoral Popliteal System. Amer. Surgeon. 31, 543, (July) 1965.

FISHER, D. A. AND MORRIS, M.D.: Idiopathic Edema and Hyperaldosteronuria: Postural Venous Plasma Pooling. Pediatrics. 35, 413, (Nov.) 1965.

FOGARTY, T. J. AND CRANLEY, J. J.: Catheter Technic for Arterial Embolectomy. Ann. Surg., 161, 325, (Nov.) 1965.

GILLIES, H. AND FRASER, F. R.: The Treatment of Lymphedema by Plastic Operation. Bul. Med. J., 1, 96, 1935.

HECKER, S. P., DRAMER, R. A. AND MEIGEN, J. R.: Clinical Value of Venography of the Lower Extremity. Ann. Int. Med., 59, 798, 1963.

HUNTER, W. C.; SNEEDEN, V. D.; ROBERTSON, T. D., AND SNYDER, G.A.C.: Thrombosis of Deep Veins of Leg: Its Clinical Significance as Exemplified in 351 Autopsies. Arch. Int. Med., 68, (July) 1941.

IPPEN, H.: Unterschenkelpigmentierungen. Zentralbloot fur Phlebologie. 2, 115, (Mav) 1965.

KINMOUTH, J. F.: Lymphangiography in Man. Method of Outlining Lymphatic Trunk at Operation. Clin. Sci. 11, 13, 1952.

MC KEE, D. M. AND EDGERTON, M. T., JR.: The Surgical Treatment of Lymphedema of the Lower Extremities. Plastic and Reconstructive Surg. 23, 480, (May) 1959.

MALAN, E. AND PUGLIONISI, A.: Congenital Angiodysplasias of the Extremities. J. Cardiovascular Surg., 5, 87, (March-April) 1964.

MALI, J. W., KUIPER, J. P., AND HAMERS, A. A.: Acro-Angiodermatitis of the Foot. Arch. Dermat., 92, 515, (Nov.) 1965.

PRESLEY, S. J., PAUL, J. AND RANKE, E. J.: Procaine in Diabetic Neuropathy. Amer. J. Med. Sci., 243, 603, 1962.

SCHATZ, I. J., ALLEN, E. V., ALLEN, C. V. AND LITIN, E. M.: Disability After Real or Alleged Venous Thrombosis. Postgraduate Med., 31, 358, 1962.

STEPHENS, G. L.: Palpable Dorsalis Pedis and Posterior Tibial Pulses. Arch. Surg., 84, 82, (June) 1962.

TANYOL, H.: The Concept of Chemo-Hemodynamics in the Pathogenesis of Primary Varicose Veins. Angiopatias (Brazilian Journal of Angiology). 3, 16, (Jan.-Mar.) 1963.

TASWELL, H. F., SOULE, E. H. AND COVENTRY, M. B.: Lymphangiosarcoma Arising in Chronic Lymphedematous Extremities: Report of 13 Cases and Review of the Literature. Brit. J. Surg., 46, 322, (Jan.) 1959.

═ Index ═